ONCOGENE AND CANCER – FROM BENCH TO CLINIC

Edited by **Yahwardiah Siregar**

Oncogene and Cancer – From Bench to Clinic
http://dx.doi.org/10.5772/3217
Edited by Yahwardiah Siregar

Contributors

Daniel Chan, Soo-Chin Lee, Cristina Marchini, Lucia Pietrella, Cristina Kalogris, Chiara Garulli, Federico Gabrielli, Elena Quaglino, Manuela Iezzi, Serenella M. Pupa, Elda Tagliabue, Augusto Amici, Zhongren Zhou, David G. Hick, Erica L. Cain, Alexander Beeser, Yasuko Kitagishi, Mayumi Kobayashi, Satoru Matsuda, Dik-Lung Ma, Victor Pui-Yan Ma, Ka-Ho Leung, Hai-Jing Zhong,Hong-Zhang He, Daniel Shiu-Hin Chan, Chung-Hang Leung, Alexey Stepanenko, Vadym Kavsan, Gabriela Anton, Adriana Plesa, Coralia Bleotu, Anca Botezatu, Mariana Anton, Lorelei Irina Brasoveanu, Mihai Stoian, Takaaki Watanabe, Denisa Ilencikova, Alexandra Kolenova, Yann Estornes, Olivier Micheau, Toufic Renno, Serge Lebecque, Laura Monica Magdalena, Lorand Savu, Ho-Hyung Woo, Setsuko K. Chambers, Gianpiero Di Leva, Michela Garofalo, Wei Liu, James M. Phang, Tiziana Triulzi, Marilena V. Iorio, Elda Tagliabue, Patrizia Casalini, Tetsuo Hirano, Leanna Cheung, Jayne E. Murray, Michelle Haber, Murray D. Norris, Gordana Konjević, Sandra Radenković, Ana Vuletić, Katarina Mirjačić Martinović, Vladimir Jurišić, Tatjana Srdić

Published by InTech

Janeza Trdine 9, 51000 Rijeka, Croatia

Publishing Process Manager Viktorija Zgela
Technical Editor InTech Prepress, Novi Sad
Cover InTech Design team

Additional hard copies can be obtained from orders@intechopen.com

Oncogene and Cancer – From Bench to Clinic, Edited by Yahwardiah Siregar
p. cm.
ISBN 978-953-51-0858-0

For EU product safety concerns:
IN TECH d.o.o., Prolaz Marije Krucifikse Kozulić 3, 51000 Rijeka, Croatia,
info@intechopen.com or visit our website at intechopen.com.

Meet the editor

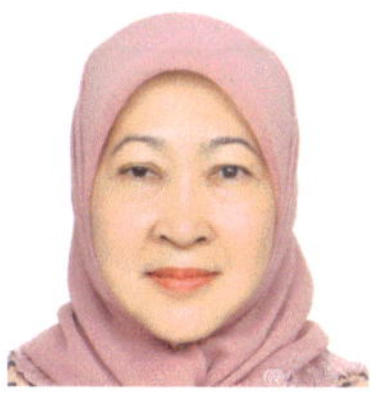

Yahwardiah Siregar was born in Bandung, Indonesia 57 years ago. During an elementary and high school and until my graduation as a medical doctor in 1981, I lived in Medan, Indonesia. I finished my Ph.D from the Medical Faculty, Eberhard-Karls University in Tübingen, Germany in 1995. I work as a medical lecturer at the Medical Faculty, Unversitas Sumatera Utara, Indonesia in the field of biochemistry and molecular biology. I am also a Head of Masters Program in Biomedical Sciences at the Medical Faculty, Universitas Sumatera Utara, Indonesia.

Contents

Preface

It took a long journey to really understand what cancer is, although many researcher are still working of finding a definite answer on how to treat cancer, and, what is more important, how to detect cancer very early, when some cells start going abnormal and transform into cancer cells.

The immune system might be the best weapon against cancer, since immune defense is programmed to recognize and destroy abnormal cells, but cancer cells may develop many defenses against immune attacks. Advances in biological processes, including apoptosis and cell proliferation, that are known to be dysregulated in tumors need to be understood in molecular mechanisms. During the last decade, scientists have shown an interest to create cancer vaccines as well as DNA vaccines using development of new biotechnological tools to elucidate an immune attack against cancer.

Recently, a new players in cancer biology have appeared: microRNAs (miRs or miRNAs), a class of small non-coding RNAs that play important roles in cell differentiation, cell growth and cell death. miRNAs can act either as oncogenes or tumor suppressors and regulate the interaction between cancer cells and the microenvironment. Understanding the function of ncRNAs by focusing on the potential involvement of specific RNA species, such as microRNAs, small nucleolar RNAs, Piwi-interacting RNA, long non-coding RNAs, in the development and progression of cancer is described in this book.

The book was written not only for medical students, but it can also be widely used by clinical and biomedical scientists, as well as by doctors studying for their postgraduate research.

My thanks are specifically aimed at Intech Open staff (Ms. Rcinic, Ms. Blecic, Mr. Greblo and Ms Zgela) who helped finish this book. I would also like to express my thankfulness to all authors who contributed a chapter to this publication. Finally, I hope this book will be useful to the health of mankind worldwide.

Yahwardiah Siregar

Section 1

HER2 Carcinogenesis: Etiology, Treatment and Prevention

Serial Changes in Expression of Proteins in Response to Neoadjuvant Chemotherapy in Breast Cancer

Daniel Chan and Soo-Chin Lee

Additional information is available at the end of the chapter

http://dx.doi.org/10.5772/54979

1. Introduction

Breast cancer is the most common malignancy and the leading cause of cancer death in women globally. There has been a sharp increase in its incidence especially in the developed world due to a combination of better detection and lifestyle changes. Breast cancer is a disorder influenced by genetic, environmental, behavioral, and reproductive factors. The most significant risk factors are gender and age. Hereditary forms of breast cancer are often related to mutations in two high-penetrance susceptibility genes namely BRCA-1 and BRCA-2 (1), and account for around 5% of all breast cancer cases. Women who are born with these mutations have 10–30-fold increased risk of developing breast cancer compared to the general population and a cumulative lifetime risk of 60–80%. Sporadic forms of breast cancer account for around 95% of cases and are a consequence of somatic mutations acquired over the lifetime; they appear to be in part related to polymorphisms in low-penetrance genes that encode proteins involved in DNA repair, cell signaling pathways, estrogen metabolism, etc. (2, 3). In the last few decades, the survival rate of breast cancer has improved due to advances in mammography and adjuvant therapy.

Histopathologically identical tumours may exhibit different biological behaviors in terms of severity, course, and response to therapy, reflecting disease heterogeneity; in addition, variability of the host immune response further contributes to differences in treatment outcomes, underscoring the need for better understanding of this disease and its relation to the host (4). At the biological level, breast cancer is a complex disease caused by multiple genetic and epigenetic alterations that ultimately lead to changes in cell processes, including cell proliferation, apoptosis, and angiogenesis, with subsequent acquisition of a malignant phenotype (5). The main genetic abnormalities that are observed include increased proto-oncogene expression, inactivation of tumour suppressor genes, chromosomal instability, alterations in DNA repair genes, telomerase reactivation, and epigenetic changes, resulting in dysregulation of cell proliferation, clonal selection, and tumour formation (6). As such one can expect breast cancer to be a heterogeneous disease and better prognostic and predictive biomarkers are clearly needed to better manage this disease.

The treatment of breast cancer continues to be challenging because of the heterogeneity of the disease. Breast cancer is staged by the TNM classification that assigns tumours to different stages based on depth of tumour invasion and presence of nodal and distant metastases. However, considering the heterogeneity in outcome of patients diagnosed with equivalent TNM stage, this classification system is suboptimal in tumour characterization or prognostication. In early-stage breast cancer, several clinicopathological factors are used to refine prognostication over and above TNM staging. These factors include histological grade, lymphovascular invasion and estrogen receptor (ER)/ progesterone (PR) status. Some of these factors have been incorporated into algorithms such as Adjuvant! Online to estimate the individual risk of cancer relapse (7-9). More recently, amplification and/or overexpression of the human epidermal growth factor receptor 2 (Her2), a therapeutic target, has been associated with worse prognosis, although its clinical utility as a prognostic marker remains uncertain (10-12). The variation in clinical outcome despite similar clinical and pathological prognostic scores seriously compromises the ability to advise women in making fully informed decisions about adjuvant systemic treatment after definitive surgery. Over the past few decades, substantial effort has been invested in the identification and validation of prognostic markers over and above ER, PR and Her2, in an attempt to improve risk stratification for breast cancer. As the evaluation of candidate prognostic markers is often limited by inadequate study design and analyses, formal recommendations for reporting tumour marker prognostic studies have been suggested, including guidelines on assay methods, study design and data analysis (13).

In recent years, gene expression microarray-based technology has resulted in the identification of breast cancer molecular subtypes and gene-expression prognostic signatures (14-16). These classification and prognostic expression signatures hold great promise, but there are concerns regarding their significance independent of ER/ PR status (17, 18). The process of validating the clinical utility of two such prognostic gene expression signatures, Oncotype DX and Mammaprint, is ongoing through the TAILORx and MINDACT trials respectively. Until these are validated prospectively, the increasing usage of these two profiling tests is unfortunately based on mainly retrospective data.

A fair proportion of breast cancers cannot be adequately resected upfront. In these situations, neoadjuvant chemotherapy is often given first. In recent times, even those tumours that are borderline resectable are often treated with neoadjuvant chemotherapy in an attempt to improve cosmetic results. Neoadjuvant chemotherapy provides prognostic information as the achievement of pathologic complete response (pCR) is associated with prolonged survival. The increasing use of neoadjuvant chemotherapy in patients with primary breast cancer makes it important to develop predictive markers of pCR, which is a surrogate marker of improved survival (19, 20). In addition, neoadjuvant chemotherapy allows the biological effect of the therapy to be evaluated as the surgically resected tumour after treatment can be examined and compared with the pre-treatment biopsy sample, providing an opportunity to study tumour biology *in vivo*. Neoadjuvant trials thus offer an excellent opportunity to study tumour DNA, RNA and protein changes and to evaluate new prognostic and predictive biomarkers of treatment response. In addition, it has the potential to reveal post-treatment biomarkers that could be complementary or even superior to the routine baseline biomarkers currently in use.

This chapter will review protein biomarkers in breast cancer. It will focus on established biomarkers, the timepoints of obtaining biomarkers, and the type of specimens on which to analyze these biomarkers. The different methods of measuring such biomarkers will also be described. In addition, several candidate protein biomarkers (*e.g.*, Topo2α, serum Her2, Cox2, MGMT, Hsp-70) will be reviewed for their possible utility as post-chemotherapy markers.

Body

Established and/or clinically relevant biomarkers	Potentially clinically relevant biomarkers	Biomarkers under evaluation
ER# PR# Her2*# Ca15-3*	Topo2α#	EGFR p53 Bcl2 MGMT Hsp-70# COX2# Osteopontin

Table 1. Biomarkers in breast cancer (*includes serum. #predictive of response.)

A. Biomarkers in breast cancer

1. Prognostic versus predictive biomarkers

A prognostic biomarker provides information about the patient's overall cancer outcome, regardless of therapy, whilst a predictive biomarker gives information about the effect of a therapeutic intervention. A predictive biomarker can also be a target for therapy. Among the genes and proteins that have proven to be of relevance in cancer are well known predictive markers such as ER, PR and Her2/neu in breast cancer, c-KIT mutations in gastrointestinal stromal tumours, EGFR mutations in non-small cell lung cancer, and BCR-ABL fusion protein in chronic myeloid leukaemia.

2. Criteria of candidate biomarkers

Several factors are important in selection and validation of candidate biomarkers. The analysis platform must be sufficiently robust to detect subtle changes between tumours.

Sample sets must be robust enough to reduce pre-analytical data biases and must reflect the intended use of the marker or marker set. Independent sample sets must be used to validate the prognostic and predictive power of biomarkers particularly when many biomarkers are assessed on small sample sets. Lastly, bioinformatics support is essential at all steps in any project. In addition, these markers would need to be validated, usually retrospectively first in existing large clinical datasets and ultimately in prospective randomized trials.

3. Gene expression biomarkers in breast cancer

The complementary DNA (cDNA) -microarray technology has made it possible to analyze the mRNA expression of numerous genes simultaneously to better characterize breast cancers, including classification and prognostication. Several studies using transcriptional profiling have classified breast cancer into different subtypes with implications in patient prognosis (21-23), frequency of genomic alterations (24, 25), and therapy response (26, 27). In breast cancer classification, the first tier of separation is between ER-negative and ER-positive tumours. Five breast cancer molecular subtypes have been identified using this technology, of which the luminal (A and B) type is ER-positive and accounts for 60% of breast tumours; the Her2 overexpressing type accounts for 15–20%; the ER and Her2 negative basal-like type accounts for 20% of the cases and has a guarded prognosis; and lastly the normal-like type, which has no definitive clinical value (28, 29). ER-positive tumours respond to endocrine therapy (*e.g.*, tamoxifen, aromatase inhibitors), and Her2 positive tumours are eligible for targeted therapy with trastuzumab or lapatinib, whereas the basal-like type has a more aggressive phenotype and while generally responsive to various chemotherapy regimens tends to acquire resistance quickly and has short survival (28-31). Currently, the advocates of this classification have suggested that the normal-like subtype might actually be an artefact of sample representation, that is, contamination of the mammary tissue by normal cells (32, 33). More recently, three other ER-negative subtypes have been described, the molecular apocrine tumour, the interferon, and lastly the claudin-low, which expresses breast epithelial stem cell markers. However, a definition of their clinical significance is still needed (34). Despite its significant contribution, the 'gene signature' described above is not a definitive classification method, but rather a developing work model that needs to be refined, considering that more subtypes have been described (5). Prognostic gene expression signatures in the form of Oncotype DX and Mammaprint have been tested in various large clinical datasets retrospectively to show prognostic value as well as value in predicting benefit from adjuvant chemotherapy, and are already in clinical use. On the other hand, predictive gene expression signatures for response to specific drug or drug regimens are still largely investigational although there have been many studies. This is because of small sample size in most studies, lack of independent validation sets in some studies, heterogeneity of the study population, a great variety of chemotherapy regimens that were evaluated in different studies, and variation in definition of response endpoint, making it difficult to pool the study results (35).

4. Protein biomarkers in breast cancer

Cancer arises from successive genetic changes, by which several cellular processes, including growth control, senescence, apoptosis, angiogenesis, and metastasis, are altered

(36). Consequently, researchers initially searched for markers by employing genomic and transcriptomic approaches, providing new biomarkers (14, 37) and expanding our insight into the genetic basis of cancer. It is however currently understood that genetic analysis alone is insufficient. Alternative splicing of mRNA combined with numerous unique post-translational protein modifications can give rise to multiple protein species (38). Hence, compared to the genome, the proteome can provide a more dynamic and accurate reflection of both the intrinsic genetic programme of the cell and the impact of its immediate environment (39).

Since proteins are the effectors of cellular behavior, interrogation of the functional proteome is likely to complement data derived from transcriptional profiling. Thus, the integrated study of the expression and activation of multiple proteins and signaling pathways has the potential to provide powerful classifiers and predictors in breast cancer (40, 41). Currently, gene-profiling technology generally requires fresh or frozen tumor tissue (other than Oncotype DX), and is cumbersome and logistically demanding, which may limit its suitability for routine use in clinical practice for some time. As such, reliable protein markers that may be readily tested on routinely available biological specimens may be more widely applicable in the clinic.

5. Established protein biomarkers in breast cancer
   i. Estrogen Receptor (ER)/ Progesterone Receptor (PR)

Assays for tumour expression of ER and PR have established utility in the clinical management of patients with both early stage and advanced breast cancer. They are routinely obtained on all tumour specimens and immunohistochemistry (IHC) is the predominant method for measuring ER and PR in clinical practice. Receptor positivity (staining of cell nuclei is considered positive) is an important indicator of hormone responsiveness and identifies tumours for which endocrine therapy is a valuable therapeutic option in both the adjuvant and advanced disease setting. Expression of ER and/or PR within tumours correlates well with low histologic grade especially in postmenopausal women. Reports have highlighted the extent of variability in ER and PR IHC assay caused by a variety of factors including differences in specimen handling, tissue fixation, antigen retrieval, and antibody type. In addition, variability in interpretation of assay results is caused by different laboratory threshold values for positive and negative. These variations have resulted in serious issues with ER reliability. In view of the controversy over what constitutes a positive test, most laboratories will report the actual percentage of positive cells. While many agree that ≥5% is considered positive, tumours with a lower percentage (1-4%), or even no staining, may show a borderline response to endocrine therapy. The American Society of Clinical Oncology (ASCO) Tumour Marker Panel in 1995 concluded that: (1) ER and PR should be measured on every primary breast cancer and metastatic lesion if it would influence treatment planning, (2) ER and PR positivity supports use of endocrine therapy regardless of menopausal status in both adjuvant and metastatic disease, and (3) ER and PR receptors are weak prognostic indicators and should not be used to determine whether to treat a patient with adjuvant therapy. Newer guidelines from a joint panel of the ASCO and the College of American Pathologists (CAP) provide recommendations to improve test accuracy and reporting of results (42). Of note, the panel now recommends that ER and PR assays be considered positive if there are at least 1% positive tumour nuclei in the sample on testing in the presence of expected reactivity of internal (normal epithelial elements) and external controls.

ii. Human epidermal growth factor receptor 2 (Her2)

Her2 is a proto-oncogene that encodes the production of Her2, a cell surface protein important in cell regulation. Abnormalities of Her2 occur in 25-30% of breast carcinomas, especially those that are poorly differentiated, lymph node positive, hormone receptor negative, flow aneuploid and/or show high proliferation rates. Her2 amplification and protein overexpression can be detected with Fluorescent In-situ hybridization (FISH) and IHC, respectively, both of which can be performed on paraffin-embedded tissue. Maximum sensitivity can be achieved by using both methods. The presence of Her2 overexpression predicts for response to anti-Her2 therapy such as trastuzumab and lapatinib. In addition, many studies have shown a positive response effect with anthracyclines in Her2 positive breast cancer, although there have been some studies recently to dispute this (43). Assay for this molecular marker is warranted as a routine part of the diagnostic work-up on all breast cancers, since Her2 overexpression is of major value in selection of anti-Her2 therapy in these patients. The bulk of available evidence supports the view that Her2 overexpression is associated with a poor prognosis. However, the value of this information in clinical practice is questionable, and guidelines from an expert panel on tumour markers in breast cancer convened by ASCO recommended against the use of Her2 in assessing prognosis (44). Given the substantial benefit of adjuvant trastuzumab in patients with Her2-overexpressing tumours, it is difficult to separate out the prognostic versus predictive utility of Her2.

Whilst the detection of tumour Her2 overexpression or amplification by IHC or FISH is standard clinical practice, the detection of serum (soluble) Her2 is a more controversial issue. In order to understand the relevance of serum Her2 we have to look at the structure of the Her2 protein. The Her2 protein is a 185-kDA transmembrane tyrosine kinase receptor with three defined domains: the intracellular tyrosine kinase portion, a short transmembrane portion, and the extracellular domain (ECD). The 105-kDa ECD (serum Her2) can be cleaved from the surface by metalloproteases and detected in the peripheral blood (45). It has been reported that trastuzumab inhibits Her2 extracellular domain cleavage; this is important considering that the remaining cleaved HER2 receptor is constitutively activated (46, 47), suggesting that the detection of sHer2 also reflects a biologic process leading to a more aggressive tumour behavior (48). Elevated levels of sHer2 have been observed in patients with primary (49) or metastatic breast cancer (50, 51). As detailed below in the specific biomarker section (E.3), there are some studies to suggest that elevated serum Her2 levels are a negative prognostic and predictive factor.

iii. Ca15-3

Ca15-3 detects circulating MUC-1 antigens in the blood. There are several studies that support the prognostic utility (52-55) of MUC-1 in early stage breast cancer. The trials showed as common finding that Ca15-3 was prognostic of disease free survival either on uni-variate or multi-variate analysis. We however do not use Ca15-3 to monitor patients with early stage breast cancer because there is no impact on the decision of chemotherapy regimen as established in a prospective clinical trial. In fact the sole approved use of this test (as per ASCO guidelines) is to monitor response to therapy in the metastatic breast cancer setting.

6. Candidate Protein Biomarkers with possible clinical application in breast cancer
   i. Topo2-alpha (Topo2α)

DNA topoisomerase 2-alpha is an enzyme that in humans is encoded by the Topo2α gene. This gene encodes a DNA topoisomerase, an enzyme that controls and alters the topologic states of DNA during transcription. This nuclear enzyme is involved in processes such as chromosome condensation, chromatid separation, and the relief of torsional stress that occurs during DNA transcription and replication. It catalyzes the transient breaking and rejoining of two strands of duplex DNA which allows the strands to pass through one another, thus altering the topology of DNA. There is increasing interest on Topo2α and anthracycline sensitivity, although the results in the past have been somewhat mixed. The BCIRG006 investigators (56) have appropriately looked for markers of benefit from anthracyclines and have suggested in a large subset analysis that Topo2α co-amplification along with Her2 amplification could indicate a subset of patients who definitely benefit from anthracyclines, and, conversely, that the majority of patients who lack Topo2α co-amplification might possibly be just as well treated with trastuzumab without anthracyclines. However, because there is no widely available and validated Topo2α test and these data have not yet been corroborated independently, Topo2α testing is currently still not routinely performed in the clinic.

7. Protein biomarkers in breast cancer under evaluation
   i. Epidermal Growth Factor Receptor (EGFR)

The epidermal growth factor receptor (EGFR; ErbB-1; Her1 in humans) is the cell-surface receptor for members of the epidermal growth factor family (EGF-family) of extracellular protein ligands. The epidermal growth factor receptor is a member of the ErbB family of receptors, a subfamily of four closely related receptor tyrosine kinases: EGFR (ErbB-1), Her2/neu (ErbB-2), Her3 (ErbB-3) and Her4 (ErbB-4). EGFR overexpression can be detected with IHC or FISH. In preclinical models of breast cancer, overexpression of EGFR leads to malignant transformation of mouse cells. It is associated with increased proliferation and resistance to apoptosis (57). One study analyzed 130 breast carcinomas using IHC analyses for the levels of nuclear and non-nuclear EGFR, and found that 37.7% of the cohort immunostained positively for nuclear EGFR and 6.9% had high levels of expression. More importantly, survival analysis revealed a significant inverse correlation between high nuclear EGFR expression and overall survival. Furthermore, expression of nuclear EGFR correlated positively with increased levels of cyclin D1 and Ki-67, both of which are indicators for cell proliferation (58). The expression of EGFR and its association with shorter survival observed in this study has also been reported in other studies (59), although its routine use in breast cancer at this time is still controversial.

ii. p53

p53 (also known as protein 53 or tumour protein 53), is a tumour suppressor protein that in humans is encoded by the TP53 gene. p53 is crucial in multicellular organisms, where it regulates the cell cycle and, thus, functions as a tumour suppressor that is involved in preventing cancer. As such, p53 has been described as "the guardian of the genome" because of its role in conserving stability by preventing genome mutation. Mutations of the p53 gene cause variant p53 proteins to have an increased half-life. These variant p53 proteins accumulate in the cell and can be detected with IHC in about 90% of cases by increased nuclear staining. One study examined a chemoresistant subgroup of breast cancers (triple negative breast cancer) and showed that p53 was possibly prognostic (60). However, although over-accumulation of p53 protein has been associated with worse survival in breast cancer patients, it also correlates with cell proliferation and thus may not be an independent prognostic factor (61). In addition, the results of its prognostic significance in breast cancer have been inconsistent, and it is therefore not routinely used in breast cancer management.

iii. Bcl2

Expression of Bcl2, an anti-apoptotic protein, has been associated with low-grade, slowly proliferating, ER positive breast tumours (62, 63). In a report (64) which pooled five studies of 11,212 women with early-stage breast cancer together for analysis, individual patient data including tumour size, grade, lymph node status, use of adjuvant endocrine therapy and/or chemotherapy, and mortality were analyzed. Bcl2, ER, PR and Her2 levels were ascertained in all tumours. A Cox model was used to explore the prognostic significance of Bcl2. The study found that in univariate analysis, ER, PR and Bcl2 positivity was associated with improved survival and Her2 positivity with worse survival. Intriguingly, in multivariate analysis, Bcl2 positivity retained independent prognostic significance (hazard ratio 0.76). Bcl2 was a powerful prognostic marker in both ER negative (HR 0.63) and ER positive disease (HR 0.56), and in both Her2 negative (HR 0.55) and Her2 positive disease (HR 0.70), regardless of the type of adjuvant therapy received. The study also looked at the addition of Bcl2 to the Adjuvant! Online prognostic model, for a subset of cases with 10-year follow-up data and showed that Bcl2 improved the survival prediction.

8. Biomarkers elucidated by high throughput methods

Serum and plasma protein profiling studies by mass spectrometry (MALDI-TOF or SELDI-TOF) have yielded numerous protein peaks that are potentially diagnostic, prognostic, or predictive in breast cancer. However, thus far, only a small percentage of reported peaks have been structurally identified. Moreover, since most studies did not investigate other cancer types or patients with benign breast disease, the specificity of reported markers for breast cancer still has to be addressed.

i. Diagnostic markers

The potential of proteomic pattern analysis was initially demonstrated in the diagnosis of ovarian cancer (65). In this study, exceptional results were seen using 5-20 specific key proteins identified, with a sensitivity and specificity of >95%, which is far superior to the sensitivities and specificities obtained with current serological cancer biomarkers. Subsequently, proteomic pattern analysis has been evaluated in a number of other cancer types, including breast, liver, and pancreatic cancers (66-68).

Two studies in breast cancer have investigated the correlation between SELDI-TOF mass spectrometry (MS) protein profiles of 105 tumour tissue lysates (69) and 27 breast cancer cell lines (26, 70). In both studies, patient subgroups identified by hierarchical clustering of SELDI-TOF MS protein profiles were analogous to the molecular breast cancer subtypes (69, 70). Of the several differentially expressed protein peaks detected, heat shock protein (Hsp) 27 and annexin V were identified as over-expressed in the luminal A type tumour tissue lysates (69), while S100-A9 (higher in basal) and a C-terminal truncated form of ubiquitin (higher in luminal) were found differentially expressed between the luminal-like and basal-like cell lines (70). Notably, subsequent IHC analysis of S100-A9 in tumour specimens of 547 early breast cancer patients confirmed its association with basal subtypes, as well as its value as an indicator of poor prognosis (70).

ii. Prognostic markers

In contrast to diagnostic studies, protein profiling studies aimed at discovering novel protein markers to prognosticate breast cancer are much more limited. One study (71) investigated the post-operative sera of 83 high-risk (mainly lymph node positive) breast cancer patients by SELDI-TOF MS and constructed a 40-protein signature that accurately predicted outcome in 83% of patients. The major components of this signature included haptoglobin alpha-1, complement component C3a, transferrin, and apolipoprotein A-I and C-I. These results should however be interpreted cautiously, as the number of proteins used for prognostication was rather high in comparison with the limited study population, indicating possible over-fitting of the data.

In another SELDI-TOF MS study performed in 60 breast cancer tissues, high levels of ubiquitin and/or low levels of ferritin light chain were found associated with a good prognosis (72). Although the results have not been confirmed by analysis of independent sample sets, ubiquitin has also been found differentially expressed in breast cancer subtypes by three other studies investigating tissue specimens (73) and cell lines (70, 74).

iii. Predictive markers

Several SELDI-TOF MS peaks (not structurally identified) were found indicative of treatment response in breast cancer cell lines to doxorubicin or paclitaxel (75). In addition, one study (76) found an increase of a 7.6kDa bovine transferrin fragment in serum-free conditioned medium of paclitaxel-resistant human breast cancer cell lines, corresponding to the increased expression of the transferrin receptor they observed in whole cell lysates. Although these results were not translated to the human *in vivo* setting, other studies have indeed reported an association between increased serum and cerebrospinal fluid transferrin levels and poor clinical outcome (71, 77). In one study, ubiquitin and S100-A6 were found to decrease in lysates of human breast cancer cell lines following chemotherapy-induced apoptosis (74); this coupled with the fact that aberrant expression of both proteins has also been reported in breast cancer tissue could make these two markers useful in predicting chemoresistant breast cancers (72, 73). In addition to these *in vitro* studies, in *vivo* studies have been performed as well (78, 79). In serum, both high molecular weight kininogen and apolipoprotein A-II were found to be significantly decreased in expression following docetaxel infusion in one particular patient with severe docetaxel side effects as compared to the other patients who tolerated the docetaxel infusion well. (79). The findings of this provocative study, if confirmed, suggest the potential of measuring protein biomarkers to predict adverse reaction to a drug.

B. Neoadjuvant chemotherapy and post-chemotherapy time point of biomarker analysis in breast cancer

Whilst the baseline pre-treatment time point is the commonest time point used in obtaining biomarkers to provide prognostic and/or predictive information, there are merits to using a post-chemotherapy time point biomarker, which may provide insights into biological effects of drugs and mechanisms of drug resistance. This however can only realistically occur in the setting of neoadjuvant or primary chemotherapy and in tumours from which serial tissue sampling can be safely obtained, such as in primary breast cancer. Neoadjuvant or primary chemotherapy in large primary breast cancers has been used with the purpose of reducing tumour volume and permitting less aggressive surgery (80). However, about 10-20% of patients do not benefit from this clinical approach (81, 82), and early identification of these patients could help avoid side effects from non-effective chemotherapy and unnecessary delay of definitive surgery.

1. Feasibility and significance of evaluating serial changes in protein expression post (neoadjuvant) chemotherapy in breast cancer

Almost a decade ago, one of the earlier studies (83) assessed the feasibility of obtaining serial core breast biopsies, and correlated rates of apoptosis, proliferation, and expression of related proteins at baseline, during, and after neoadjuvant single agent chemotherapy for locally advanced breast cancer with treatment response. The study recruited women with a histologically confirmed unresected T3 or T4 infiltrating carcinoma of the breast. The first 20 patients received three cycles of doxorubicin

90mg/m^2 followed by three cycles of paclitaxel 250mg/m^2, or the reverse. Nine women received four cycles of each (doxorubicin 60mg/m^2 and paclitaxel 175mg/m^2). The end points studied included: clinical and pathological response, serial apoptotic [terminal deoxynucleotidyl transferase (Tdt)-mediated nick end labeling] and proliferation rates, and expression of ER, HER2, Bcl2, and p53 by IHC. Twelve patients (42%) had a clinical complete response (cCR), and 16 (55%) had a clinical partial response. Five women (17%) had pCR, 7 (24%) had microscopic residual disease, and 17 (58%) had macroscopic residual disease. Higher baseline apoptosis and proliferation were associated with a statistically significant improved pCR rate. In addition, among 14 evaluable patients, apoptosis increased in women who had a cCR to the first agent but not in women without a cCR. The study however did not show any serial changes in ER, Her2, Bcl2 or p53. The authors concluded that it was feasible to obtain serial core biopsies that are informative for studies of apoptosis and IHC in patients undergoing neoadjuvant chemotherapy.

2. Limitations of post-chemotherapy biomarker analysis

While feasible, for the most part, post-chemotherapy biomarker analysis is likely to be less well accepted by patients. This is because of all the accompanied logistical and patient discomfort issues with repeated biopsies. There would also be the issue of sampling error: biopsy and analysis of a chemotherapy-induced necrotic part of the tumour versus a still viable part or even chemo-resistant part of the tumour may reveal completely different profiles. It is also unclear at this point in time if any predictive biomarker for response obtained after treatment would be superior to standard clinical or radiological measurement of response. Having said that, many of the above issues also plague baseline biomarker analysis; a good example would be that of the recently recognized issue of Her2 heterogeneity in breast cancer (84).

C. Specimen sources for measuring changes in protein expression

1. Blood/ plasma/ serum

Since whole blood is considered to provide a dynamic reflection of physiological and pathological status, human plasma and serum represent the most extensively studied biological matrices in the quest for (breast) cancer biomarkers (85). Besides the usual circulatory proteins, it also contains specific tumour-secreted proteins, normal tissue- and plasma-proteins digested by tumour-secreted proteases, and proteins produced by local and distant responses to the tumour (86, 87). Several proteomic studies on plasma or serum utilizing MALDI-TOF MS and SELDI-TOF MS peaks have been reported to differentiate patients with breast cancer from those with benign breast disease and/or healthy controls (78, 88, 89)

Blood plasma is the liquid component of blood in which the blood cells in whole blood are normally suspended. It makes up about 55% of the total blood volume, and is the intravascular fluid part of extracellular fluid, comprising mostly water (93% by volume) and contains dissolved proteins, glucose, clotting factors, mineral ions, hormones and carbon dioxide. Blood plasma is prepared by centrifuging a tube of fresh blood containing an anti-coagulant until the blood cells fall to the bottom of the tube. The blood plasma is then drawn off. In contradistinction, blood serum is blood plasma with the clotting factors removed by letting a collected tube of blood clot and the ensuing liquid portion aliquoted off. This would thus require less equipment than collecting blood plasma. Serum contains all proteins not used in blood clotting (coagulation) and all the electrolytes, antibodies, antigens, hormones and any exogenous substances. Plasma specimens may thus be analyzed for biomarkers related to the coagulation cascade, unlike serum specimens where the coagulation factors would have been consumed in the clotting process.

The commonest clinical use of blood instead of tissue biopsy to assess a tumour's status serially in breast cancer would be the use of Ca15-3 (Section A5) as a surrogate for tumour response in metastatic breast cancer. The serial decrease in Ca15-3 in response to treatment is often congruent with the imaging findings of a response to chemotherapy even though it is based on expert panel (ASCO) recommendations rather than rigorous prospective data.

The most promising use of blood instead of tissue biopsy for measuring serial changes in protein expression would be in the area of Her2 oncoprotein. Other blood markers (e.g. osteopontin) showing serial changes of possible prognostic significance are discussed below. (Section E)

2. Tumour tissue

Tumour tissue can be collected fresh, 'snap' frozen in liquid nitrogen, or in formalin and then fixed in paraffin. The former is much more labour and logistics intensive while the latter has the potential problems of protein degradation from the fixation process. As it stands now most protein biomarker analysis are done on paraffin-fixed tissue due to the low cost and ease of transport. Fresh or fresh frozen tissue can be subject to MALDI/SELDI-TOF analysis but paraffin-fixed tissue can essentially only be used for IHC assessment.

3. Cerebrospinal fluid (CSF)

Besides blood, CSF has also been explored for cancer biomarkers (77, 90). CSF contains less total protein than serum and provides a low fluid-volume-to-organ ratio, thereby augmenting biomarker discovery (91). As collection of CSF by invasive lumbar puncture is not applicable to healthy controls, the studies thus far only have been for diagnosis of metastatic disease in the leptomeninges or for prognosis rather than for primary diagnostic purposes in breast cancer. In one study which aimed to search for markers indicative of leptomeningeal metastases, CSF samples of 106 breast cancer patients were digested with trypsin (77); the resulting peptides were then analysed by MALDI-TOF MS and a 164 peak classifier with 77% accuracy in determining leptomeningeal disease was constructed. The discriminative tryptic peptides were derived of several proteins (90), three of which (i.e. apolipoprotein A-I, haptoglobin and transferrin) have also been found to be associated with clinical outcome in serum (71).

4. Urine

Urine has also been looked at as a source of biomarkers for breast cancer due to its ease of collection. One study looked at matrix metalloproteinase-9 (MMP-9) and a disintegrin and metalloprotease 12 (ADAM12) and found that they could predict women who were at increased risk of developing breast cancer (92).

5. Nipple aspirate

Nipple aspirate and nipple ductal lavage have been investigated as a source of biomarkers; the rationale being that tumour cells could secrete proteins into the ducts. One study looked at nipple aspirate and ductal lavage specimens in patients with and without breast cancer, and found that elevated human neutrophil peptide in high risk cancer-free women, defined as those with estimated 5-year Gail risk of >1.6% or history of lobular carcinoma in situ, could predict early onset breast cancer better than current detection methods (93).

6. Tumour lysates

Tumour lysates are harvested from fresh or fresh frozen tumour samples. They are homogenized in a lysis buffer with protease inhibitors to prevent protein degradation. The sample is then centrifuged and the supernatant decanted to obtain the tumour lysate, which can be used for MALDI-TOF or SELDI-TOF, reverse phase protein array (RRPA; see below), and other high throughput proteomic analyses.

7. Circulating tumour cells (CTCs)

It has been appreciated in the past several years that tumour cells are shed from the primary tumour/ metastases and circulate in the blood stream. Intense research is ongoing to determine the utility of the detection of these cells in prognostication and prediction of therapy. One study showed that captured CTCs are amenable to biomarker analyses such as Her2 status, quantitative RT-PCR for breast cancer subtype markers, KRAS mutation detection and EGFR staining by immunofluorescence. The study was able to determine Her2 status by immunofluorescence and FISH in CTCs from metastatic breast cancer patients, although concordance with tumor Her2 status was only 89% (94).

D. Methods of measuring protein expression and its changes

1. Enzyme-Linked ImmunoSorbent Assay (ELISA)/ antibody microarray

In ELISA, an unknown amount of antigen is affixed to a surface, and then a specific antibody is applied over the surface so that it can bind to the antigen. This antibody is linked to an enzyme, and, in the final step, a substance containing the enzyme's substrate is added. The subsequent reaction produces a detectable signal, most commonly a color change in the substrate.

Performing an ELISA involves at least one antibody with specificity for a particular antigen. The sample with an unknown amount of antigen is immobilized on a solid support either non-specifically (via adsorption to the surface) or specifically (via capture by another antibody specific to the same antigen, in a "sandwich" ELISA). After the antigen is immobilized, the detection antibody is added, forming a complex with the antigen. The detection antibody can be covalently linked to an enzyme, or can itself be detected by a secondary antibody that is linked to an enzyme through bioconjugation. Between each step, the plate is typically washed with a mild detergent solution to remove any proteins or antibodies that are not specifically bound. After the final wash step, the plate is developed by adding an enzymatic substrate to produce a visible signal, which indicates the quantity of antigen in the sample. The commonest medical use of ELISA is for assaying antigens/ substances that can be found in the serum component of blood or bodily fluids (*e.g.*, human immunodeficiency virus).

An antibody microarray is a specific form of ELISA-based protein microarray; a collection of antibodies are fixed on a solid surface such as glass, plastic or silicon chip, for the purpose of detecting antigens. The antibody microarray is often used for detecting protein expression from cell lysates and special biomarkers from serum or urine for diagnostic applications.

2. Tumour Immunohistochemistry (IHC)

Immunohistochemistry, which is the most practical method for assessing protein expression changes, not only provides a semi-quantitative assessment of protein abundance but also reveals cellular localization. Because no special processing of tissue samples is needed and labour intensive and expensive diagnostic techniques are avoided, IHC is perhaps the most readily adaptable technique to clinical practice. Inter-observer reproducibility of immunohistochemical scoring is sometimes problematic, although this can generally be resolved by re-evaluation and discussion to reach consensus. Analysis of protein expression using IHC has identified molecular subtypes in breast cancer that are similar to those derived from gene expression arrays (95). The most powerful use of IHC is that of a tissue microarray (TMA), which analyzes simultaneously a new protein marker or a group of 'protein signature' markers in hundreds to thousands of cylindrical fragments of clustered tumour samples collected from original paraffin blocks (96).

3. Proteomics: MALDI-TOF/ SELDI-TOF

Proteomic-pattern profiling is a recent approach to protein biomarker discovery. Given that mRNA information does not always accurately reflect the function of proteins which are the functional components within organisms, the use of proteomic patterns to enable tumour diagnosis or sub-classification seems more promising. The rationale is that proteins produced by cancer cells or their microenvironment may eventually enter the circulation and that the patterns of expression of these proteins could be assessed by mass spectrometry (MS) in combination with mathematical algorithms for diagnostic purposes. The search for novel protein biomarkers has for the longest time been dominated by two-dimensional gel electrophoresis (97), a significant disadvantage of which is its lack of real high-throughput capability. However, recent advances in analytical technologies, such as protein microarrays and mass spectrometry, have enabled large-scale proteomic analyses (98).

Technologies such as differential in-gel electrophoresis, two-dimensional polyacrylamide gel electrophoresis and multidimensional protein identification technology, can be used for high-throughput protein profiling. Due to their relative ease of sample preparation, high analytical sensitivity and speed of data acquisition, two MS-based technologies in particular, matrix-assisted laser desorption/ionisation time-of-flight (MALDI-TOF) MS (99) and its variant surface-enhanced laser desorption/ionisation (SELDI-) TOF MS (100) have been widely deployed for cancer biomarker discovery (101). In both platforms, biological samples (*e.g.*, serum, tissue lysate) are co-crystallised with an energy absorbing matrix on a sample probe surface. Subsequent irradiation with brief laser pulses sublimates and ionises the proteins out of their crystalline matrix, after which an electric field migrates the charged proteins to the time-of-flight mass analyser. The proteins are then separated based on their mass, as the time to detector impact (TOF) is proportional to the protein mass per charge. The two platforms differ in their sample probe surfaces. In MALDI, the probe surface merely presents the sample to the mass spectrometer, warranting off-line sample fractionation and clean-up to produce usable MS signals. In contrast, the probe surfaces utilised by SELDI are comprised of various chromatographic surfaces, enabling their active role in sample fractionation.

The technology that has received considerable attention involves the use of a minute amount of biological sample added to a 'protein-chip', which is subsequently analyzed by MALDI or SELDI-TOF-MS to generate a proteomic signature (102). These patterns reflect part of the tissue or body fluid proteome, but without knowledge of the actual identity of the proteins. In addition to the issue of protein identification, there are also problems related to the other aspects of this technology. Validation and the consistency of bioinformatics analysis is of great importance to ascertain reproducibility and prevent systematic bias and overfitting of data. This is highlighted by a study (103), in which the potential markers for breast cancer and lymph node status reported by two studies (104, 105) could not be confirmed following analysis of an independent sample set. The shortcomings also include bias from artefacts related to the clinical sample collection and storage, the inherent qualitative control issues of mass spectrometric analysis, failure to identify well-established cancer biomarkers, bias when identifying high-abundance molecules within the serum, and disagreement between peaks generated by different laboratories (106, 107). Another limitation concerns possible bioinformatic artifacts; one study (108) showed that even signals that are detected that are actually a result of 'noise' can also achieve a high level of discrimination between patients with cancer and those without, further highlighting the lack of specificity of some of the signals detected. As such, despite a significant period since the first report of this technology, no independent validation studies have been published, and no product has yet reached the clinic.

4. Isobaric Tags for Relative and Absolute Quantification (iTRAQ)

iTRAQ is based on the labeling of the N-terminus and side chain amines of peptides from digested proteins with tags of varying mass. One such method commercialized by Applied Biosystems® is called iTRAQ and uses four amine specific (4-plex) isobaric reagents to label the primary amines of peptides from four different biological samples. In recent times, an eight amine specific set of reagents (8-plex) has also been available. These samples are then pooled and usually fractionated by nano liquid chromatography and analyzed by tandem mass spectrometry. A database search is then performed using the fragmentation data to identify the labeled peptides and hence the corresponding proteins. The fragmentation of the attached tag generates a low molecular mass reporter ion that can be used to relatively quantify the peptides and the proteins from which they originated. iTRAQ reagents therefore allow simultaneous identification and quantification of proteins in four or eight different samples using tandem mass spectrometry.

5. Reverse Phase Protein Array (RPPA)

The principle of RPPA involves the spotting of patient samples in an array format onto a nitrocellulose support. Hundreds of patient specimens can be spotted onto the same array, allowing a large number of samples to be compared simultaneously under identical conditions. Each array is incubated with one particular antibody, and signal intensity proportional to the amount of analyte in the sample spot is generated. Signal detection is commonly performed by fluorescence, chemiluminescence or colorimetric methods, and the results are quantified by scanning and analyzed by software such as P-SCAN® and ProteinScan®.

RPPA is possibly a useful tool to identify and validate proteins and phospho-proteins in cancer (109, 110). The aim of one such study was to determine whether functional proteomics using RPPA improves breast cancer classification and prognostication and also whether it can predict pCR in patients receiving neoadjuvant taxane and anthracycline-taxane-based chemotherapy. Six breast cancer subgroups were identified by a 10-protein biomarker panel in the 712 tumour training set, that were associated with different recurrence-free survival. A prognosis score constructed using the 10 protein-signature (ER, PR, Bcl2, GATA3, CCNB1, CCNE1, EGFR, Her2, Her2p1248 and EIG121) in the training set was associated with relapse free survival in both the training and test sets. In addition, there was a significant association between the prognostic score and likelihood of pCR to neoadjuvant chemotherapy in yet another independent sample set.

E. Serial changes in expression of various established protein biomarkers in response to neoadjuvant chemotherapy

1. ER/PR

The most obvious candidate biomarker for which one would expect extensive data on with regards to serial changes post chemotherapy would be ER and PR. Much as it would have been hoped that the data on this would be consistent, the fact is that various trials showed a spectrum of findings. In a relatively recent meta-analysis (111), it was found that discordance in ER and PR between core needle biopsy and subsequent resection material was more evident in the patients treated with neoadjuvant chemotherapy (around 15%) than the reported discordance in patients not treated with neoadjuvant chemotherapy (around 2%). Although the studies reviewed were quite heterogeneous with respect to study methodology, design and outcome measures, the discordances could only partly be explained by the study design confounders and are instead more likely due to the direct effect of the chemotherapy. A change of hormone receptor status in up to a third of patients after neoadjuvant chemotherapy was reported in several studies (112-114). In general, studies that reported a good concordance of hormone receptor status before and after neoadjuvant chemotherapy had a relatively smaller number of patients compared to the studies that found significant changes. The small sample size might have prevented these trials from showing statistical significance. Intriguingly, PR was found to be more discordant compared to ER.

Various postulations regarding the mechanisms resulting in a change in the receptor status caused by chemotherapy have been put forth. The targeting of chemosensitive tumour cells leaves resistant tumour cells behind, which may have different ER status (positive or negative) from the sensitive tumour cells that were eradicated. Lower circulating levels of estrogens caused by ovarian insufficiency during or after chemotherapy in premenopausal women (115) might cause downregulation of the estrogen and/or progesterone receptor of the tumour leading to estrogen-independent growth.

In spite of the likely true observed phenomenon of serial changes in ER/PR status post chemotherapy, however, little is known about the predictive or prognostic value of a changed receptor status. A few investigators tried to correlate changes to treatment response, but discordant conclusions were drawn (116, 117). A positive switch of the hormone receptor status could be an indicator for a better outcome and indeed was significantly correlated with better disease-free and overall survival in patients who were treated with adjuvant endocrine therapy compared to those with a positive switch who were not (118). In clinical practice, the likely utility of repeating the ER/PR status post chemotherapy is to evaluate if there is any hormone receptor positivity necessitating endocrine therapy.

2. Tumor Her2

In one study (119), the authors evaluated the correlation among patients' characteristics, immunohistochemical expression of hormonal receptors (ER and PR), p53, p21 and Her2 protein expression and the clinical and pathological response to a neoadjuvant combination of docetaxel and epirubicin chemotherapy. There was a reduction in p53 protein expression, as well as in p21 protein expression after neoadjuvant chemotherapy. However, neoadjuvant taxane and anthracycline did not change Her2 expression in patients with locally advanced breast carcinoma. The tissue Her2 stable phenotype observed in this study during neoadjuvant chemotherapy has also been reported by other groups (112, 117, 120). Recent studies have focused on the role of tumour Her2 as a predictive factor of response to neoadjuvant chemotherapy (112) but have failed to observe a correlation between tumour baseline Her2 positivity and the clinical or pathological response to neoadjuvant chemotherapy. This is in contradistinction to serum Her2 which will be detailed below.

3. Serum Her2

There have been several studies showing serial changes in serum Her2 (sHer2) following neoadjuvant chemotherapy. One study within a large clinical trial (121) sought to use serum markers to optimize treatment strategies in breast cancer. The authors investigated serum

Her2 levels (sHer2) in 175 breast cancer patients participating in the GeparQuattro trial. This study incorporated neoadjuvant chemotherapy approaches in Her2-positive and negative patients (epirubicin/cyclophosphamide prior to randomization to either docetaxel alone, docetaxel in combination with capecitabine or docetaxel followed by capecitabine) and the addition of trastuzumab treatment for patients with Her2-positive tumours. sHer2 levels were measured by ELISA before and after initiation of neoadjuvant chemotherapy in 90 Her2 positive and 85 Her2 negative patients. Median pre-chemotherapy sHer2 levels were higher in patients with positive Her2 status of the primary tumour than in patients with negative tumor Her2 status (14.9ng/ml versus 7.7ng/ml). A pre-chemotherapy sHer2 cut-off level of 10ng/ml had the best sensitivity and specificity in differentiating between Her2 positive and Her2 negative tumours. In Her2 positive patients, the authors found a significant positive association between pCR and elevated baseline sHer2 levels (above 15ng/ml) and a more than 20% decrease of sHer2 levels during neoadjuvant chemotherapy, which was of borderline significance in multivariate analysis (odds ratio=3.29). In Her2 negative patients, the authors observed no association between sHer2 levels and pCR. The authors thus hypothesized that monitoring sHer2 levels in the presence of anti-Her2 treatment might be an adjunct to clinical evaluation during neoadjuvant chemotherapy in Her2 positive disease.

Two smaller published reports investigated the correlation between treatment-induced changes in sHer2 and pathologic complete response from neoadjuvant chemotherapy plus trastuzumab. One study evaluated sHer2 levels in a trastuzumab-based neoadjuvant setting in 16 patients. In this small group of patients, the authors could show that a decrease of sHer2 levels was associated with response to therapy (122). In the other study which monitored sHer levels serially over 6 months, 39 patients were treated with neoadjuvant chemotherapy including 29 patients who received a trastuzumab combination. A 9% decrease in sHer2 levels from week 3 to week 6 after initiation of therapy (but not earlier or later) was predictive of pCR (123). This study also illustrated that time dependency of post chemotherapy biomarkers could be an important issue. In this study, the mean sHer2 baseline values were not different between the pCR group and the group with residual disease suggesting that post-chemotherapy evaluation could be superior to baseline evaluation.

In contrast, Quaranta *et al.* could not find a correlation between serum positivity for Her2 (using a cutoff of 10ng/ml as per the GeparQuattro trial) and tissue positivity for Her2 levels in an unselected patient group of 108 patients (124). In addition, no clear relationship was found between baseline sHer2 levels and tumour response to trastuzumab-based treatment in a recently published meta-analysis (125). In an abstract of a small study presented at ASCO 2011, Lee *et al* investigated the correlation between the response of advanced breast cancers to neoadjuvant chemotherapy and the change of serum Her2 and short-term disease free survival. Twenty-two locally advanced Her2 IHC 3+ or FISH amplified breast cancer patients were treated with neoadjuvant doxorubicin or trastuzumab. Serum Her2 levels were measured by chemiluminescence immunoassay before and after neoadjuvant chemotherapy. The cutoff value was 10.2mg/ml which is similar to that of the GeparQuattro trial. Mean serum Her2 before chemotherapy was 15.8± 1.6ng/ml, and that after chemotherapy was 10.6 ± 0.38ng/ml. The change of serum Her2 in the CR group was higher than that in the PR group (13.26 ± 14.1ng/ml and 2.74±3.2ng/ml respectively). However, at a mean follow-up of 41 months, the change of serum Her2 before and after chemotherapy was not correlated with disease recurrence or with disease free interval.

Several groups have postulated that monitoring changes in sHer2 levels after a specific time-period after trastuzumab treatment might be valuable for identifying a patient population that might benefit from additional treatment regimens with other Her2 targeted therapies and certainly merits confirmation in further large prospective trials (126).

F. Serial changes in expression of various candidate protein biomarkers in response to neoadjuvant chemotherapy

1. COX-2

Cyclooxygenases (COX-1 and COX-2) are rate-limiting enzymes in the formation of prostaglandins from arachidonic acid. COX-1 is considered to be constitutively expressed while COX-2 is highly inducible by various factors and is associated with tumourigenesis (127-129). Several studies have shown the unfavourable prognostic significance of COX-2 expression in breast cancer (130, 131). A few retrospective breast cancer studies have also suggested that tumour expression of COX-2 may be associated with more aggressive breast cancer phenotypes, poorer response to chemotherapy and inferior survival (130, 132). One study compared serial tumour samples from individual breast cancer patients before and after exposure to sequential cycles of doxorubicin and docetaxel and examined changes in tumour expression of COX-2 by IHC. The study also correlated any significant changes in biomarker expression with tumour clinical response and progression-free survival. There was a statistically significant progressive downward trend in COX-2 expression with increasing cycles of chemotherapy for the entire cohort. Subgroup analysis found that this decrease in COX-2 expression to be predominant in clinical responders but not in non-responders. COX-2-positive tumours at baseline showed a statistically significant reduction in COX-2 expression with chemotherapy. This downward trend was most marked between the third and sixth cycle of chemotherapy rather than after one cycle of chemotherapy suggesting that this change did not occur early during chemotherapy. Tumours that were COX-2 positive both at baseline and after treatment had the worst outcome, while those that were COX-2 negative both at baseline and after treatment had the best outcome with a median progression free survival (PFS) of 25 versus 47 months. Another significant finding is related to ER status and COX-2 overexpression. For ER-positive and COX-2-positive tumours at baseline, a change to COX-2 negativity resulted in a statistically significant improvement in PFS compared with tumours that remained COX-2 positive (52 versus 27 months). As for ER-negative and COX-2-positive tumours at baseline, the PFS is generally poor regardless of whether the tumour remained COX-2 positive or became negative after chemotherapy. The study also showed that COX-2-positive tumours at baseline correlated with more advanced tumour size, presence of metastases and inferior PFS as compared with COX-2-negative tumours. That neoadjuvant chemotherapy resulted in a reduction in COX-2 expression in breast tumours is consistent with findings previously observed in breast cancer cell lines after chemotherapy (133). Furthermore, this reduction in COX-2 expression was seen mainly in clinical responders, a phenomenon that is also documented in other cancers (134). Another interesting finding in this study was that in patients with ER-positive and COX-2-positive tumours at baseline, post-chemotherapy COX-2 positivity had a significant negative influence on PFS, suggesting that COX-2 could play an important role in hormone-dependent breast cancers.

The interest in COX-2 expression in cancer arises from the fact that this over-expression occurs in many human malignancies including colon and lung cancer (131, 135, 136), and the possibility of using widely available COX-2 inhibitors, *e.g.*, nonsteroidal anti-inflammatory drugs, together with conventional anticancer therapy to enhance treatment efficacy. This is based on the premise that many of the COX-2-regulated genes that contribute to tumour progression may also be determinants of tumour sensitivity to treatment (137). Although the potential chemopreventive properties of selective COX-2 inhibitors are being actively investigated, little is known about the utility of these agents in the treatment of cancer. However, there is emerging data from breast, pancreatic and lung cancer studies showing potential benefit of combining COX-2 inhibitors with chemotherapy (137-139). In particular, a recent study involving patients with heavily pretreated breast cancer showed that the combination of chemotherapy and a selective COX-2 inhibitor resulted in a statistically significant doubling of time to progression for COX-2-positive tumours compared with COX-2 negative ones. At this point in time, there have not been confirmatory studies on COX2 serial changes post chemotherapy in breast cancer but this appears to be an area worth exploring. In particular, post-chemotherapy COX-2 expression may serve as a biomarker for COX-2 inhibition as a therapeutic strategy that warrants evaluation.

2. Topo2α

A seminal study (140) analyzed the value of Topo2*α* in predicting clinical response to anthracycline-based neoadjuvant chemotherapy in breast cancers and its potential changes after chemotherapy. The study also looked at p53 and Her2 the latter being commonly coexpressed with Topo2α. Forty-one patients with primary breast cancer and treated with neoadjuvant anthracycline-based chemotherapy were included in the study. Topo2α, Her2 and p53 expression were measured by IHC in pre- and post-chemotherapy tumour specimens and the results were correlated with clinical response. Topo2α was overexpressed in 16 of 41 (31%) tumours before treatment, and this baseline overexpression was significantly associated with clinical response. Of note, Topo2α overexpression, but not Her2 or p53, was lost in specimens after chemotherapy, although this change did not correlate with clinical response. The observed link between baseline Topo2α expression and clinical response to neoadjuvant anthracycline-based chemotherapy, together with its loss after chemotherapy, suggests that Topo2α deserves further testing in a prospective setting as a predictive marker for chemotherapy response.

3. MGMT

O6-Methylguanine-DNA methyltransferase (MGMT) rapidly reverses alkylation (including methylation) at the O6 position of guanine by transferring the alkyl-group to the active site of the enzyme, constituted by a cysteine. An inactivated MGMT gene allows accumulation of O6-alkylguanine that is the most cytotoxic lesion of alkylating agents, which subsequent to incorrect pairing with thymidine triggers mismatch repair, thereby inducing DNA damage and eventually cell death. There has been one recent trial published by a Japanese group showing the possible utility of MGMT in breast cancer (141). The study evaluated thirty-two basal like breast cancer patients receiving neoadjuvant chemotherapy with an anthracycline and taxane-based regimen. The immunoreactivities of MGMT, MLH1, MSH2 and BRCA1 before and after neoadjuvant chemotherapy were evaluated. pCR was achieved in 10 of 32 cases (31%), and cancer-related and disease-free survival rates were significantly higher in the pCR group than in the non-pCR group. In biopsy samples before neoadjuvant chemotherapy, attenuated expression of MGMT, MLH1, MSH2 and BRCA1 was observed in 12/32 (38%), 0/32 (0%), 5/32 (16%) and 28/32 (88%) cases, respectively. On evaluation of predictors of pCR, including patient characteristics (age, menopausal status, clinical and pathological stages) and immunohistochemical patterns, pre-chemotherapy reduced expression of MGMT was found to be the only factor significantly predictive of pCR. Paired biopsy samples before neoadjuvant chemotherapy and surgical tumour material after neoadjuvant chemotherapy were available for 19 cases of non-pCR. In these 19 cases, decrease in expression of MGMT during neoadjuvant chemotherapy was more frequently observed in those with tumour shrinkage (i.e. > 60%) as compared to those with no decrease, although the difference was not statistically significant possibly due to the small sample size. If these results can be validated, baseline MGMT expression may be used as a predictor of pCR to neoadjuvant chemotherapy, while decrease in MGMT expression with chemotherapy may have additional predictive value for treatment response.

4. Heat shock protein 70

Recently one group has shown using proteomic analysis (2-dimensional gel electrophoresis and mass spectrometry) of fourteen matched pairs of ER positive tumour tissues before and after neoadjuvant treatment with an aromatase inhibitor (AI) that ten proteins were differentially expressed before and after AI treatment. Among the identified proteins, treatment-induced reduction in heat shock protein 70 (Hsp-70) expression was the most significantly correlated with both clinical and pathological responses (142). This downregulation of Hsp-70 with chemotherapy was subsequently confirmed by IHC. These findings suggest that Hsp-70 may represent a potential novel predictive marker to endocrine therapy response (143).

5. Osteopontin

Osteopontin has been reported to be a malignancy-associated protein measurable in tumour tissue and blood. In a prospective clinical study that measured serial plasma osteopontin levels in women with metastatic breast cancer throughout the course of their disease, serial elevation of osteopontin was found to be prognostic (144).

One hundred fifty-eight women with newly diagnosed metastatic breast cancer were enrolled in the study. Plasma osteopontin was measured using an ELISA assay, at baseline and every 3 to 12 weeks during and after therapy until death. Multivariate time-dependent survival analyses were conducted using models that right censored patient outcomes 3, 6, and 12 months after the last known osteopontin measurement. Osteopontin was measured in 1,378 samples (median, 9 per patient). Ninety-nine patients had elevated baseline osteopontin (median, 177 ng/ml; range, 1-2,648 ng/ml). In univariate analysis, elevated baseline osteopontin was associated with shorter survival ($p = 0.02$). In a multivariate model incorporating standard prognostic factors, baseline osteopontin was only marginally significantly associated with survival duration (relative risk, 1.001; $p = 0.038$). However, in a multivariate model incorporating standard prognostic factors and changes in sequential osteopontin levels, an osteopontin increase of >250 ng/mL at any time was the variable with the most prognostic value for poor survival (relative risk, 3.26; $p=0.0003$).

This study is a further proof of concept that serial changes (and not just a baseline value) in a blood biomarker (and not just a tumour biomarker) can be prognostic in breast cancer.

6. Serial changes in protein profiles identified by high-throughput assays

The study of serial changes in protein profiles in tumour and/or serum induced by chemotherapy has been assessed in a high throughput fashion. In a proteomics study, comparison of protein profiles using MALDI-TOF analysis of sera acquired before and after preoperative chemotherapy for breast cancer was performed (145). The study analyzed pre- and post-chemotherapy protein profiles of sera from 39 Her2-postive breast cancer patients who received 6 months of preoperative chemotherapy using liquid chromatography-MALDI-TOF/MS technology, and detected qualitative and quantitative differences in pair-wise comparison of pre- and post chemotherapy samples that were different in the 21 patients who achieved pathological complete response compared with the 18 patients with residual disease. 2329 and 3152 peaks were identified as differentially expressed in the pre-chemotherapy samples of the responders and non-responders respectively. Comparison of paired pre- and post-chemotherapy samples identified 34 (32 decreased, 2 increased) and 304 peaks (157 decreased, 147 increased) that significantly changed after treatment in responders and non-responders, respectively. The top 11 most significantly altered peptide peaks with the greatest change in intensity were also identified. These peaks matched eight different known proteins in an NCBInr database search by MASCOT® software, including α-2-macroglobulin, complement 3, hemopexin, and serum amyloid P in the responder group and chains C and A of apolipoprotein A-I, hemopexin precursor, complement C, and amyloid P component in the non-responding group. All proteins decreased after therapy, except chain C apolipoprotein A and hemopexin precursor that increased. These results suggest that changes in serum protein levels occur in response to chemotherapy and these changes to a certain extent appear different in patients who are highly sensitive to chemotherapy compared with those who are more resistant.

7. Negative studies of post chemotherapy changes in biomarkers

Publication bias would tend to result in under-reporting of negative findings of changes in biomarkers post-chemotherapy. In the few negative trials published, some of them conflict with the findings of the other trials mentioned above. For example, in a study of 97 patients who received neoadjuvant anthracycline-based chemotherapy (146), the authors failed to find any post-chemotherapy change in ER, Her2, p53, Ki67 or Bcl2 as assessed by IHC. This is in contradistinction to the study by Dawson *et al* (64) who found changes in Bcl2. One possible reason for the failure to find a change in the biomarkers post-chemotherapy is the small sample size in this trial.

G. The future of protein biomarkers in breast cancer

Studies of protein biomarkers in breast cancer still rely heavily on IHC and with a possible emerging role of ELISA. Newer technologies on the horizon could facilitate the discovery of novel biomarkers in a high throughput fashion, and there are a few interesting developments attempting to push the frontier in proteomics.

1. SILAC

SILAC (stable isotope labeling by/with amino acids in cell culture) is a MS-based methodology (used for quantitative proteomics) that detects differences in protein abundance using non-radioactive labeling. SILAC has emerged as a very powerful method to study cell signaling, post translation modifications, protein-protein interaction and regulation of gene expression.

2. Peptidomics

The low-molecular-weight plasma (serum proteome) has been the focus of recent attempts to find new biomarkers (147). Peptides are critical for many physiological processes, such as blood glucose (insulin) regulation. It has been suggested that "the low molecular-weight region of the blood proteome contains precious diagnostic information (148). The low-molecular-weight serum proteome has been characterized by ultrafiltration, enzymatic digestion, and liquid chromatography coupled to tandem mass spectrometry (149, 150), or via a top-down proteomics approach (whereby the intact peptide is distinguished directly by its fragment ions) (151) or by means of pattern profiling (152). Informative diagnostic peptides that are generated after proteolysis of high-abundance proteins by the coagulation and complement enzymatic cascades can be identified by mass spectrometry. These proteomic patterns were claimed to distinguish not only healthy controls from patients with cancer (153) but also between various types of cancer (152). However, one major concern is that these peptides present in the serum are derived from a small number of highly abundant proteins. One study showed that peptides in serum are affected by collection conditions. Improper collection could give rise to artefacts and serum is not ideal for proteomic experiments as it contains substantial endoproteolytic and exoproteolytic enzymatic activity (154). These findings raise concerns regarding peptidomics data generated by profiling technologies, with some investigators suggesting that peptidomic profiling might represent nothing more than peptides cleaved during coagulation or functions inherent to plasma or serum, including immune modulation, inflammatory response and protease inhibition (155). In addition, many of the issues associated with mass-spectrometry- based protein profiling technologies also apply to peptidomics. Thus, while this technology looks promising, more confirmatory data is required and awaited.

3. Cancer-biomarker-family approach

The basis for the 'cancer biomarker family' approach is that if a member of a protein family is already an established biomarker, then other members of that family might also be candidate cancer biomarkers. As an example, Prostate Specific Antigen (PSA) is a member of the human tissue kallikrein family. Kallikreins are secreted enzymes with trypsin-like or chymotrypsin-like serine protease activity. This enzyme family consists of 15 genes clustered in tandem on chromosome 19q13.4.63. PSA (KLK3) and KLK2 currently have important clinical applications as prostate cancer biomarkers (156). Other members of the human kallikrein family have been implicated in the process of carcinogenesis and are being investigated as biomarkers for diagnosis and prognosis. For example, KLK6 has been studied as a novel biomarker for ovarian cancer (157), and it was found that elevated serum levels of KLK6 was associated with late-stage tumour, high grade and serous histology and chemo-resistance. Similarly, KLK3, KLK5 and KLK14 have been shown to be increased in the serum of patients with breast cancer, thereby potentially serving as diagnostic markers. The fact that these proteins are serine proteases could implicate them in tumour progression through extracellular matrix degradation.

4. Secreted protein approach

Examination of tissues or biological fluids near to the tumour site of origin could facilitate identification of candidate biomarker molecules. The mounting evidence that tumour growth is dependent on the malignant potential of the tumour cells as well as on the microenvironment surrounding the tumour (*e.g.*, stroma, inflammatory cells, etc) further supports this approach (158). A number of technologies can be employed for analysis of these samples, but for systematic characterization of proteins in complex mixtures, mass spectrometry is the preferred technology. In the case of breast cancer, breast tissue, nipple aspirate fluid, breast cyst fluid and tumour interstitial fluid can all be explored. The tumour interstitial fluid that perfuses the tumour microenvironment in invasive ductal carcinomas of the breast has been examined by proteomic approaches (159). Over 250 proteins were identified, many of which were relevant to processes such as cell proliferation and invasion. The identification of secreted proteins in tissues or other biological fluids does not necessarily imply that the proteins will be detectable in the sera of cancer patients though, as this will depend on the stability of the protein, its clearance, its association with other serum proteins and the extent of post-translational modifications.

20–25% of all proteins are secreted and/ or undergo aberrant secretion of membrane-bound proteins that have a secretable/ cleavable extracellular domain. Alterations in the signal peptide of proteins as a result of single nucleotide polymorphisms can result in unusual secretion patterns (160). Moreover, elevation of molecules in biological fluids can result from a change in the polarity of cancer cells, which can lead to the release of cancer-associated glycoproteins into the circulation. Increased expression of proteases that cleave the extracellular domain portion of membrane proteins can also cause increased circulating levels. One currently used secreted marker in breast cancer is that of CA15-3; it being a soluble form of MUC1, which is an antigenic focus on breast cancer. It is hoped that in the years to come, more of such secreted proteins can be discovered so as to facilitate breast cancer monitoring.

2. Conclusion

Biomarkers guide physicians in counseling patients with regard to their prognosis and also provide information to physicians with respect to the optimal treatment for a particular patient/ patient group. The latter scenario (predictive biomarkers) is an area in which the natural history of the patient can be affected positively and thus are deemed to be more important.

The baseline status of the predictive protein biomarkers ER, PR and Her2 are the most important in current breast cancer management. While post chemotherapy protein biomarkers in breast cancer is not currently used in routine clinical practice, evaluation of serial changes in expression of proteins in response to neoadjuvant chemotherapy has been shown to be feasible and in some studies shown to be a better biomarker than the baseline biomarker. It is achievable using an ELISA or IHC platform, which are technologies that are readily available in almost all clinical practices. However, the logistical challenges of obtaining serial tumour samples, reproducibility of the expression profile and patients' compliance could be major factors that may limit widespread application of studying serial changes of protein expression in tumor routinely. There is also the issue of intra and inter-individual variability when examining for the presence of prognostic and/or predictive serial changes in any putative biomarkers. In fact such an issue already exists with regard to Her2 testing by FISH; the clinical significance of genetic heterogeneity (i.e. in certain tumours, only a fraction of the cells are positive for the oncoprotein) of Her2 is still being investigated (84, 161).

Although newer technologies (*e.g.*, MALDI-TOF, etc.) are promising, the inability to identify all 'peaks' and the reproducibility issues at this point in time are major limitations. However, development of methods that allows rapid characterization of identified protein peaks holds promise for more widespread use of these technologies in the near future.

Author details

Daniel Chan and Soo-Chin Lee
National University Cancer Institute Singapore

3. References

[1] King MC, Marks JH and Mandell JB: Breast and ovarian cancer risks due to inherited mutations in BRCA1 and BRCA2. Science 302: 643-646, 2003.

[2] Mitrunen K and Hirvonen A: Molecular epidemiology of sporadic breast cancer. The role of polymorphic genes involved in oestrogen biosynthesis and metabolism. Mutat Res 544: 9-41, 2003.

[3] Zhang Y, Newcomb PA, Egan KM, *et al*: Genetic polymorphisms in base-excision repair pathway genes and risk of breast cancer. Cancer Epidemiol Biomarkers Prev 15: 353-358, 2006.

[4] van 't Veer LJ, Dai H, van de Vijver MJ, *et al*: Expression profiling predicts outcome in breast cancer. Breast Cancer Res 5: 57-58, 2003.

[5] Reis-Filho JS and Lakhani SR: Breast cancer special types: why bother? J Pathol 216: 394-398, 2008.

[6] Rodenhiser D and Mann M: Epigenetics and human disease: translating basic biology into clinical applications. Cmaj 174: 341-348, 2006.

[7] Ravdin PM, Siminoff LA, Davis GJ, *et al*: Computer program to assist in making decisions about adjuvant therapy for women with early breast cancer. J Clin Oncol 19: 980-991, 2001.

[8] Blamey RW, Ellis IO, Pinder SE, *et al*: Survival of invasive breast cancer according to the Nottingham Prognostic Index in cases diagnosed in 1990-1999. Eur J Cancer 43: 1548-1555, 2007.

[9] Blamey RW, Pinder SE, Ball GR, *et al*: Reading the prognosis of the individual with breast cancer. Eur J Cancer 43: 1545-1547, 2007.

[10] Paik S, Hazan R, Fisher ER, *et al*: Pathologic findings from the National Surgical Adjuvant Breast and Bowel Project: prognostic significance of erbB-2 protein overexpression in primary breast cancer. J Clin Oncol 8: 103-112, 1990.

[11] Yamauchi H, Stearns V and Hayes DF: When is a tumor marker ready for prime time? A case study of c-erbB-2 as a predictive factor in breast cancer. J Clin Oncol 19: 2334-2356, 2001.

[12] Chia S, Norris B, Speers C, *et al*: Human epidermal growth factor receptor 2 overexpression as a prognostic factor in a large tissue microarray series of node-negative breast cancers. J Clin Oncol 26: 5697-5704, 2008.

[13] McShane LM, Altman DG, Sauerbrei W, Taube SE, Gion M and Clark GM: Reporting recommendations for tumor marker prognostic studies (REMARK). J Natl Cancer Inst 97: 1180-1184, 2005.

[14] van 't Veer LJ, Dai H, van de Vijver MJ, *et al*: Gene expression profiling predicts clinical outcome of breast cancer. Nature 415: 530-536, 2002.

[15] Sorlie T, Tibshirani R, Parker J, *et al*: Repeated observation of breast tumor subtypes in independent gene expression data sets. Proc Natl Acad Sci U S A 100: 8418-8423, 2003.

[16] Paik S, Tang G, Shak S, *et al*: Gene expression and benefit of chemotherapy in women with node-negative, estrogen receptor-positive breast cancer. J Clin Oncol 24: 3726-3734, 2006.

[17] Cardoso F, Van't Veer L, Rutgers E, Loi S, Mook S and Piccart-Gebhart MJ: Clinical application of the 70-gene profile: the MINDACT trial. J Clin Oncol 26: 729-735, 2008.

[18] Sparano JA and Paik S: Development of the 21-gene assay and its application in clinical practice and clinical trials. J Clin Oncol 26: 721-728, 2008.

[19] Tewari M, Krishnamurthy A and Shukla HS: Predictive markers of response to neoadjuvant chemotherapy in breast cancer. Surg Oncol 17: 301-311, 2008.

[20] Symmans WF, Peintinger F, Hatzis C, *et al*: Measurement of residual breast cancer burden to predict survival after neoadjuvant chemotherapy. J Clin Oncol 25: 4414-4422, 2007.

[21] Ayers M, Symmans WF, Stec J, *et al*: Gene expression profiles predict complete pathologic response to neoadjuvant paclitaxel and fluorouracil, doxorubicin, and cyclophosphamide chemotherapy in breast cancer. J Clin Oncol 22: 2284-2293, 2004.

[22] Paik S, Shak S, Tang G, *et al*: A multigene assay to predict recurrence of tamoxifen-treated, node-negative breast cancer. N Engl J Med 351: 2817-2826, 2004.

[23] Hu Z, Fan C, Oh DS, *et al*: The molecular portraits of breast tumors are conserved across microarray platforms. BMC Genomics 7: 96, 2006.

[24] Fan C, Oh DS, Wessels L, *et al*: Concordance among gene-expression-based predictors for breast cancer. N Engl J Med 355: 560-569, 2006.

[25] Bergamaschi A, Kim YH, Wang P, *et al*: Distinct patterns of DNA copy number alteration are associated with different clinicopathological features and gene-expression subtypes of breast cancer. Genes Chromosomes Cancer 45: 1033-1040, 2006.

[26] Neve RM, Chin K, Fridlyand J, *et al*: A collection of breast cancer cell lines for the study of functionally distinct cancer subtypes. Cancer Cell 10: 515-527, 2006.

[27] Hess KR, Anderson K, Symmans WF, *et al*: Pharmacogenomic predictor of sensitivity to preoperative chemotherapy with paclitaxel and fluorouracil, doxorubicin, and cyclophosphamide in breast cancer. J Clin Oncol 24: 4236-4244, 2006.

[28] Perou CM, Sorlie T, Eisen MB, *et al*: Molecular portraits of human breast tumours. Nature 406: 747-752, 2000.

[29] Sorlie T, Perou CM, Tibshirani R, *et al*: Gene expression patterns of breast carcinomas distinguish tumor subclasses with clinical implications. Proc Natl Acad Sci U S A 98: 10869-10874, 2001.

[30] Reis-Filho JS and Tutt AN: Triple negative tumours: a critical review. Histopathology 52: 108-118, 2008.

[31] Hugh J, Hanson J, Cheang MC, *et al*: Breast cancer subtypes and response to docetaxel in node-positive breast cancer: use of an immunohistochemical definition in the BCIRG 001 trial. J Clin Oncol 27: 1168-1176, 2009.

[32] Parker JS, Mullins M, Cheang MC, *et al*: Supervised risk predictor of breast cancer based on intrinsic subtypes. J Clin Oncol 27: 1160-1167, 2009.

[33] Peppercorn J, Perou CM and Carey LA: Molecular subtypes in breast cancer evaluation and management: divide and conquer. Cancer Invest 26: 1-10, 2008.

[34] Weigelt B, Baehner FL and Reis-Filho JS: The contribution of gene expression profiling to breast cancer classification, prognostication and prediction: a retrospective of the last decade. J Pathol 220: 263-280, 2010.

[35] Tan SH and Lee SC: Clinical implications of chemotherapy-induced tumor gene expression in human breast cancers. Expert Opin Drug Metab Toxicol 6: 283-306, 2010.

[36] Reis-Filho JS and Lakhani SR: The diagnosis and management of pre-invasive breast disease: genetic alterations in pre-invasive lesions. Breast Cancer Res 5: 313-319, 2003.

[37] Wang Y, Klijn JG, Zhang Y, *et al*: Gene-expression profiles to predict distant metastasis of lymph-node-negative primary breast cancer. Lancet 365: 671-679, 2005.

[38] Banks RE, Dunn MJ, Hochstrasser DF, *et al*: Proteomics: new perspectives, new biomedical opportunities. Lancet 356: 1749-1756, 2000.

[39] Aebersold R, Anderson L, Caprioli R, Druker B, Hartwell L and Smith R: Perspective: a program to improve protein biomarker discovery for cancer. J Proteome Res 4: 1104-1109, 2005.

[40] Abramovitz M and Leyland-Jones B: A systems approach to clinical oncology: focus on breast cancer. Proteome Sci 4: 5, 2006.

[41] Garcia M, Millat-Carus R, Bertucci F, Finetti P, Birnbaum D and Bidaut G: Interactome-transcriptome integration for predicting distant metastasis in breast cancer. Bioinformatics 28: 672-678, 2012.

[42] Hammond ME, Hayes DF, Dowsett M, *et al*: American Society of Clinical Oncology/College Of American Pathologists guideline recommendations for immunohistochemical testing of estrogen and progesterone receptors in breast cancer. J Clin Oncol 28: 2784-2795, 2010.

[43] Yao L, Liu Y, Li Z, *et al*: HER2 and response to anthracycline-based neoadjuvant chemotherapy in breast cancer. Ann Oncol 22: 1326-1331, 2010.

[44] Harris L, Fritsche H, Mennel R, *et al*: American Society of Clinical Oncology 2007 update of recommendations for the use of tumor markers in breast cancer. J Clin Oncol 25: 5287-5312, 2007.

[45] Codony-Servat J, Albanell J, Lopez-Talavera JC, Arribas J and Baselga J: Cleavage of the HER2 ectodomain is a pervanadate-activable process that is inhibited by the tissue inhibitor of metalloproteases-1 in breast cancer cells. Cancer Res 59: 1196-1201, 1999.

[46] Molina MA, Codony-Servat J, Albanell J, Rojo F, Arribas J and Baselga J: Trastuzumab (herceptin), a humanized anti-Her2 receptor monoclonal antibody, inhibits basal and activated Her2 ectodomain cleavage in breast cancer cells. Cancer Res 61: 4744-4749, 2001.

[47] Hudelist G, Kostler WJ, Attems J, *et al*: Her-2/neu-triggered intracellular tyrosine kinase activation: in vivo relevance of ligand-independent activation mechanisms and impact upon the efficacy of trastuzumab-based treatment. Br J Cancer 89: 983-991, 2003.

[48] Molina MA, Saez R, Ramsey EE, *et al*: NH(2)-terminal truncated HER-2 protein but not full-length receptor is associated with nodal metastasis in human breast cancer. Clin Cancer Res 8: 347-353, 2002.

[49] Schwartz MK, Smith C, Schwartz DC, Dnistrian A and Neiman I: Monitoring therapy by serum HER-2/neu. Int J Biol Markers 15: 324-329, 2000.

[50] Muller V, Witzel I, Luck HJ, *et al*: Prognostic and predictive impact of the HER-2/ neu extracellular domain (ECD) in the serum of patients treated with chemotherapy for metastatic breast cancer. Breast Cancer Res Treat 86: 9-18, 2004.

[51] Esteva FJ, Cheli CD, Fritsche H, *et al*: Clinical utility of serum HER2/neu in monitoring and prediction of progression-free survival in metastatic breast cancer patients treated with trastuzumab-based therapies. Breast Cancer Res 7: R436-443, 2005.

[52] Ebeling FG, Stieber P, Untch M, *et al*: Serum CEA and CA 15-3 as prognostic factors in primary breast cancer. Br J Cancer 86: 1217-1222, 2002.

[53] Gion M, Boracchi P, Dittadi R, *et al*: Prognostic role of serum CA15.3 in 362 node-negative breast cancers. An old player for a new game. Eur J Cancer 38: 1181-1188, 2002.
[54] Kumpulainen EJ, Keskikuru RJ and Johansson RT: Serum tumor marker CA 15.3 and stage are the two most powerful predictors of survival in primary breast cancer. Breast Cancer Res Treat 76: 95-102, 2002.
[55] Martin A, Corte MD, Alvarez AM, *et al*: Prognostic value of pre-operative serum CA 15.3 levels in breast cancer. Anticancer Res 26: 3965-3971, 2006.
[56] Slamon D, Eiermann W, Robert N, *et al*: Adjuvant trastuzumab in HER2-positive breast cancer. N Engl J Med 365: 1273-1283, 2011.
[57] Di Fiore PP, Pierce JH, Fleming TP, *et al*: Overexpression of the human EGF receptor confers an EGF-dependent transformed phenotype to NIH 3T3 cells. Cell 51: 1063-1070, 1987.
[58] Lo HW, Xia W, Wei Y, Ali-Seyed M, Huang SF and Hung MC: Novel prognostic value of nuclear epidermal growth factor receptor in breast cancer. Cancer Res 65: 338-348, 2005.
[59] Rimawi MF, Shetty PB, Weiss HL, *et al*: Epidermal growth factor receptor expression in breast cancer association with biologic phenotype and clinical outcomes. Cancer 116: 1234-1242, 2010.
[60] Chae BJ, Bae JS, Lee A, *et al*: p53 as a specific prognostic factor in triple-negative breast cancer. Jpn J Clin Oncol 39: 217-224, 2009.
[61] Lacroix M, Toillon RA and Leclercq G: p53 and breast cancer, an update. Endocr Relat Cancer 13: 293-325, 2006.
[62] Silvestrini R, Veneroni S, Daidone MG, *et al*: The Bcl-2 protein: a prognostic indicator strongly related to p53 protein in lymph node-negative breast cancer patients. J Natl Cancer Inst 86: 499-504, 1994.
[63] Lipponen P, Pietilainen T, Kosma VM, Aaltomaa S, Eskelinen M and Syrjanen K: Apoptosis suppressing protein bcl-2 is expressed in well-differentiated breast carcinomas with favourable prognosis. J Pathol 177: 49-55, 1995.
[64] Dawson SJ, Makretsov N, Blows FM, *et al*: BCL2 in breast cancer: a favourable prognostic marker across molecular subtypes and independent of adjuvant therapy received. Br J Cancer 103: 668-675, 2010.
[65] Petricoin EF, Ardekani AM, Hitt BA, *et al*: Use of proteomic patterns in serum to identify ovarian cancer. Lancet 359: 572-577, 2002.
[66] Paradis V, Degos F, Dargere D, *et al*: Identification of a new marker of hepatocellular carcinoma by serum protein profiling of patients with chronic liver diseases. Hepatology 41: 40-47, 2005.
[67] Rosty C, Christa L, Kuzdzal S, *et al*: Identification of hepatocarcinoma-intestine-pancreas/pancreatitis-associated protein I as a biomarker for pancreatic ductal adenocarcinoma by protein biochip technology. Cancer Res 62: 1868-1875, 2002.
[68] Li J, Zhang Z, Rosenzweig J, Wang YY and Chan DW: Proteomics and bioinformatics approaches for identification of serum biomarkers to detect breast cancer. Clin Chem 48: 1296-1304, 2002.

[69] Brozkova K, Budinska E, Bouchal P, *et al*: Surface-enhanced laser desorption/ionization time-of-flight proteomic profiling of breast carcinomas identifies clinicopathologically relevant groups of patients similar to previously defined clusters from cDNA expression. Breast Cancer Res 10: R48, 2008.

[70] Goncalves A, Charafe-Jauffret E, Bertucci F, *et al*: Protein profiling of human breast tumor cells identifies novel biomarkers associated with molecular subtypes. Mol Cell Proteomics 7: 1420-1433, 2008.

[71] Goncalves A, Esterni B, Bertucci F, *et al*: Postoperative serum proteomic profiles may predict metastatic relapse in high-risk primary breast cancer patients receiving adjuvant chemotherapy. Oncogene 25: 981-989, 2006.

[72] Ricolleau G, Charbonnel C, Lode L, *et al*: Surface-enhanced laser desorption/ionization time of flight mass spectrometry protein profiling identifies ubiquitin and ferritin light chain as prognostic biomarkers in node-negative breast cancer tumors. Proteomics 6: 1963-1975, 2006.

[73] Sanders ME, Dias EC, Xu BJ, *et al*: Differentiating proteomic biomarkers in breast cancer by laser capture microdissection and MALDI MS. J Proteome Res 7: 1500-1507, 2008.

[74] Leong S, Christopherson RI and Baxter RC: Profiling of apoptotic changes in human breast cancer cells using SELDI-TOF mass spectrometry. Cell Physiol Biochem 20: 579-590, 2007.

[75] Mian S, Ball G, Hornbuckle J, *et al*: A prototype methodology combining surface-enhanced laser desorption/ionization protein chip technology and artificial neural network algorithms to predict the chemoresponsiveness of breast cancer cell lines exposed to Paclitaxel and Doxorubicin under in vitro conditions. Proteomics 3: 1725-1737, 2003.

[76] Dowling P, Maurya P, Meleady P, *et al*: Purification and identification of a 7.6-kDa protein in media conditioned by superinvasive cancer cells. Anticancer Res 27: 1309-1317, 2007.

[77] Dekker LJ, Boogerd W, Stockhammer G, *et al*: MALDI-TOF mass spectrometry analysis of cerebrospinal fluid tryptic peptide profiles to diagnose leptomeningeal metastases in patients with breast cancer. Mol Cell Proteomics 4: 1341-1349, 2005.

[78] Pusztai L, Gregory BW, Baggerly KA, *et al*: Pharmacoproteomic analysis of prechemotherapy and postchemotherapy plasma samples from patients receiving neoadjuvant or adjuvant chemotherapy for breast carcinoma. Cancer 100: 1814-1822, 2004.

[79] Heike Y, Hosokawa M, Osumi S, *et al*: Identification of serum proteins related to adverse effects induced by docetaxel infusion from protein expression profiles of serum using SELDI ProteinChip system. Anticancer Res 25: 1197-1203, 2005.

[80] Beriwal S, Schwartz GF, Komarnicky L and Garcia-Young JA: Breast-conserving therapy after neoadjuvant chemotherapy: long-term results. Breast J 12: 159-164, 2006.

[81] Bonadonna G, Veronesi U, Brambilla C, *et al*: Primary chemotherapy to avoid mastectomy in tumors with diameters of three centimeters or more. J Natl Cancer Inst 82: 1539-1545, 1990.

[82] Schwartz GF, Meltzer AJ, Lucarelli EA, Cantor JP and Curcillo PG, 2nd: Breast conservation after neoadjuvant chemotherapy for stage II carcinoma of the breast. J Am Coll Surg 201: 327-334, 2005.

[83] Stearns V, Singh B, Tsangaris T, *et al*: A prospective randomized pilot study to evaluate predictors of response in serial core biopsies to single agent neoadjuvant doxorubicin or paclitaxel for patients with locally advanced breast cancer. Clin Cancer Res 9: 124-133, 2003.

[84] Vance GH, Barry TS, Bloom KJ, *et al*: Genetic heterogeneity in HER2 testing in breast cancer: panel summary and guidelines. Arch Pathol Lab Med 133: 611-612, 2009.

[85] Hanash SM, Pitteri SJ and Faca VM: Mining the plasma proteome for cancer biomarkers. Nature 452: 571-579, 2008.

[86] Conrads TP, Zhou M, Petricoin EF, 3rd, Liotta L and Veenstra TD: Cancer diagnosis using proteomic patterns. Expert Rev Mol Diagn 3: 411-420, 2003.

[87] Grizzle WE, Semmes OJ, Bigbee W, *et al*: the need for review and understanding of SELDI/MALDI mass spectroscopy data prior to analysis. Cancer Inform 1: 86-97, 2005.

[88] Callesen AK, Vach W, Jorgensen PE, *et al*: Combined experimental and statistical strategy for mass spectrometry based serum protein profiling for diagnosis of breast cancer: a case-control study. J Proteome Res 7: 1419-1426, 2008.

[89] Shin S, Cazares L, Schneider H, *et al*: Serum biomarkers to differentiate benign and malignant mammographic lesions. J Am Coll Surg 204: 1065-1071; discussion 1071-1063, 2007.

[90] Rompp A, Dekker L, Taban I, *et al*: Identification of leptomeningeal metastasis-related proteins in cerebrospinal fluid of patients with breast cancer by a combination of MALDI-TOF, MALDI-FTICR and nanoLC-FTICR MS. Proteomics 7: 474-481, 2007.

[91] Good DM, Thongboonkerd V, Novak J, *et al*: Body fluid proteomics for biomarker discovery: lessons from the past hold the key to success in the future. J Proteome Res 6: 4549-4555, 2007.

[92] Pories SE, Zurakowski D, Roy R, *et al*: Urinary metalloproteinases: noninvasive biomarkers for breast cancer risk assessment. Cancer Epidemiol Biomarkers Prev 17: 1034-1042, 2008.

[93] Li J, Zhao J, Yu X, *et al*: Identification of biomarkers for breast cancer in nipple aspiration and ductal lavage fluid. Clin Cancer Res 11: 8312-8320, 2005.

[94] Punnoose EA, Atwal SK, Spoerke JM, *et al*: Molecular biomarker analyses using circulating tumor cells. PLoS One 5: e12517, 2010.

[95] Callagy G, Cattaneo E, Daigo Y, *et al*: Molecular classification of breast carcinomas using tissue microarrays. Diagn Mol Pathol 12: 27-34, 2003.

[96] Bertucci F and Goncalves A: Clinical proteomics and breast cancer: strategies for diagnostic and therapeutic biomarker discovery. Future Oncol 4: 271-287, 2008.

[97] Hondermarck H, Vercoutter-Edouart AS, Revillion F, *et al*: Proteomics of breast cancer for marker discovery and signal pathway profiling. Proteomics 1: 1216-1232, 2001.

[98] Engwegen JY, Gast MC, Schellens JH and Beijnen JH: Clinical proteomics: searching for better tumour markers with SELDI-TOF mass spectrometry. Trends Pharmacol Sci 27: 251-259, 2006.

[99] Hortin GL: The MALDI-TOF mass spectrometric view of the plasma proteome and peptidome. Clin Chem 52: 1223-1237, 2006.

[100] Merchant M and Weinberger SR: Recent advancements in surface-enhanced laser desorption/ionization-time of flight-mass spectrometry. Electrophoresis 21: 1164-1177, 2000.

[101] Simpson RJ, Bernhard OK, Greening DW and Moritz RL: Proteomics-driven cancer biomarker discovery: looking to the future. Curr Opin Chem Biol 12: 72-77, 2008.

[102] Wulfkuhle JD, Paweletz CP, Steeg PS, Petricoin EF, 3rd and Liotta L: Proteomic approaches to the diagnosis, treatment, and monitoring of cancer. Adv Exp Med Biol 532: 59-68, 2003.

[103] Gast MC, Bonfrer JM, van Dulken EJ, *et al*: SELDI-TOF MS serum protein profiles in breast cancer: assessment of robustness and validity. Cancer Biomark 2: 235-248, 2006.

[104] Vlahou A, Laronga C, Wilson L, *et al*: A novel approach toward development of a rapid blood test for breast cancer. Clin Breast Cancer 4: 203-209, 2003.

[105] Laronga C, Becker S, Watson P, *et al*: SELDI-TOF serum profiling for prognostic and diagnostic classification of breast cancers. Dis Markers 19: 229-238, 2003.

[106] Karsan A, Eigl BJ, Flibotte S, *et al*: Analytical and preanalytical biases in serum proteomic pattern analysis for breast cancer diagnosis. Clin Chem 51: 1525-1528, 2005.

[107] Banks RE, Stanley AJ, Cairns DA, *et al*: Influences of blood sample processing on low-molecular-weight proteome identified by surface-enhanced laser desorption/ionization mass spectrometry. Clin Chem 51: 1637-1649, 2005.

[108] Baggerly KA, Morris JS, Edmonson SR and Coombes KR: Signal in noise: evaluating reported reproducibility of serum proteomic tests for ovarian cancer. J Natl Cancer Inst 97: 307-309, 2005.

[109] Hennessy BT, Lu Y, Gonzalez-Angulo AM, *et al*: A Technical Assessment of the Utility of Reverse Phase Protein Arrays for the Study of the Functional Proteome in Non-microdissected Human Breast Cancers. Clin Proteomics 6: 129-151, 2010.

[110] Cowherd SM, Espina VA, Petricoin EF, 3rd and Liotta LA: Proteomic analysis of human breast cancer tissue with laser-capture microdissection and reverse-phase protein microarrays. Clin Breast Cancer 5: 385-392, 2004.

[111] van de Ven S, Smit VT, Dekker TJ, Nortier JW and Kroep JR: Discordances in ER, PR and HER2 receptors after neoadjuvant chemotherapy in breast cancer. Cancer Treat Rev 37: 422-430, 2011.

[112] Burcombe RJ, Makris A, Richman PI, *et al*: Evaluation of ER, PgR, HER-2 and Ki-67 as predictors of response to neoadjuvant anthracycline chemotherapy for operable breast cancer. Br J Cancer 92: 147-155, 2005.

[113] Hirata T, Shimizu C, Yonemori K, *et al*: Change in the hormone receptor status following administration of neoadjuvant chemotherapy and its impact on the long-term outcome in patients with primary breast cancer. Br J Cancer 101: 1529-1536, 2009.

[114] Jain V, Landry M and Levine EA: The stability of estrogen and progesterone receptors in patients receiving preoperative chemotherapy for locally advanced breast carcinoma. Am Surg 62: 162-165, 1996.

[115] Bines J, Oleske DM and Cobleigh MA: Ovarian function in premenopausal women treated with adjuvant chemotherapy for breast cancer. J Clin Oncol 14: 1718-1729, 1996.

[116] Frassoldati A, Adami F, Banzi C, Criscuolo M, Piccinini L and Silingardi V: Changes of biological features in breast cancer cells determined by primary chemotherapy. Breast Cancer Res Treat 44: 185-192, 1997.

[117] Kasami M, Uematsu T, Honda M, *et al*: Comparison of estrogen receptor, progesterone receptor and Her-2 status in breast cancer pre- and post-neoadjuvant chemotherapy. Breast 17: 523-527, 2008.

[118] Dowsett M and Dunbier AK: Emerging biomarkers and new understanding of traditional markers in personalized therapy for breast cancer. Clin Cancer Res 14: 8019-8026, 2008.

[119] Tiezzi DG, Andrade JM, Ribeiro-Silva A, Zola FE, Marana HR and Tiezzi MG: HER-2, p53, p21 and hormonal receptors proteins expression as predictive factors of response and prognosis in locally advanced breast cancer treated with neoadjuvant docetaxel plus epirubicin combination. BMC Cancer 7: 36, 2007.

[120] Taucher S, Rudas M, Mader RM, *et al*: Influence of neoadjuvant therapy with epirubicin and docetaxel on the expression of HER2/neu in patients with breast cancer. Breast Cancer Res Treat 82: 207-213, 2003.

[121] Witzel I, Loibl S, von Minckwitz G, *et al*: Monitoring serum HER2 levels during neoadjuvant trastuzumab treatment within the GeparQuattro trial. Breast Cancer Res Treat 123: 437-445, 2010.

[122] Kostler WJ, Steger GG, Soleiman A, *et al*: Monitoring of serum Her-2/neu predicts histopathological response to neoadjuvant trastuzumab-based therapy for breast cancer. Anticancer Res 24: 1127-1130, 2004.

[123] Mazouni C, Hall A, Broglio K, *et al*: Kinetics of serum HER-2/neu changes in patients with HER-2-positive primary breast cancer after initiation of primary chemotherapy. Cancer 109: 496-501, 2007.

[124] Quaranta M, Daniele A, Coviello M, *et al*: c-erbB-2 protein level in tissue and sera of breast cancer patients: a possibly useful clinical correlation. Tumori 92: 311-317, 2006.

[125] Lennon S, Barton C, Banken L, *et al*: Utility of serum HER2 extracellular domain assessment in clinical decision making: pooled analysis of four trials of trastuzumab in metastatic breast cancer. J Clin Oncol 27: 1685-1693, 2009.

[126] Ali SM, Leitzel K, Lipton A, Carney WP and Kostler WJ: Value of serum human epidermal growth factor receptor 2 (HER2)/neu testing for early prediction of response to HER2/neu-directed therapies is still an open one and deserves further study in large prospective trials. J Clin Oncol 27: e273; author reply e274-275, 2009.

[127] Tsujii M, Kawano S, Tsuji S, Sawaoka H, Hori M and DuBois RN: Cyclooxygenase regulates angiogenesis induced by colon cancer cells. Cell 93: 705-716, 1998.

[128] Gately S: The contributions of cyclooxygenase-2 to tumor angiogenesis. Cancer Metastasis Rev 19: 19-27, 2000.

[129] Sheng H, Shao J, Morrow JD, Beauchamp RD and DuBois RN: Modulation of apoptosis and Bcl-2 expression by prostaglandin E2 in human colon cancer cells. Cancer Res 58: 362-366, 1998.

[130] Spizzo G, Gastl G, Wolf D, *et al*: Correlation of COX-2 and Ep-CAM overexpression in human invasive breast cancer and its impact on survival. Br J Cancer 88: 574-578, 2003.

[131] Rolland PH, Martin PM, Jacquemier J, Rolland AM and Toga M: Prostaglandin in human breast cancer: Evidence suggesting that an elevated prostaglandin production is a marker of high metastatic potential for neoplastic cells. J Natl Cancer Inst 64: 1061-1070, 1980.

[132] de Azambuja E, Cardoso F, de Castro G, Jr., *et al*: Ki-67 as prognostic marker in early breast cancer: a meta-analysis of published studies involving 12,155 patients. Br J Cancer 96: 1504-1513, 2007.

[133] Loo WT, Sasano H and Chow LW: Effects of capecitabine and vinorelbine on cell proliferation, metabolism and COX2 and p16 expression in breast cancer cell lines and solid tumour tissues. Biomed Pharmacother 61: 596-600, 2007.

[134] Ferrandina G, Ranelletti FO, Martinelli E, Paglia A, Zannoni GF and Scambia G: Cyclo-oxygenase-2 (Cox-2) expression and resistance to platinum versus platinum/paclitaxel containing chemotherapy in advanced ovarian cancer. BMC Cancer 6: 182, 2006.

[135] Sano H, Kawahito Y, Wilder RL, *et al*: Expression of cyclooxygenase-1 and -2 in human colorectal cancer. Cancer Res 55: 3785-3789, 1995.

[136] Hida T, Yatabe Y, Achiwa H, *et al*: Increased expression of cyclooxygenase 2 occurs frequently in human lung cancers, specifically in adenocarcinomas. Cancer Res 58: 3761-3764, 1998.

[137] Uchida K, Schneider S, Yochim JM, *et al*: Intratumoral COX-2 gene expression is a predictive factor for colorectal cancer response to fluoropyrimidine-based chemotherapy. Clin Cancer Res 11: 3363-3368, 2005.

[138] Lipton A, Campbell-Baird C, Witters L, Harvey H and Ali S: Phase II trial of gemcitabine, irinotecan, and celecoxib in patients with advanced pancreatic cancer. J Clin Gastroenterol 44: 286-288, 2010.

[139] O'Kane SL, Eagle GL, Greenman J, Lind MJ and Cawkwell L: COX-2 specific inhibitors enhance the cytotoxic effects of pemetrexed in mesothelioma cell lines. Lung Cancer 67: 160-165, 2010.

[140] Martin-Richard M, Munoz M, Albanell J, *et al*: Serial topoisomerase II expression in primary breast cancer and response to neoadjuvant anthracycline-based chemotherapy. Oncology 66: 388-394, 2004.

[141] Nakai K, Mitomi H, Alkam Y, *et al*: Predictive value of MGMT, hMLH1, hMSH2 and BRCA1 protein expression for pathological complete response to neoadjuvant chemotherapy in basal-like breast cancer patients. Cancer Chemother Pharmacol 2010.

[142] Yiu CC, Sasano H, Ono K and Chow LW: Changes in protein expression after neoadjuvant use of aromatase inhibitors in primary breast cancer: a proteomic approach to search for potential biomarkers to predict response or resistance. Expert Opin Investig Drugs 19 Suppl 1: S79-89, 2010.

[143] Yiu CC, Chanplakorn N, Chan MS, *et al*: Down-regulation of heat-shock protein 70 (HSP-70) correlated with responsiveness to neoadjuvant aromatase inhibitor therapy in breast cancer patients. Anticancer Res 30: 3465-3472, 2010.

[144] Bramwell VH, Doig GS, Tuck AB, *et al*: Serial plasma osteopontin levels have prognostic value in metastatic breast cancer. Clin Cancer Res 12: 3337-3343, 2006.

[145] Mazouni C, Baggerly K, Hawke D, *et al*: Evaluation of changes in serum protein profiles during neoadjuvant chemotherapy in HER2-positive breast cancer using an LC-MALDI-TOF/MS procedure. Proteomics 10: 3525-3532, 2010.

[146] Faneyte IF, Schrama JG, Peterse JL, Remijnse PL, Rodenhuis S and van de Vijver MJ: Breast cancer response to neoadjuvant chemotherapy: predictive markers and relation with outcome. Br J Cancer 88: 406-412, 2003.

[147] Lopez MF, Mikulskis A, Kuzdzal S, *et al*: High-resolution serum proteomic profiling of Alzheimer disease samples reveals disease-specific, carrier-protein-bound mass signatures. Clin Chem 51: 1946-1954, 2005.

[148] Liotta LA, Ferrari M and Petricoin E: Clinical proteomics: written in blood. Nature 425: 905, 2003.

[149] Tirumalai RS, Chan KC, Prieto DA, Issaq HJ, Conrads TP and Veenstra TD: Characterization of the low molecular weight human serum proteome. Mol Cell Proteomics 2: 1096-1103, 2003.

[150] Harper RG, Workman SR, Schuetzner S, Timperman AT and Sutton JN: Low-molecular-weight human serum proteome using ultrafiltration, isoelectric focusing, and mass spectrometry. Electrophoresis 25: 1299-1306, 2004.

[151] Rai DK, Green BN, Landin B, Alvelius G and Griffiths WJ: Accurate mass measurement and tandem mass spectrometry of intact globin chains identify the low proportion variant hemoglobin Lepore-Boston-Washington from the blood of a heterozygote. J Mass Spectrom 39: 289-294, 2004.

[152] Villanueva J, Shaffer DR, Philip J, *et al*: Differential exoprotease activities confer tumor-specific serum peptidome patterns. J Clin Invest 116: 271-284, 2006.

[153] Lopez MF, Mikulskis A, Kuzdzal S, *et al*: A novel, high-throughput workflow for discovery and identification of serum carrier protein-bound peptide biomarker candidates in ovarian cancer samples. Clin Chem 53: 1067-1074, 2007.

[154] Koomen JM, Li D, Xiao LC, *et al*: Direct tandem mass spectrometry reveals limitations in protein profiling experiments for plasma biomarker discovery. J Proteome Res 4: 972-981, 2005.

[155] Diamandis EP: Peptidomics for cancer diagnosis: present and future. J Proteome Res 5: 2079-2082, 2006.

[156] Rittenhouse HG, Finlay JA, Mikolajczyk SD and Partin AW: Human Kallikrein 2 (hK2) and prostate-specific antigen (PSA): two closely related, but distinct, kallikreins in the prostate. Crit Rev Clin Lab Sci 35: 275-368, 1998.

[157] Diamandis EP, Scorilas A, Fracchioli S, *et al*: Human kallikrein 6 (hK6): a new potential serum biomarker for diagnosis and prognosis of ovarian carcinoma. J Clin Oncol 21: 1035-1043, 2003.

[158] Liotta LA and Kohn EC: The microenvironment of the tumour-host interface. Nature 411: 375-379, 2001.

[159] Celis JE, Gromov P, Cabezon T, *et al*: Proteomic characterization of the interstitial fluid perfusing the breast tumor microenvironment: a novel resource for biomarker and therapeutic target discovery. Mol Cell Proteomics 3: 327-344, 2004.
[160] Jarjanazi H, Savas S, Pabalan N, Dennis JW and Ozcelik H: Biological implications of SNPs in signal peptide domains of human proteins. Proteins 70: 394-403, 2008.
[161] Brunelli M, Manfrin E, Martignoni G, *et al*: Genotypic intratumoral heterogeneity in breast carcinoma with HER2/neu amplification: evaluation according to ASCO/CAP criteria. Am J Clin Pathol 131: 678-682, 2009.

Chapter 2

HER2-Driven Carcinogenesis: New Mouse Models for Novel Immunotherapies

Cristina Marchini, Lucia Pietrella, Cristina Kalogris, Chiara Garulli, Federico Gabrielli, Elena Quaglino, Manuela Iezzi, Serenella M. Pupa, Elda Tagliabue and Augusto Amici

Additional information is available at the end of the chapter

http://dx.doi.org/10.5772/53880

1. Introduction

The immune system might well be the best weapon against cancer, since immune defense is programmed to recognize and destroy abnormal cells infected by viruses or affected by transforming genetic or epigenetic alterations. If properly activated, a specific immune attack can be amplified and maintained long-term. These powerful mechanisms must be harnessed to fight against invading microorganisms and against cancer cells, which subvert the circuits that normally control cell proliferation and survival by displaying an anarchic behavior.

Even at the start of the 20th century, the physician Paul Ehrlich proposed the potential ability of the immune system to continually survey and destroy newly arising cancer cells [1]. This hypothesis represented the first version of the immune surveillance theory, formulated in 1957 by Burnet [2, 3]. However, this theory was long-discredited by evidence that while the immune system can fight tumors, it is often unable to eradicate them. In the last decade, many cancer immunologists have shown renewed interest in immune surveillance theory, with the goal of generating novel immunotherapics against cancer, such as cancer vaccines. Advances in cancer biology, increased knowledge of immune mechanisms, and the availability of new animal models that recapitulate several human cancers have all helped to elucidate the critical issues that influence the efficacy of an immune attack against cancer [4]. This information is crucial for the rational design of cancer vaccines.

Cancer cells elaborate many defenses against immune attack. For example, they try to evade recognition by T cells and, in turn, T cell-mediated cytotoxicity, one of the major mechanisms to control tumor growth, by decreasing the expression of glycoproteins of the major histocompatibility complex (MHC) on the cell membrane [5]. In fact, the T-cell receptor (TCR) recognizes antigen only when it is displayed on the surface of the target cell as peptide fragments by the class I and class II molecules of the MHC. Moreover, the increasing instability of the genome of transformed cells favors the emergence of clones with low immunogenicity no longer expressing tumor antigens. Thus, tumors can evade immune recognition, an ability that appears to increase as a tumor grows. Finally, cancer cells suppress immune reactivity through direct release of transforming growth factor (TGF)-beta, interleukin (IL)-10, and indoleamine 2,3-dioxygenase (IDO), or through the activation of myeloid-derived suppressor cells, tumor-associated macrophages and dendritic cells to secrete these molecules. As a consequence, a tumor favors the activation and the expansion of adaptive regulatory T (Treg) cells, leading to the generation of a tolerogenic environment [6].

In these conditions, the choice of antigen is a crucial factor in deriving a cancer vaccine. Recently, Lollini et al. [7] defined the "oncoantigens" as ideal targets since these antigens are indispensible for tumor progression and thus cannot be lost, and since, depending on their localization, they can be targeted by both cytotoxic cells and antibodies. Among oncoantigens, HER2 represents a very attractive target in light of its direct association with the malignant transformation of epithelial cells and its shared presence in several human carcinomas. Indeed, vaccines targeting HER2, designed as whole cells, peptides, as well as DNA expression plasmids, are able to hamper cancer progression when used at early stages of the disease [8]. However, the promising results obtained in preclinical models are difficult to reproduce in advanced cancers, when the immune system is already severely weakened. New molecular strategies are required to generate effective cancer vaccines able to awaken the immune responses against established tumors.

1.1. HER2 protein structure and function

HER2, also known as ErbB2 or neu in rat, is a 185-kd transmembrane receptor with tyrosine kinase activity and initially identified in a rat glioblastoma model. HER2 belongs to the epidermal growth factor receptor (EGFR) family, which also includes HER1 (EGFR, ErbB1), HER3 (ErbB3) and HER4 (ErbB4). Each of these receptors consists of an extracellular binding domain (ECD), a single transmembrane-spanning domain, and a long cytoplasmic tyrosine kinase domain. The ECD is about 630 amino acids long and contains four subdomains arranged as a tandem repeat of a two-domain unit. The first and third subdomains (I/L1 and III/L2) have a β-barrel conformation, and the second and fourth subdomains (II/CR1 and IV/CR2) are cysteine-rich [9] (Figure 1).

Generally, binding of ligand to the extracellular region induces receptor dimerization and activation of the cytoplasmic kinase, which in turn lead to autophosphorylation and initiation of downstream signaling events. Among the EGFR family members, HER2 and HER3 are exceptional since HER3 is kinase-inactive and HER2 has no identified ligand. Although HER2 is the only receptor without a known ligand, it is the preferred partner in heterodimer formation with other HER members.

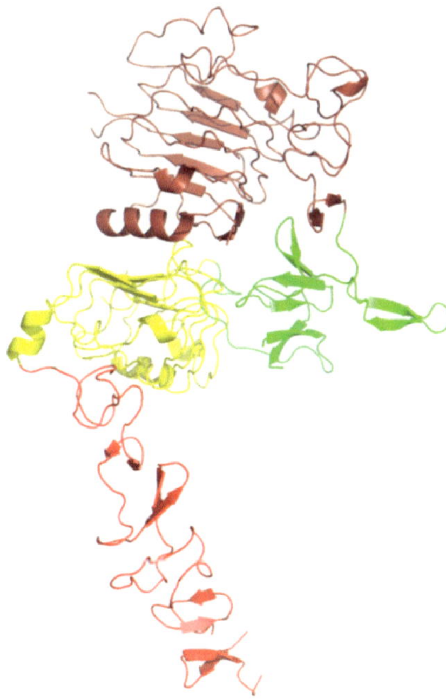

Figure 1. The structure of HER2. Ribbon diagram of HER2 ECD: Subdomains I (dark red), II (green), III (yellow) and IV (red), are indicated. Adapted from Cho H.S. et al., 2003 [9].

Crystallographic studies have helped to elucidate the structural basis for the differences in HER receptor function. There are two conformations of the ECD, the closed configuration and the open configuration. In the closed configuration, a dimerization arm located on domain II makes an intramolecular contact with a pocket on domain IV, preventing its association with the dimerization arms of other HER receptors and maintaining the receptor in an auto-inhibited form. Binding of its native ligand to the receptor brings domains I and III close together, switching the receptor's conformation to the open configuration (active state), in which the dimerization arm is free to participate in receptor dimerization. Unlike the three other HER receptors, HER2 can adopt a fixed conformation resembling a ligand-activated state but permitting it to dimerize in the absence of a ligand (Figure 2). The constitutive open structure of HER2 helps to explain its readiness to interact with the ligand-activated HER receptors [10].

Receptor homo- and heterodimerization leads to the activation of downstream signaling pathways associated with cell proliferation, differentiation, survival and angiogenesis. Activation of the kinase domains by receptor dimerization and the subsequent transphosphorylation of tyrosine residues in the carboxy-terminal tails creates binding sites for several key proteins. These specific proteins activate intracellular signaling pathways, including the mitogen-activated protein kinases (Ras/Raf/MEK/MAPK) pathway, which mainly regulates cell proliferation, and the phosphoinositide 3-kinase (PI3K)–activated Akt (PI3K/Akt) pathway, which is important for cell survival [10].

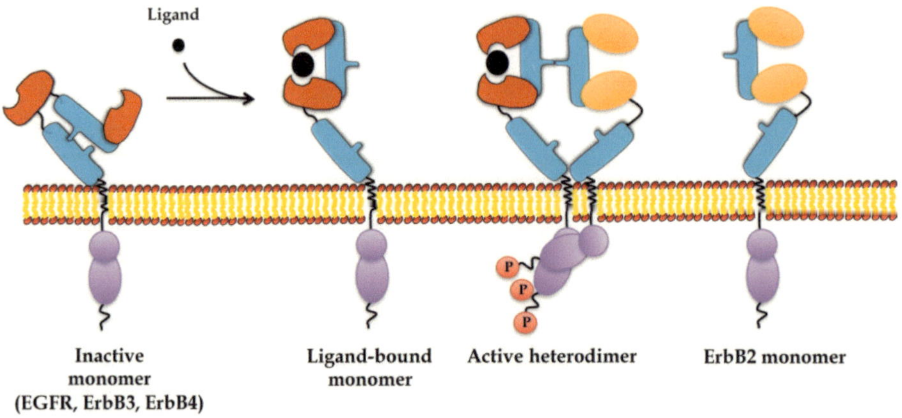

Figure 2. Schematic overview of the structural basis for HER receptor dimerization and activation. In the ligand-free state, HER1, HER3, and HER4 have a closed conformation. Binding of ligand, involving subdomains I and III, creates an extended conformation, allowing for receptor homo- and heterodimerization. Receptor dimerization leads to C-terminal tyrosine phosphorylation, creating phosphotyrosine binding sites for binding of adaptors, signaling molecules and regulatory proteins. HER2 is unique in that it is fixed in the active conformation ready to interact with other HER receptors. Adapted from Wieduwilt M. J. and Moasser M. M., 2008 [10].

The HER signaling network normally governs cellular programs during development and post-natal life, but its deregulation is directly involved in the pathogenesis of several human tumors. Overexpression of HER2, enhancing and prolonging signals that trigger cell transformation, has a causal role in the promotion of carcinogenesis. The absence of the auto-inhibited conformation explains, at least in part, this HER2 transforming potential. Amplification and/or overexpression of HER2 have been reported in malignancies, such as breast, ovarian, prostate, colorectal, pancreatic and gastric cancers [11].

1.2. Role of HER2 oncogene in breast carcinoma

Breast cancer, one of the most common malignancies worldwide, is a heterogeneous disease that can be classified according to the expression of the estrogen receptor, progesterone receptor, and HER2. The resulting subgroups differ not only in clinical behavior and prognosis, but also in the predicted response to targeted therapies against these receptors and the pathways they activate. Amplification of the HER2 gene and overexpression at the messenger RNA or protein level occurs in about 20-30% of patients with early stage breast cancer and predicts a poor prognosis [12]. Further support for the involvement of HER2 in the initiation and progression of breast cancer comes from studies on transgenic mice, although careful analysis of these transgenic mouse models suggests that overexpression of HER2, primarily due to gene amplification, is necessary but not sufficient to induce transformation. The expression of the oncoprotein induces tumors only when accompanied by genetic alterations, which include point mutations, deletions, and insertions. These alterations are invariably located in the juxtamembrane region of HER2 and lead to an unbalanced number of cysteines, potentially affecting cysteine-mediated dimerization [13].

Evidence for the insufficiency of wild-type HER2 expression, alone and without additional mutations, to induce full malignant transformation was reported by Finkle et al. [14], who found that transgenic mice overexpressing human HER2 under the murine mammary tumor virus (MMTV) promoter developed mammary tumors in a stochastic manner and after a long latency. Interestingly, those authors found sequence anomalies, including in-frame small deletions, in the juxtamembrane region of wild-type HER2 in more than half of the analyzed mammary tumors. The majority of these mutations affected the conserved cysteine residues and could function as a second hit in the transformation process, implying that additional genetic changes beyond HER2 overexpression are required for mammary tissue transformation and tumor formation. Accordingly, somatic mutations confined to the juxtamembranous region of neu have been associated with the induction of mammary tumors in neu protooncogene transgenic mice described by Siegel et al. [15]. The relatively long latency period for the progression of these tumors seems to reflect the acquisition of activating mutations in the transgene.

Interestingly, an alternative splice form of the human HER2 gene, Δ16HER2, containing an in-frame deletion in the same region mutated in rat neu or human HER2 protooncogene transgenic mice, has been described [16]. This oncogenic isoform is clinically important and commonly coexpressed with HER2 in human breast tumors, as reported by Castiglioni et al. [17] and Mitra et al. [18], who detected Δ16HER2 transcripts in human breast carcinomas in about 10% of total HER2 transcripts. This deletion removes the relevant cysteine residues in HER2, disrupting the disulfide bond structure of the protein and leaving the remaining unpaired cysteine residues available for intermolecular bonding. Consequently, Δ16HER2, which can be defined as a normal byproduct of HER2, forms stable homodimers maintained by intermolecular disulfide bonds (Figure 3).

Δ16HER2 has increased transforming potency as compared with the wild-type HER2, as first demonstrated *in vitro* [17, 18]. Ectopic expression of Δ16HER2, but not wild-type HER2, promoted receptor dimerization and significantly enhanced the proliferation of murine NIH3T3 fibroblasts and human MCF-7 breast tumor cells. In addition, Δ16HER2 expression potentiated MCF-7 cell migration and invasion, whereas HER2 did not. In analysis of anchorage-independent growth as an *in vitro* test for tumorigenesis, both HER2 wild-type- and Δ16HER2-transfected MCF-7 cells showed enhanced colony formation in soft agar medium, but the Δ16HER2-expressing cells formed significantly larger colonies [18]. We obtained similar results with human embryonic kidney HEK293 cells stably transfected with wild-type HER2 or Δ16HER2 (Figure 4). *In vivo* analyses showed that the Δ16HER2 variant is tumorigenic *per se* since athymic mice injected with Δ16HER2-expressing HEK293 transfectants developed tumors, whereas mice injected with HEK293 control cells ectopically overexpressing only wild-type HER2 did not [17]. The predicted enhanced oncogenic potential of Δ16HER2-expressing cells *in vivo* is supported by analysis of our new mouse model transgenically expressing the human Δ16HER2 under the transcriptional control of the MMTV promoter; all of the transgenic females developed multifocal mammary tumors with a rapid onset, suggesting that the Δ16HER2 splice variant represents the transforming form of the HER2 oncoprotein [19].

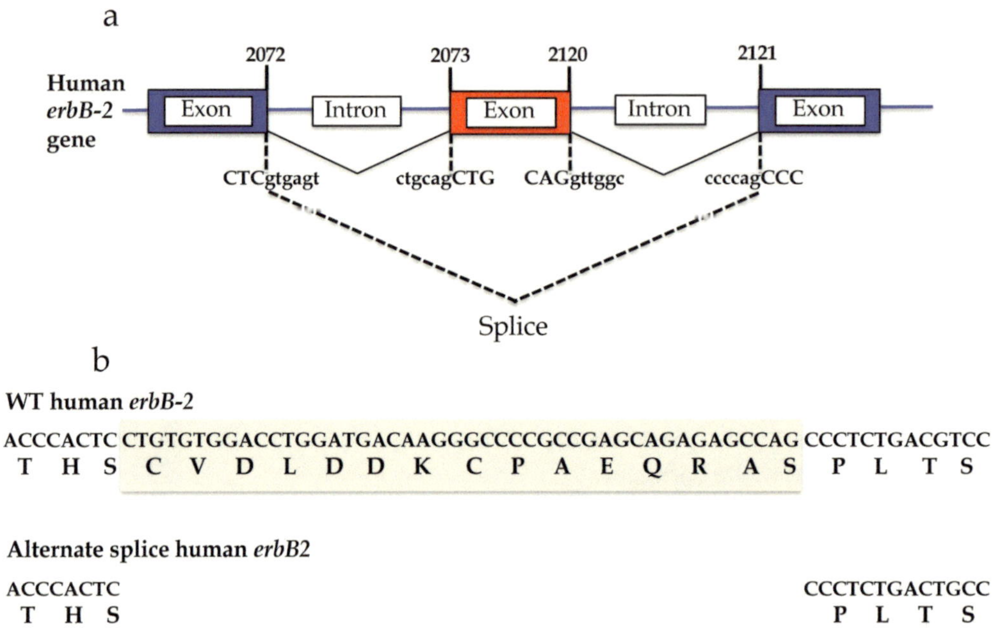

Figure 3. Δ16HER2 splice variant. a. Schematic representation of the small region of the human HER2 genomic locus indicating the exon-intron boundaries and the alternative splicing that eliminates exon 16. The values indicated above the schematic represent nucleotide numbers corresponding to the cDNA. b. Alignment of the wild-type and alternatively spliced Δ16HER2 mRNAs; the grey box indicates sequences removed by the splicing event.

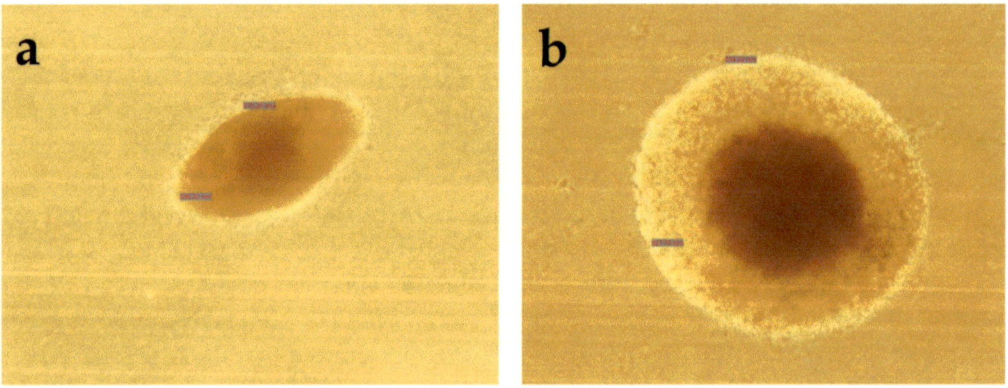

Figure 4. Anchorage-independent growth of stable transfected HEK293 cells. Cells expressing Δ16HER2 (b) form larger colonies than cells expressing wild-type HER2 (a).

The key role of the cysteine residues in the HER2 juxtamembrane region has been also demonstrated by Pedersen et al. [20], who described a subtype of HER2-positive tumors expressing a series of carboxy-terminal fragments collectively known as p95HER2. These fragments arise through at least two different mechanisms: proteolytic shedding of the ECD of the full-length receptor; and translation of the mRNA encoding HER2 from internal initiation codons [21]. One of these fragments, 611-CTF, which contains a transmembrane domain and a short extracellular region including the sequence deleted in Δ16HER2, is hyperactive because of its ability to form homodimers maintained by intermolecular disulfide bonds. Despite lacking the majority of the ECD, this HER2 fragment drives breast cancer progression *in vivo*, as shown by the development of aggressive mammary tumors in mice transgenically expressing 611-CTF and suggesting a causal role for p95HER2 fragments in tumorigenesis based on their ability to constitutively homodimerize [20].

Together, these findings demonstrate that the overexpression of full-length HER2 alone is not sufficient to drive malignant transformation of mammary glands.

1.3. Mouse models for HER2-positive breast cancer

The first direct evidence for the involvement of HER2 in the initiation and progression of breast cancer came from analysis of transgenic mice with MMTV promoter-targeted overexpression of activated neu (the rat homolog of HER2) in the mammary gland. Activated neu (neu-NT) is a mutated form with valine instead of glutamic acid at residue 664 in the transmembrane domain of the protein. Although the endogenous mouse HER2 promoter has recently been used to control mammary-specific expression of activated neu-NT [22], MMTV-based mouse models have greatly increased our knowledge of the mechanisms that control HER2-mediated mammary tumor progression (Figure 5). In 1988, Leder and co-workers [23] generated the first transgenic mice that developed mammary tumors due to MMTV-driven expression of neu-NT. The short latency (11-13 weeks) and the high multiplicity of mammary tumors arising in those MMTV-neu-NT mice suggested that overexpression of the activated neu variant could drive mammary carcinogenesis in a single step.

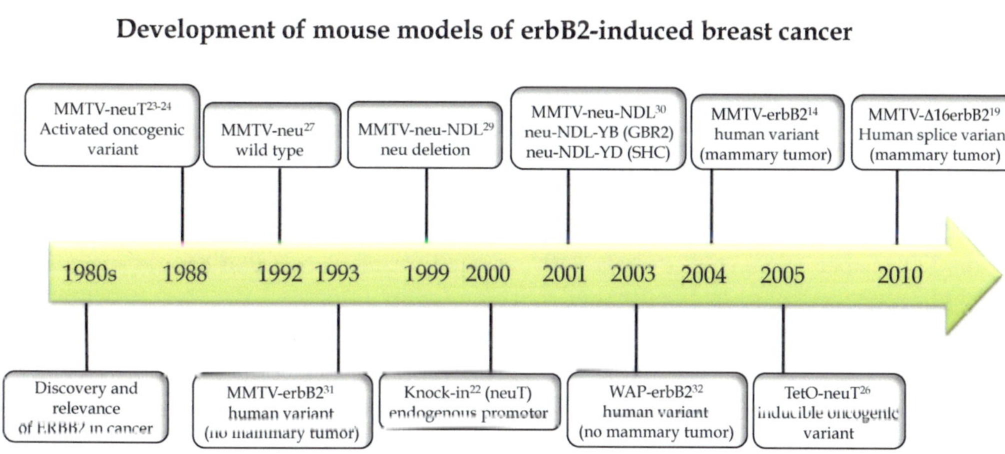

GRB2, growth factor receptor-bound protein 2; MMTV, mouse mammary tumour virus; NDL, NEU deletion; TetO, tetracycline operator.

Figure 5. Timeline. Several mouse models transgenic for the rat or human HER2 been generated over the past 24 years, increasing our knowledge of the mechanisms that control HER2-mediated mammary tumour progression. Adapted from Ursini-Siegel et al., 2007 [33].

However only 1 year later, Jolicoeur's laboratory developed a second MMTV-neu-NT transgenic mouse model in which mammary tumor development was stochastic and with a significantly longer latency, suggesting that mammary epithelial cells require many genetic events in concert with neu-NT overexpression to undergo transformation [24]. The differences between these two transgenic mouse models probably reflect the ability of the transgene to integrate randomly into the mouse genome, which, in turn, influences transgene expression levels. In fact, transgenic animals generated even with the same construct may exhibit different tumor multiplicity and latency depending on the site of integration and on the transgene copy number. Nonetheless, subsequent studies of additional MMTV-neu-NT transgenic mice clearly demonstrated that overexpression of activated neu is sufficient to efficiently transform mammary epithelial cells [25]. To assess the dependence of cancer cells in advanced tumors or metastases on an initiating oncogenic event for maintenance of the transformed state, an inducible transgenic model for neu was obtained, using the tetracycline regulatory system to conditionally express activated neu in the mammary epithelium [26]. In these MMTV-rtTA/TetO-neu-NT mice, neu-initiated tumorigenesis is reversible: upon induction with doxycycline, multiple invasive mammary carcinomas developed that regressed to a clinically undetectable state following transgene deinduction. Interestingly, most animals eventually developed neu-independent recurrent tumors long after the apparently complete regression of their tumors, indicating that neu-induced mammary tumors typically progress to a neu-independent state [26].

Although rapid onset of multifocal mammary tumors has been observed in the majority of activated neu transgenic mice, this mutation has never been observed in human cancers, which present only amplification of the HER2 gene copy number and consequent overexpression of HER2 protein on the cell membrane. In wild-type neu-expressing mice under the MMTV promoter, focal mammary tumors arise next to hyperplastic mammary tissue after a long latency period (17-48 weeks) [27], suggesting that genetic alterations in addition to those inducing HER2 overexpression are required for mammary transformation. Notably, tumors in these transgenic mice arose only when the oncoprotein carried mutations in the ECD involving small deletions that promote neu transforming activity through formation of intermolecular covalent cysteine bonds [15, 28]. Accordingly, mammary epithelium-specific expression of two activated neu receptors harboring distinct in-frame neu deletions (NDL) (MMTV-neu-NDL mice) led to rapid induction of mammary tumors [29]. Other transgenic animals with mutated forms of neu that couple specifically with Grb2 (neu-NDL-YB) or Shc (neu-NDL-YD) adaptor proteins have been generated to address the significance of HER2-coupled unique downstream signaling pathways in induction of mammary cancers [30].

More recently, after initial failed attempts [31], transgenic mice with wild-type human HER2 have been generated. A transgenic mouse expressing human HER2 under the whey acidic protein promoter was obtained, but no mammary neoplastic transformation was ever detected in any animal [32]. While another human wild-type HER2 transgenic model under the MMTV promoter did develop HER2-overexpressing breast tumors, but with a long latency of about 28.6 weeks [14]. Sequencing of the human HER2 transcripts from primary mammary tumors developed in these transgenic mice identified an in-frame 15-bp deletion in the wild-type HER2 juxtamembrane region, potentially affecting cysteine-mediated dimerization [14].

Overall, these results point to the role of HER2-activating mutations that change the number of cysteines in mammary tumorigenesis. In this context, expression of the alternatively spliced Δ16HER2 isoform, which is constitutively active by virtue of its ability to form disulfide-bridged homodimers, might be required to obtain an oncogenic phenotype. HER2 gene amplification in primary human breast cancer might increase the levels of this oncogenic variant above a critical threshold, allowing it to contribute to breast cancer progression.

1.4. Δ16HER2 mice

The value of Δ16HER2 transgenic mouse models in addressing the biological importance of this oncogenic variant in breast cancer progression and in response to targeted therapies was suggested in 2007 by Ursini-Siegal et al. [33]. Indeed, we recently generated a mouse line transgenically expressing human Δ16HER2, established using a bicistronic vector containing an IRES sequence between the human Δ16HER2 and the firefly luciferase gene to ensure their coordinated expression driven by the same MMTV promoter (Figure 6) [19]. Luciferase was chosen as a reporter gene since it is rapidly detectable by optical imaging in live organisms and simultaneously allows accurate quantitation in tissue extracts and immunohistochemical detection using specific antibodies. In addition, a restriction enzyme PCR-based technique [34, 35] confirmed integration of the transgene at a single site on murine chromosome 5, inside an intergenic region containing neither genes nor regulatory sequences such that the insertion itself does not affect tumorigenesis. Quantitative PCR analysis revealed a transgene copy number of 5 [36] (Figure 6).

In steps to characterize Δ16HER2 mice, we found that the founder female developed 8 spontaneous mammary tumors starting at 18 weeks of age and, as expected, readily visualized by bioluminescence analysis even one month before tumors became palpable, suggesting that luciferase expression might be predictive of tumor onset. Whole-mount and histological analysis of the mammary glands confirmed the presence of small neoplastic masses (Figure 7a). Immunohistochemical analysis of these non-palpable tumors revealed HER2 protein expression (Figure 7c), with larger tumors displaying heterogeneous membrane staining for the human transgene, while small tumors showed homogeneous distribution of HER2 in the tumor parenchyma. In all cases, HER2 expression was detected only in the mammary gland and in strict correlation with tumor development. HER2 expression also correlated with that of PCNA, a marker for mitotic activity in transformed epithelial cells (Figure 7d).

Because the MMTV promoter is hormonally regulated and tumor development in founder females might be enhanced by increased transgene expression in the mammary gland during pregnancy and lactation, we monitored spontaneous mammary tumor development by palpation in virgin female F2 transgenic mice; all of these mice developed multiple asynchronous mammary tumors (4-5 tumors/mouse) at 12 to 19 weeks of age (Figure 8c), each reaching 1-1.5 cm^3 within a short time-frame (Figure 8d). Histologically, these fast-growing tumors were classified as invasive HER2-positive adenocarcinomas. Indeed,

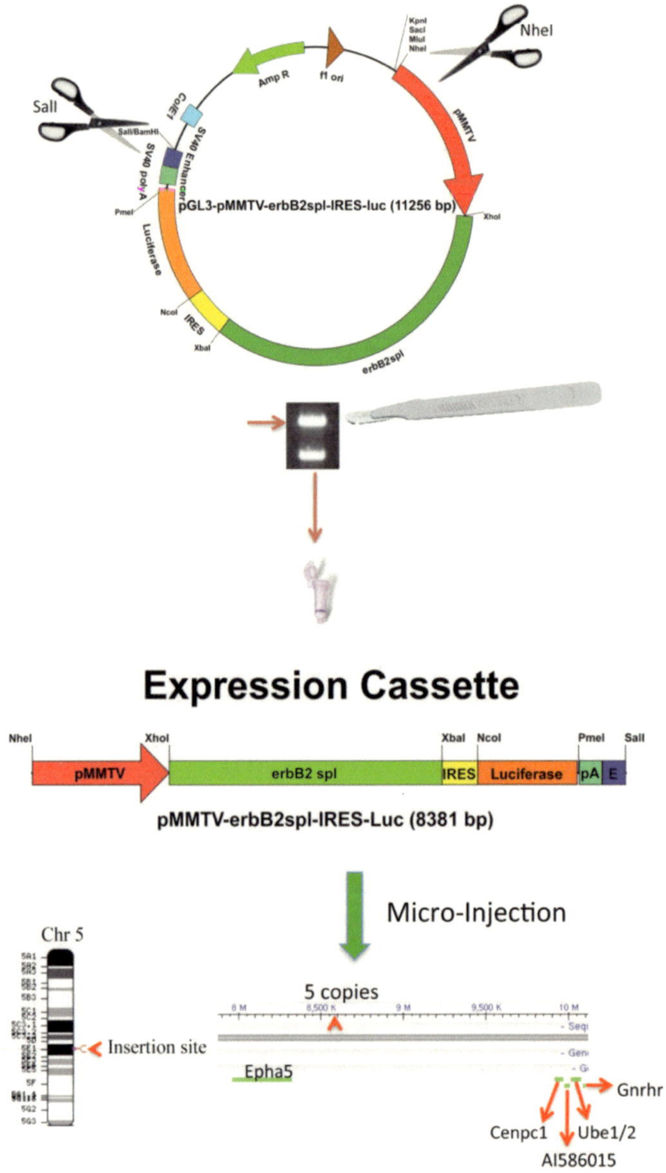

Figure 6. Bicistronic vector for Δ16HER2 mice generation. Schematic representation of the MMTV-driven human Δ16HER2-LUC transgene, with the MMTV LTR promoter (pMMTV, red), the human Δ16HER2 cDNA (green), the internal ribosome entry site (IRES, yellow), the luciferase cDNA (LUC, orange), and the termination signal from the SV40 (Poly A). Relevant restriction sites are indicated. The MMTV- Δ16HER2-IRES-LUC expression cassette (8381 bp) was isolated from the plasmid backbone by NheI and SalI digestions, purified, and microinjected into fertilized eggs from FVB females. The transgene randomly integrated at a single site (at 85.72 Mb) on murine chromosome 5 region E-1 (NT109320.4) inside an intergenic region (NCBI Build m37.1). The insertion occurred exactly 1.17 Mb downstream of the non-histone chromosomal protein HMG-17-like gene and 718 Kb upstream of the centromere protein C1 gene. Quantitative PCR analysis revealed a transgene copy number of 5.

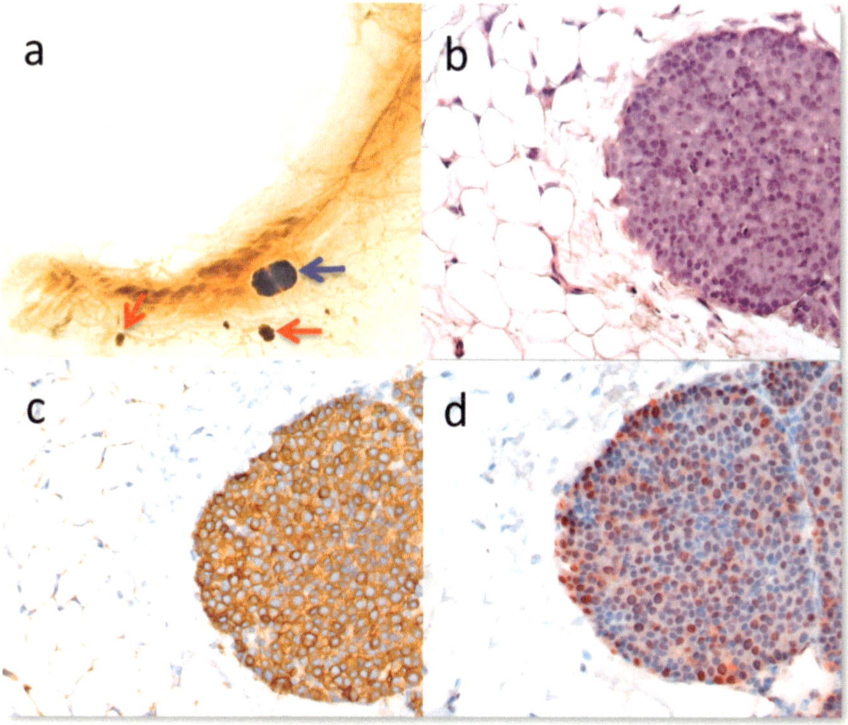

Figure 7. **Analysis of non-palpable tumors in Δ16HER2 transgenic mice.** a. Whole-mount analysis of an inguinal mammary gland of a 14 week old mouse reveals non-palpable tumors (red arrows); blue arrow indicates a limph node. Hematoxylin-eosin (b) and immunohistochemical staining for HER2 (c) and PCNA (d) of non palpable mammary tumors at 14 weeks. Magnification: a, X6; b-d, X400.

immunohistochemical analysis confirmed the concurrent expression of the human Δ16HER2 oncogene and the luciferase gene, and revealed the specific staining of epithelial cells but not of stromal cells or adipocytes, while non-neoplastic mammary ducts were negative. Tumors consisted of cells with round nuclei and eosinophilic cytoplasm growing in solid sheets and packets traversed by delicate fibrovascular septa. Growth of these unencapsulated tumors compressed the surrounding tissues (Figure 8b). Subsequent monitoring of all generations following F2 revealed similar results, indicating that formation of Δ16HER2-overexpressing mammary tumors is a reproducible phenotype in these transgenic mice. Furthermore, transgenic Δ16HER2 females bearing primary mammary tumors developed lung metastases starting at 25 weeks of age and present in 100% of mice at 36 weeks, suggesting particularly aggressive tumor behavior upon expression of the Δ16HER2 splice variant. The histological features of these pulmonary metastatic lesions were consistent with a primary breast tumor origin, with robust staining for HER2 demonstrating high-level transgene expression (Figure 9).

Western analysis using lysates of cells isolated *ex vivo* from Δ16HER2 mice revealed a protein expression profile consistent with the immunohistochemical data, but also the presence of some phosphorylated Δ16HER2 dimers with a higher activation status in the

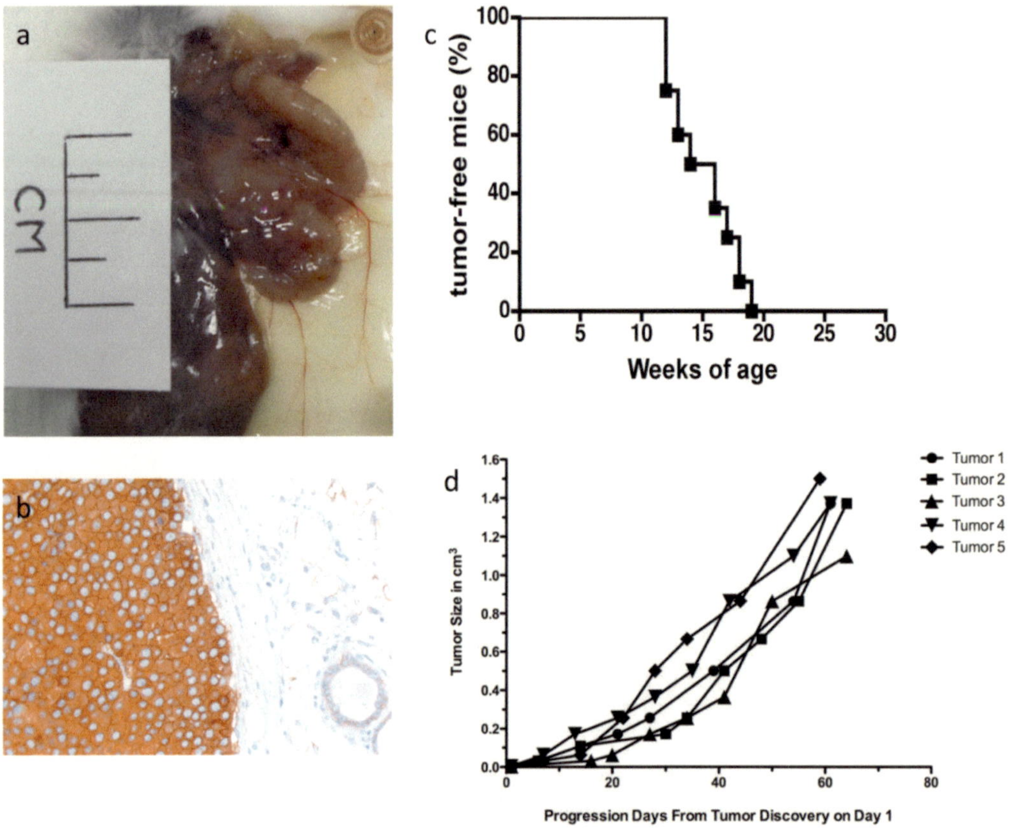

Figure 8. Characterization of tumorigenesis in Δ16HER2 mice. a. Primary breast tumors just before their removal from a Δ16HER2 transgenic female mouse. b. Immunohistochemical detection of HER2, revealing strong and uniform expression of HER2 protein in the mammary tumor, while the normal duct (right) is negative. Magnification: X400. c. Kaplan-Meier disease-free survival plot for F2 generation Δ16HER2-LUC transgenic mice. Mammary tumor incidence is 100% and tumor onset is from 11 to the 19 weeks (n=20). d. Tumor growth curves of five different tumors. Tumor volume was calculated as $0.5 x d_1^2 x d_2$, where d_1 and d_2 are the smaller and larger diameters, respectively.

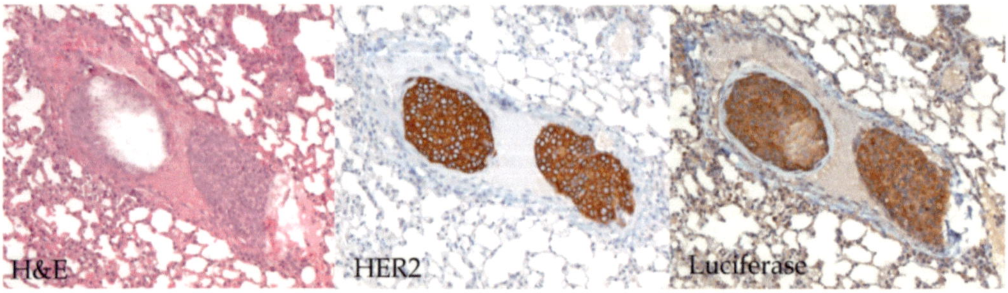

Figure 9. Pulmonary metastases. Hematoxylin-eosin (left) and immunohistochemical staining for HER2 (middle) and luciferase (right) in intravascular lung metastases in Δ16HER2 transgenic mice. Tumor cell aggregates are strongly positive for both human HER2 and luciferase staining. Magnification: X400.

dimeric than the monomeric form. These findings suggest a mechanism through which the disulfide-bonded Δ16HER2 homodimer amplifies HER2 transforming potential. The same analysis showed that Src kinase and several other protein mediators involved in the signaling cascade were consistently activated (phosphorylated), implicating this pathway in neoplastic transformation and tumor progression dynamics.

In vitro analyses to elucidate the oncogenic mechanisms involving the Δ16HER2 splice variant will benefit from the availability of Δ16HER2-positive cell lines derived from surgically excised primary breast tumors and lung metastases from Δ16HER2 transgenic mice. Preliminary data from our ongoing efforts to establish such lines show that these cells maintain transgene expression even after repeated passages.

Overall, the higher tumor incidence as well as the shorter latency period in Δ16HER2 transgenic mice as compared with that in the MMTV-wild-type HER2 transgenic mice described by Finkle et al. [14], together with the higher metastatic potential of the splice variant, strongly supports the candidacy of Δ16HER2 as the transforming form of the HER2 oncoprotein. Indeed, despite some similarities between the two different experimental models, i.e., use of the same mouse strain (FVB) to derive the transgenic lines, use of the same MMTV promoter, and the development of rapidly growing adenocarcinomas, these transgenic experimental systems appear to differ greatly in some features that determine tumor aggressiveness. Not only do Δ16HER2 females develop asynchronous mammary adenocarcinomas with a higher tumor incidence and a significantly shorter average latency compared to wild-type HER2 transgenic females (15.1 vs 28.6 weeks), but transgene expression in the model described by Finkle et al was detected in tumor tissue as well as in normal mammary gland and several other epithelial tissues, whereas our transgenic mice revealed strong staining for the Δ16HER2 human transgene exclusively in tumor mammary tissue, suggesting that overexpression of Δ16HER2 in the mammary gland is sufficient to induce malignant transformation in a single step. It is also noteworthy that only 5 transgene copies can drive neoplastic transformation of mammary epithelial cells compared to a relatively high number of wild-type HER2 transgene copies (30-50) necessary to induce mammary adenocarcinomas in about 80% of MMTV-wild-type HER2 transgenic mice. Since the Δ16HER2 splice variant represents about 10% of total HER2 transcript in human breast carcinoma, it is plausible that malignant transformation ensues when Δ16HER2 reaches a critical threshold in mammary cells presenting HER2 gene amplification.

1.5. HER2 as target of immunotherapies

The crucial role of HER2 in epithelial transformation as well as its selective overexpression in cancer tissues makes it an ideal target for cancer immunotherapy. Notwithstanding the clinically approved use of the anti-HER2 monoclonal antibody Trastuzumab, a number of concerns, including resistance, considerable costs associated with repeated treatments, and side effects, make active immunotherapies that generate polyclonal and long-lasting immune responses desirable alternative approaches.

1.5.1. Involvement of Δ16HER2 in Trastuzumab resistance

Trastuzumab, a humanized monoclonal antibody against the ectodomain of HER2, was the first rationally designed anti-HER2 therapy approved by the US Food and Drug Administration for the clinical treatment of HER2-overexpressing breast cancer. Trastuzumab uses multiple mechanisms to interfere with HER2 downstream signaling and inhibit tumor growth, including HER2 receptor downregulation and blocking cleavage of the HER2 ECD, which otherwise leads to activation of the HER2 receptor [37]. In particular, the cytostatic effect of Trastuzumab is associated with the reduction of the signaling by the PI3K/Akt pathway and the upregulation of the cyclin-dependent kinase inhibitor p27kip1, as demonstrated by Western analysis of breast tumor cell lines treated with Trastuzumab *in vitro* [38]. The consequences of these Trastuzumab actions are G1 arrest, reduction in cell proliferation, and apoptosis. Trastuzumab also has cytotoxic properties, such as antibody-dependent cell-mediated cytotoxicity (ADCC) against HER2-overexpressing tumor cells. ADCC is mainly due to natural killer (NK) cells which express the Fcγ receptor that binds the Fc domain of the IgG1 Trastuzumab [38].

Overall, Trastuzumab is clinically effective, but a significant proportion of HER2-overexpressing breast cancer patients either do not respond to initial Trastuzumab treatment (*de novo* resistance) or eventually become resistant after continuous treatment (acquired resistance). In fact, an objective response (complete + partial) when Trastuzumab is used alone is observed in only about 26% of patients with HER2-positive tumors, and many of the initial responders develop resistance in less than 6 months [39]. While higher response rates (50–80%) have been reported when Trastuzumab is used in combination with standard chemotherapy for metastatic disease, primary and acquired resistance to this reagent remains a significant clinical problem.

Understanding the molecular mechanisms of Trastuzumab resistance is crucial for the development of new therapeutic strategies and for improved survival of HER2-positive breast cancer patients. Several mechanisms have been proposed in Trastuzumab resistance [38], including steric hindrance of HER2-antibody interaction by membrane-associated glycoproteins [40], PTEN deficiency (phosphatase and tensin homolog deleted on chromosome 10) [41], increased PI3K/Akt pathway activation [42], and HER2 crosstalk with other HER members or with insulin-like growth factor-I receptor (IGF-IR) [43]. In the latter context, Huang et al. [43] showed that a heterotrimeric complex of IGF-IR, HER2 and HER3 forming exclusively in Trastuzumab-resistant cells plays a key role in resistance, since knockdown of HER3 or IGF-IR by short hairpin RNA–mediated strategies upregulates p27kip1, inactivates downstream receptor signaling, and resensitizes resistant cells.

While these mechanisms may explain Trastuzumab resistance in tumors expressing only the full-length HER2 receptor, there is increasing recognition that HER2 altered forms, including p95HER2 fragments and the Δ16HER2 splice variant commonly coexpressed with wild-type protein in human tumors, play a significant role in Trastuzumab resistance. In a series of patients with HER2–positive advanced breast cancer and treated with Trastuzumab, Scaltriti et al. [44] reported that the presence of p95HER2 fragments, which lack the Trastuzumab binding domain but retain kinase activity, was associated with clinical resistance to Trastuzumab, whereas tumors expressing only the full-length receptor exhibited a high response rate to Trastuzumab. Analysis of cell lines expressing either full-length HER2 or p95HER2 confirmed the ineffectiveness of Trastuzumab on cells expressing p95HER2 fragments [44]. Using a similar experimental approach, Mitra and coworkers [18] found that ectopic expression of Δ16HER2, but not wild-type HER2, promotes Trastuzumab resistance in NIH3T3 fibroblasts and MCF-7 breast tumor cells; both Δ16HER2-expressing cell types were refractory to Trastuzumab treatment, as shown in both cell proliferation and invasion assays, and displayed sustained oncogenic signaling. It seems likely that Δ16HER2 expression above a critical threshold in wild-type HER2-overexpressing human breast cancer contributes to Trastuzumab resistance, consistent with clinical evidence of an inverse correlation between increased HER2 FISH ratios (>8) and Trastuzumab responsiveness [45].

Although the Trastuzumab binding site is amino-terminal to the exon 16 deletion of Δ16HER2, Trastuzumab resistance might reflect the inefficient targeting of the splice variant receptor by the antibody because of the stable disulfide-bonded HER2 homodimers or the activation of alternative compensatory signaling pathways. In fact, Δ16HER2 harbors an in-frame deletion which promotes constitutive dimerization of the receptor and the coupling of Δ16HER2 to unique oncogenic signaling pathways mediated by Src kinase. Indeed, Mitra and coworkers [18] proposed Src kinase as the "master regulator" of Δ16HER2 protein signal transduction, based on the cooperation between Δ16HER2 and Src kinase as demonstrated by the ability of the Src family inhibitor dasatinib to induce Src inactivation, destabilization of Δ16HER2, and suppression of tumorigenicity. Consistent with this proposal, a recent study by Zhang et al [46] identified Src activation as a key convergence point of several Trastuzumab resistance mechanisms, since targeting Src in combination with Trastuzumab resensitized multiple resistant cell lines and eliminated Trastuzumab-resistant tumors *in vivo*. The association between Src-mediated transduction pathways and the transforming ability of ΔHER16 in our transgenic model [19] points to the value of this model in preclinical studies to elucidate the *in vivo* mechanisms underlying Trastuzumab resistance as well as the role of this variant in HER2-targeted drug responsiveness. Moreover, Δ16HER2 transgenic mice may recapitulate the clinical spectrum of Trastuzumab resistance associated with HER2-positive tumors and thus serve in testing innovative immunotherapies.

1.5.2. DNA vaccines

The idea of generating DNA vaccines comes from the pioneer work of Wolff and colleagues [47], who first showed that direct injection of naked DNA into the muscles of mice led to expression of the encoded reporter proteins. DNA vaccines are simple circles of DNA derived primarily from bacterial plasmids and contain a cDNA encoding the full-length or truncated target antigen, a strong viral promoter to drive antigen expression in mammalian cells, and a polyadenylation signal (usually from bovine growth hormone or from SV40) to terminate transcription. In addition, DNA vaccines contain sequences necessary for the cloning procedures (a multiple cloning site) and for plasmid production in bacteria,

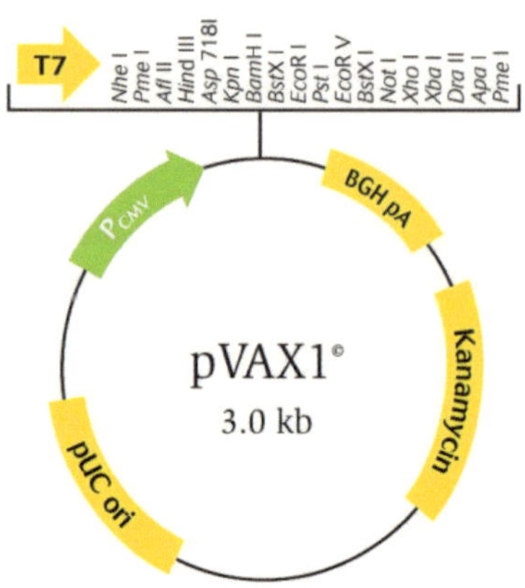

Figure 10. DNA vaccine backbone. pVAX1 (Invitrogen) is a 3.0 kb plasmid vector designed for use in the development of DNA vaccines and approved for such use by the US Food and Drug Administration. Features of the vector allow high-copy number replication in *E. coli* and high-level transient expression of the protein of interest in most mammalian cells. The vector contains the following elements: human cytomegalovirus immediate-early (CMV) promoter for high-level expression in a wide range of mammalian cells; bovine growth hormone (BGH) polyadenylation signal for efficient transcription termination and polyadenylation of mRNA; kanamycin resistance gene for selection in *E. coli;* and origin of bacterial replication (pUC ori) (http://products.invitrogen.com:80/ivgn/product/V26020).

consisting of the origin of replication (usually from *E. coli*) and an antibiotic-resistance gene to permit selective amplification of the vaccine [48] (Figure 10).

After purification (Figure 11), the DNA vaccine is commonly delivered into the skin or muscle using the biolistic system, in which compressed helium propels DNA-coated microparticles through a gene gun [49], or by simple intradermal or i.m. injection. While both delivery methods permit the introduction of DNA vaccines, the efficacy of DNA vaccination is strongly increased if it is followed by an *in vivo* short electric pulse, i.e., electroporation [50], which enhances DNA transfection into normal tissues by inducing transient permeability of biological membranes through the opening of microscopic pores.

Once DNA vaccines enter mammalian cells, antigen synthesis and presentation occur [48], with professional antigen-presenting cells (APCs), such as dendritic cells, presenting the transcribed and translated antigen in the context of major histocompatibility complex (MHC) and costimulatory molecules. If DNA vaccine-coded antigens are processed as endogenous intracytoplasmic proteins, the peptide fragments are presented on cell surface MHC I molecules to cytolytic T lymphocytes (CD8+ T cells). If the antigens are secreted from the cells, they can be taken up by APCs, processed through the exogenous pathway, and presented by MHC II molecules for the activation of specific helper T cells (CD4+ T cells) which produce 'helpful' cytokines. For antibody responses, B cells recognize and respond to extracellularly exposed antigens, both secreted and transmembrane proteins [48]. Through these mechanisms, DNA vaccines can elicit both cellular and humoral responses, and this combined immunity may be more effective than either arm alone.

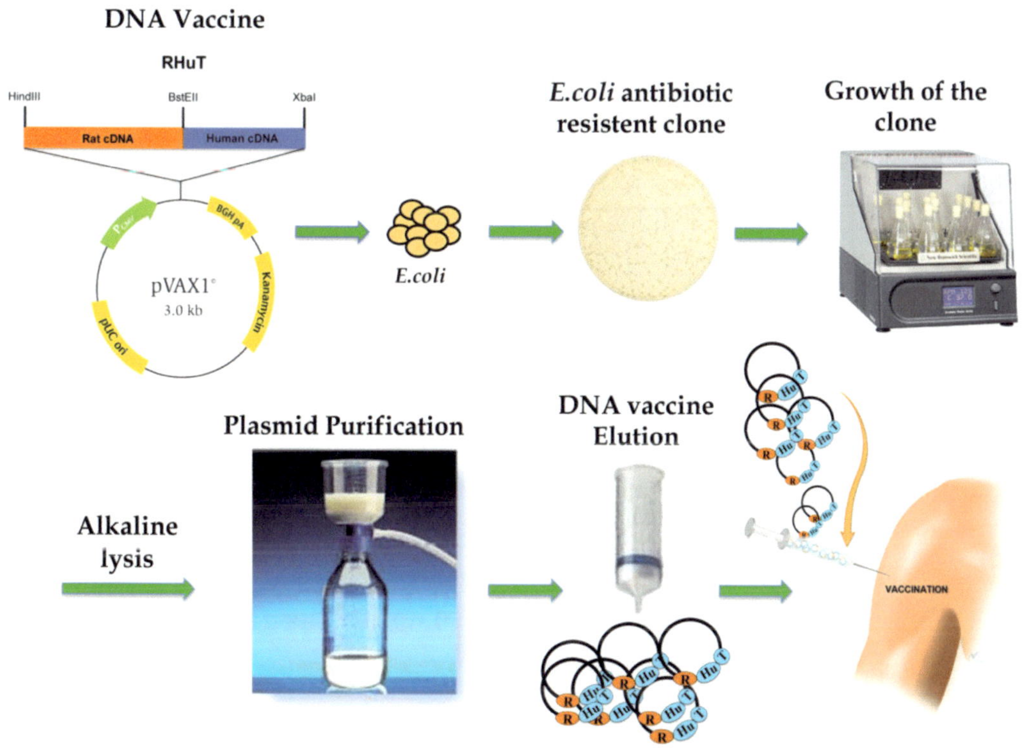

Figure 11. DNA vaccines production in bacteria. Once the antigen of interest is cloned into the plasmid, the vaccine is introduced into bacterial cells, where it replicates as the bacterium multiplies. The presence of a "relaxed origin of replication" and an antibiotic-resistance gene allows efficient plasmid replication in bacterial cells and their selection, two key aspects for high-scale plasmid production. Finally, the vaccine, i.e., RHuT, can be purified using commercial kits.

The ability to induce cytotoxic responses is a distinctive property of DNA vaccines, representing the only approach other than the use of live viruses for the activation of CD8+ T cells. In addition, unlike mammalian DNA, bacterial plasmids are rich in unmethylated CpG dinucleotides, which act as a "danger signal" that warns of bacterial infection and activates the innate immune response through recognition of CpG motifs by Toll-like receptor 9 expressed on B cells and APCs. Thus, DNA vaccines are effective even when administrated without adjuvants [51].

DNA vaccines also have further distinct advantages over other vaccine prototypes, such as stability and ease of manipulation. Since the subcellular localization of the recombinant antigen dictates the type and the intensity of the immune response, it is possible to change the intracellular fate of a protein to induce selective immune responses [52, 53]. For example, signal (leader) sequences can be added or deleted from an antigen to modulate its immunogenic performance. Signal peptides, consisting of amino-terminal extensions that direct the insertion of proteins into the membrane of the endoplasmic reticulum, can be removed from secreted or membrane proteins to target them into the cytoplasm to improve antigen presentation by the MHC class I pathway and thereby enhance cytotoxic T cell induction. To optimize cytotoxic responses, an antigen can also be ubiquitinated; when expressed in fusion with a target protein, ubiquitin can promote rapid proteasomal degradation of the protein, leading to MHC I peptide presentation [54]. Alternatively, CD4+ T-cell responses can be enhanced by a DNA vaccine designed to direct endogenously synthesized proteins to the lysosomal compartment of APCs, where the proteins are degraded into peptides that can be eventually loaded into the pockets of MHC class II molecules. For this purpose, a fusion construct of the full-length protein and the 20-amino acid C-terminal tail of lysosomal integral membrane protein-II (LIMP-II) has been used [55]. To favor the antibody response, signal sequences, usually of 16 to 30 amino acid residues comprising a central hydrophobic core and a C-terminal region with the cleavage site for signal peptidase, can be cloned in-frame with the sequence encoding a cytoplasmic protein, driving it toward the plasma membrane.

Recently, we have conceived a new kind of DNA vaccine that combines antigen expression with the silencing of molecules involved in the immunosuppression exerted by growing cancers. This double action is associated with two distinct modules: one is the conventional antigen expression cassette, while the other generates short hairpin (sh)RNA under the control of a polymerase III promoter [56, 57]. The RNA interference with synthesis of negative immune regulators, such as IDO or IL-10, is expected to ensure optimal presentation of the encoded antigen by APCs.

1.5.3. DNA vaccination targeting HER2

While the success of vaccination in preventing infectious diseases is uncontested, the derivation of efficient vaccines against cancer represents a more difficult challenge. Although cancer cells express antigens in a way that distinguishes them immunologically from normal cells, most tumors are only weakly immunogenic because most tumor antigens are "self" proteins and generally tolerated by the host. Thus, an effective cancer vaccine must activate the immune system to react against tumor–associated molecules and, in some cases, overcome immunological tolerance to such molecules. This implies a vaccine-stimulated immune reaction in patients showing no or only a weak pre-existing immune response against the tumor antigen [58].

The HER2 oncoantigen is considered an ideal target for DNA vaccination because it is directly involved in cancer progression and because it plays a causal role in the transformed phenotype, restricting the emergence of antigen-loss variants. HER2 overexpression in several carcinomas with an aggressive course, unlike its expression in normal tissues, ensures a specific anti-cancer response and minimal risk of an autoimmune attack on healthy tissues. Finally, HER2 is exposed on the cell membrane and can thus be readily targeted by antibodies and cell-mediated immunity [5]. On the other hand, HER2 is a “self” molecule, such that triggering a response to it must circumvent tolerance mechanisms.

An abundance of experiments in preclinical models demonstrates the promise of DNA vaccination as an effective approach to prevent the development of HER2-positive tumors, eliciting immune protection against spontaneous mammary carcinomas in mice transgenic for the rat HER2 oncogene as well as in transplantable rat and human HER2-expressing tumors [59-65]. As we specifically documented [63], anti-HER2 antibody production after vaccination represents the main mechanism responsible for the anti-tumor response. In fact, anti-HER2 antibodies are able to downmodulate the expression of this growth factor receptor causally implicated in carcinogenesis. Indirect reactions, such as ADCC and complement-mediated cytotoxicity, are also crucial in preventing the onset of a tumor and controlling its progression.

As mentioned above, DNA vaccines are easily manipulated to optimize immune activation using recombinant DNA technologies. In one of the first studies of HER2-targeted DNA vaccination, the plasmid encoding the extracellular and transmembrane (EC-TM) domains of this molecule proved to be far superior to plasmids encoding only the extracellular domain (secreted form) or the full-length protein [59]. Most subsequent studies, performed in both wild-type BALB/c mice and cancer-prone BALB-neuT transgenic mice, confirmed the unique ability of this vaccine to trigger protective immunity toward rat HER2-positive tumors [60-63]. BALB-neuT mice transgenically expressing the rat activated neu oncogene under the control of the MMTV promoter are genetically predestined to develop lethal invasive carcinomas in the mammary glands at high multiplicity (all mammary glands are affected) and with relatively short latency [66]. About 50% of BALB-neuT mice electroporated with EC-TM plasmid when the mammary glands display atypical hyperplasia, at 10 and 12 weeks of age, remained free of autochthonous mammary tumors up to at least 1 year of age, whereas all unvaccinated mice succumbed to mammary cancer within 22–27 weeks [62].

In efforts to define the minimal antigen portion still able to elicit protective immunity, we carried out molecular dissection of the HER2 molecule through sequential deletions of multiples of 240 bp, corresponding to 80 amino acids, starting from the amino-terminal of the extracellular sequence [63]. The resulting seven cut-down fragments were cloned into a recipient expression vector downstream of the leader sequence, which drives the proteins through the endoplasmic reticulum toward the plasma membrane (Figure 12).

A first series of DNA vaccination experiments with these seven cut-down plasmids was performed in wild-type BALB/c mice transplanted with syngeneic rat HER2-positive adenocarcinoma cells, established from a mammary tumor of BALB-neuT mice (TUBO cells). Significant protection was obtained in mice immunized with the first four cut-down plasmids, while protection declined in mice immunized with shorter fragments. In particular, EC4-TM, which lacks almost half of the EC domain and exposes only 344 amino acids, protected all vaccinated mice through the induction of anti-rat HER2 antibodies at levels comparable to those in mice vaccinated with the whole EC-TM [63]. However, in wild-type BALB/c mice, vaccination triggered a strong immune response because the rat HER2 protein target is a foreign, xenogeneic antigen. It is much more difficult to induce immunoprotection in cancer-prone BALB-neuT mice, which are tolerant to rat HER2 protein because they express the transgene in the thymus early in life [67]. In those mice, only electroporation with EC-TM or EC4-TM led to a significant delay in the progression of mammary lesions, whereas the other cut-down plasmids were completely ineffective.

Interestingly, EC4-TM induced a stronger ADCC response than did the whole EC-TM, suggesting that EC4-TM provides accessible critical determinants that may be partially masked in the whole EC-TM [63]. Together, the results of these experiments suggest that the first 390 amino acids of HER2 are those responsible for triggering the protective immunity induced by EC-TM vaccination.

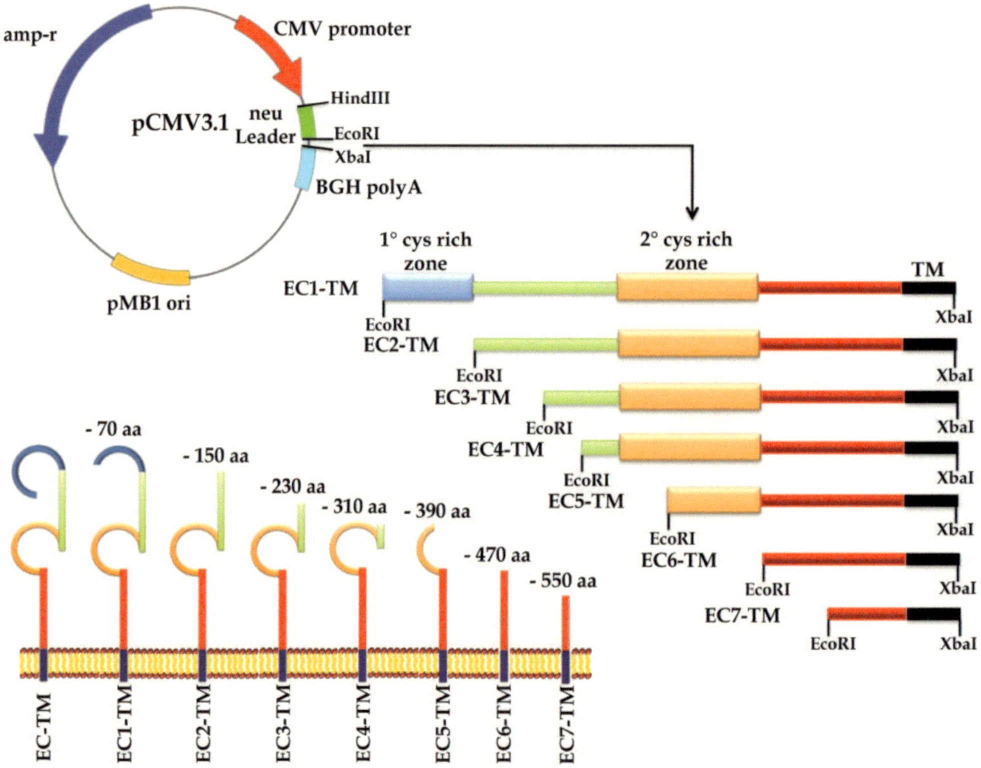

Figure 12. HER2 cut-down vaccines. The seven cut-down HER2 DNA fragments were inserted downstream of the leader sequence using EcoRI and XbaI restriction enzymes. The truncated protein encoded by the first cut-down plasmid (EC1-TM) displays an EC domain lacking the first 70 NH_2-terminal residues. All the other truncated proteins, encoded respectively by the EC2-TM, EC3-TM, EC4-TM, EC5-TM, EC6-TM, and EC7-TM cut-down plasmids, display EC domains progressively shortened by 80 NH_2-terminal residues. All of these truncated proteins have an identical TM domain.

In a strategy aimed at breaking the tolerance to HER2 and further improving the elicited protection in BALB-neuT mice, we constructed two new DNA vaccines, RHuT and HuRT, encoding rat and human HER2 chimeric proteins. Containing both syngeneic and xenogeneic portions of the protein antigen, they ensure specificity as well as a tolerance break [64, 65]. In particular, HuRT was derived by cloning the human cDNA fragment encoding the first 390 amino-terminal residues into the rat EC5-TM cut-down plasmid to regenerate the whole EC domain. Almost symmetrically, RHuT encodes a protein in which the 410 amino-terminal residues are from the rat HER2 and the remaining residues from human HER2 (Figure 13 and Figure 14).

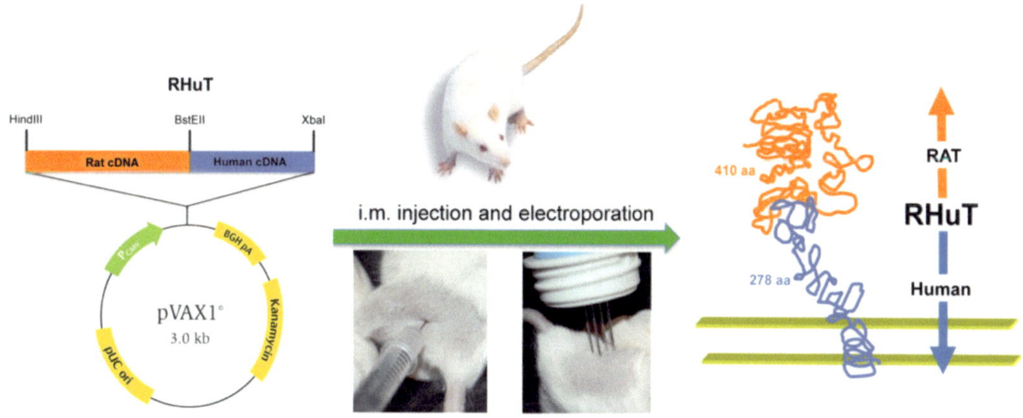

Figure 13. RHuT electroporation. RHuT encodes for a chimeric protein in which the 410 NH_2-terminal residues are from the rat HER2 extracellular domain and the remaining residues from the human protein. After i.m. injection of 50 µg of DNA plasmid, two low voltage pulses of 150V of 25 ms with a 300 µs interval were applied through the insertion of Cliniporator needles (Igea, Carpi, Italy) into the mouse quadriceps muscles.

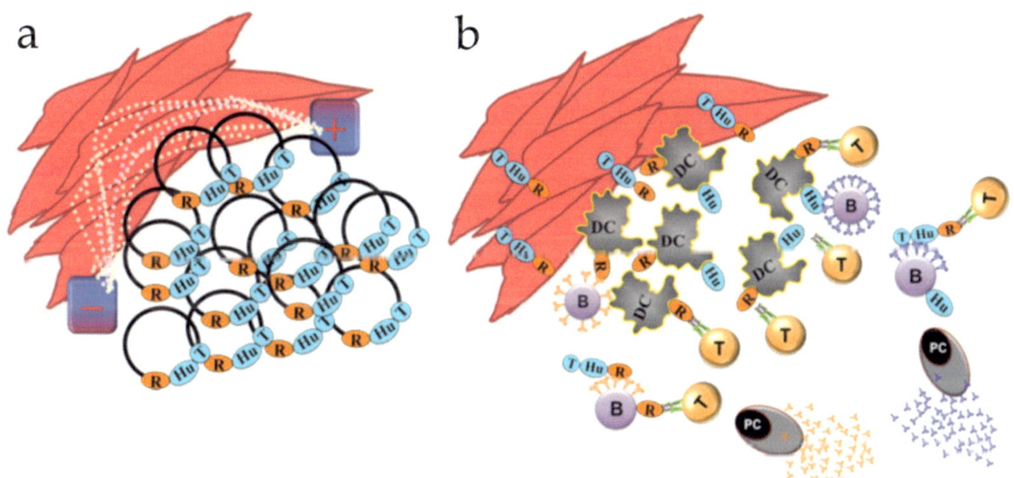

Figure 14. Presentation of xenogeneic peptides by dendritic cells (DC) contributes to an antibody response to both the tolerated and non-tolerated moieties of the antigen. Following DNA electroporation (a) with RHuT plasmid encoding for a rat (orange) and human (blue) chimeric HER2 protein, T cells (T) recognizing the xenogeneic peptides proliferate. The expanded T cells interact and provide helper signals to B cells, leading to the production of antibodies (Y) to both the xenogeneic and tolerated moieties by plasmacells (PC). Adapted from Iezzi M. et al, 2012 [68].

Chimeric vaccines displayed superior performance in tolerant BALB neu-T mice [64, 65]. While control mice vaccinated with empty pVAX plasmid developed HER2-positive mammary tumors within 27 weeks of age, all mice electroporated at 10 weeks and at 12 weeks of age with RHuT or fully rat EC-TM (RRT) remained tumor-free at 40 weeks. However, 10 weeks later, the protection of mice vaccinated with RRT decreased to about

50%, while 80% of RHuT vaccinated mice remained tumor-free (Figure 15a). In both cases, the tumor rejection pattern correlated with higher titers of anti-rat HER2 antibodies (Figure 15b). In addition, RHuT protection could be further extended by repeated boosting to maintain immunological memory [64].

Preclinical data obtained with RHuT provided the rationale for its use in an ongoing phase I clinical trial (EudraCT 2011-001104-34) approved by Italian Ministry of Health in HER2-positive head-and-neck cancers (protocol code: IOV-HN-1-2011). Moreover, preliminary data have shown that chimeric vaccines used in Δ16HER2 transgenic mice are also able to counteract the aggressive breast carcinogenesis driven by the Δ16HER2 splice variant.

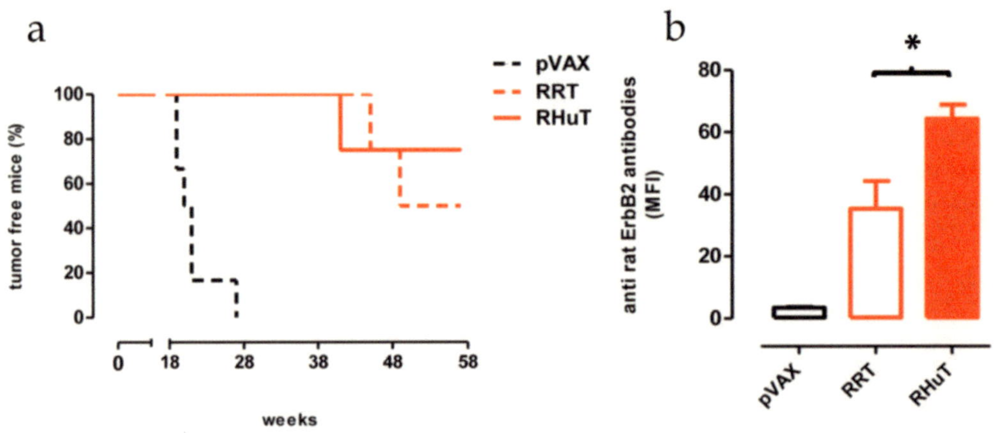

Figure 15. Vaccination with RHuT effectively protects Balb-neuT mice from HER2-driven mammary carcinogenesis. a. Mammary tumor incidence of BALB-neuT vaccinated mice with RHuT (dotted red line, n = 7 mice), RRT (continuous red line, n = 8 mice), and empty control pVAX (dotted black line, n = 6 mice). Differences in tumor incidence were analyzed by the log-rank (Mantel-Cox) test. b. Mouse sera collected 2 weeks after the second vaccination were analyzed for anti-rat HER2 antibody titer by flow cytometry (b). Data are mean MFI ± SEM (* p = 0.02, Student's t test).

2. Conclusions

Breast cancer remains one of the major causes of morbidity and mortality in Western Countries, despite progress in both knowledge and treatment. A deeper understanding of the underlying biology of breast cancer is necessary for the identification of new molecular targets and development of novel targeted therapeutics.

In the last three decades, a large number of transgenic mice have been generated that demonstrate the direct involvement of the HER2 receptor in mammary carcinogenesis. In these cancer-prone mice transgenically expressing the rat or human HER2 molecule, the development of autochthonous tumors recapitulates several of the molecular and genetic features of human cancer progression. Some of these animal models support the hypothesis that overexpression of HER2 alone is not sufficient to generate mammary tumors and requires activating mutations.

Emerging evidence indicates that the Δ16HER2 splice variant plays a key role in tumor progression and refractoriness to Trastuzumab treatment. Currently, a new mouse model transgenic for the human Δ16HER2 isoform is available. While no single genetically engineered mouse can offer a complete model of the wide assortment of human neoplasms found in human breast cancer, the Δ16HER2 mouse represents a novel tool to test the ability of drugs and vaccines to inhibit the progression of HER2-driven cancer and to investigate Trastuzumab resistance.

Among targeted therapies being developed for breast cancer, anti-HER2 cancer vaccines seem particularly promising.

However, the generation of an effective vaccine able to trigger a long-lasting immunity that prevents tumor recurrence in cancer patients implies the understanding of how tolerance, immunity and immunosuppression regulate antitumor immune responses. Equally important for the rational design of cancer vaccines is the development of new biotechnological tools for the identification of the most immunogenic portions of a molecule and for the selection of the key epitopes within a protein.

In Steven Spielberg's "War of the Worlds", mankind prevailed over extraterrestrial invaders thanks to immunity, because "For neither do men live nor die in vain." The challenge is to redirect the powerful mechanisms of the immune response, so effective against outside invaders such as microorganisms, against an inside enemy, i.e., cancer.

Author details

Cristina Marchini*, Lucia Pietrella, Cristina Kalogris, Chiara Garulli, Federico Gabrielli and Augusto Amici*
Department of Bioscience and Biotechnology, University of Camerino, Camerino (MC), Italy

Serenella M. Pupa and Elda Tagliabue
Molecular Targeting Unit, Department of Experimental Oncology and Molecular Medicine, Fondazione IRCCS, Istituto Nazionale dei Tumori, AmadeoLab, Milan; Italy

Elena Quaglino
Molecular Biotechnology Center, University of Turin, Turin, Italy

Manuela Iezzi
Aging Research Centre, G. d'Annunzio University, Chieti, Italy

Acknowledgement

The experimental data herein were obtained through grants from the Italian Association for Cancer Research (AIRC, IG11889) and the Italian Ministry for the Universities and Research. We thank Prof. Guido Forni for being a beacon in our scientific life.

* Corresponding Authors

3. References

[1] Ehrlich P. (1909). Über den jetzigen Stand der Karzinomforschung. Ned. Tijdschr. Geneeskd. 5: 273-290.

[2] Burnet F.M. (1957). Cancer-a Biological Approach. BMJ. 1: 841–847.

[3] Burnet F.M. (1970). The concept of immunological surveillance. Prog. Exp. Tumor Res. 13: 1-27.

[4] Finn O.J. (2003). Cancer vaccines: between the idea and the reality. Nat Rev Immunol 3:630-641.

[5] Lollini P.L. and Forni G. (2003). Cancer immunoprevention: tracking down persistent tumor antigens. Trends in Immunology. 24 (2): 62-66.

[6] Cavallo F., De Giovanni C., Nanni P., Forni G., Lollini P.L. (2011). 2011: The immune hallmarks of cancer. Cancer Immunol. Immunother. 60: 319-326.

[7] Lollini P.L., Cavallo F., Nanni P., Forni G. (2006). Vaccines for tumour prevention. Nat Rev Cancer 6: 204-216.

[8] Ladjemi M.Z., Jacot W., Charde`s T., Pe`legrin A., Navarro-Teulon I. (2010). Anti-HER2 vaccines: new prospects for breast cancer therapy. Cancer Immunol. Immunother. 59: 1295-1312.

[9] Cho H.S., Mason K., Ramyar K.X., Stanley A.M., Gabelli S.B., Denney D.W. Jr., Leahy D.J. (2003). Structure of the extracellular region of HER2 alone and in complex with the Herceptin Fab. Nature. 421: 756-760.

[10] Wieduwilt M. J., Moasser M. M. (2008). The epidermal growth factor receptor family: Biology driving targeted therapeutics Cell Mol Life Sci. 65 (10): 1566 - 1584.

[11] Hynes N.E., Stern D.F. (1994). The biology of erbB-2/neu/HER-2 and its role in cancer. Biochem Biophys Acta Rev Cancer. 1198: 165-84.

[12] Slamon D.J., Clark G.M., Wong S. G., Levin W.J., Ullrich A., McGuire W.L. (1987). Human breast cancer: correlation of relapse and survival with amplification of the HER-2/neu oncogene. Science. 235 (4785): 177-182.

[13] Siegel P.M., Muller W.J. (1996). Mutations affecting conserved cysteine residues within the extracellular domain of Neu promote receptor dimerization and activation. Proc Natl Acad Sci U S A. 93: 8878-8883.

[14] Finkle D., Quan Z.R., Asghari V., Kloss J., Ghaboosi N., Mai E., Wong W.L., Hollingshead P., Schwall R., Koeppen H., Erickson S. (2004) HER2-targeted therapy reduces incidence and progression of midlife mammary tumors in female murine mammary tumor virus huHER2-transgenic mice. Clin Cancer Res. 10: 2499-2511.

[15] Siegel P.M., Dankort D.L., Hardy W.R., Muller W.J. (1994) Novel activating mutations in the neu proto-oncogene involved in induction of mammary tumors. Mol Cell Biol 14: 7068-7077.

[16] Kwong K.Y., Hung M.C. (1998). A novel splice variant of HER2 with increased transformation activity. Molecular Carcinogenesis. 23: 62-68.

[17] Castiglioni F, Tagliabue E, Campiglio M, Pupa SM, Balsari A, Menard S. (2006) Role of exon-16-deleted HER2 in breast carcinomas. Endocr Relat Cancer 13: 221-232.

[18] Mitra D, Brumlik MJ, Okamgba SU, Zhu Y, Duplessis TT, Parvani J.G., Lesko S.M., Brogi E., Jones F.E. (2009) An oncogenic isoform of HER2 associated with locally disseminated breast cancer and trastuzumab resistance. Mol Cancer Ther 8: 2152-2162.

[19] Marchini C., Gabrielli F., Iezzi M., Zenobi S., Montani M., Pietrella L., Kalogris C., Rossini A., Ciravolo V., Castagnoli L., Tagliabue E., Pupa S.M., Musiani P., Monaci P., Menard S., Amici A. (2011) The Human Splice Variant Δ16HER2 Induces Rapid Tumor Onset in a Reporter Transgenic Mouse. PLoS One. 6(4): e18727.

[20] Pedersen K., Angelini P.D., Laos S., Bach-Faig A., Cunningham M.P., Ferrer-Ramón C., Luque-García A., García-Castillo J., Parra-Palau J.L., Scaltriti M., Ramón y Cajal S., Baselga J., Arribas J. (2009) A naturally occurring HER2 carboxy-terminal fragment promotes mammary tumor growth and metastasis. Mol Cell Biol 29: 3319-3331.

[21] Arribas J., Baselga J., Pedersen K., Parra-Palau J.L. (2011) p95HER2 and Breast Cancer. Cancer Res. 71(5): 1515-1519.

[22] Andrechek E.R., Hardy W.R., Siegel P.M., Rudnicki M.A., Cardiff R.D., Muller W.J. (2000) Amplification of the neu/erbB-2 oncogene in a mouse model of mammary tumorigenesis. Proc. Natl Acad. Sci. USA 97: 3444-3449.

[23] Muller W.J., Sinn E., Pattengale P.K., Wallace R., Leder P. (1988) Single-step induction of mammary adenocarcinoma in transgenic mice bearing the activated c-neu oncogene. Cell 54: 105-115.

[24] Bouchard L., Lamarre L., Tremblay P. J., Jolicoeur, P. (1989) Stochastic appearance of mammary tumors in transgenic mice carrying the MMTV/c-neu oncogene. Cell 57: 931-6.

[25] Guy C. T., Cardiff R. D., Muller W. J. (1996) Activated neu induces rapid tumor progression. J. Biol. Chem. 271: 7673-7678.

[26] Moody S.E., Sarkisian C.J., Hahn K.T., Gunther E.J., Pickup S., Dugan K.D., Innocent N., Cardiff R.D., Schnall M.D., Chodosh L.A. (2002) Conditional activation of Neu in the mammary epithelium of transgenic mice results in reversible pulmonary metastasis. Cancer Cell 2: 451–461.

[27] Guy C.T., Webster M.A., Schaller M., Parsons T.J., Cardiff R.D., Muller W.J.(1992) Expression of the neu proto oncogene in the mammary epithelium of transgenic mice induces metastatic disease. Proc. Natl Acad. Sci. USA 89: 10578-10582.

[28] Siegel P. M., Muller W. J. (1996) Mutations affecting conserved cysteine residues within the extracellular domain of Neu promote receptor dimerization and activation. Proc. Natl Acad. Sci. USA 93: 8878–8883.

[29] Siegel P. M., Ryan E. D., Cardiff R. D., Muller, W. J. (1999) Elevated expression of activated forms of Neu/ErbB-2 and ErbB-3 are involved in the induction of mammary tumors in transgenic mice: implications for human breast cancer. EMBO J. 18: 2149–2164.

[30] Dankort D., Maslikowski B., Warner N., Kanno N., Kim H., Wang Z., Moran M.F., Oshima R.G., Cardiff R.D., Muller W.J. (2001) Grb2 and Shc adapter proteins play distinct roles in Neu (ErbB-2)-induced mammary tumorigenesis: implications for human breast cancer. Mol. Cell. Biol. 21: 1540-1551.

[31] Stocklin E., Botteri F., Groner B. (1993) An activated allele of the c-erbB-2 oncogene impairs kidney and lung function and causes early death of transgenic mice. J. Cell Biol. 122, 199-208.

[32] Piechocki M.P., Ho Y.S., Pilon S., Wei W.Z. (2003) Human ErbB-2 (Her-2) transgenic mice: a model system for testing Her-2 based vaccines. J Immunol 171: 5787-5794.

[33] Ursini-Siegel J., Schade B., Cardiff R.D., Muller W.J. (2007) Insights from transgenic mouse models of ERBB2-induced breast cancer. Nature Reviews Cancer 7: 389-397.

[34] Bryda EC, Bauer BA (2010) A restriction enzyme-PCR-based technique to determine transgene insertion sites. Methods Mol Biol 597: 287-299.

[35] Bryda EC, Pearson M, Agca Y, Bauer BA (2006) Method for detection and identification of multiple chromosomal integration sites in transgenic animals created with lentivirus. Biotechniques 41: 715-719.

[36] Shepherd C.T., Moran Lauter A.N., Scott M.P. (2009) Determination of transgene copy number by real-time quantitative PCR. Methods Mol Biol 526: 129-134.

[37] Arteaga C.L., Sliwkowski M.X., Osborne C.K., Perez E.A., Puglisi F., Gianni L. (2011) Treatment of HER2-positive breast cancer: current status and future perspectives. Nat Rev Clin Oncol. 9(1): 16-32.

[38] Fiszman G.L., Jasnis M.A. (2011) Molecular Mechanisms of Trastuzumab Resistance in HER2 Overexpressing Breast Cancer. Int J Breast Cancer 2011: 352182-352194.

[39] Vogel C.L., Cobleigh M.A., Tripathy D., Gutheil J.C., Harris L.N., Fehrenbacher L., Slamon D.J., Murphy M., Novotny W.F., Burchmore M., Shak S., Stewart S.J., Press M. (2002) Efficacy and safety of trastuzumab as a single agent in first-line treatment of HER2-overexpressing metastatic breast cancer. J. Clin. Oncol. 20: 719-726.

[40] Nagy P., Friedlander E., Tanner M., Kapanen A.I., Carraway K.L., Isola J., Jovin T.M. (2005) Decreased accessibility and lack of activation of ErbB2 in JIMT-1, a Herceptin-resistant, MUC4-expressing breast cancer cell line. Cancer Res 65:473–82.

[41] Nagata Y., Lan K.H., Zhou X., Tan M., Esteva F.J., Sahin A.A., Klos K.S., Li P., Monia B.P., Nguyen N.T., Hortobagyi G.N., Hung M.C., Yu D. (2004) PTEN activation contributes to tumor inhibition by trastuzumab, and loss of PTEN predicts trastuzumab resistance in patients. Cancer Cell. 6(2): 117-27.

[42] Berns K., Horlings H.M., Hennessy B.T., Madiredjo M., Hijmans E.M., Beelen K., Linn S.C., Gonzalez-Angulo A.M., Stemke-Hale K., Hauptmann M., Beijersbergen R.L., Mills G.B., van de Vijver M.J., Bernards R. (2007) A functional genetic approach identifies the PI3K pathway as a major determinant of trastuzumab resistance in breast cancer. Cancer Cell. 12(4): 395-402.

[43] Huang X., Gao L., Wang S., McManaman J.L., Thor A.D., Yang X., Esteva F.J., Liu B. (2010) Heterotrimerization of the growth factor receptors erbB2, erbB3, and insulin-like growth factor-I receptor in breast cancer cells resistant to herceptin. Cancer Res. 70(3): 1204-14.

[44] Scaltriti M., Rojo F., Ocaña A., Anido J., Guzman M., Cortes J, Di Cosimo S., Matias-Guiu X., y Cajal S.R., Arribas J., Baselga J. (2007) Expression of p95HER2, a Truncated Form of the HER2 Receptor, and Response to Anti-HER2 Therapies in Breast Cancer. J Natl Cancer Inst. 99: 628-38

[45] Dowsett M., Procter M., McCaskill-Stevens W., de Azambuja E., Dafni U., Rueschoff J., Jordan B., Dolci S., Abramovitz M., Stoss O., Viale G., Gelber R.D., Piccart-Gebhart M., Leyland-Jones B. (2009) Disease-free survival according to degree of HER2 amplification for patients treated with adjuvant chemotherapy with or without 1 year of trastuzumab: the HERA Trial. J Clin Oncol. 27(18): 2962-9.

[46] Zhang S., Huang W.C., Li P., Guo H., Poh S.B., Brady S.W., Xiong Y., Tseng L.M., Li S.H., Ding Z., Sahin A.A., Esteva F.J., Hortobagyi G.N., Yu D. (2011) Combating trastuzumab resistance by targeting SRC, a common node downstream of multiple resistance pathways Nature Medicine 17: 461-469.

[47] Wolff J.A., Malone R.W., Williams P., Chong W., Acsadi G., Jani A., Felgner P.L. (1990) Direct gene transfer into mouse muscle in vivo. Science. 247: 1465-1468.

[48] Liu MA. (2003) DNA vaccines: a review. J Intern Med. 253(4): 402-10.

[49] Fynan E.F., Webster R.G., Fuller D.H., Haynes J., Santoro J.C., Robinson H.L. (1993) DNA vaccines: protective immunizations by parenteral, mucosal, and gene-gun inoculations. Proc Natl Acad Sci U S A. 90: 11478-82

[50] Bodles-Brakhop A.M., Heller R., Draghia-Akli R. (2009) Electroporation for the delivery of DNA-based vaccines and immunotherapeutics: Current clinical developments. Mol. Ther. 17: 585-592.

[51] Krieg A.M. (2002) CpG motifs in bacterial DNA and their immune effects. Annu. Rev. Immunol. 20: 709-760.

[52] Piechocki M.P., Pilon S.A., and Wei W.Z. (2001) Complementary antitumor immunity induced by plasmid DNA encoding secreted and cytoplasmic human ErbB-2. J. Immunol. 167: 3367-3374.

[53] Sominskaya I., Alekseeva E., Skrastina D., Mokhonov V., Starodubova E., Jansons J., Levi M., Prilipov A., Kozlovska T., Smirnov V., Pumpens P., Isaguliants M.G. (2006) Signal sequences modulate the immunogenic performance of human hepatitis C virus E2 gene. Molecular Immunology. 43: 1941-1952.

[54] Rodriguez F., J. Zhang, and J. L. Whitton (1997) DNA immunization: ubiquitination of a viral protein enhances CTL induction, and antiviral protection, but abrogates antibody induction. J. Virol. 71: 8497-8503.

[55] Rodriguez F., Harkins S., Redwine J.M., De Pereda J.M., Whitton J.L. (2001) CD4+ T Cells Induced by a DNA Vaccine: Immunological Consequences of Epitope-Specific Lysosomal Targeting. J. Virol. 75 (21): 10421–10430.

[56] Macagno M., Bolli E., Marchini C., Amici A., Riganti C., Bosia A., Forni G., Cavallo F. (2010) Indoleamine 2,3-Dioxygenase (IDO) silencing for improved antitumour vaccination. European Journal Cancer SUPPLEMENTS, 8(5): 75.

[57] Bolli E., Macagno M., Arigoni M., Marchini C., Amici A., Forni G., Cavallo F. (2010) Cyclooxygenase-2 (COX2) gene silencing with siRNA could enhance DNA vaccination to inhibit established ErbB-2 carcinomas. European Journal Cancer SUPPLEMENTS, 8(5): 76.

[58] Lollini P.L., Nicoletti G., Landuzzi L., Cavallo F., Forni G., De Giovanni C., Nanni P. (2011) Vaccines and other immunological approaches for cancer immunoprevention. Current Drug Targets. 12: 1957-1973.

[59] Amici A., Smorlesi A., Noce G., Santoni G., Cappelletti P., Capparuccia L., Coppari R., Lucciarini R., Petrelli F., and Provinciali M. (2000) DNA vaccination with full-length or truncated neu induces protective immunity against the development of spontaneous mammary tumors in HER-2/neu transgenic mice. Gene Ther. 7: 703-706.

[60] Rovero S., Amici A., Di Carlo E., Bei R., Nanni P., Quaglino E., Porcedda P., Boggio K., Smorlesi A., Lollini P.L., Landuzzi L., Colombo M.P., Giovarelli M., Musiani P., Forni, G. (2000) DNA Vaccination against rat Her-2/Neu p185 more effectively inhibits carcinogenesis than transplantable carcinomas in transgenic BALB/c mice. J. Immunol. 165: 5133-5142.

[61] Curcio C., Di Carlo E., Clynes R., Smyth M.J., Boggio K., Quaglino E., Spadaro M., Colombo M.P., Amici. A., Lollini P-L., Musiani P., and Forni G. (2003) Nonredundant roles of antibody, cytokines and perforin in the eradication of established Her-2/neu carcinomas. J. Clin. Invest. 111 (8): 1161-1170.

[62] Quaglino E., Iezzi M., Mastini C., Amici A., Pericle F., Di Carlo E., Pupa S.M., De Giovanni C., Spadaro M., Curcio C., Lollini P.L., Musiani P., Forni G., Cavallo F. (2004) Electroporated DNA vaccine clears away multifocal mammary carcinomas in her-2/neu transgenic mice. Cancer Res. 64: 2858-2864.

[63] Rolla S., Marchini C., Malinarich S., Quaglino E., Lanzardo S., Montani M., Angeletti M., Ramadori G., Forni G., Cavallo F., and Amici A. (2008) Protective immunity against neu-positive carcinomas elicited by electroporation of plasmids encoding decreasing fragments of rat neu extracellular domain. Hum. Gene Ther. 19: 229-239.

[64] Quaglino E., Mastini C., Amici A., Marchini C., Iezzi M., Lanzardo S., De Giovanni C., Montani M., Lollini P.L., Masucci G., Forni G., Cavallo F. (2010) A Better Immune Reaction to Erbb-2 Tumors Is Elicited in Mice by DNA Vaccines Encoding Rat/Human Chimeric Proteins. Cancer Res. 70: 2604-2612.

[65] Jacob J.B., Quaglino E., Radkevich-Brown O., Jones R.F., Piechocki M.P., Reyes J.D., Weise A., Amici A., Wei W.Z. (2010) Combining human and rat sequences in HER-2 DNA vaccines blunts immune tolerance and drives antitumor immunity. Cancer Res. 70: 119-128.

[66] Quaglino E., Mastini C., Forni G., Cavallo F. (2008) ErbB2 transgenic mice: a tool for investigation of the immune prevention and treatment of mammary carcinomas. Curr. Protoc. Immunol. 20:Unit 20.9.1-20.9-10.

[67] Rolla S., Nicoló C., Malinarich S., Orsini M., Forni G., Cavallo F., Ria F. (2006) Distinct and non-overlapping T cell receptor repertoires expanded by DNA vaccination in wild-type and HER-2 transgenic BALB/c mice. J. Immunol. 177: 7626-7633.

[68] Iezzi M., Quaglino E., Amici A., Lollini P.L., Forni G., Cavallo F. (2012) DNA vaccination against oncoantigens. A promise. OncoImmunology 1 (3): 1-10.

Chapter 3

HER2 Amplification or Overexpression in Upper GI Tract and Breast Cancer with Clinical Diagnosis and Treatment

Zhongren Zhou and David G. Hick

Additional information is available at the end of the chapter

http://dx.doi.org/10.5772/53921

1. Introduction

EGFR and HER2 family with signal pathway and carcinogenesis: The human epidermal growth factor receptors (HER-2) gene is localized to chromosome 17q and encodes a transmembrane tyrosine kinase receptor protein. Numerous studies were done from basic mechanism of HER family for cell proliferation and oncogenesis, HER2 overexpression or amplification in various solid tumors to clinical treatment of breast cancer, gastro-esophageal cancer by trastuzumab in many recent reviews [1-8].

HER2 belongs to a family including epidermal growth factor receptor (EGFR), HER2, HER3 and HER4, which are a group of transmembrane glycoproteins, collectively named receptor tyrosine kinases (RTKs), whose cytoplasmic domains harbor an enzymatic activity, namely tyrosine-specific phosphorylation [9]. The family of epidermal growth factor molecules, which comprises different ligands sharing a 50–60 amino acid receptor binding domain, bind with subtype RTKs. Each receptor consists of an extracellular ligand-binding domain, a transmembrane domain, and a tyrosine kinase portion [10]. Upon ligand binding, the otherwise inactive monomeric receptors form active homodimers or heterodimers, thereby leading to receptor phosphorylation and signaling via various biochemical pathways (Fig.1), such as the mitogen-activated protein kinase (MAPK), the phosphatidylinositol 3-kinase (PI3K), phospholipase C-γ, and transcription factors like the signal transducers and activators of transcription (STATs) or SMAD proteins [1]. These modules of cellular activation and the respective growth factors (GFs)s are co-opted in several phases of tumor progression.

HER-2 gene amplification in breast cancer has been associated with increased cell proliferation, cell motility, tumor invasiveness, progressive regional and distant metastases, accelerated angiogenesis, and reduced apoptosis [11]. Overexpression of HER2 in human

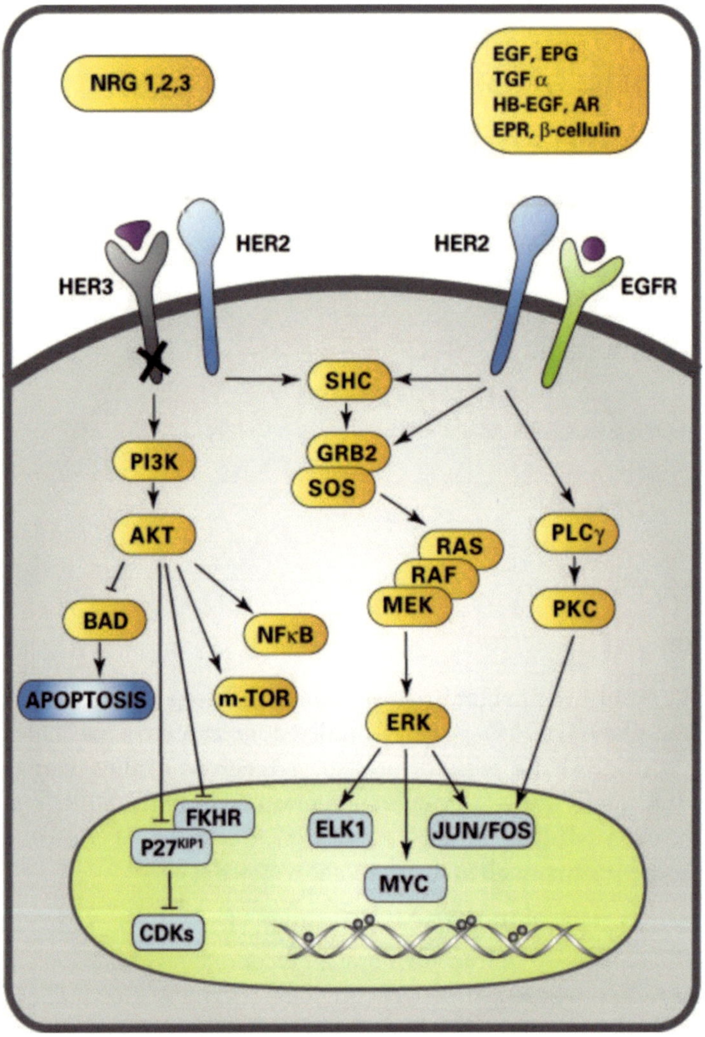

Figure 1. Signal transduction pathways instigated by HER2, co-receptors and EGF-like growth factors. Heterodimers of HER2/ErbB-2 and either EGFR/ErbB-1 or the kinase-defective ErbB-3/HER3 (note the letter X that symbolizes a defective cytoplasm-facing kinase domain) are shown, along with the growth factor ligands they bind. All ligands share an epidermal growth factor (EGF) motif of 50–60 amino acids. They include, in addition to EGF, epiregulin (EPG), transforming growth factor alpha (TGF-alpha), heparin-binding epidermal growth factor-like factor (HB-EGF), amphiregulin (AR), epiregulin (EPR) and betacellulin. Another group includes four classes of neuregulins (NRGs). Note that HER2 is unable to bind a ligand. Nevertheless, HER2 takes part in signaling via its own constitutive phosphorylation, as well as by trans-activation of its heterodimerization partners. Tyrosine phsphorylated receptors are coupled to several biochemical cascades, including the phosphoinositide-3-kinase (PI3K) pathway and the extracellular signal-regulated kinase (ERK), which belongs to the MAPK family. Activation of ERK/MAPK is mediated via the RAS-RAF-MEK pathway and leads to cellular proliferation via the activation of a number of nuclear targets, including the AP1 (FOS and JUN) complex, MYC, which regulates cell cycle progression, and ELK1, a member of the ETS family of transcription factors. SHC and GRB2 are adaptor proteins sharing the ability to bind each other, as well

as tyrosine phosphorylated receptors. The EGFR/HER2 heterodimer also couples to phospholipase C (PLC) and the downstream protein kinase C. On the other hand, ErbB-3/HER3-containing heterodimers strongly activate another kinase, AKT, via a lipid kinase, PI3K, leading to activation of mTOR (mechanistic target of rapamycin). Activation of AKT blocks signaling via BAD, a BH3-only protein, which contributes to tissue homeostasis by regulating initiation of apoptosis. Activation of AKT inhibits FKHR and the cyclin-dependent kinase inhibitor $p27^{KIP}$. The forkhead box O1 (FKHR, FOXO1) transcription factor is a member of the FOXO family of transcription factors, involved in tumor suppression and cell death. (From Emde A, et al. Crit Rev Oncol/Hematol (2010), http://dx.doi.org/10.1016/j.critrevonc.2010.09.002, Permitted by Elsevier Limited).

mammary epithelial cells induces proliferative advantage, transformed characteristics, tumorigenic growth, and induces proliferative and anti-apoptotic changes that mimic early stages of epithelial cell transformation [12]. HER2 amplification is also seen in early in situ ductal carcinomas without any evidence of invasive disease [13, 14]. HER2 status is maintained during progression to invasive disease, nodal metastasis and distant metastasis [14, 15]. HER2 overexpression has been shown to activate multiple signaling complexes, which results in a striking dysregulation of the global transcriptome [1].

Clinical treatment targeting on HER2 receptor: It took a long journey to develop monoantibody to target HER2. Murine origin of mAb to HER2 limits their clinical application since immunoglobulin molecules are immunogenic. When injected into humans, it shortens their half-lives in circulation. Winter and colleagues (1988) generated a mouse–human chimeric antibody [16]. Later transgenic mice whose immunoglobulin loc have been genetically inactive, was used to produce the first fully human antibody, Panitumumab, an antibody to EGFR. Then, trastuzumab which carry all human immunoglobulin genes, a monoclonal antibody to HER2, was approved for clinical use in lymphoma and in breast cancer [17]. So far, only two drugs that target HER2, Trastuzumab and a kinase inhibitor called Lapatinib/Tykerb, are approved for clinical application in breast cancer, but several novel drugs are in development (see figure 2).

Trastuzumab, monoclone antibody on HER2: Trastuzumab, a monoclonal antibody that targets HER2, induces antibody-dependent cellular cytotoxicity, inhibits HER2-mediated signaling and prevents cleavage of the extracellular domain of HER2 [12]. Based on multi-centers and countries clinical trial for HER2 positive breast cancer, [18,19,20] trastuzumab was significantly improve the prognosis of breast cancer. Therefore, it was initially approved for treatment of patients with HER2 overexpressing metastatic breast cancer. Because Trastuzumab also enhances the efficacy of adjuvant chemotherapy in operable or locally advanced HER2-positive tumors [21], the antibody currently represents the standard of care for patients with early or advanced stages of HER2 overexpressing breast cancer.

Since breast cancer showed better prognosis with trastuzumab treatment for HER2 positive breast cancer patients and similar HER2 positive cancers were identified in gastric and gastro-esophageal cancer, clinical trial ToGA was performed in gastric carcinoma. ToGA (Trastuzumab for Gastric Cancer) was an open-label, international, phase 3, randomized controlled trial undertaken in 122 centers in 24 countries [22]. Clinical trial ToGA used trastuzumab combined with standard chemotherapy for HER2 positive gastric cancer and gastro-esophageal junction cancer which demonstrated a significant improvement of gastric cancer survival. Now, trastuzumab is approved for treatment of gastric cancer in European, United States, Japan and other multiple countries.

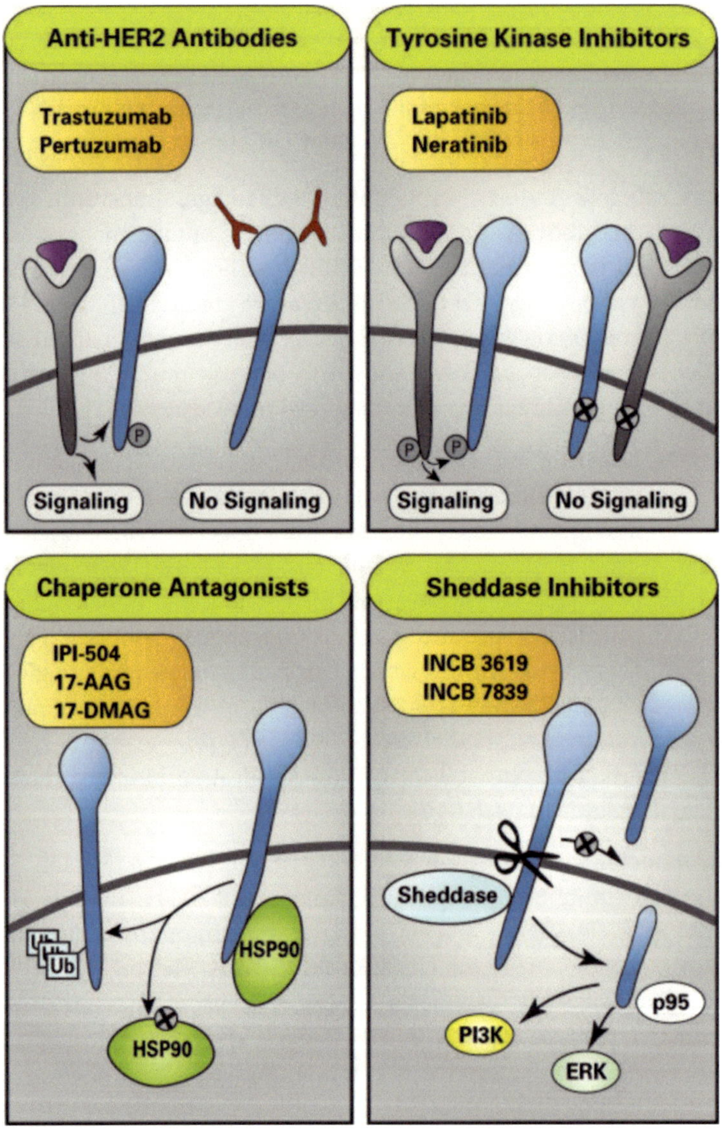

Figure 2. Clinically approved and experimental therapeutic strategies targeting ErbB-2/HER2 in carcinomas. Trastuzumab, a humanized monoclonal antibody directed against the extracellular domain of HER2, is approved for the treatment of HER2-overexpressing breast cancer. The antibody recruits immune effector mechanisms and can induce apoptosis, block angiogenesis and inhibit tumor cell proliferation. Similarly, Pertuzumab is able to prevent heterodimerization of HER2 with other family members. Unlike the ultimate specificity of Trastuzumab and Pertuzumab to HER2, tyrosine kinase inhibitors like the reversible inhibitor Lapatinib (approved for treatment of breast cancer) and the irreversible inhibitor Neratinib variably inhibit a broad range of tyrosine kinases. The drug has

completed phase II clinical trials. HSP90 is a molecular chaperone required for proper folding of protein kinases like HER2. Hence, HSP90 inhibitors, such as 17-AAG, which block the ATP/ADP binding pocket of HSP90 and target HER2 for proteasomal degradation are in clinical trials. A naturally occurring truncated form of HER2, p95-HER2, has been implicated as a mechanism conferring resistance to Trastuzumab. Its formation is mediated by processing of the membrane bound HER2 by matrix metalloproteinases (MMPs) of the ADAM (*a disintegrin and metalloproteinase*) family. INCB3619 and INCB7839 are potent inhibitors of ADAM10 and ADAM17. ADAM10 is the principle sheddase for different molecules associated with tumor cell proliferation, whereas ADAM17 is the main sheddase for the EGFR ligands TGF-alpha, AR, NRGs, and HB-EGF. These similar inhibitors may effectively block truncation of HER2 and onset of patient resistance to Trastuzumab, but clinical testing has not been completed. (From Emde A, et al. Crit Rev Oncol/Hematol (2010), http://dx.doi.org/10.1016/j.critrevonc.2010.09.002, Permitted by Elsevier Limited).

The clinical efficacy of Trastuzumab likely entails a combination of immunological and non-immunological mechanisms [1]. The ability of Trastuzumab to elicit antibody-dependent cellular cytotoxicity critically influences the efficacy of Trastuzumab-based therapies. Non-immunological mechanisms of Trastuzumab action include the inhibition of HER2 activation and downstream signaling. Alternatively, Trastuzumab may act by removing HER2 from the cell surface. Because it binds to an epitope near the cleavage site of HER2's extracellular domain, Trastuzumab inhibits HER2 activation by metalloproteinase-mediated shedding of the extracellular domain. The resulting interference with HER2-mediated downstream signaling processes shuts down cell proliferation, angiogenesis, invasive growth, resistance to apoptosis, and DNA repair, thus sensitizing tumor cells to conventional therapeutic modalities such as chemotherapy, endocrine treatment and radiotherapy.

Lapatinib, small molecule kinase inhibitor: Lapatinib, binding either reversibly or irreversibly to the nucleotide-binding cleft of their target kinases, is a highly specific, reversible inhibitor that blocks the catalytic action of both HER2 and EGFR[23]. Experiments in vitro and xenograft models, established the ability of Lapatinib to inhibit both the intact form of HER2 and the truncated intracellular form (p95-HER2), which is not recognized by Trastuzumab.

Similar to Trastuzumab, Lapatinib combined with chemotherapy was found to be better effect than capecitabine alone in HER2-positive women with advanced breast cancer that progressed after treatment with regimens that included Trastuzumab, an anthracycline and a taxane [24]. In addition, Lapatinib demonstrated clinical activity and was well tolerated as first-line monotherapy in HER2-amplified, locally advanced or metastatic breast cancer [25, 26]. Recently, laptinib showed a synergistic effect with trastuzumab in vitro and in vivo to inhibit HER2 amplified human gastric cancer cells and animal model [23]. Clinical phase II trial of lapatinib as first line therapy in patients with advanced or metastatic cancer showed well tolerated, which will be another potential drug to target HER2 receptors.

Lapatinib response correlated with EGFR and HER2 expression levels in patients' tumors, and associated with increased pre-treatment expression of phosphorylated-HER2 (p-

HER2)[27]. Lapatinib is able to induce apoptosis of Trastuzumab-resistant breast cancer cells via alteration of IGF-1 signaling, [28, 29] and also block NRG-induced p95-HER2/HER3 heterodimers formation [30].

2. HER2 in gastric adenocarcinoma

Gastric cancer is the fourth most common cancer worldwide and the second most common cause of cancer-related death in the world [31, 32]. The incidence of gastric cancer varies substantially worldwide, with the highest rates (>20 per 100,000) occurring in Japan, China, Eastern Europe, and South America, but the lowest rates (<10 per 100,000) finding in North America, southern Asia, North and East Africa, Australia, and New Zealand. In addition, it is more common in men than in women (10.9 vas 5.5 per 100,000). Although the survival of gastric cancer is improved in recently years in Western countries the 5 year survival is still around 5-20%. The multimodality treatments including surgery and neoadjuvent chemotherapy have a limited effect on the overall survival. In breast cancer, HER2 overexpression and amplification were reported around 25% and associate with poorer prognosis [2]. Trastuzumab treatment of HER2 positive breast cancer patient improved survival. HER2 overexpression and amplification were reported in gastric and gastro-esophageal junction (GEJ) tumors from 6-43%. In addition, trastuzumab were found to inhibit tumor growth in gastric carcinoma cell lines, animal model and xenograft models [33-35]. Recently international large scale phase III clinical trial called ToGA showed that trastuzumab added to standard chemotherapy significantly improved the response rate, median progression-free survival, and overall survival of gastric adenocarcinoma[22]. Trastuzumab combined with standard chemical therapy (such as capecitabine or 5-fluorouracil and cisplatin) now is approved by European Medicines Agency, United States and Japan etc. for the treatment of patients with HER2 overexpression or amplification. Thus clinical tests for HER2 overexpression and amplification in gastric adenocarcinoma patients become a key to recruit eligible patients for clinical treatment and evaluation of treatment effect.

IHC studies on HER2 overexpression: HER 2 overexpression was reported from 7-34% by many studies [3]. For clinical trial and treatment, it is very important to develop a standard HER2 test to recruit eligible patients for trastuzumab treatment. Before clinical trial ToGA, Hofmann and colleagues (2008)[36] first set up an IHC criteria based on HER2 IHC test on 168 gastric and GEJ resection patients (see Table 2). Based on the standard HER2 test on the breast cancer, they further proposed that strong incompletely membranous stain with basolateral "U" shape in gastric cancer was positive for HER2 overexpression. In addition, the HER2 expression showed higher heterogeneity about 4.8% in gastric samples than about 1.4% in breast cancer. They modified breast criteria in several points including incomplete membranous stain pattern and percentage of cells (≥ 10% cut off), which improved the concordance level between IHC and FISH tests to 93.5%. For ToGA clinical trial, Bang et al [22] reported that HER2 positive rate was a 22.1%. In addition, they found that HER2-

Gastric Cancer	**Breast Cancer**	**Score/classification**
IHC score criteria		
No reactivity or membranous reactivity in <10% of cells; Biopsy specimens < 5 Cells	No reactivity or membranous reactivity in <10% of cells	**0/negative**
Faint/barely perceptible membranous reactivity in ≥10% of cells; biopsy specimens≥5 Cells	Faint membranous reactivity in >10% of cells;	**1+/negative**
Weak to moderate complete or basolateral membranous activity in ≥10% of tumor cells; biopsy specimens≥5 Cells	Weak to moderate complete membrane staining in >10% of tumor cells	**2+/equivocal**
Moderate to strong complete or basal/lateral membranous activity in ≥10% of resection tumor cells; biopsy specimens≥5 Cells	Strong complete membrane staining in >10% of tumor cells	**3+/positive**
FISH HER2/CEP 17		
≥ 2 At least 20 evaluable, non-overlapping cells in the invasive component	**> 2.2** At least 20 evaluable, non-overlapping cells in the invasive component	**Amplification**
	1.8 2.2	**Equivocal**
<2 At least 20 evaluable, non-overlapping cells in the invasive component	**<1.8** At least 20 evaluable, non-overlapping cells in the invasive component	**negative**

Table 1. Consensus panel recommendations on HER2 scoring for gastric cancer

positive rate were higher in GEJ cancer than in gastric cancer (33% vs 21%) and in intestinal than diffuse or mixed cancer (32.2% vs 6.1% vs 20.4%). The concordance between IHC and FISH was 87.5%. Ruschoff and colleaguesl[37, 38](2010, 2012) further validate the HER2 test procedure to determine whether pathologists from different sits were able to reproduce the method of gastric cancer HER2 status evaluation as it was used by Ruschoff within the ToGA study. They validated the HER2 status testing procedure in terms of inter-laboratory and inter observe consensus for IHC scoring a series of 547 gastric cancer tissue samples on a tissue microarray. They published a practical approach of HER2 test in gastric carcinoma. Based on multiple laboratories and 8 pathologists HER2 test results, they further confirmed the HER2 positive rate of 22.8% which is close to 22.1% from Hoffman's score system. In addition, they compared Daco (HecepTest) and Ventana (Pathway HER2 antibody, 4B5). They found that HercepTest had a higher inter-laboratory discordance than 4B5. Furthermore, Ruschoff and a group of international pathologist reviewed previous HER2 studies; they built up new detailed criteria for gastric and gastro-esophageal HER2 tests (see Table 3; Ruschoff 2012). In their practical procedure for gastric cancer HER2 test, the surgical specimen cutoff is complete, basolateral, or lateral membranous reactivity in ≥10% of cells; the biopsy specimen cutoff is complete, basolateral, or lateral membranous reactivity in ≥5 clustered cells; the borderline cutoff is immunohistochemistry 1+/immunohistochemistry 2+ or focal staining in <10% cells which recommend for FISH or SISH tests. This new score system further improved Hoffmann's score system, but it still need further proved in future HER2 tests, especially the results mostly based on European laboratories. The large scale HER2 studies in Asia are need to build up an optimal HER2 test system in gastric cancer since the incidence of gastric cancer is much higher in Asian countries.

a. Immunohistochemistry

Testing recommendations

- Representative surgical samples or an adequate number of viable biopsy specimens (ideally six to eight) are required
  - If few biopsies are available, all viable specimens should be tested
- Immunohistochemistry should be the initial HER2 testing methodology for gastric cancer and bright-field methodologies are preferred wherever possible

  HER2-positive per European Medicines Agency license: immunohistochemistry 3+ or immunohistochemistry 2+/fluorescence *in situ* hybridization-positive or immunohistochemistry 2+/silver *in situ* hybridization-positive

  Borderline immunohistochemistry 1+/immunohistochemistry 2+ cases and samples with focal and intense membranous reactivity in <10% cells may also be retested with fluorescence *in situ* hybridization or silver *in situ* hybridization (scores for both assays should be indicated separately on the report)
- Validated immunohistochemistry HER2 assays should be used

Scoring recommendations

- Due to the tumor heterogeneity (focal areas of positivity) and incomplete membrane staining commonly seen in gastric cancer, the gastric cancer-specific scoring criteria should be adhered to:
  - Surgical specimen cutoff: complete, basolateral, or lateral membranous reactivity in ≥10% of cells
  - Biopsy specimen cutoff: complete, basolateral, or lateral membranous reactivity in ≥5 clustered cells
- The 'magnification rule' should be used in conjunction with the scoring criteria
- Borderline cases (immunohistochemistry 1+/immunohistochemistry 2+ or focal staining in <10% cells) that score fluorescence *in situ* hybridization-positive or silver *in situ* hybridization-positive may be considered HER2-positive (scores for both assays should be indicated separately on the report)

b. In situ hybridization

Testing recommendations

- Tumor samples classified as immunohistochemistry 2+ should be retested by fluorescence in situ hybridization or silver in situ hybridization to assess HER2 status

- Silver *in situ* hybridization is a more suitable methodology than fluorescence *in situ* hybridization for assessing HER2 status in gastric tumor samples as it is a bright-field methodology and thus allows for rapid identification of HER2-positive tumor foci within a heterogeneous sample

Validated *in situ* hybridization HER2 assays should be used

Scoring recommendations

- The definition of fluorescence *in situ* hybridization or silver *in situ* hybridization positivity in gastric or gastro–esophageal junction cancer is a HER2:chromosome 17 ratio of ≥2.0
- The entire case should be screened for amplified regions (particularly important for fluorescence *in situ* hybridization samples where a bright-field image is not available)
- At least 20 evaluable, non-overlapping cells in the invasive component should be counted initially
- In borderline amplification cases, ~20 additional cells should be recounted or scoring should be performed in an alternative area of tissue

The overall *HER2* gene count is important:

  - >6 *HER2* gene copies using single probe: considered positive
  - Four to six *HER2* gene copies: dual probe test advised and the ratio should be recalculated by counting an additional 20 cells

Ensuring quality and timely HER2 testing results

- The use of validated immunohistochemistry and *in situ* hybridization tests is strongly recommended and appropriate controls should be included in each run
- Turnaround time from initial diagnosis to reporting of results should ideally not exceed 5 working days and a multidisciplinary approach is required
- Centralized testing is recommended wherever possible and all laboratories should participate in validated quality assurance programs

Table 2. Human epidermal growth factor receptor 2 (HER2) testing recommendations in gastric cancer, (a) immunohistochemistry and (b) *in situ* hybridization (From Ruschoff J, Hanna W, Bilous M, et al. HER2 testing in gastric cancer: a practical approach. Mod Pathol 2012)

HER2 immunohistochemistry features	**Score**
No reactivity or very faint membranous stain in <10% of cells; biopsy specimens<5 Cells	**0**
Faint membranous stain in >10% of cells; biopsy specimens≥5 Cells	**1+**
Weak to moderate complete or baso/lateral membranous stain in >10% of tumor cells; biopsy specimens≥5 Cells	**2+/positive**
Strong complete or basal/lateral membranous stain in >10% of tumor cells; biopsy specimens≥5 Cells	**3+/positive**
HER2 FISH/chromogenic in situ hybridization test	
Ratio of average *HER2*/CEP17 ≥2.0	**Positive**
Ratio of average *HER2*/CEP17 <2.0	**Negative**

Table 3. Modified score criteria of HER2 immunohistochemical stain and FISH/chromogenic in situ hybridization for esophageal adenocarcinoma

Recently, in Asia, several IHC HER2 tests focused on comparing the HER2 antibodies from various companies. Cho and colleagues [39] used four different HER2 antibodies compared to standard FISH test. They found the various positive rates with HercepTest (14%), A0485 (16%), 4B5 (14%), and CB11 (9%). The sensitivity and specificity of IHC compared to FISH was 78.9%/96% for HercepTest, 86.5%/94.4% for A0485, 76.3%/95.6% for 4B5 and 60.5%/98.4% for CB11. Compare to FISH, there was no significantly differences in the sensitivity and specificity among the four IHC tests. However, CB11 had a highest specificity (98%), but a lowest sensitivity (61%). Park et al [39] (2012) compared HercepTest with 4B5, only 41 cases showed discrepancies, yielding a 96.1% concordance rate. However, HER2 positive rate with both methods are very low: HecepTEST, 5.9% and 4B5, 6.4%.

In addition, the standard breast HER2 test was compared with modified gastric carcinoma HER2 test (Table2). Sever studies used breast cancer score rule [40-42]. Barros-Silva et al. [40] found 3.9% as IHC2+ and 5.4% as IHC3+ from resection 463 gastric adenocarcinomas using the breast cancer scoring rules. Using breast cancer scoring, Park et al. (2012)[41] found that HER2 positive rate are very low with two antibodies: HecepTEST, 5.9% and 4B5, 6.4%. The similar result also was presented in TMA data which were classified as IHC2+ (1.6%) or IHC3+ (3.2%) if breast cancer scoring was applied[42]. As the same group also tested gastric cancer TMAs using gastric cancer specific scoring [36]the corresponding rates were 4% IHC2+ and 13% for IHC3+, demonstrating an about fourfold increase of HER2 positivity rate[42]. Therefore, Rushcoff concluded that it is supposed that application of breast cancer scoring to gastric cancer may produce an up to 50% false-negative rate if IHC is used as the primary test platform as favored by EMEA[37].

FISH, CISH and SISH studies on HER2 amplification: HER2 amplification was first reported in gastric cancer in 1986[43]. Since then, HER2 amplification in gastric cancer was extensively studied (see Table 3). Kimura et al. [44] first set criteria of FISH test as HER2/CEP17 ≥ 2.0 which is modified from breast standard HER2 FISH test with 83% of concordance between IHC 2+ and 3+ samples. Hoffman et al.[36] proved that these FISH criteria for gastric cancer showed a higher concordance (93%) between HER2 amplification and overexpression in gastric cancer. Ruschoff et al. [38, 45] (2010, 2012) further validate the HER2 test procedure to determine whether pathologists from different sits were able to reproduce the method of gastric cancer HER2 status evaluation as it was used by Ruschoff within the ToGA study. HER2 amplification was determined by FISH assays, using either HER2 FISH pharmDX™ (Dako Denmark A/S) or PathVysion® (Abbott Laboratories, Des Plaines, IL, USA). Automated brightfield dual-color silver in situ hybridization (SISH) assay (BDISH; Inform™, Ventana Medical Systems SA) was used to determine gene amplification at three of the participating sites. Based on their experience and previous studies, a new practical procedure for HER2 FISH, CISH or SISH tests were established. The positivity of HER2 FISH, CISH or SISH tests in gastric or gastro-esophageal junction cancer is a HER2/Chromosome 17 ratio ≥ 2.0 and > 6 *HER2* gene copies using single probe. At least 20 evaluable, non-overlapping cells in the invasive component should be counted initially. If the results are borderline (four to six *HER2* gene copies or HER2/Chromosome 17 ratio 1.8-2.2), [20] additional cells should be recounted or scoring should be performed in an alternative area of tissue. However, they also concluded that silver *in situ* hybridization is a more suitable methodology than fluorescence *in situ* hybridization for assessing HER2 status in gastric tumor samples as it is a bright-field methodology and thus allows for **rapid** identification of HER2-positive tumor foci within a heterogeneous sample.

Comparing FISH and SISH methods for HER2 test in gastric cancer was also reported by several studies. Park et al [41] (2012) compared both SISH and FISH HER2 tests in Korea gastric adenocarcinoma 588 cases. They found only 9 cases with discrepancy, yielding a 98.3% concordance rate. Garcia-Garcia et al [46] (2011) compared both SISH and FISH HER2 tests in Spanish gastric adenocarcinoma in 166 cases. They found 96% concordance rate. Long et al [47] (2011) compared both SISH and FISH HER2 tests in China gastric adenocarcinoma 80 cases. They found only one case with discrepancy, yielding a 99% concordance rate. From above studies, FISH and SISH showed similar positive rates. The only difference between two methods is that SISH is much easier to count the HER2 signals.

HER2 amplification or overexpression in primary tumor vs metastatic tumor was also reported. Bozzetti et al [18] (2011) tested HER2 status with both FISH and IHC. The found that concordance of HER2 status between primary and metastatic tumor is 98.2% by FISH and 94.9% by IHC. They concluded that HER2 status is maintained in most cases unchanged during the metastatic process.

HER2 amplification or overexpression correlating with patient survival and clinicopathological features: In breast cancer, HER2 amplification or overexpression is clearly associated with poorer prognosis and aggressive disease. However, the prognosis of HER2 amplification or overexpression in gastric cancer is controversial. In addition, the association of HER2 positive gastric cancer with clinicopathological features are also not consistent.

Yonemura et al [49] (1991) first reported HER2 overexpression in 260 primary gastric cancer. Patients with erbB-2 protein-positive tumors had 5-fold greater relative risk of death, as compared with those with erbB-2 protein-negative tumors. erbB-2 protein expression was associated with serosal invasion, lymph node metastasis, and lymphatic invasion. Later, their results were confirmed by Nakajima et al (1999). Nakajima et al. [50](1999) also reported HER2 overexpression in 16.4% of gastric cancer, which was associated with significantly poorer survival. However, Kim et al. [51] (1994) studied the HER2 overexpression in 152 Korea gastric carcinoma patients. They reported that the survival analysis of 104 patients with stage III gastric carcinoma revealed no significant association between c-erbB-2 staining status and survival duration. The 5-year survival rates of the c-erbB-2 positive group and its negative group were 21% and 28%, respectively. In addition, there was little association between staining of c-erbB-2 protein and clinicopathological findings such as age, sex, location, histology, gross type, lymph node status, depth of invasion, and stage. However, other Korea studies found HER2 positive gastric cancer had a poor prognosis [41,52]. Park et al [41] reported that HER-2/neu overexpression and amplification in 182 gastric cancer Korea patients was examined with IHC. Twenty-nine of 182 patients expressed the HER-2/neu protein by IHC. Tumors with HER-2/neu amplification were associated with poor mean survival rates (922 vs 3243 days) and 5-year survival rates (21.4% vs 63.0%; P < 0.05). Age, TNM stage, and amplification of HER-2/neu were found to be independently related to survival by multivariate analysis. In another Korea study with 1,414 cases and 595 tissue microarray cases, HER2-positivity was detected in 12.3% of whole-tissue sections and 17% of TMAs [53]. They found that HER2-positivity was correlated with age, histological type, lymphovascular invasion, and lymph node metastasis. Multivariate analyses of the differentiated gastric carcinoma subgroup revealed that HER2-positivity was an independent poor prognostic.

Zhang et al (2009) studied the HER2 and HER3 overexpression in Chinese gastric cancer with 102 cases. Overexpression of HER2 and HER3 was detected around 18.6% and 13.7%. HER2 and HER3 overexpression was correlated with a significantly worse survival (p = 0.046 and 0.024, respectively). The overexpression rates of HER2 and HER3 in phase III-IV (TNM stage) disease were significantly higher than that in phase I-II disease (24.0% vs. 7.7%, p < 0.05 and 22.0% vs. 5.8%, p < 0.05, respectively). They proposed that HER3 may become another molecular target.

In European and United States, Tanner et al [54] (2005) found that HER2 amplification was present in 12.2% of the 131 gastric cancer and 24% of the 100 GEJ adenocarcinomas in Finland which was associated with poor carcinoma-specific survival. In contrast, Kunz [55](2012) reported that twelve of 99 (12%) gastric carcinomas were positive for HER2 and seven of 70 (10%) gastroesophageal junction carcinomas were positive for HER2. HER2 status or primary tumor site did not correlate with patient survival.

Recently, Jorgensen and Hersom [56] (2012) reviewed previous studies with more than 100 patients and analysis of association between the HER2 status and survival or relevant clinicopathological characteristics. Forty-two publications with a total of 12,749 patients fulfilled the two criteria and were reviewed in detail. The majority of the publications (71%) showed that a HER2-postive status measured either by IHC or ISH was associated with poor survival and/or clinicopathological characteristics, such as serosal invasion, lymph node metastases, disease stage, or distant metastases. Based on the current analysis a clear trend towards a potential role for HER2 as a negative prognostics factor in gastric cancer was shown, suggesting that HER2 overexpression and/or amplification is a molecular abnormality that might be linked to the development of gastric cancer

Trastuzumab or other HER2 related medication on treatment of HER2 amplification gastric adenocarcinoma: Trastuzumab, a monoclonal antibody that targets HER2, induces antibody-dependent cellular cytotoxicity, inhibits HER2-mediated signaling, and prevents cleavage of the extracellular domain of HER2[12]. Trastuzumab were found to inhibit tumor growth in gastric carcinoma cell lines, animal model and xenograft models[23, 33, 57, 58]. Fujimoto-Ouchi (2007) used trastuzumab as a single agent inhibited the tumor growth in both of the HER2-overexpressing models but not in the HER2-negative models, GXF97 and MKN-45. In any combination with capecitabine, cisplatin, irinotecan, docetaxel, or paclitaxel, trastuzumab showed more potent antitumor activity than the anticancer agents alone. A three-drug combination of capecitabine, cisplatin, and trastuzumab showed remarkable tumor growth inhibition. Since breast cancer showed better prognosis with trastuzumab treatment for HER2 positive breast cancer patients, clinical trial was also performed in gastric carcinoma. ToGA (Trastuzumab for Gastric Cancer) was an open-label, international, phase 3, randomised controlled trial undertaken in 122 centers in 24 countries[22]. Patients with gastric or gastro-esophageal junction cancer were eligible for inclusion if their tumors showed overexpression of HER2 protein by immunohistochemistry or gene amplification by fluorescence in-situ hybridization. Participants were randomly assigned in a 1:1 ratio to receive a chemotherapy regimen consisting of capecitabine plus cisplatin or fluorouracil plus cisplatin given every 3 weeks for six cycles or chemotherapy in combination with intravenous trastuzumab. 594 patients were randomly assigned to study treatment (trastuzumab plus chemotherapy, n=298; chemotherapy alone, n=296). Median follow-up was 18·6 months in the trastuzumab plus chemotherapy group and 17·1 months in the chemotherapy alone group. Median overall survival was 13·8 months in those assigned to trastuzumab plus chemotherapy compared with 11·1 months in those assigned to chemotherapy alone (hazard ratio 0·74).

Although the survival improvement about 3 months, it is a great breakthrough for gastric carcinoma treatment since the survival of these cancer has not change for a decade. After ToGA clinical trial, trastuzumab combined with standard chemical therapy (such as capecitabine or 5-fluorouracil and cisplatin) now is approved by European Medicines Agency, United States and Japan etc. for the treatment of patients with HER2 overexpression or amplification. In addition, laptinib showed a synergistic effect with trastuzumab in vitro and in vivo to inhibit HER2 amplified human gastric cancer cells and animal model [23]. Clinical phase II trial of lapatinib as first line therapy in patients with advanced or metastatic cancer showed well tolerated, which will be another potential drug to target HER2 receptors[59].

3. HER2 in esophageal adenocarcinoma

EAC incidence has increased 6 folds in United States and Western countries in the last three decades and the prognosis is usually very poor with 5-year survival rates ranging from 14-22%[60-63]. While surgical treatment of EAC can offer cure, many patients first present as a disseminated disease and require systemic therapy. Current chemotherapy regimens provide only minimal survival benefit, predominantly when used in combination with surgery or radiation. Recently clinical trial (ToGA) in Asian and European countries showed that anti-HER2 monoclonal antibody trastuzumab treatment significantly improved the survival of patients with gastric adenocarcinoma and HER2 overexpression and amplification. The clinical trial of trastuzumab to treat esophageal adenocarcinoma patients are approved in United States and European countries. Here is a comprehensive review of HER2 overexpression and amplification in esophageal adenocarcinoma.

IHC studies on HER2 overexpression: In esophageal adenocarcinoma, *HER2* overexpression and amplification recently has been reported at frequencies similar to those observed in breast cancer. Based on most reports from English literature, the frequency of

HER-2 immunohistochemistry shows an average of 12%. The current problems for IHC test for HER2 overexpression is the standard score criteria of the intensity of IHC stain. Recently, Zhou and his colleagues (2011) set up a new score criteria which is modified from Hoffman's gastric adenocarcinoma score system (Table 3). In our modified score criteria, IHC 2+ will be counted as positive HER2 overexpression since all IHC 2+ case had HER2 amplification with CISH test. However, the recent Mayo Clinic study reported that only 15% of IHC2+ cases showed HER2 amplification with FISH tests with breast HER2 criteria. It is difficult to compare their criteria since there are no pictures in their reports.

FISH and CISH studies on HER2 amplification: In esophageal adenocarcinoma, HER2 amplification recently has been extensively studies. Reichelt *et al.* found that 15% (16/110) of tumors had *HER2* gene amplification with FISH. Similarly, Brien *et al.* showed that 19% (12/63) of esophageal adenocarcinomas had *HER2* gene amplification. In addition, with 3-dimentional FISH method in thick slides (16 μm, n=124), Rauser et al. [64] found that *HER2* amplification was 10.5% in high-level amplification (≥ 6.0 signals) and 60% in low-level copy number change (≥ 2.5-4.0 signals). However, in thin slides (4 μm, n=123), *HER2* amplification was found in 9 % in high-level amplification (≥ 6.0 signals) and 6 % in low-level copy number change (≥ 2.5-4.0 signals). However, there is a huge difference between traditional FISH in thin section (6%) and three-dimensional FISH in thick section (60%) to detect the low-level *HER2* amplification. They considered that the tumor cell nuclei were truncated due to standardized thin tissue sectioning. Therefore, three dimension FISH need to be further evaluated to help better understand any prognostic significance. In our study, we found that *HER2* amplification was 18% (21/116) detected by CISH and 16.4% (19/116) by high definition microarray in cases of esophageal adenocarcinoma. In addition we found no evidence of *HER2* amplification in low grad dysplasia, Barrett's esophagus, columnar cell metaplasia or normal esophageal squamous epithelium. Thus, the frequency of *HER2* amplification in esophageal adenocarcinoma appears to be consistent between studies with a range of 15-19% and this event appears not to occur prior to the development of high grade dysplasia. Radu et al[65] (2012) compared HER2 antibodies with FISH tests. They used CAP definition of HER2 amplification to evaluate the FISH results. They found that the very high HER2 amplification rate (30/103, 29%) with HER2/CEP17 ≥ 2.2 and (32/102, 31%) with HER2/CEP17 ≥ 2.0. From their slides, they used 5 μm instead of 3-4 μm routine section. Actually the similar phenomenon was reported in esophageal adenocarcinoma cases [64]. Using 16 μm *vs* 4 μm sections for HER2 FISH tests, they found that 16 μm sections showed higher HER2 amplification than 4 μm. Higher HER2 amplification from Radu may be caused by thicker section.

HER2 amplification or overexpression correlating with patient survival and clinicopathological factors: In esophageal adenocarcinoma, the relationship between *HER2* amplification and prognosis is limited and controversial [66, 67]. Brien et al. [66] found that patients with *HER2* amplification (n=11) had shorter survival durations than did patients without amplification (n=43). In contrast, Reichelt et al.[67] found no survival difference between the *HER2* amplification (n=16) and no *HER2* amplification groups (n=90)(p=0.953).

In addition, Rauser et al.[28] found that *HER2* gene amplification was associated with increased disease-specific mortality on 3-dimensional fluorescence in situ hybridization (FISH) analysis in thick slides (16 μm), but not on FISH and immunohistochemical analyses in thin (4 μm) sections. Our results [68] indicate no association of *HER2* amplification with patient survival in a large cohort studies (total 232 patients) by both CISH and high density DNA microarrays methods although HER2 amplification group shows better prognosis (23 months vs 25 months). However, Yoon et al[69] (2012) found that HER2 amplification significantly associated with improved overall survival (n=713) with 35% of HER2 positive patients alive at 5 years as compared with 26% of HER2 negative patients. It is interesting that they divided the HER2 positive EAC into two groups: EAC with and without adjacent BE. They found that HER2 positive EAC with BE significantly associated with disease specific survival and overall survival, but HER2 positive EAC without BE was not significantly associated with disease-specific-survival and overall survival. The prognosis of HER2 positive EAC patients still cannot be concluded. At present, we can say HER2 positive EAC patients do not show worse prognosis.

The association between *HER2* amplification and these clinicopathological factors were controversial. First, Brien [66] 2000 reported that HER2 amplification was not significantly associated with any clinicopathological features such as depth of tumor invasion, lymph node metastasis, differentiation and pathological stage. Reichelt et al [67] (2007) found that HER2 amplification was not associated with pathological staging (TNM) and grade. In our study [68], 21 of 116 EAC patients had *HER2* amplification. Nineteen were male, and 2 female (M:F ratio, 10:1), with a mean age of 63 years (range, 51 to 74 years). The remaining patients (85 males and 10 females [M:F ratio, 9:1]; mean age, 65 years [34 to 85 years]) had no amplification. A Fisher's exact test shows that there is no significant association between *HER2* and gender (p=1.0), age (p =0.188,), the stage (p =0.325), and the number of metastatic lymph nodes (p =0.234). However, the frequency of HER2 amplification was found to be significantly higher (p=0.004) in moderately differentiated tumors (13/22) compared with poor or well differentiated tumors (1/6 and 7/61 respectively). Yoon [69](2012) study supported our finding that HER2 amplification cases were significantly associated with better differentiation, but HER2 amplification cases were not associated with age and gender. However, they also showed that HER2 amplification was associated with lower depth of tumor invasion (T stage), fewer malignant nodes, and absence of signet ring cells.

In summary, the association of HER2 amplification with survival and clinicopathological features is not very clear. At least HER2 amplification was not associated with worse prognosis in most large cohort studies. In addition, the HER2 amplification may be associated better differentiation, but not associated with age and sex. The large, multi-institute study is needed to confirm current studies.

Trastuzumab or other HER2 related medication on treatment of HER2 amplification esophageal adenocarcinoma: Safran et al [70, 71] (2004, 2007) first reported clinical trial with trastuzumab, paclitaxel, cisplatin and radiation for locally advanced esophageal adenocarcinoma patients with HER2 overexpression. They took patients with histologically documented EAC with T3, T4 or lymph nodal disease. They used IHC 2+ and 3+ with more than 10% cells as HER2 positive overexpression and set FISH ratio greater than 2 as HER2 amplification. The median survival for all 19 patients is 24 months, which is similar to prior studies. Esophagitis, nausea, dehydration, and neutropenia were the most common toxicity. However, toxicity was modest with only 2 patients (10%) having grade 3-4 esophagitis. Therefore, trastuzumab does not increase toxicities when added to chemoradiation for patients with esophageal cancer.

ToGA clinical trials in patients with gastric adenocarcinoma (trial *vs* control: 236 *vs* 243 patients) and gastroesophageal junction adenocarcinoma (trial *vs* control: 58 *vs* 48 patients) have shown a significant survival benefit for patients treated with a combination of trastuzumab and standard chemotherapy.[22,72] Now Safran and colleagues started Phase III clinical trial to study Radiotherapy, Paclitaxel, and Carboplatin with versus without Trastuzumab in patients with HER2-overexpressing esophageal adenocarcinoma (RTOG-1010, and NCI web site: http://www.cancer.gov/ncicancerbulletin/062811/page6). Their primary goal is to determine whether trastuzumab increases disease-free survival when combined with radiotherapy, paclitaxel, and carboplatin followed by surgery in patients with HER2-overexpressing esophageal adenocarcinoma. It is interesting to follow up their results.

4. HER2 in breast cancers

Among new breast cancer patients, 15% to 20% will develop tumors that harbor a genomic alteration involving the *HER2* gene locus. This alteration results in amplification of an amplicon on chromosome 17 that contains the HER2 proto-oncogene[73, 74]. Gene amplification is the primary mechanism that drives HER2 receptor protein over-expression in this important subset of breast cancers. HER2 over-expression resulting from gene amplification dramatically increases the likelihood of receptor activation and signaling, contributing to a more aggressive tumor biology and is associated with worse clinical outcome including higher rates of early, predominantly visceral and central nervous system recurrence and mortality. [75, 76] In addition to the prognostic impact, HER2 over-expression in breast cancer is highly correlated with a younger age at presentation, higher tumor grade as well as a higher tumor burden compared with HER2 negative disease [77]. HER2 over-expression in breast cancer was recognized early on as being an ideal target for therapy, given the location of the receptor on the surface of tumor cells and its role in driving the clinical course of disease for the subset of patients with the HER2 alteration [78], [79]. The drug Trastuzumab was developed as a targeted biologic therapeutic against the HER2 receptor protein. Trastuzumab is a humanized monoclonal antibody that combines the mouse recognition sequence of a monoclonal antibody (clone 4D5) against an extracellular epitope of the receptors with a human IgG1[74]. Trastuzumab demonstrates a high affinity and specificity for the HER2 receptor and in preclinical studies was shown to be effective at inhibiting the growth of HER2 over-expressing breast cancer cells.[80]

In numerous clinical trials, targeting HER2 has been shown to be remarkably effective against HER2 positive breast cancer in both the metastatic and the adjuvant settings, particularly in combination with cytotoxic chemotherapy. Treatment with the drug Trastuzumab has been shown to improve response rates, time to progression, and even survival when used alone[18] or added to chemotherapy in metastatic setting .[78] The success of therapeutically targeting HER2 in the metastatic setting led to several international, prospective randomized trials that have demonstrated that adjuvant trastuzumab reduces the relative risk of recurrence by half and mortality by one third in early-stage breast cancer.[81-84] The data from these clinical trials highlights the importance of accurate HER2 testing for every newly diagnosed breast cancer patient in order to help select those patients who will be the most suitable candidates for HER2 targeted therapy. [85]

Clinical assays to assess the HER2 status include IHC, which detects protein over-expression, or FISH, which detects gene amplification. [85-87] Both assays have been clinically validated in the above mentioned prospective randomized clinical trials and have received FDA approval for predicting a clinical response and patient benefit from HER2-targeted treatment. Published data from these clinical trials suggest that only those patients whose breast cancer demonstrates protein over-expression and/or gene amplification by the above assays are likely to benefit from therapy with Trastuzumab. [88] Since the results of HER2 assays stand alone in determining which breast cancer patients will be the most appropriate for HER2-targeted therapy, accurate, reliable and reproducible results are a high priority for ensuring optimal patient treatment.

The ASCO/CAP task force, has published recommendations for HER2 testing, in which the panel has concluded that both tests were equally efficient in identifying patients who are candidates for HER2-targeted therapy, as long as the assays have been properly validated and all aspects of the testing is performed in a highly standardized fashion with a rigorous quality assurance program. [89] This task force also recognized the importance of standardizing pre-analytical variables including tissue handling and fixation to improve the quality of clinical samples for predictive factor analysis. [90] The IHC and FISH methodologies for evaluating the HER2 status in breast cancer are complementary in nature. [91] These tests examine different aspects of the biology that underlies HER2 driven breast tumors. FISH evaluates the status of the *HER2* gene in the nucleus and is a surrogate for protein expression, while IHC directly evaluates over-expression of the receptor protein at the surface of the cell. In the majority of HER2-positive cancers, HER2 protein over-expression is the result of gene amplification, thus *HER2* gene/protein status should be highly correlated in most cases. Consequently, HER2 gene/protein discordant results in the majority of cases are related to technical issues. However, unusual *HER2* genotypes such as polysomy for chromosome 17 and genomic heterogeneity can lead to discrepant non-correlating cases that may be clinically important. [92, 93] For such cases, the assessment of both the gene and the protein may be necessary in order to sort out the most appropriate HER2 status for the purpose of determining therapy.

Despite the remarkable clinical efficacy of HER2 targeted therapy, not all patients respond and de novo as well as acquired resistance remains an important clinical issue. Currently there are no clinically validated factors that can be used to predict resistance to HER2 targeted therapy in breast cancer. Preclinical data and more recent clinical studies have suggested a number of potential mechanisms of resistance including reduction of antibody affinity and binding due to steric hindrance from MUC4 over-expression, constitutively active downstream signaling involving p27 Kip1, PTEN, PI3K, mTOR, and Akt as well as cross-talk with other signaling pathways including EGFR and IGFR-1, that can by-pass HER2-blockade. [94, 95]

		HER2 amplified		**HER2 non-amplified**		*p* value
Age		63 (51-74)		65 (34-85)		0.188
Gender		MALE	FEMALE	MALE	FEMALE	1.0
		19	2	85	10	
		POS	NEG	POS	NEG	
Lymph node METASTASIS		13	8	69	26	0.234
pStaging						0.325
	I	3		10		
	II	8		25		
	III	10		60		
Median survival (months)		25 (7-71)		23 (0.03-108)		0.19
Differentiation						0.004
	poor	7		61		
	moderate	13		22		
	well	1		6		

Table 4. Association *of HER2* amplified group and *non-HER2* amplified group with multiple clinical factors (From Hu Y, Bandla S, Godfrey TE, et al. HER2 amplification, overexpression and score criteria in esophageal adenocarcinoma. Mod Pathol 2011;24:899-907)

Author details

Zhongren Zhou and David G. Hick
University of Rochester Medical Center, USA

5. References

[1] Emde A, Kostler WJ, Yarden Y. Therapeutic strategies and mechanisms of tumorigenesis of HER2-overexpressing breast cancer. *Crit Rev Oncol Hematol* 2010 http://dx.doi.org/10.1016/j.critrevonc.2010.09.002.

[2] Ross JS. Update on HER2 testing for breast and upper gastrointestinal tract cancers. *Biomark Med* 2011; 5(3):307-18.

[3] Albarello L, Pecciarini L, Doglioni C. HER2 testing in gastric cancer. *Adv Anat Pathol* 2011; 18(1):53-9.

[4] Fornaro L, Lucchesi M, Caparello C, *et al.* Anti-HER agents in gastric cancer: from bench o bedside. *Nat Rev Gastroenterol Hepatol* 2011; 8(7):369-83.

[5] Hicks DG, Whitney-Miller C. HER2 testing in gastric and gastroesophageal junction cancers: a new therapeutic target and diagnostic challenge. *Appl Immunohistochem Mol Morphol* 2011; 19(6):506-8.

[6] Tsang RY, Finn RS. Beyond trastuzumab: novel therapeutic strategies in HER2-positive metastatic breast cancer. *Br J Cancer* 2012; 106(1):6-13.

[7] Rexer BN, Arteaga CL. Intrinsic and Acquired Resistance to HER2-Targeted Therapies n HER2 Gene-Amplified Breast Cancer: Mechanisms and Clinical Implications. *Crit Rev Oncog* 2012; 17(1):1-16.

[8] Petrelli F, Barni S. Role of HER2-neu as a prognostic factor for survival and relapse in pT1a-bN0M0 breast cancer: a systematic review of the literature with a pooled-analysis. *Med Oncol* 2012.

[9] Witsch E, Sela M, Yarden Y. Roles for growth factors in cancer progression. *Physiology Bethesda)* 2010; 25(2):85-101.

[10] Olayioye MA, Neve RM, Lane HA, Hynes NE. The ErbB signaling network: receptor heterodimerization in development and cancer. *EMBO J* 2000; 19(13):3159-67.

[11] Moasser MM. The oncogene HER2: its signaling and transforming functions and its role in human cancer pathogenesis. *Oncogene* 2007; 26(45):6469-87.

[12] Moulder SL, Yakes FM, Muthuswamy SK, *et al.* Epidermal growth factor receptor (HER1) tyrosine kinase inhibitor ZD1839 (Iressa) inhibits HER2/neu (erbB2)-overexpressing breast cancer cells in vitro and in vivo. *Cancer Res* 2001; 61(24):8887-95.

[13] Liu E, Thor A, He M, *et al.* The HER2 (c-erbB-2) oncogene is frequently amplified in in situ carcinomas of the breast. *Oncogene* 1992; 7(5):1027-32.

[14] Park K, Han S, Kim HJ, Kim J, Shin E. HER2 status in pure ductal carcinoma in situ and in the intraductal and invasive components of invasive ductal carcinoma determined by fluorescence in situ hybridization and immunohistochemistry. *Histopathology* 2006; 48(6):702-7.

[15] Carlsson J, Nordgren H, Sjostrom J, *et al.* HER2 expression in breast cancer primary tumours and corresponding metastases. Original data and literature review. *Br J Cancer* 2004; 90(12):2344-8.

[16] Riechmann L, Clark M, Waldmann H, Winter G. Reshaping human antibodies for therapy. *Nature* 1988; 332(6162):323-7.

[17] Ben-Kasus T, Schechter B, Sela M, Yarden Y. Cancer therapeutic antibodies come of age: targeting minimal residual disease. *Mol Oncol* 2007; 1(1):42-54.

[18] Cobleigh MA, Vogel CL, Tripathy D, *et al.* Multinational study of the efficacy and safety of humanized anti-HER2 monoclonal antibody in women who have HER2-overexpressing metastatic breast cancer that has progressed after chemotherapy for metastatic disease. *J Clin Oncol* 1999; 17(9):2639-48.

[19] Vogel CL, Cobleigh MA, Tripathy D, *et al.* Efficacy and safety of trastuzumab as a single agent in first-line treatment of HER2-overexpressing metastatic breast cancer. *J Clin Oncol* 2002; 20(3):719-26.

[20] Slamon D, Pegram M. Rationale for trastuzumab (Herceptin) in adjuvant breast cancer trials. *Semin Oncol* 2001; 28(1 Suppl 3):13-9.

[21] Untch M, Rezai M, Loibl S, *et al.* Neoadjuvant treatment with trastuzumab in HER2-positive breast cancer: results from the GeparQuattro study. *J Clin Oncol* 2010; 28(12):2024-31.

[22] Bang YJ, Van Cutsem E, Feyereislova A, *et al.* Trastuzumab in combination with chemotherapy versus chemotherapy alone for treatment of HER2-positive advanced gastric or gastro-oesophageal junction cancer (ToGA): a phase 3, open-label, randomised controlled trial. *Lancet* 2010; 376(9742):687-97.

[23] Wainberg ZA, Anghel A, Desai AJ, *et al.* Lapatinib, a dual EGFR and HER2 kinase inhibitor, selectively inhibits HER2-amplified human gastric cancer cells and is synergistic with trastuzumab in vitro and in vivo. *Clin Cancer Res* 2010; 16(5):1509-19.

[24] Geyer CE, Forster J, Lindquist D, *et al.* Lapatinib plus capecitabine for HER2-positive advanced breast cancer. *N Engl J Med* 2006; 355(26):2733-43.

[25] Baselga J, Bradbury I, Eidtmann H, *et al.* Lapatinib with trastuzumab for HER2-positive early breast cancer (NeoALTTO): a randomised, open-label, multicentre, phase 3 trial. *Lancet* 2012; 379(9816):633-40.

[26] Gravalos C, Gomez-Martin C, Rivera F, *et al.* Phase II study of trastuzumab and cisplatin as first-line therapy in patients with HER2-positive advanced gastric or gastroesophageal junction cancer. *Clin Transl Oncol* 2011; 13(3):179-84.

[27] Spector NL, Xia W, Burris H, 3rd, *et al.* Study of the biologic effects of lapatinib, a reversible inhibitor of ErbB1 and ErbB2 tyrosine kinases, on tumor growth and survival pathways in patients with advanced malignancies. *J Clin Oncol* 2005; 23(11):2502-12.

[28] Nahta R, Yuan LX, Du Y, Esteva FJ. Lapatinib induces apoptosis in trastuzumab-resistant breast cancer cells: effects on insulin-like growth factor I signaling. *Mol Cancer Ther* 2007; 6(2):667-74.

[29] Nahta R, Shabaya S, Ozbay T, Rowe DL. Personalizing HER2-targeted therapy in metastatic breast cancer beyond HER2 status: what we have learned from clinical specimens. *Curr Pharmacogenomics Person Med* 2009; 7(4):263-74.

[30] Xia W, Liu LH, Ho P, Spector NL. Truncated ErbB2 receptor (p95ErbB2) is regulated by heregulin through heterodimer formation with ErbB3 yet remains sensitive to the dual EGFR/ErbB2 kinase inhibitor GW572016. *Oncogene* 2004; 23(3):646-53.

[31] Kamangar F, Dores GM, Anderson WF. Patterns of cancer incidence, mortality, and prevalence across five continents: defining priorities to reduce cancer disparities in different geographic regions of the world. *J Clin Oncol* 2006; 24(14):2137-50.

[32] Patel SH, Kooby DA. Gastric adenocarcinoma surgery and adjuvant therapy. *Surg Clin North Am* 2011; 91(5):1039-77.

[33] Tanner M, Hollmen M, Junttila TT, *et al.* Amplification of HER-2 in gastric carcinoma: association with Topoisomerase IIalpha gene amplification, intestinal type, poor prognosis and sensitivity to trastuzumab. *Ann Oncol* 2005; 16(2):273-8.

[34] Matsui Y, Inomata M, Tojigamori M, *et al.* Suppression of tumor growth in human gastric cancer with HER2 overexpression by an anti-HER2 antibody in a murine model. *Int J Oncol* 2005; 27(3):681-5.

[35] Tanaka S, Mori M, Akiyoshi T, *et al.* Coexpression of Grb7 with epidermal growth factor receptor or Her2/erbB2 in human advanced esophageal carcinoma. *Cancer Res* 1997; 57(1):28-31.

[36] Hofmann M, Stoss O, Shi D, *et al.* Assessment of a HER2 scoring system for gastric cancer: results from a validation study. *Histopathology* 2008; 52(7):797-805.

[37] Ruschoff J, Dietel M, Baretton G, *et al.* HER2 diagnostics in gastric cancer-guideline validation and development of standardized immunohistochemical testing. *Virchows Arch* 2010; 457(3):299-307.

[38] Ruschoff J, Hanna W, Bilous M, *et al.* HER2 testing in gastric cancer: a practical approach. Mod Pathol 2012 25(5):637-50.

[39] Cho EY, Srivastava A, Park K, *et al.* Comparison of four immunohistochemical tests and FISH for measuring Her2 expression in gastric carcinomas. *Pathology* 2012; 44(3):216-20.

[40] Barros-Silva JD, Leitao D, Afonso L, *et al.* Association of ERBB2 gene status with histopathological parameters and disease-specific survival in gastric carcinoma patients. *Br J Cancer* 2009; 100(3):487-93.

[41] Park YS, Hwang HS, Park HJ, *et al.* Comprehensive analysis of HER2 expression and gene amplification in gastric cancers using immunohistochemistry and in situ hybridization: which scoring system should we use? *Hum Pathol* 2012; 43(3):413-22.

[42] Tapia C, Glatz K, Novotny H, *et al.* Close association between HER-2 amplification and overexpression in human tumors of non-breast origin. *Mod Pathol* 2007; 20(2):192-8.

[43] Yamamoto T, Ikawa S, Akiyama T, *et al.* Similarity of protein encoded by the human c-erb-B-2 gene to epidermal growth factor receptor. *Nature* 1986; 319(6050):230-4.

[44] Kimura M, Tsuda H, Morita D, *et al.* Usefulness and limitation of multiple endoscopic biopsy sampling for epidermal growth factor receptor and c-erbB-2 testing in patients with gastric adenocarcinoma. *Jpn J Clin Oncol* 2005; 35(6):324-31.

[45] Ruschoff J, Nagelmeier I, Baretton G, *et al.* [Her2 testing in gastric cancer. What is different in comparison to breast cancer?]. *Pathologe* 2010; 31(3):208-17.

[46] Garcia-Garcia E, Gomez-Martin C, Angulo B, *et al.* Hybridization for human epidermal growth factor receptor 2 testing in gastric carcinoma: a comparison of fluorescence in-situ hybridization with a novel fully automated dual-colour silver in-situ hybridization method. *Histopathology* 2011; 59(1):8-17.

[47] Long XY, Bu H, Wei B, *et al.* [Dual-color silver-enhanced in-situ hybridization and fluorescence in-situ hybridization for determination of HER2 gene status in gastric carcinoma]. *Zhonghua Bing Li Xue Za Zhi* 2011; 40(5):300-3.

[48] Bozzetti C, Negri FV, Lagrasta CA, *et al.* Comparison of HER2 status in primary and paired metastatic sites of gastric carcinoma. *Br J Cancer* 2011; 104(9):1372-6.

[49] Yonemura Y, Ninomiya I, Ohoyama S, *et al.* Expression of c-erbB-2 oncoprotein in gastric carcinoma. Immunoreactivity for c-erbB-2 protein is an independent indicator of poor short-term prognosis in patients with gastric carcinoma. *Cancer* 1991; 67(11):2914-8.

[50] Nakajima M, Sawada H, Yamada Y, *et al.* The prognostic significance of amplification and overexpression of c-met and c-erb B-2 in human gastric carcinomas. *Cancer* 1999; 85(9):1894-902.

[51] Kim JP, Oh ST, Hwang TS, Chi JG. The prognostic significance of c-erbB-2 and p53 protein expressions in gastric carcinoma--a multivariate analysis of prognostic factors. *J Korean Med Sci* 1994; 9(3):248-53.

[52] Kim JW, Im SA, Kim M, *et al.* The Prognostic Significance of HER2 Positivity for Advanced Gastric Cancer Patients Undergoing First-line Modified FOLFOX-6 Regimen. *Anticancer Res* 2012; 32(4):1547-53.

[53] Kim KC, Koh YW, Chang HM, *et al.* Evaluation of HER2 protein expression in gastric carcinomas: comparative analysis of 1,414 cases of whole-tissue sections and 595 cases of tissue microarrays. *Ann Surg Oncol* 2011; 18(10):2833-40.

[54] Tanner SM, Li Z, Perko JD, *et al.* Hereditary juvenile cobalamin deficiency caused by mutations in the intrinsic factor gene. *Proc Natl Acad Sci U S A* 2005; 102(11):4130-3.

[55] Kunz PL, Mojtahed A, Fisher GA, *et al.* HER2 expression in gastric and gastroesophageal junction adenocarcinoma in a US population: clinicopathologic analysis with proposed approach to HER2 assessment. *Appl Immunohistochem Mol Morphol* 2012; 20(1):13-24.

[56] Jorgensen JT, Hersom M. HER2 as a Prognostic Marker in Gastric Cancer - A Systematic Analysis of Data from the Literature. *J Cancer* 2012; 3:137-44.

[57] Fujimoto-Ouchi K, Sekiguchi F, Yasuno H, *et al.* Antitumor activity of trastuzumab in combination with chemotherapy in human gastric cancer xenograft models. *Cancer Chemother Pharmacol* 2007; 59(6):795-805.

[58] Yamashita-Kashima Y, Iijima S, Yorozu K, *et al.* Pertuzumab in combination with trastuzumab shows significantly enhanced antitumor activity in HER2-positive human gastric cancer xenograft models. *Clin Cancer Res* 2011; 17(15):5060-70.

[59] Wainberg ZA, Lin LS, DiCarlo B, *et al.* Phase II trial of modified FOLFOX6 and erlotinib in patients with metastatic or advanced adenocarcinoma of the oesophagus and gastro-oesophageal junction. *Br J Cancer* 2011; 105(6):760-5.

[60] Gamliel Z, Krasna MJ. Multimodality treatment of esophageal cancer. *Surg Clin North Am* 2005; 85(3):621-30.

[61] Luketich JD, Alvelo-Rivera M, Buenaventura PO, *et al.* Minimally invasive esophagectomy: outcomes in 222 patients. *Annals of surgery* 2003; 238(4):486-94; discussion 94-5.

[62] Swanson SJ, Batirel HF, Bueno R, *et al.* Transthoracic esophagectomy with radical mediastinal and abdominal lymph node dissection and cervical esophagogastrostomy for esophageal carcinoma. *Ann Thorac Surg* 2001; 72(6):1918-24; discussion 24-5.

[63] Pohl H, Welch HG. The role of overdiagnosis and reclassification in the marked increase of esophageal adenocarcinoma incidence. *J Natl Cancer Inst* 2005; 97(2):142-6.

[64] Rauser S, Weis R, Braselmann H, *et al.* Significance of HER2 low-level copy gain in Barrett's cancer: implications for fluorescence in situ hybridization testing in tissues. *Clin Cancer Res* 2007; 13(17):5115-23.

[65] Radu OM, Foxwell T, Cieply K, *et al.* HER2 Amplification in Gastroesophageal Adenocarcinoma: Correlation of Two Antibodies Using Gastric Cancer Scoring Criteria, H Score, and Digital Image Analysis With Fluorescence In Situ Hybridization. *Am J Clin Pathol* 2012; 137(4):583-94.

[66] Brien TP, Odze RD, Sheehan CE, McKenna BJ, Ross JS. HER-2/neu gene amplification by FISH predicts poor survival in Barrett's esophagus-associated adenocarcinoma. *Human pathology* 2000; 31(1):35-9.

[67] Reichelt U, Duesedau P, Tsourlakis M, *et al.* Frequent homogeneous HER-2 amplification in primary and metastatic adenocarcinoma of the esophagus. *Mod Pathol* 2007; 20(1):120-9.

[68] Hu Y, Bandla S, Godfrey TE, *et al.* HER2 amplification, overexpression and score criteria in esophageal adenocarcinoma. *Mod Pathol* 2011; 24(7):899-907.

[69] Yoon HH, Shi Q, Sukov WR, *et al.* Association of HER2/ErbB2 expression and gene amplification with pathologic features and prognosis in esophageal adenocarcinomas. *Clin Cancer Res* 2012; 18(2):546-54.

[70] Safran H, Dipetrillo T, Akerman P, *et al.* Phase I/II study of trastuzumab, paclitaxel, cisplatin and radiation for locally advanced, HER2 overexpressing, esophageal adenocarcinoma. *Int J Radiat Oncol Biol Phys* 2007; 67(2):405-9.

[71] Safran H, DiPetrillo T, Nadeem A, *et al.* Trastuzumab, paclitaxel, cisplatin, and radiation for adenocarcinoma of the esophagus: a phase I study. *Cancer Invest* 2004; 22(5):670-7.

[72] Jorgensen JT. Target HER2 treatment in advanced gastric cancer *Oncology* 2010; 78(1):26-33.

[73] Hicks DG, Tubbs RR. Assessment of the HER2 status in breast cancer by fluorescence in situ hybridization: a technical review with interpretive guidelines. *Hum Pathol* 2005; 36(3):250-61.

[74] Ross JS. Breast cancer biomarkers and HER2 testing after 10 years of anti-HER2 therapy. *Drug News Perspect* 2009; 22(2):93-106.

[75] Winstanley J, Cooke T, Murray GD, *et al.* The long term prognostic significance of c-erbB-2 in primary breast cancer. *Br J Cancer* 1991; 63(3):447-50.

[76] Hicks DG, Yoder BJ, Short S, *et al.* Loss of breast cancer metastasis suppressor 1 protein expression predicts reduced disease-free survival in subsets of breast cancer patients. *Clin Cancer Res* 2006; 12(22):6702-8.

[77] Crowe JP, Patrick RJ, Rybicki LA, *et al.* A data model to predict HER2 status in breast cancer based on the clinical and pathologic profiles of a large patient population at a single institution. *Breast* 2006; 15(6):728-35.

[78] Slamon DJ, Leyland-Jones B, Shak S, *et al.* Use of chemotherapy plus a monoclonal antibody against HER2 for metastatic breast cancer that overexpresses HER2. *N Engl J Med* 2001; 344(11):783-92.

[79] Slamon DJ, Clark GM, Wong SG, *et al.* Human breast cancer: correlation of relapse and survival with amplification of the HER-2/neu oncogene. *Science* 1987; 235(4785):177-82.

[80] Yarden Y. Biology of HER2 and its importance in breast cancer. *Oncology* 2001; 61 Suppl 2:1-13.

[81] Slamon DJ, Romond EH, Perez EA. Advances in adjuvant therapy for breast cancer. *Clin Adv Hematol Oncol* 2006; 4(3 Suppl 7):suppl 1, 4-9; discussion suppl 10; quiz 2 p following suppl

[82] Joensuu H, Kellokumpu-Lehtinen PL, Bono P, *et al.* Adjuvant docetaxel or vinorelbine with or without trastuzumab for breast cancer. *N Engl J Med* 2006; 354(8):809-20.

[83] Romond EH, Perez EA, Bryant J, *et al.* Trastuzumab plus adjuvant chemotherapy for operable HER2-positive breast cancer. *N Engl J Med* 2005; 353(16):1673-84.

[84] Piccart-Gebhart MJ, Procter M, Leyland-Jones B, *et al.* Trastuzumab after adjuvant chemotherapy in HER2-positive breast cancer. *N Engl J Med* 2005; 353(16):1659-72.

[85] Hicks DG, Kulkarni S. Trastuzumab as adjuvant therapy for early breast cancer: the importance of accurate human epidermal growth factor receptor 2 testing. *Arch Pathol Lab Med* 2008; 132(6):1008-15.

[86] Tubbs RR, Hicks DG, Cook J, *et al.* Fluorescence in situ hybridization (FISH) as primary methodology for the assessment of HER2 Status in adenocarcinoma of the breast: a single institution experience. *Diagn Mol Pathol* 2007; 16(4):207-10.

[87] Powell WC, Hicks DG, Prescott N, *et al.* A new rabbit monoclonal antibody (4B5) for the immunohistochemical (IHC) determination of the HER2 status in breast cancer: comparison with CB11, fluorescence in situ hybridization (FISH), and interlaboratory reproducibility. *Appl Immunohistochem Mol Morphol* 2007; 15(1):94-102.

[88] Yoder BJ, Tso E, Skacel M, *et al.* The expression of fascin, an actin-bundling motility protein, correlates with hormone receptor-negative breast cancer and a more aggressive clinical course. *Clin Cancer Res* 2005; 11(1):186-92.

[89] Wolff AC, Hammond ME, Schwartz JN, *et al.* American Society of Clinical Oncology/College of American Pathologists guideline recommendations for human epidermal growth factor receptor 2 testing in breast cancer. *Arch Pathol Lab Med* 2007; 131(1):18-43.

[90] Hicks DG, Kushner L, McCarthy K. Breast cancer predictive factor testing: the challenges and importance of standardizing tissue handling. *J Natl Cancer Inst Monogr* 2011; 2011(42):43-5.

[91] Hicks DG, Kulkarni S. HER2+ breast cancer: review of biologic relevance and optimal use of diagnostic tools. *Am J Clin Pathol* 2008; 129(2):263-73.

[92] Downs-Kelly E, Yoder BJ, Stoler M, *et al.* The influence of polysomy 17 on HER2 gene and protein expression in adenocarcinoma of the breast: a fluorescent in situ hybridization, immunohistochemical, and isotopic mRNA in situ hybridization study. *Am J Surg Pathol* 2005; 29(9):1221-7.

[93] Vance GH, Barry TS, Bloom KJ, *et al.* Genetic heterogeneity in HER2 testing in breast cancer: panel summary and guidelines. *Arch Pathol Lab Med* 2009; 133(4):611-2.

[94] Khoury T, Mojica W, Hicks D, *et al.* ERBB2 juxtamembrane domain (trastuzumab binding site) gene mutation is a rare event in invasive breast cancers overexpressing the ERBB2 gene. *Mod Pathol* 2011; 24(8):1055-9.

[95] Gallardo A, Lerma E, Escuin D, *et al.* Increased signalling of EGFR and IGF1R, and deregulation of PTEN/PI3K/Akt pathway are related with trastuzumab resistance in HER2 breast carcinomas. *Br J Cancer* 2012; 106(8):1367-73.

Section 2

DNA Repair Mechanism and Cancer

Chapter 4

Emerging Roles of Atypical Dual Specificity Phosphatases in Cancer

Erica L. Cain and Alexander Beeser

Additional information is available at the end of the chapter

http://dx.doi.org/10.5772/54485

1. Introduction

The dual specificity phosphatases (DUSPs) are a subfamily within the protein tyrosine phosphatase (PTP) family, with the unique property of being able to hydrolyze phospho-serine or phospho-threonine residues and phospho-tyrosine residues [1]. All DUSPs share the characteristic Class I PTP consensus sequence, D…HC(X)$_5$RS/T, with C representing the essential catalytic cysteine [1]. Unlike other PTPs, DUSPs lack the phospho-tyrosine recognition domain, resulting in a shallower catalytic cleft, most likely enabling DUSPs to dephosphorylate all three residues (S/T/Y) [1]. In addition to protein substrates, the DUSP subfamily contains members that dephosphorylate additional substrates including lipids, nucleic acids, and sugars [2].

DUSPs are regulators of multiple signaling pathways driving fundamental cell processes such as growth, proliferation, apoptosis, and migration, and as such they are often deregulated in a variety of diseases [2]. DUSPs can be further classified on substrate specificity and sequence homology, but all DUSPs share a highly conserved prototypical DUSP domain initially characterized in the Vaccinia virus's VH1 gene [3]. The best-characterized DUSPs include the MAP kinase phosphatases (MKP's), which directly antagonize the activating dual phosphorylation of mitogen activated protein kinases, and PTEN that functions to dephosphorylate phosphatidyl-inositol 3,4,5 triphosphate (PIP3), the product of PI3 kinase (PI3K) [2]. As these signaling pathways are intimately implicated in cancer initiation and progression, it is not surprising that their cognate phosphatases also functionally contribute to disease progression [2,4].

In addition to DUSPs described above, the DUSP subfamily contains a distinct subgroup described as the atypical DUSPs [2,5]. In humans there are at least 16 DUSPs classified as atypical (Table 1) based on the lack of sequence similarity to better-characterized DUSPs and/or due to their substrate specificity [2,5]. Physiological substrates for several atypical

Atypical DUSPs	
Name	**Aliases**
Laforin	EPM2A (epilepsy, progressive myoclonus type 2A)
STYX	Serine/threonine/tyrosine interacting protein
DUSP3	VHR (VH1 related)
DUSP11	PIR1 (phosphatase that interacts with RNA-ribonucleoprotein complexes)
DUSP12	hYVH1 (human YVH1)
DUSP13A	MDSP (muscle-restricted DUSP), SKRP4 (stress activated protein kinase pathway-regulating phosphatase-4), BEDP (branching-enzyme interacting DUSP)
DUSP13B	TMDP (testis-and skeletal muscle-specific DUSP)
DUSP14	MKP-L (MKP-1 like protein tyrosine phosphatases), MKP6
DUSP15	VHY (VH1-like member Y)
DUSP18	DUSP20, LMWDSP20 (low-molecular-weight DUSP20)
DUSP19	DUSP17, SKRP1
DUSP21	LMWDSP21
DUSP22	LMWDSP2, JSP1 (JNK-stimulating phosphatases 1), JKAP (JNK pathway-associated phosphatase), MKPX, VHX
DUSP23	DUSP25, LDP3 (low molecular mass DUSP3), VHZ
DUSP26	DUSP24, LDP4, MKP8, NEAP (neuroendrocrine associated phosphatase), SKRP3
DUSP27	DUPD1 (DUSP and pro-isomerase domain containing 1

Table 1. The atypical DUSPs and their various aliases.

DUSPs include proteins (MAPKs), nucleic aids (RNA), and phosphorylated carbohydrates (amylopectin and glycogen), but for many atypical DUSPs physiological substrates are unknown [2,5]. However, even for cases where phosphatase-substrate relationships are known, they are somewhat complicated by the fact that several DUSPs appear to function independently of their phosphatase activity and instead function as scaffolds in signal transduction pathways [6-8].

Several atypical DUSPs have been implicated in apoptosis and proliferation [2,5], but how the DUSPs contribute to these processes is largely also unknown. Emerging roles for atypical DUSPs in malignancy are beginning to be inferred from high throughput sequencing/ genomic approaches, which have demonstrated that, like MKP's and lipid phosphatases, the atypical DUSP genes are differentially expressed in a variety of cancers and may contribute to cancer initiation and/or progression [2,4,5]. The following sections present a current synthesis of what is known about how the atypical DUSPs function, and will focus specifically on how these proteins may contribute to cancer initiation and progression. Current gaps in knowledge on the function of these proteins in both normal and cancer cell biology is highlighted to hopefully inspire new research on these poorly understood proteins.

2. Atypical DUSPs currently implicated in cancer

2.1. Laforin

Due to alternative splicing of mRNA encoded by the *epm2a* gene, at least two isoforms of Laforin have been described that differ in their subcellular localization and phosphatase activity [9]. The major isoform encodes for a 331 amino acid protein containing a catalytically active DUSP domain and a N-terminal carbohydrate-binding module (CBM). Loss of function mutations of the major isoform are causative for Lafora's disease, a fatal form of progressive myoclonus epilepsy that is thought to occur as a result of deregulated glycogen metabolism [10-13] with the accumulation of insoluble complex carbohydrates [14]. Laforin regulates glycogen metabolism, in part, by its ability to directly dephosphorylate phosphorylated carbohydrates including glycogen [14]. Loss of epm2a or mutations in epm2a that prevent glycogen binding or alter its phosphatase activity, contribute to Lafora's disease [14,15]. Laforin also regulates glycogen metabolism in a phosphatase independent manner by functioning as an adapter protein to promote the ubiquitination of proteins involved in glycogen metabolism by recruiting Malin, an E3 ubiquitin ligase [16]. Proteins regulating glycogen metabolism are often complexed with glycogen, as Laforin can bind glycogen and independently recruit Malin this provides an additional regulatory mechanism [16]. As a result, mutations in epm2a that disrupt the ability to bind Malin also contribute to Lafora's disease [16]. Over the last several years, studies have revealed additional potential role(s) for Laforin in cancer development and/or progression where it most likely functions as a tumor suppressor, but may also contribute to cancer by promoting cell survival [17,18]. Here, we focus on potential roles of the major isoform in cancer, as it is the most studied.

A role for Laforin as a tumor suppressor was demonstrated by the observation that immunocompromised mice lacking Laforin produce spontaneous lymphomas [19]. Additionally, Laforin mRNA and protein levels were reduced in murine and human primary lymphomas [19]. In addition to the roles of Laforin in glycogen metabolism and Lafora's disease, Laforin regulates glycogen synthase kinase 3 (GSK3β) activity, a key signaling protein in the β-catenin/WNT signaling pathway [20] by removal of the inhibitory phosphate at Ser9 [21]. Cells lacking Laforin display decreased GSK3β activity resulting in increased cyclin D1 stability, and increased WNT signaling [21,22]. As both cyclin D1 expression and WNT signaling have been implicated in a variety of cancers [20], the ability of Laforin to regulate GSK3β to inhibit cyclin D1 and WNT signaling is a possible mechanism by which Laforin may function as a tumor suppressor. In addition to a GSK3β-dependent role in promoting cell cycle progression [21,22], Laforin additionally possesses pro-survival attributes and may be a potential therapeutic target in lymphomas where low Laforin expression promotes apoptosis induced by energy deprivation, while lymphomas with high Laforin expression are resistant [18]. Laforin's ability to promote cell survival could be related to glycogen metabolism, or alternatively due to its indirect regulation of the WNT signaling pathway via activation of GSK3β [18,19].

Laforin additionally has a role in stress induced proteostasis [23-26]. Knock down of Laforin in human embryonic kidney (HEK293) cells and the neuroblastoma cell line, SH-SY5Y, resulted in increased apoptosis induced by endoplasmic reticulum (ER) stress [24]. Laforin also promotes autophagy by inhibiting the mammalian target of rapamycin (mTOR) pathway by a currently unknown mechanism to further protect cells from ER stress [25]. In addition to targeting genes involved in glycogen metabolism, recruitment of Malin further promotes ubiquitination of misfolded and aggregated proteins, thereby facilitating their protoosomal degradation [27]. Laforin also interacts with heat shock factor 1 (HSF1), an essential transcription factor in the heat shock response [26] and is necessary for up-regulation of HSF1-dependent gene expression and for protection from thermal stress in COS7 cells [26]. Accordingly, increased Laforin expression may allow cancer cells to survive in conditions where proteostasis has been perturbed.

2.2. DUSP3/VHR

Despite the ability of DUSP3 (alternatively named VHR for VH-1 related) to dephosphorylate the ERK1/2 and JNK MAPKs, it is generally not considered a MKP as it lacks the MAPK binding domain characteristic of MKPs [2,28,29]. Nevertheless, as a functional MAPK phosphatase, it is not surprising that DUSP3 is implicated in cancer, where it has been alternatively described as having both oncogenic [30-32] and tumor suppressive [33,34] properties.

dusp3 is up-regulated in cervical cancer cell lines and primary cervical cancers [30], and in HeLa cells, knock-down of *dusp3* inhibited proliferation by increasing the phosphorylation levels of ERK1/2 and JNK [31,35]. *dusp3* is also over-expressed in primary prostate tumors where it may function as a pro-survival phosphatase [32]. In prostate cancer cells (LNCaP), DUSP3 functions as an inhibitor of apoptosis, where *dusp3* knock-down resulted in increased JNK phosphorylation and increased apoptosis when treated with thapsigargin, an inducer of ER stress, or 12-*0*-tetradecanoylophorbol-13-acetate (TPA) [31].

DUSP3 may also inhibit tumor growth by regulating proliferation, particularly in the context of breast cancer cells expressing the oncogene, *brca1-iris. brca1-iris* is a splice variant of the breast cancer type 1 susceptibility (*brca1*) locus that promotes cell proliferation, cell migration, and invasion [34,36]. Over-expression of *brca1-iris* in breast cancer cell lines MCF7 and SKBR3 promoted proliferation through up-regulation of cyclin D1, and over-expression of *dusp3* was sufficient to suppress cyclin D1 expression [34]. *dusp3* expression is also down-regulated in primary non-small cell lung cancer (NSCLC) tumors [34]. A tumor suppressive function for DUSP3 in NSCLC is supported experimentally, as in both the NSCLC H1299 cell line and mouse xenographs, over-expression of *dusp3* suppressed growth of cells and tumors respectively [32]. Further supporting a tumor suppressor function for DUSP3, its expression suppressed phospholipase C (PLC) - protein kinase C (PKC) signaling [36]. The ErbB tyrosine kinase receptor, known to act upstream of PLC-gamma was subsequently identified as a direct DUSP3 substrate [37]. Increased ErbB tyrosine kinase activity drives several cancer-relevant properties including proliferation, cell motility, and invasion [36]. *dusp3* over-expression removed the activating phosphate from Y992 of ErbB, preventing ErbB kinase activity [33]. As the ErbB family of proto-oncogenes is strongly associated with cancers in a kinase dependent manner [37], the ability of DUSP3 to inhibit its activity may have important implications for cancer therapies.

If DUSP3 functions as a tumor suppressor or oncogene, modulators of DUSP3 function(s) could be attractive anti-cancer drug targets. The ZAP70 cytoplasmic tyrosine kinase, a key component in signaling machinery downstream of the T-cell antigen receptor, directly phosphorylates DUSP3 on tyrosine 138 (Y138) and increases it's ability to temper Erk1/2 and JNK signaling and reduce expression of a NFAT-AP1 dependent luciferase reporter, as VHR^{Y138F} functions as a dominant negative [38]. This observation is consistent with Y138 increasing the catalytic activity VHR, but this hypothesis is technically difficult to confirm due to VHR's ability to auto-dephosphorylate [38]. ZAP70 has been implicated in cancer as it is a prognostic marker for chronic lymphocytic leukemia (CLL) and B-cell acute lymphoblastic leukemia (B-ALL) where increased ZAP70 expression correlates with poor clinical outcome [39,40]. Besides being a prognostic marker, ZAP70 contributes to cancer by promoting survival and migration in both CLL and B-ALL [41,42] but whether ZAP70's modulation of DUSP3 has importance in B-ALL and CLL remains unknown. ZAP70 is not the only tyrosine kinase to target DUSP3 at tyrosine 138. TYK2, the non receptor tyrosine kinase of the Janus kinase family that regulates the expression of type 1 interferons and interleukin 12 [43] also targets this site [44]. Phosphorylation of DUSP3 by TYK2 was required for DUSP3 to dephosphorylate and inhibit signal transducer and activator of transcription 5 (STAT5) [44]. The ability of DUSP3 to inhibit STAT5 transcriptional activity may have consequences in cancer cell biology, since STAT5 activity is known to promote cancer by transcriptionally regulating genes involved in proliferation and survival [45], therefore loss of DUSP3 activity could possibly result in increased STAT5 activity thereby promoting cancer development. Furthermore, TYK2 has a suggested role in breast cancer metastasis, as analysis of 140 tissue samples from 70 breast cancer patients revealed that TYK2 protein levels are reduced in tumors that have metastasized to the regional lymph nodes [46]. Additionally, knock-down of *tyk2* in the MCF10A breast epithelial cell line decreased cell migration and invasion [46]. Whether loss of TYK2 promotes metastasis, migration, and invasion due to reduced DUSP3 activity remains to be determined

DUSP3's activity is additionally activated by the pseudokinase, Vaccinia-related kinase 3 (VRK3) [47], whose expression is down-regulated in colorectal cancer [48]. VRK3 inhibits ERK1/2 signaling by the formation of a VRK3-DUSP3-ERK1/2 complex where VRK3 is able to enhance the activity of DUSP3 towards ERK1/2 in a kinase independent manner [47]. It would be interesting to examine whether tumors with decreased *vrk3* expression also have decreased DUSP3 activity. Since VRK3 promotes DUSP3's activity towards ERK1/2, one would expect tumors with decreased VRK3 to have increased ERK1/2 signaling, and these investigations could further indicate a potential tumor suppressor for DUSP3.

2.3. DUSP11

Due to interactions with ribonucleoprotein (RNP) complexes and RNA splicing factors and its ability to dephosphorylate RNA trinucleotides, DUSP11 is thought to have a role in RNA splicing [49]. DUSP11 also associates with SAM68 (SRC-associated protein in mitotic cells), an ERK1/2 phosphorylated splicing factor that promotes the alternative splicing of cluster of differentiation 44 *(CD44)* mRNA encoding a glycoprotein involved in cell-cell interactions, cell adhesion, and migration [50,51]. Alternatively spliced isoforms of CD44 include up to 10 variant exon sequences (V1 to V10) that are though to contribute to human organismal complexity from a relatively restricted number of genes [50]. The v5 exon splice variant of CD44 is suggested to promote metastatic cancers [50,51] and this alternative splicing event is thought to be under the control of Ras singaling pathway through recruitement of SAM68. As forced overexpression of Sam68 leads to increased inclusion of the V5-exon sequence in CD44 and Dusp11 associated with SAM68, and variants of SAM68 that cannot be phosphrylated by ERK abrogate the inclusion of the V5-exon variant, it suggests that SAM68 function is under control of Ras signaling pathways in response to extracellular cues, but whether DUSP11 can counteract the ERK1/2 dependent phosphorylation of SAM68 similar to Sam68 varaints lacking all candidate ERK1/2 phosphorylation sites remains to be determined experimentally. As alternative splicing affects the activities of many oncogenes and tumor suppressors, DUSP11's role in splicing may extend beyond CD44, which could have important implications for cancer [52].

dusp11 is also a transcriptional target of the p53 tumor suppressor [53]. p53 is a potent tumor suppressor that induces cell cycle arrest, senescence, and apoptosis in response to DNA damage and oncogene activation, and is one of the most commonly mutated genes in cancer [54]. The ability of p53 to up-regulate *dusp11* may provide a link between p53 function and to the splicing machinery [53].

DUSP11 regulates proliferation as over-expression of *dusp11* in U20S and mouse embryonic fibroblasts resulted in inhibition of proliferation in a manner dependent on DUSP11's phosphatase activity [53]. Additionally, knock-down of *dusp11* increased proliferation in both untreated and UV or Doxorubicin DNA damaged U20S cells where DUSP11 most likely inhibits proliferation in response to genotoxic stress in a p53 dependent manner [53]. Loss of growth arrest in response to DNA damage in cells lacking *dusp11* could result in genomic instability, which can promote cancer development and/or progression [55].

2.4. DUSP12

dusp12 is up-regulated or amplified in a variety of cancers including neuroblastoma, retinoblastoma, intracranial ependymoma, and chronic myelogenous leukemia [56-59]. Additionally, *dusp12* is one of only two candidate genes for the target of a 1q21-1q23 amplification found in invasive liposarcomas [60] leading to the hypothesis that *dusp12* is an oncogene. Within the atypical DUSPs, DUSP12 is unique in that it contains an evolutionarily conserved cysteine-rich domain (CRD) at the C-terminus that binds zinc [61], but whose biological function remains obscure.

DUSP12 was initially identified as a pro-survival phosphatase from a high throughput siRNA screen in HeLa cells [62] as knock-down of *dusp12* induced spontaneous apoptosis [62]. Later, it was demonstrated that transient over-expression of *dusp12* in HeLa rendered cells resistant to apoptotic stimuli including heat shock, oxidative stress, and FAS death receptor activation, but not against the DNA damage inducing agent, cisplatin [63]. In HeLa cells, the ability of DUSP12 to protect cells from apoptosis was dependent on phosphatase activity [63].

DUSP12 interacts with the heat shock protein 70 (HSP70) and the requirement of the enzymatic activity to protect cells from apoptosis activity raises the possibility that HSP70 may be a direct substrate for DUSP12. However, if DUSP12 does regulate HSP70, it does not appear to regulate HSP70's chaperone function as demonstrated by *in vitro* folding assays [63]. Conversely, HSP70 was able to promote DUSP12's phosphatase activity against the phospho-tyrosine analog, 6,8-di-fluoro-4-methylumbeliferyl phosphate (DiFMUP), in a manner that is most likely not a chaperone:substrate interaction as DUSP12 binds the ATPase domain of HSP70 [63]. The C-terminal CRD was also required for DUSP12 to protect from apoptosis [63]. As oxidation of catalytic cysteines is a common mechanism to post-translationally regulate DUSP's [64], it was later demonstrated that the zinc binding ability of the C-terminus protected DUSP12's phosphatase activity during oxidizing conditions *in vitro* [65].

DUSP12 also has a role in cell cycle regulation. Transient over-expression of *dusp12* in HEK293 cells resulted in an increase in the percentage of cells in the G2/M phase and polyploidy and knock-down resulted in cell cycle arrest and senescence [66]. Since, *dusp12* is amplified in several cancers [56,57,60], it is possible that DUSP12 may promote cancer by increasing genomic instability. Unlike the pro-survival properties described above, DUSP12's effect on the cell cycle was independent of its phosphatase activity and required the CRD domain [66]. The CRD function is also likely regulated post-translationally: replacement of serine 335 with alanine (S335A) elicited cell cycle profiles similar to wild type DUSP12, whereas the phosphomimetic S335E variant led to a significant increase in the percentage of G2/M cells (29.8 % for S335A vs. 36.6 % for S335E) [66]. This alteration also affects subcellular localization from the cytoplasm (WT and S335E) to the nuclear compartment (S335A), but does not affect DUSP12's phosphatase activity *in vitro* [66]. To the best of our knowledge this is the only study demonstrating phosphorylation dependent regulation of DUSP12 and the kinases and/or phosphatases responsible remain unknown. Additionally, The S335 kinases may be restricted to mammals, as the S335 site is not well conserved in other organisms [66].

To determine whether DUSP12 has oncogenic properties, we examined the oncogenic potential of DUSP12 in a cell culture model [67]. Unlike the cell cycle effects in HEK293 cells transiently over-expressing *dusp12* described above, we observed no difference in proliferation in HEK293 cells stably over-expressing *gfp-dusp12* (hereafter referred to as *dusp12* over-expression) [67]. Despite the lack of effect on proliferation, we did find that *dusp12* over-expression protected cells from apoptosis induced by both staurosporine and thapsigargin [67]. We additionally observed, that *dusp12* over-expression increased cell motility in scratch wound and transmigration assays [67]. *dusp12* over-expression also up-regulated the expression of two validated oncogenes; integrin alpha 1 (*itga1*) and the hepatocyte growth factor receptor, *c-met* [67]. ITGA1, a component of the cellular receptor for collagen, promotes proliferation, invasion, and angiogenesis of cancer cells [68-70], but whether it is responsible for the DUSP12 dependent motility remains to be determined. The c-MET proto-oncogene is a well established regulator of growth, survival, and migratory signaling [71], but it seems unlikely that c-MET is responsible for the pro-survival and migratory function of DUSP12 overexpression, since we failed to observed increased c-MET activation in cells over-expressing *dusp12* [67]. This was not wholly unexpected as c-MET frequently requires its ligand, HGF, to be supplied in an autocrine or paracrine manner in order to function [72]. The ability of elevated DUSP12 to promote c-MET and ITGA1 expression has potential implications in cancer where, in the right tumor microenvironment, DUSP12-dependent up-regulation could co-opt the oncogenic potential of these validated oncogenes [73].

Although it is clear that DUSP12 regulates several important cancer-relevant processes, how DUSP12 accomplishes this is largely unknown. Insights into DUSP12's cellular function(s) can be obtained by investigating the budding yeast DUSP12 ortholog, Yvh1p. *YVH1* transcription is up-regulated by nitrogen starvation and low temperatures and *yvh1Δ* yeast strains exhibit a severe growth phenotype, display defects in sporulation, glycogen accumulation, and ribosome biogenesis [74-78]. Expression of the Yvh1p CRD domain in isolation was able to suppress all the mutant phenotypes of *yvh1Δ* strains, suggesting that neither phosphatase activity nor the N-terminal phosphatase domain is required for its cellular function in yeast [76]. The DUSP12 CRD has been alternatively described as a LIM-domain, a zinc-finger and a RING-variant domain due to its ability to coordinate zinc, but how it contributes to biological function is not clear [61]. However, either full-length human DUSP12 or a variant rendered catalytically inactive (C115S) were able to suppress the *yvh1Δ* phenotypes, suggesting that these proteins are functional orthologs [61]. It is important to note that to date, unlike human DUSP12, phosphatase-dependent function(s) of Yvh1p have yet to be characterized, suggesting that, DUSP12 has acquired additional cellular functions than those described in yeast.

Recent independent genetic screens in yeast have revealed that Yvh1p is a critical factor in ribosome biogenesis [77,78]. Ribosome biogenesis is an extremely complex process that is regulated both spatially and temporally [79]. Ribosomal RNA is transcribed and processed in the nucleolus and the pre-40S and pre-60S subunits, are assembled in the nucleus [79]. The pre-40S and pre-60S subunits are exported into the cytoplasm where additional maturation occurs including the binding of multiple translation initiation factors to the small ribosomal subunit to form a 48S complex [79]. Upon recognition of the Met initiation anticodon, the translation initiation factors are expelled to facilitate the joining of the large 60S ribosomal subunit to form a translationally competent 80S ribosome [79]. Defects within specific steps or association of proteins with defined complexes within this multistep process can be inferred from polysome analyses as each complex in endowed with a unique sedimentation coefficient within sucrose gradients [80]. Polysome analysis in yeast demonstrated that Yvh1p associates with pre-60S ribosomes and loss of *YVH1* results in an increase in half-mers (consisting of a 48S small subunit that fails to join to a large 60S ribosomal subunit) [81]. The production of translationally incompetent half-mers likely results from defects in cytoplasmic 60S maturation [80,81]. In addition to specific temporal associations of initiation factors with the 40S subunit, the nuclear pre-60S subunits associate with Mrt4p, which is subsequently displaced by the P0/P1/P2 ribosomal stalk proteins upon export of the complex into the cytoplasm [78, 82]. The addition of the ribosomal stalk to the cytoplasmic 60S ribosomal subunits is one of the last essential steps prior to large subunit joining [82]. In *yvh1* null yeast strains Mrt4p remained associated with the cytoplasmic 60S subunits preventing the assemblage of the P0/P1/P2 proteins that form the ribosomal stalk [78]. Further supporting a genetic interaction between *YVH1* and *MRT4*, specific mutations of *mtr4* suppressed all *yvh1Δ* phenotypes, suggesting that the pleiotropic phenotypes associated with *yvh1Δ* strains may be an indirect consequence of aberrant ribosome maturation [83].

A similar role for DUSP12 regulating ribosome biogenesis in humans is borne from observations that knock-down of human *dusp12* in HeLa cells promoted the mislocalization of the ribosome factors MRTO4 and eIF6, a translation initiation factor that also binds to the 60S subunit preventing its association with the 40S subunit [84]. In addition, siRNA knock-down of the ribosome factor P0 in HeLa cells resulted in exclusion of DUSP12 from the nucleus [84], its initially characterized sub-cellular localization [61]. As was described in yeast, the reported pleiotropic roles for human DUSP12 may also be an indirect consequence of defects in the production of translationally competent ribosomes, as several proteins affecting ribosome biogenesis are known oncogenes [85] and many other oncogenes are selectively regulated at the translational level [86].

2.5. DUSP18

dusp18 mRNA is expressed in a variety of primary tumors and cancer cell lines [87]. The crystal structure of DUSP18 demonstrates that the phosphatase domain adopts a structure similar to the phosphatase domain of DUSP3/VHR with some minor modifications, including alterations in charge distribution within the active site pocket, suggesting the possibility that it may have distinct substrate specificity profile [88]. Additionally, DUSP18 contains a C-terminal motif (CT) that specifically interacts with the catalytic domain, which may be responsible for Dusp18's elevated thermostability, with a temperature optimum of 55°C [89]. DUSP18 localizes to the nuclear and cytoplasmic compartments as well as the intermembrane space of the mitochondria [90,91] although it appears that the mitrochondrial localization is native as reports of DUSP18 localizing to the cytoplasm and nucleus was due to over-expression of *dusp18* with an N-terminal tag that disrupted the mitochondrial localization [91]. Like components of the intrinsic pathway of apoptosis, mitochondrial DUSP18 can be released into the cytoplasm in response to apoptotic signals [91]. DUSP18 selectively dephosphorylates the JNK stress activated MAPK *in vitro* and *in vivo* [87,90,91], but since JNK is not thought to be mitochondrially resident, it seems unlikely that DUSP18 interacts with JNK under normal conditions [91]. However, due to the ability of intrinsic apoptosis to release DUSP18 from mitochondria, it is possible that DUSP18 may be able to interact with and dephosphorylate JNK under apoptotic conditions. The JNK

MAPK is a well-established regulator of tumorigenesis, and regulates processes such as cell proliferation [92], apoptosis [93], and inflammation [94].

2.6. DUSP22

DUSP22 expression is down-regulated in breast cancer and lymphomas [95, 96], and is used as a prognostic marker for B cell chronic lymphocytic leukemia patients [97]. In anaplastic lymphoma kinase (ALK)-negative anaplastic large cell lymphomas, the commonly found t(6;7)(p25.3;q32.3) translocation disrupts the *dusp22* gene [96]. Down-regulation of *dusp22* in cancer suggests a possible tumor suppressive role for DUSP22, but exactly how DUSP22 may function in cancer and normal cell biology awaits further characterization.

There are conflicting reports concerning the ability of DUSP22 to dephosphorylate MAPKs [97-100], but most studies indicate DUSP22 as a regulator of JNK [99-101]. Over-expression of both JNK and DUSP22 in COS7 suppressed JNK phosphorylation [99]. However, other reports have identified a phosphatase-dependent role for DUSP22 in promoting JNK activity [100,101]. Glutathione S-transferase (GST) pull downs and immunoprecipitations revealed that DUSP22 can bind the JNK activating kinase, MKK7, but not JNK itself, and the association with MKK7 activates MKK7's phosphorylation of JNK [99]. Exactly how DUSP22 activates MKK7 and JNK activity is unclear but the requirement is biologically significant as mouse embryonic stem cells lacking DUSP22 were unable to activate JNK in response to cytokines [100].

Another reported substrate of DUSP22 is the estrogen receptor (ERα) an important prognostic marker for breast cancer regulating proliferation and apoptosis [102,103]. DUSP22 most likely functions within a negative feedback loop to regulate ERα, as activation of ERα induces *dusp22* mRNA expression and DUSP22 dephosphorylates and inhibits ERα's transcriptional activity in breast cancer cells [102]. Additionally, *dusp22* expression is down-regulated in breast cancers, specifically those containing the 8p11-12 amplicon [95]. This amplicon contains the potential oncogene, *ppapdc1b,* which is thought to be responsible for DUSP22 down-regulation as siRNA knock-down of *ppapdc1b* increases *dusp22* expression [95]. The oncogenic ability of *ppapdc1b,* in part, may be due to its ability to down-regulate *dusp22* expression to allow for increased estrogen receptor activity, as it was reported that all 11 tumor samples analyzed that contain the 8p11-12 amplicon, had ER-positive statuses [95].

DUSP22 may also regulate metastasis as it dephosphorylates tyrosines 576/577 and 397 of focal adhesion kinase (FAK) [104]. FAK is a key regulator of integrin-mediated attachment and FAK inhibition results in detachment and apoptosis in some cell lines [105]. *dusp22* over-expression inhibited cell migration and reduced FAK phosphorylation while *dusp22* knock-down promoted cell migration and FAK phosphorylation in H1299 cells [104]. DUSP22 is myristoylated [106], which may allow for its co-localization with FAK at actin filament enriched regions of lamelapodia [104]. The subcellular localization of DUSP22 likely contributes to its biological function as myristoylation-deficient variants of DUSP22 do not display altered enzymatic activity *in vitro,* but unlike wild-type DUSP22, induced cell detachment and apoptosis when over-expressed [106].

2.7. DUSP23

DUSP23 dephosphorylates ERK1/2 *in vitro,* but DUSP23 is an activator of JNK and p38 in COS7 cells [6]. In addition, the regulation of JNK and p38 is phosphatase independent, and the MAPKKs for JNK and p38, MKK4 and MKK6, also have increased phosphorylation when *dusp23* is over-expressed and the cells are treated with sorbitol, suggesting that DUSP23 may act as a scaffold to promote MKK binding to JNK and p38 [6].

The *dusp23* gene is highly methylated and decreased *dusp23* mRNA expression is observed in neuroblastoma [107]. Interestingly, *dusp23* mRNA levels were lower in tumors from deceased patients than patients exhibiting no clinical symptoms, suggesting that DUSP23 levels could be a prognostic marker for neuroblastomas [107]. The generality of *dusp23* functioning as a tumor suppressor is called into question by observations that it is amplified in many other cancers, including breast, colon, lung, squamous carcinoma, pancreatic, brain, esophageal, stomach, bladder, kidney, skin, ovary, prostate, and testicular cancers [108], and selective over-expression of *dusp23* in MCF7 cells increased proliferation while knock-down of *dusp23* decreased proliferation [108].

2.8. DUSP26

A role for *dusp26* in cancer is borne by observations that it is located on an 8p12 amplicon found in anaplastic thyroid carcinoma tissue [109] and differential expression of *dusp26* has additionally been observed in glioblastoma tissues, neuroblastoma, brain, and ovarian cancer cell lines, where *dusp26* is down-regulated [110,111]. Additionally, knock-down of *dusp26* in immortalized ovarian epithelia HOSE17.1 cells increased both colony formation and proliferation [111]. Over-expression of *dusp26* in immortalized breast epithelial MCF10A, cells suppressed colony formation and acinar growth in 3D culture [111]. Alternatively, in anaplastic thyroid carcinoma primary tumors and cell lines, over-expression of *dusp26* promoted colony formation, while knock-down of *dusp26* expression reduced proliferation [109]. Defining a more precise role for DUSP26 is further complicated by the fact that different groups have come to opposing conclusions regarding *dusp26* expression in neuroblastoma cell lines [111,112]

The cellular function of DUSP26 is also unclear as the substrates for DUSP26 are debated. DUSP26 can dephosphorylate the tumor suppressor p53 at Ser20 and Ser37, inhibiting p53-mediated apoptosis induced by genotoxic stress [112], suggesting a pro-survival role. In addition to p53, several other *in vitro* DUSP26 substrates have been described, including p38 [109]. In HEK293T cells, over-expression of *dusp26* resulted in reduction of p38 activity and p38-mediated apoptosis [113]. The small molecule inhibitor NSC-87877 functions as an *in vitro* DUSP26 inhibitor with an IC_{50} of 16.7 uM that additionally prevented the DUSP26-dependent dephosphorylation of p38 in HEK293 cells [114]. However, in COS7 cells, over-expression of *dusp26* increased both JNK and p38 activities [6], and in the rat neuronal cell line, PC12, and epithelial cells DUSP26 had no affect on MAPKs [17,112] questioning the generality of DUSP26 functioning as a p38 phosphatase.

DUSP26 is also implicated in regulating the kinesin superfamily 3 (KIF3) microtubule-directed protein motor complex by dephosphorylating the kinesin-associated protein 3 (KAP3) [111]. The KIF3 motor complex has been implicated in cancer due to its ability to traffic cancer relevant proteins including, adenamaous polyposis coli (APC), β-catenin, cadherins, and the polarity complex, PAR3 [115,116]. Consistent with DUSP26 functioning as a positive regulator of KIF3, over-expression of *dusp26* in the mouse fibroblast cell line, NIH3T3, increased cell-to-cell adhesion and intracellular transport of N-cadherin and β-catenin to the cell surface [111].

3. Less well-characterized atypical DUSPs.

The previous sections discussed the atypical DUSPs that have been described in the literature as having a relationship, however tenuous or controversial, to tumor suppressive and/or oncogenic properties and are often supported by genetic/genomic analyses of primary tumors samples. Although the previous sections should reaffirm that the function(s) of many of the atypical DUSPs are likely both cell type and context dependent, we nevertheless undertook a comparison of the expression profiles of all the atypical DUSPs in tumors of the prostate to normal prostate tissue using the cBio Cancer Genomics Portal (http://www.cbioportal.org/) and microarray data deposited by the Memorial Sloan-Kettering Cancer (MSKCC) Center's Prostate Oncogenome Project [117]. Comparison of the transcriptome of 85 tumors to normal prostate tissue revealed that many atypical DUSPs have aberrant expression in prostate cancer (Table 2). In at least two cases this difference

Gene	Down	Up	Total
EPM2A	13%	0%	13%
STYX	2%	7%	9%
DUSP3	40%	0%	40%
DUSP11	4%	5%	8%
DUSP12	1%	15%	16%
DUSP13	0%	5%	5%
DUSP14	6%	11%	16%
DUSP15	4%	0%	4%
DUSP18	40%	4%	44%
DUSP19	1%	1%	2%
DUSP21	0%	7%	7%
DUSP22	15%	2%	18%
DUSP23	11%	8%	19%
DUSP26	1%	2%	4%
DUSP27	2%	5%	7%
Androgen Receptor (AR)	2%	7%	9%

Table 2. Using the cBio Cancer Genomics protal (http://www.cbioportal.org/), and microarray data deposited by MSKCC Prostate Oncogenome Project [117]. we compared the expression of atypical DUSPs in tumors to normal prostate tissue using a Z score threshold of +/- 2. The androgen receptor (AR) is included for comparison as a gene already implicated in cancer progression [117]

was reflected clinically as patients harboring tumors with aberrant *dusp22* or *dusp23* expression had faster disease relapse than those harboring tumors with normal *dusp22* or *dusp23* expression (Figure 1). Although differential expression of any particular gene in prostate cancer may not functionally contribute to the initiation or progression of the disease, this analysis serves as an example of one way to potentially identify cancer-relevant markers. The following sections describe what is currently known about the remaining atypical DUSPs that, to date, have not been specifically associated with cancer.

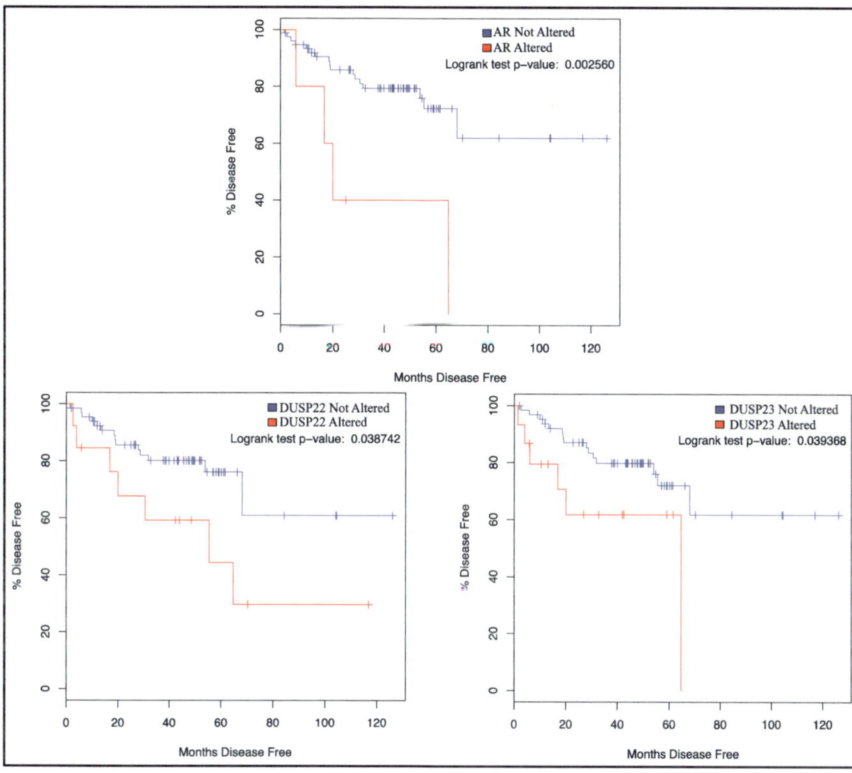

Figure 1. Kaplan-Meyer analysis of disease free survival for patients with altered expression of the androgen receptor or atypical DUSPs. This graph was generated by the cBio Cancer Genomics Portal (http://www.cbioportal.org/) using data deposited by the MSKCC Prostate Oncogenome Project [117]. Microarray expression data from tumors compared to normal prostate was used in this analysis with a Z-score threshold of +/- 2.

3.1. STYX

The prototypical pseudophosphatase, STYX, contains a substitution of the catalytic cysteine for glycine, rendering it catalytically inactive [118]. As this mutation abrogates catalysis, but not substrate binding, pseudophosphatases are though to function as substrate traps preventing dephosphorylation of the target protein(s) [119]. In mice, *styx* expression is restricted to the testis, and is essential for spermatogenesis, as STYX knock-out male mice are infertile [118].

3.2. DUSP13A/B

The *dusp13* gene encodes for two similar protein products via alternative reading frames [120,121]. Designated DUSP13A and DUSP13B, the proteins are expressed in the muscle and testis respectively [121,122]. Both proteins have phosphatase activity *in vitro,* with DUSP13B exhibiting higher activity than DUSP13A [122]. Interestingly, both DUSP13A and B regulate apoptosis, but by different mechanisms. Knock-down of DUSP13A in mouse embryonic fibroblasts reduced apoptosis signal regulating kinase 1 (ASK1) kinase activity and intrinsic apoptosis induced by *ask1* over-expression [7]. Furthermore, autophosphorylation assays of ASK1 with increasing amounts of DUSP13A demonstrated that DUSP13A increases ASK1 autophosphorylation in a phosphatase independent manner [7]. In contrast to DUSP13A, DUSP13B appears to be pro-survival [123]. Over-expression of DUSP13B in COS7 cells resulted in reduced phosphorylation of the stress activated MAPKs, JNK and p38 [123]. Over-expression of DUSP13B resulted in reduced activity of the down-stream JNK effector AP-1 in a phosphatase dependent manner [123]. AP-1 activity is associated with a large number of cellular processes including transformation, proliferation, differentiation, and is specifically implicated in apoptosis [124].

3.3. DUSP14

dusp14 is located on a chromosomal region that is amplified in gastric cancer, but it may not be the target for the genetic amplification, as *dusp14* expression is not increased [125]. *In vitro,* DUSP14 dephosphorylates all three MAPK isoforms, leading to its alternate designations of MKP-L (MKP1-Like) and MKP-6 [126]. However, DUSP14 is classified as an atypical DUSP as it lacks the characteristic MAPK binding domain found in the MKP DUSP subfamily [2]. In T-cells, expression of the catalytically inactive DUSP14 C111S variant enhanced ERK1/2 and JNK phosphorylation, suggesting that *in vivo,* p38 is not a DUSP14 substrate [126]. Additionally, in β pancreatic cells, knock-down of *dusp14* expression or the expression of a dominant negative DUSP14 variant resulted in increased ERK1/2 phosphorylation and cell proliferation [127]. Elucidating a role for DUSP14 may be aided by the discovery of the PTP inhibitor IV, an inhibitor of DUSP14 *in vitro* that increases hydrogen peroxide induced JNK activation in a concentration dependent manner [128].

3.4. DUSP15

The DUSP15 crystal structure reveals it lacks the MAPK substrate recognition domain and it has a unique additional alpha helix located at the back end of the active site suggesting that DUSP15 has unique substrate recognition mechanisms [129]. DUSP15 displays phosphatase activity against the artificial substrate pNPP *in vitro* [130], but physiological substrates for DUSP15 have yet to be reported. DUSP15 contains an N-terminal myristoylation signal, resulting in targeting of the protein to plasma membrane [90] and in mice DUSP15 has been identified as a candidate gene in a quantitative trait locus (QTL) thought to harbor genes that control for the predisposition to growth and fatness in mice [131].

3.5. DUSP19

Like DUSP13A, DUSP19 is thought to facilitate ASK1 activation leading to MKK7 activation and in turn activating JNK as DUSP19 directly binds MKK7, but not JNK *in vitro*, and co-immunoprecipitates with ASK1 and MKK7 [8,132]. The proposed model for how DUSP19 differentially regulates JNK activation is that at high levels of DUSP19 ASK1 is sequestered by DUSP19 thereby inhibiting MKK7 and JNK activation, while at low levels DUSP19 functions as a scaffold to promote the activation of MKK7 by ASK1 [8,132].

3.6. DUSP21

Similar to DUSP18, DUSP21 contains a highly conserved mitochondrial localization signal, however DUSP21 localizes to the peripheral membrane of the inner membrane of the mitochondria, which is the opposing side to which DUSP18 is found [91]. DUSP21 exhibits activity against synthetic MAPK peptides *in vitro*, but cell based assays fail to demonstrate that DUSP21 has activity against any cellular MAPKs [90].

3.7. DUSP27

Substrates for the newest atypical DUSP, DUSP27, are unknown but solution of the DUSP27 3D structure suggests that it may have substrates other than the MAPKs [133]. The catalytic site can accommodate dually-phosphorylated residues separated by two amino acids, which differs from the catalytic site of DUSPs that can dephosphorylate the characteristic MAPK activation loop (T-X-Y) [133].

4. Conclusion

Although many atypical DUSPs display differential expression in tumor samples, significant amounts of work will be required to determine whether and how these differences contribute to malignancy, especially with the common discrepancy between *in vitro* and *in vivo* results. Due to the central localization of the MAPK signaling cascade and the role of MKPs in malignancy, much of the initial work has been to evaluate if and how atypical DUSPs affect MAPK signaling. The MAPK pathway however represents a doubled edged sword, although it is strongly associated with disease, it is difficult to modulate pharmacologically due to complex crosstalk and feedback loops. We envision that specific inhibitors for atypical DUSPs, particularly those that do not target MAPK isoforms but other cancer relevant substrates, could have important therapeutic value. Even in the event that these inhibitors fail to function as therapeutics, we think that selective inhibitors will be instrumental in advancing the elucidation of the cellular functions, substrates, and expression of the atypical DUSPs. Even in instances where the mechanism of oncogenesis remains unknown, we anticipate that continued large-scale expression profiling of the atypical DUSPs may be increasingly used to for clinical benefit to patients through the identification of potential novel biomarkers.

Author details

Erica L. Cain and Alexander Beeser*
Division of Biology, Kansas State University, Manhattan, Kansas, USA

5. References

[1] Denu JM and Dixon JE (1995) A catalytic mechanism for the dual-specific phosphatases. Proc. Natl. Acad. Sci. U. S. A. 92(13):5910-5914.
[2] Patterson KI, Brummer T, O'Brien PM, Daly RJ (2009) Dual-specificity phosphatases: critical regulators with diverse cellular targets. Biochem. J. 418:475-489.
[3] Barford D, Das AK, Egloff MP (1998) The structure and mechanism of protein phosphatases: insights into catalysis and regulation. Annu. Rev. Biophys. Biomol. Struct. 127:133-164.
[4] Jeffrey KL, Camps M, Rommel C, Mackay CR (2007) Targeting dual-specificity phosphatases: manipulating MAP kinase signalling and immune responses. Nat. Rev. Drug. Discov. 6(5):391-403.
[5] Bayon Y and Alonso A (2010) Atypical DUSPs: 19 phosphatases in search of a role. In: Lazo PA, editor. Emerging Signaling Pathways in Tumor Biology. Kerala: Transworld Research Network. pp. 185-208.
[6] Takagaki K, Satoh T, Tanuma N, Masuda K, Takekawa M, Shima H, et al. (2004) Characterization of a novel low-molecular-mass dual-specificity phosphatase-3 (LDP-3) that enhances activation of JNK and p38. Biochem. J. 383(Pt. 3):447-455.
[7] Park JE, Park BC, Kim HA, Song M, Park SG, Lee do H, et al. (2010) Positive regulation of apoptosis signal-regulating kinase 1 by dual-specificity phosphatase 13A. Cell Mol. Life Sci. 67(15):2619-2629.
[8] Zama T, Aoki R, Kamimoto T, Inoue K, Ikeda Y, Hagiwara M (2002) Scaffold role of a mitogen-activated protein kinase phosphatase, SKRP1, for the JNK signaling pathway. J. Biol. Chem. Jun 28;277(26):23919-23926.
[9] Dubey D, Parihar R, Ganesh S (2012) Identification and characterization of novel splice variants of the human EPM2A gene mutated in Lafora progressive myoclonus epilepsy. Genomics. 99(1):36-43.
[10] Ganesh S, Suzuki T, Yamakawa K (2002) Alternative splicing modulates subcellular localization of laforin. Biochem. Biophys. Res. Commun. 291(5):1134-1137.
[11] Ianzano L, Young EJ, Zhao XC, Chan EM, Rodriguez MT, Torrado MV, et al. (2004) Loss of function of the cytoplasmic isoform of the protein laforin (EPM2A) causes Lafora progressive myoclonus epilepsy. Hum. Mutat. 23(2):170-176.
[12] Ganesh S, Puri R, Singh S, Mittal S, Dubey D (2006) Recent advances in the molecular basis of Lafora's progressive myoclonus epilepsy. J. Hum. Genet. 51(1):1-8.
[13] Singh S, Satishchandra P, Shankar SK, Ganesh S (2008) Lafora disease in the Indian population: EPM2A and NHLRC1 gene mutations and their impact on subcellular localization of laforin and malin. Hum. Mutat. 29(6):E1-12.

* Corresponding Author

[14] Worby CA, Gentry MS, Dixon JE (2006) Laforin, a dual specificity phosphatase that dephosphorylates complex carbohydrates. J. Biol. Chem. 281(41):30412-30418.

[15] Wang J, Stuckey JA, Wishart MJ, Dixon JE (2002) A unique carbohydrate binding domain targets the lafora disease phosphatase to glycogen. J. Biol. Chem. 277(4):2377-2380.

[16] Worby CA, Gentry MS, Dixon JE (2008) Malin decreases glycogen accumulation by promoting the degradation of protein targeting to glycogen (PTG). J. Biol. Chem. 283(7):4069-4076.

[17] Wang JY, Lin CH, Yang CH, Tan TH, Chen YR (2006) Biochemical and biological characterization of a neuroendocrine-associated phosphatase. J. Neurochem. 98(1):89-101.

[18] Wang Y, Liu Y, Wu C, McNally B, Liu Y, Zheng P (2008) Laforin confers cancer resistance to energy deprivation-induced apoptosis. Cancer Res. 68(11):4039-4044.

[19] Wang Y, Liu Y, Wu C, Zhang H, Zheng X, Zheng Z, et al. (2006) Epm2a suppresses tumor growth in an immunocompromised host by inhibiting Wnt signaling. Cancer Cell.10(3):179-190.

[20] Polakis P (2012) Wnt Signaling in Cancer. Cold Spring Harb. Perspect. Biol. Mar 20 DOI: 10.1101/cshperspect.a008052.

[21] Liu Y, Wang Y, Wu C, Liu Y, Zheng P (2006) Dimerization of Laforin is required for its optimal phosphatase activity, regulation of GSK3beta phosphorylation, and Wnt signaling. J. Biol. Chem. 281(46):34768-34774.

[22] Liu R, Wang L, Chen C, Liu Y, Zhou P, Wang Y, et al. (2008) Laforin negatively regulates cell cycle progression through glycogen synthase kinase 3beta-dependent mechanisms. Mol. Cell Biol. 28(23):7236-7244.

[23] Liu Y, Wang Y, Wu C, Liu Y, Zheng P (2009) Deletions and missense mutations of EPM2A exacerbate unfolded protein response and apoptosis of neuronal cells induced by endoplasm reticulum stress. Hum. Mol. Genet. 18(14):2622-2631.

[24] Vernia S, Rubio T, Heredia M, Rodriguez de Cordoba S, Sanz P (2009) Increased endoplasmic reticulum stress and decreased proteasomal function in lafora disease models lacking the phosphatase laforin. PLoS One. 4(6):e5907.

[25] Aguado C, Sarkar S, Korolchuk VI, Criado O, Vernia S, Boya P, et al. (2010) Laforin, the most common protein mutated in Lafora disease, regulates autophagy. Hum. Mol. Genet. 19(14):2867-2876.

[26] Sengupta S, Badhwar I, Upadhyay M, Singh S, Ganesh S (2011) Malin and laforin are essential components of a protein complex that protects cells from thermal stress. J. Cell Sci. 124(Pt 13):2277-2286.

[27] Garyali P, Siwach P, Singh PK, Puri R, Mittal S, Sengupta S, et al. (2009) The malin-laforin complex suppresses the cellular toxicity of misfolded proteins by promoting their degradation through the ubiquitin-proteasome system. Hum. Mol. Genet. 18(4):688-700.

[28] Todd JL, Tanner KG, Denu JM (1999) Extracellular regulated kinases (ERK) 1 and ERK2 are authentic substrates for the dual-specificity protein-tyrosine phosphatase VHR. A novel role in down-regulating the ERK pathway. J. Biol. Chem. 274(19):13271-13280.

[29] Todd JL, Rigas JD, Rafty LA, Denu JM (2002) Dual-specificity protein tyrosine phosphatase VHR down-regulates c-Jun N-terminal kinase (JNK). Oncogene. 21(16):2573-2583.

[30] Henkens R, Delvenne P, Arafa M, Moutschen M, Zeddou M, Tautz L, et al. (2008) Cervix carcinoma is associated with an up-regulation and nuclear localization of the dual-specificity protein phosphatase VHR. BMC Cancer. 8:147.

[31] Wu S, Vossius S, Rahmouni S, Miletic AV, Vang T, Vazquez-Rodriguez J, et al. (2009) Multidentate small-molecule inhibitors of vaccinia H1-related (VHR) phosphatase decrease proliferation of cervix cancer cells. J. Med. Chem. 52(21):6716-6723.

[32] Arnoldussen YJ, Lorenzo PI, Pretorius ME, Waehre H, Risberg B, Maelandsmo GM, et al. (2008) The mitogen-activated protein kinase phosphatase vaccinia H1-related protein inhibits apoptosis in prostate cancer cells and is overexpressed in prostate cancer. Cancer Res. 68(22):9255-9264.

[33] Wang JY, Yeh CL, Chou HC, Yang CH, Fu YN, Chen YT, et al. (2011) Vaccinia H1-related phosphatase is a phosphatase of ErbB receptors and is down-regulated in non-small cell lung cancer. J. Biol. Chem. 286(12):10177-10184.

[34] Hao L, and ElShamy WM (2007) BRCA1-IRIS activates cyclin D1 expression in breast cancer cells by downregulating the JNK phosphatase DUSP3/VHR. Int. J. Cancer. 121(1):39-46.

[35] Rahmouni S, Cerignoli F, Alonso A, Tsutji T, Henkens R, Zhu C, et al. (2006) Loss of the VHR dual-specific phosphatase causes cell-cycle arrest and senescence. Nat. Cell Biol. 8(5):524-531.

[36] ElShamy WM and Livingston DM (2004) Identification of BRCA1-IRIS, a BRCA1 locus product. Nat. Cell Biol. 6(10):954-967.

[37] Howe LR and Brown PH (2011) Targeting the HER/EGFR/ErbB family to prevent breast cancer. Cancer Prev. Res. (Phila). 4(8):1149-1157.

[38] Alonso A, Rahmouni S, Williams S, van Stipdonk M, Jaroszewski L, Godzik A, et al. (2003) Tyrosine phosphorylation of VHR phosphatase by ZAP-70. Nat. Immunol. 4(1):44-48.

[39] Sagatys EM, Zhang L (2012) Clinical and laboratory prognostic indicators in chronic lymphocytic leukemia. Cancer Control. 19(1):18-25.

[40] Chiaretti S, Guarini A, De Propris MS, Tavolaro S, Intoppa S, Vitale A, et al. (2006) ZAP-70 expression in acute lymphoblastic leukemia: association with the E2A/PBX1 rearrangement and the pre-B stage of differentiation and prognostic implications. Blood. 107(1):197-204.

[41] Deaglio S, Vaisitti T, Aydin S, Bergui L, D'Arena G, Bonello L, et al. (2007) CD38 and ZAP-70 are functionally linked and mark CLL cells with high migratory potential. Blood. 110(12):4012-4021.

[42] Richardson SJ, Matthews C, Catherwood MA, Alexander HD, Carey BS, Farrugia J, et al. (2006) ZAP-70 expression is associated with enhanced ability to respond to migratory and survival signals in B-cell chronic lymphocytic leukemia (B-CLL). Blood. 107(9):3584-3592.

[43] Shimoda K, Kato K, Aoki K, Matsuda T, Miyamoto A, Shibamori M, et al. (2000) Tyk2 plays a restricted role in IFN alpha signaling, although it is required for IL-12-mediated T cell function. Immunity. 13(4):561-571.

[44] Hoyt R, Wei Z, Cerignoli F, Alonso A, Mustelin T, and David M (2007) Cutting Edge: Selective Tyrosine Dephosphorylation of Interferon-Activated Nuclear STAT5 by the VHR Phosphatase. J. Immunol. 179(6):3402-3406.

[45] Silva, CM (2004) Role of STATs as downstream signal transducers in Src family kinase-mediated tumorigenesis. Oncogene. 23:8017-8023.
[46] Sang QX, Man YG, Sung YM, Khamis ZI, Zhang L, Lee MH, et al. (2012) Non-receptor tyrosine kinase 2 reaches its lowest expression levels in human breast cancer during regional nodal metastasis. Clin. Exp. Metastasis. 29(2):143-153.
[47] Kang TH and Kim KT (2006) Negative regulation of ERK activity by VRK3-mediated activation of VHR phosphatase. Nat. Cell Biol. 8(8):863-869.
[48] Hennig EE, Mikula M, Rubel T, Dadlez M, Ostrowski J (2012) Comparative kinome analysis to identify putative colon tumor biomarkers. J. Mol. Med. (Berl). 90(4):447-456.
[49] Yuan Y, Li DM, Sun H (1998) PIR1, a novel phosphatase that exhibits high affinity to RNA . ribonucleoprotein complexes. J, Biol. Chem. 273(32):20347-20353.
[50] Matter N, Herrlich P, Konig H (2002) Signal-dependent regulation of splicing via phosphorylation of Sam68. Nature. 420(6916):691-695.
[51] Arch R, Wirth K, Hofmann M, Ponta H, Matzku S, Herrlich P, et al. (1992) Participation in normal immune responses of a metastasis-inducing splice variant of CD44. Science. 257(5070):682-685.
[52] Blair CA and Zi X (2011) Potential molecular targeting of splice variants for cancer treatment. Indian J. Exp. Biol. 49(11):836-839.
[53] Caprara G, Zamponi R, Melixetian M, Helin K (2009) Isolation and characterization of DUSP11, a novel p53 target gene. J. Cell Mol. Med. 13(8B):2158-2170.
[54] Suzuki K and Matsubara H (2011) Recent advances in p53 research and cancer treatment. J. Biomed. Biotechnol. 2011:978312.
[55] Hanahan D, Weinberg RA (2011) Hallmarks of cancer: the next generation. Cell. 144(5):646-674.
[56] Hirai M, Yoshida S, Kashiwagi H, Kawamura T, Ishikawa T, Kaneko M, et al. (1999) 1q23 gain is associated with progressive neuroblastoma resistant to aggressive treatment. Genes Chromosomes Cancer. 25:261-269.
[57] Gratias S, Schuler A, Hitpass LK, Stephan H, Rieder H, Schneider S, et al. (2005) Genomic gains on chromosome 1q in retinoblastoma: consequences on gene expression and association with clinical manifestation. Int. J. Cancer. 116:555-563.
[58] Mendrzyk F, Korshunov A, Benner A, Toedt G, Pfister S, Radlwimmer B, et al. (2006) Identification of Gains on 1q and Epidermal Growth Factor Receptor Overexpression as Independent Prognostic Markers in Intracranial Ependymoma. Clin. Cancer Res. 12:2070-2079.
[59] Biernacki MA, Marina O, Zhang W, Liu F, Bruns I, Cai A, et al. (2010) Efficacious immune therapy in chronic myelogenous leukemia (CML) recognizes antigens that are expressed on CML progenitor cells. Cancer Res. 70(3):906-915.
[60] Kresse SH, Berner JM, Meza-Zepeda LA, Gregory SG, Kuo WL, Gray JW, et al. (2005) Mapping and characterization of the amplicon near APOA2 in 1q23 in human sarcomas by FISH and array CGH. Mol. Cancer. 4:39.
[61] Muda M, Manning ER, Orth K, Dixon JE (1999) Identification of the Human YVH1 Protein-tyrosine Phosphatase Orthologue Reveals a Novel Zinc Binding Domain Essential for *in Vivo* Function. J. of Biol. Chem. 274:23991-23995.

[62] MacKeigan JP, Murphy LO, Blenis J (2005) Sensitized RNAi screen of human kinases and phosphatases identifies new regulators of apoptosis and chemoresistance. Nat. Cell Biol. 7:591-600.

[63] Sharda PR, Bonham CA, Mucaki EJ, Butt Z, Vacratsis PO (2009) The dual-specificity phosphatase hYVH1 interacts with Hsp70 and prevents heat-shock-induced cell death. Biochem. J. 418(2):391-401.

[64] Denu JM and Tanner KG (1998) Specific and reversible inactivation of protein tyrosine phosphatases by hydrogen peroxide: evidence for a sulfenic acid intermediate and implications for redox regulation. Biochemistry. 37(16):5633-5642.

[65] Bonham CA and Vacratsis PO (2009) Redox regulation of the human dual specificity phosphatase YVH1 through disulfide bond formation. J. Biol. Chem. 21;284(34):22853-22864.

[66] Kozarova A, Hudson JW, Vacratsis PO (2011) The dual-specificity phosphatase hYVH1 (DUSP12) is a novel modulator of cellular DNA content. Cell Cycle. 10(10):1669-1678.

[67] Cain EL, Braun SE, Beeser A (2011) Characterization of a human cell line stably over-expressing the candidate oncogene, dual specificity phosphatase 12. PLoS One. 6(4):e18677.

[68] Lochter A, Navre M, Werb Z, Bissell MJ (1999) a1 and a2 Integrins Mediate Invasive Activity of Mouse Mammary Carcinoma Cells through Regulation of Stromelysin-1 Expression. Mol. Biol. Cell. 10:271-282.

[69] Pozzi A, Wary KK, Giancotti FG, Gardner HA (1998) Integrin a1b1 Mediates a Unique Collagen-dependent Proliferation Pathway In Vivo. J. Cell Biol. 142:587-594.

[70] Senger DR, Perruzzi CA, Streit M, Koteliansky VE, de Fougerolles AR, Detmar M (2002) The alpha1beta1 and alpha2beta1 Integrins Provide Critical Support for Vascular Endothelial Growth Factor Signaling, Endothelial Cell Migration, and Tumor Angiogenesis. Am. J. Pathol. 160:195-204.

[71] Birchmeier C, Birchmeier W, Gherardi E, Vande Woude GF (2003) Met, metastasis, motility and more. Nat. Rev. Mol. Cell Biol. 4:915-925.

[72] Fukuda T, Ichimura E, Shinozaki T, Sano T, Kashiwabara K, Oyama T, et al. (1998) Coexpression of HGF and c-MET/HGF receptor in human bone and sof tissue tumors. Pathol. Int. 48:757-762.

[73] Mueller MM, Fusenig NE (2004) Friends or foes - bipolar effects of the tumour stroma in cancer. Nat. Rev. Cancer. 4(11):839-849.

[74] Guan K, Hakes DJ, Wang Y, Park HD, Cooper TG, Dixon JE (1992) A yeast protein phosphatase related to the vaccinia virus VH1 phosphatase is induced by nitrogen starvation. Proc. Natl. Acad. Sci. U. S. A. 89:12175-12179.

[75] Sakumoto N, Mukai Y, Uchida K, Kouchi T, Kuwajima J, Nakagawa Y, et al. (1999) A series of protein phosphatase gene disruptants in Saccharomyces cerevisiae. Yeast. 15(15):1669-1679.

[76] Beeser AE and Cooper TG (2000) The Dual-Specificity Protein Phosphatase Yvh1p Regulates Sporulation, Growth, and Glycogen Accumulation Independently of Catalytic Activity in *Saccharomyces cerevisiae* via the Cycle AMP-Dependent Protein Kinase Cascade. J. Bacteriol. 182:3517-3528.

[77] Kemmler S, Occhipiniti L, Veisu M, Panse VG (2009) Yvh1 is required for a late maturation step in the 60S biogenesis pathway. J. Cell Biol. 186:863-880.

[78] Lo K, Li Z, Wang F, Marcotte EM, Johnson AW (2009) Ribosome stalk assembly requires the dual-specificity phosphatase Yvh1 for the exchange of Mrt4 with P0. J. Cell Biol. 186:849-862.

[79] Kressler D, Hurt E, Bassler J (2010) Driving ribosome assembly. Biochim. Biophys. Acta. 1803(6):673-683.

[80] Rotenberg MO, Moritz M, Woolford JL, Jr (1988) Depletion of Saccharomyces cerevisiae ribosomal protein L16 causes a decrease in 60S ribosomal subunits and formation of half-mer polyribosomes. Genes Dev. 2(2):160-172.

[81] Liu Y and Chang A (2009) A mutant plasma membrane protein is stabilized upon loss of Yvh1, a novel ribosome assembly factor. Genetics. 181(3):907-915.

[82] Tchorzewski M, Krokowski D, Rzeski W, Issinger OG, Grankowski N (2003) The subcellular distribution of the human ribosomal "stalk" components: P1, P2 and P0 proteins. Int. J. Biochem. Cell Biol. 35(2):203-211.

[83] Sugiyama M, Nugroho S, Iida N, Sakai T, Kaneko Y, Harashima S (2011) Genetic interactions of ribosome maturation factors Yvh1 and Mrt4 influence mRNA decay, glycogen accumulation, and the expression of early meiotic genes in Saccharomyces cerevisiae. J. Biochem. 150(1):103-111.

[84] Lo KY, Li Z, Bussiere C, Bresson S, Marcotte EM, Johnson AW (2010) Defining the pathway of cytoplasmic maturation of the 60S ribosomal subunit. Mol. Cell. 30;39(2):196-208.

[85] Silvera D, Formenti SC, Schneider RJ (2010) Translational control in cancer. Nat. Rev. Cancer. 10(4):254-266.

[86] Calkhoven CF, Muller C, Leutz A (2002) Translational control of gene expression and disease. Trends Mol. Med. 8(12):577-583.

[87] Wu Q, Huang S, Sun Y, Gu S, Lu F, Dai J, et al. (2006) Dual specificity phosphotase 18, interacting with SAPK, dephosphorylates SAPK and inhibits SAPK/JNK signal pathway in vivo. Front Biosci. 11:2714-2724.

[88] Jeong DG, Cho YH, Yoon TS, Kim JH, Son JH, Ryu SE, Kim SJ (2006) Structure of human DSP18, a member of the dual-specificity protein tyrosine phosphatase family. Axta. Crystallogr. D. Biol. Crystallogr. 62:582-588

[89] Wu Q, Gu S, Dai J, Dai J, Wang L, Li Y, et al. (2003) Molecular cloning and characterization of a novel dual-specificity phosphatase18 gene from human fetal brain. Biochim. Biophys. Acta. 1625(3):296-304.

[90] Hood KL, Tobin JF, Yoon C (2002) Identification and characterization of two novel low-molecular-weight dual specificity phosphatases. Biochem. Biophys. Res. Commun. 298(4):545-551.

[91] Rardin MJ, Wiley SE, Murphy AN, Pagliarini DJ, Dixon JE (2008) Dual specificity phosphatases 18 and 21 target to opposing sides of the mitochondrial inner membrane. J. Biol. Chem. 283(22):15440-15450.

[92] Rennefahrt U, Illert B, Greiner A, Rapp UR, Troppmair J (2004) Tumor induction by activated JNK occurs through deregulation of cellular growth. Cancer. Lett. 215(1): 113-124.

[93] Whitfield J, Neame SJ, Paquet L, Bernard O, Ham J (2001) Dominant-negative c-Jun promotes neuronal survival by reducing BIM expression and inhibiting mitochondrial cytochrome c release. Neuron. 29(3):629-643.

[94] Han Z, Boyle DL, Chang L, Bennett B, Karin M, Yang L, et al. (2001) c-Jun N-terminal kinase is required for metalloproteinase expression and joint destruction in inflammatory arthritis. J Clin. Invest. 108(1):73-81.
[95] Bernard-Pierrot I, Gruel N, Stransky N, Vincent-Salomon A, Reyal F, Raynal V, et al. (2008) Characterization of the recurrent 8p11-12 amplicon identifies PPAPDC1B, a phosphatase protein, as a new therapeutic target in breast cancer. Cancer Res. 68(17):7165-7175.
[96] Feldman AL, Dogan A, Smith DI, Law ME, Ansell SM, Johnson SH, et al. (2011) Discovery of recurrent t(6;7)(p25.3;q32.3) translocations in ALK-negative anaplastic large cell lymphomas by massively parallel genomic sequencing. Blood. 117(3):915-919.
[97] Jantus Lewintre E, Reinoso Martin C, Montaner D, Marin M, Jose Terol M, Farras R, et al. (2009) Analysis of chronic lymphotic leukemia transcriptomic profile: differences between molecular subgroups. Leuk. Lymphoma. 50(1):68-79.
[98] Alonso A, Merlo JJ, Na S, Kholod N, Jaroszewski L, Kharitonenkov A, et al. (2002) Inhibition of T cell antigen receptor signaling by VHR-related MKPX (VHX), a new dual specificity phosphatase related to VH1 related (VHR). J. Biol. Chem. 277(7):5524-5528.
[99] Aoyama K, Nagata M, Oshima K, Matsuda T, Aoki N (2001) Molecular cloning and characterization of a novel dual specificity phosphatase, LMW-DSP2, that lacks the cdc25 homology domain. J. Biol. Chem. 276(29):27575-27583.
[100] Chen AJ, Zhou G, Juan T, Colicos SM, Cannon JP, Cabriera-Hansen M, et al. (2002) The dual specificity JKAP specifically activates the c-Jun N-terminal kinase pathway. J. Biol. Chem. 277(39):36592-36601.
[101] Shen Y, Luche R, Wei B, Gordon ML, Diltz CD, Tonks NK (2001) Activation of the Jnk signaling pathway by a dual-specificity phosphatase, JSP-1. Proc. Natl. Acad. Sci. U. S. A. 98(24):13613-13618.
[102] Sekine Y, Ikeda O, Hayakawa Y, Tsuji S, Imoto S, Aoki N, et al. (2007) DUSP22/LMW-DSP2 regulates estrogen receptor-alpha-mediated signaling through dephosphorylation of Ser-118. Oncogene. 26(41):6038-6049.
[103] Chen GG, Zeng Q, Tse GM (2008) Estrogen and its receptors in cancer. Med. Res. Rev. 28(6):954-974.
[104] Li JP, Fu YN, Chen YR, Tan TH (2010) JNK pathway-associated phosphatase dephosphorylates focal adhesion kinase and suppresses cell migration. J. Biol. Chem. 2010 285(8):5472-5478.
[105] Martin GS (2003) Cell signaling and cancer. Cancer Cell. 4(3):167-174.
[106] Schwertassek U, Buckley DA, Xu CF, Lindsay AJ, McCaffrey MW, Neubert TA, et al. (2010) Myristoylation of the dual-specificity phosphatase c-JUN N-terminal kinase (JNK) stimulatory phosphatase 1 is necessary for its activation of JNK signaling and apoptosis. FEBS. J. 277(11):2463-2473.
[107] Caren H, Djos A, Nethander M, Sjoberg RM, Kogner P, Enstrom C, et al. (2011) Identification of epigenetically regulated genes that predict patient outcome in neuroblastoma. BMC Cancer. 11:66.
[108] Tang JP, Tan CP, Li J, Siddique MM, Guo K, Chan SW, et al. (2010) VHZ is a novel centrosomal phosphatase associated with cell growth and human primary cancers. Mol. Cancer. 9:128.

[109] Yu W, Imoto I, Inoue J, Onda M, Emi M, Inazawa J (2007) A novel amplification target, DUSP26, promotes anaplastic thyroid cancer cell growth by inhibiting p38 MAPK activity. Oncogene. 26(8):1178-1187.

[110] Tanuma N, Nomura M, Ikeda M, Kasugai I, Tsubaki Y, Takagaki K, et al. (2009) Protein phosphatase Dusp26 associates with KIF3 motor and promotes N-cadherin-mediated cell-cell adhesion. Oncogene. 28(5):752-761.

[111] Patterson KI, Brummer T, Daly RJ, O'Brien PM (2010) DUSP26 negatively affects the proliferation of epithelial cells, an effect not mediated by dephosphorylation of MAPKs. Biochim. Biophys. Acta. 1803(9):1003-1012.

[112] Shang X, Vasudevan SA, Yu Y, Ge N, Ludwig AD, Wesson CL, et al. (2010) Dual-specificity phosphatase 26 is a novel p53 phosphatase and inhibits p53 tumor suppressor functions in human neuroblastoma. Oncogene. 29(35):4938-4946.

[113] Vasudevan SA, Skoko J, Wang K, Burlingame SM, Patel PN, Lazo JS, et al. (2005) MKP-8, a novel MAPK phosphatase that inhibits p38 kinase. Biochem. Biophys. Res. Commun. 330(2):511-518.

[114] Song M, Park JE, Park SG, Lee do H, Choi HK, Park BC, Ryu SE, Kim JH, Cho S (2009) NSC-87877, Inhibitor of SHP-1/2 PTPs, inhibits dual-specificity phosphatase 26 (DUSP26). Biochem. Biophys. Res. Commun. 381(4):491-495.

[115] Jimbo T, Kawasaki Y, Koyama R, Sato R, Takada S, Haraguchi K, et al. (2002) Identification of a link between the tumour suppressor APC and the kinesin superfamily. Nat. Cell Biol. 4(4):323-327.

[116] Nishimura T, Kato K, Yamaguchi T, Fukata Y, Ohno S, Kaibuchi K (2004) Role of the PAR-3-KIF3 complex in the establishment of neuronal polarity. Nat. Cell Biol. 6(4): 328-334.

[117] Taylor BS, Schultz N, Hieronymus H, Gopalan A, Xiao Y, Carver BS, et al. (2010) Integrative genomic profiling of human prostate cancer. Cancer Cell. 18(1):11-22.

[118] Wishart MJ and Dixon JE (2002) The archetype STYX/dead-phosphatase complexes with a spermatid mRNA-binding protein and is essential for normal sperm production. Proc. Natl. Acad. Sci. U. S. A. 99(4):2112-2117.

[119] Wishart MJ and Dixon JE (1998) Gathering STYX: phosphatase-like form predicts functions for unique protein-interaction domains. Trends Biochem. Sci. 23(8):301-306.

[120] Alonso A, Sasin J, Bottini N, Friedberg I, Friedberg I, Osterman A, et al. (2004) Protein tyrosine phosphatases in the human genome. Cell. 117(6):699-711.

[121] Chen HH, Luche R, Wei B, Tonks NK (2004) Characterization of two distinct dual specificity phosphatases encoded in alternative open reading frames of a single gene located on human chromosome 10q22.2. J. Biol. Chem. 279(40):41404-41413.

[122] Nakamura K, Shima H, Watanabe M, Haneji T, Kikuchi K (1999) Molecular cloning and characterization of a novel dual-specificity protein phosphatase possibly involved in spermatogenesis. Biochem. J. 344 Pt 3:819-825.

[123] Katagiri C, Masuda K, Nomura M, Tanoue K, Fujita S, Yamashita Y, et al. (2011) DUSP13B/TMDP inhibits stress-activated MAPKs and suppresses AP-1-dependent gene expression. Mol. Cell Biochem. 352(1-2):155-162.

[124] Ameyar M, Wisniewska M, Weitzman JB (2003) A role for AP-1 in apoptosis: the case for and against. Biochimie. 85(8):747-752.

[125] Varis A, Wolf M, Monni O, Vakkari ML, Kokkola A, Moskaluk C, et al. (2002) Targets of gene amplification and overexpression at 17q in gastric cancer. Cancer Res. 62(9):2625-2629.

[126] Marti F, Krause A, Post NH, Lyddane C, Dupont B, Sadelain M, et al. (2001) Negative-feedback regulation of CD28 costimulation by a novel mitogen-activated protein kinase phosphatase, MKP6. J. Immunol. 166(1):197-206.

[127] Klinger S, Poussin C, Debril MB, Dolci W, Halban PA, Thorens B (2008) Increasing GLP-1-induced beta-cell proliferation by silencing the negative regulators of signaling cAMP response element modulator-alpha and DUSP14. Diabetes. 57(3):584-593.

[128] Park JE, Park BC, Song M, Park SG, Lee do H, Park SY, et al. (2009) PTP inhibitor IV protects JNK kinase activity by inhibiting dual-specificity phosphatase 14 (DUSP14). Biochem. Biophys. Res. Commun. 387(4):795-799.

[129] Yoon TS, Jeong DG, Kim JH, Cho YH, Son JH, Lee JW, et al. (2005) Crystal structure of the catalytic domain of human VHY, a dual-specificity protein phosphatase. Proteins. 61(3):694-697.

[130] Alonso A, Narisawa S, Bogetz J, Tautz L, Hadzic R, Huynh H, et al. (2004) VHY, a novel myristoylated testis-restricted dual specificity protein phosphatase related to VHX. J. Biol. Chem. 279(31):32586-32591.

[131] Jerez-Timaure NC, Eisen EJ, Pomp D (2005) Fine mapping of a QTL region with large effects on growth and fatness on mouse chromosome 2. Physiol. Genomics 21(3):411-422.

[132] Zama T, Aoki R, Kamimoto T, Inoue K, Ikeda Y, Hagiwara M (2002) A novel dual specificity phosphatase SKRP1 interacts with the MAPK kinase MKK7 and inactivates the JNK MAPK pathway. Implication for the precise regulation of the particular MAPK pathway. J. Biol. Chem. 277(26):23909-23918.

[133] Friedberg I, Nika K, Tautz L, Saito K, Cerignoli F, Friedberg I, et al. (2007) Identification and characterization of DUSP27, a novel dual-specific protein phosphatase. FEBS Lett. 581(13):2527-2533.

Chapter 5

DNA Repair Molecules and Cancer Therapeutical Responses

Yasuko Kitagishi, Mayumi Kobayashi and Satoru Matsuda

Additional information is available at the end of the chapter

http://dx.doi.org/10.5772/53532

1. Introduction

Cells are equipped with the multiple DNA repair mechanisms to deal with DNA damage and transduce the signal downward, which provokes a process to inhibit cell cycle progression and to induce DNA repair [1, 2]. The main DNA damage recognition molecule is ataxia telangiectasia-mutated (ATM), which is a checkpoint kinase that phosphorylates a number of proteins including p53 and BRCA1 in response to DNA damage (**Figure 1**), and thus induce the response to it [3, 4]. Mutations in the ATM have been associated with increased risk of developing a cancer. In addition, it is well known that mutations in the p53 and BRCA1 tumor suppressor genes account for a certain amount of cancers. The p53 protein is a key transcription factor that regulates several signaling pathways involved in the cellular response to genome stress and DNA damage. Through the stress-induced activation, p53 triggers the expression of target genes that protect the genetic integrity of cells [5, 6]. Normal cells show an exquisite balance among these various mechanisms of DNA repair.

Genomic instability is often linked to DNA repair deficiencies. Standard DNA repair pathways available in mammalian cells include homologous repair, nonhomologous end joining, single strand annealing and so on. Those are different pathways that repair DNA double strand breaks (DSBs) [7]. The DNA repair is essential for the survival of both normal and cancer cells. An elaborate set of signaling pathways detect the DSBs and mediate either survival on the DNA repair or apoptotic cell death [8, 9]. The DNA damaging agents for cancer therapies are potent inducers of cell death triggered by the apoptosis. Recent advances in basic science have led to a better understanding of the molecular events important in the pathogenesis of cancer. In the present review, we summarize the function of prominent DNA repair molecules and the tumor suppressor gene products, p53 and

BRCA1 (**Figure 2**), at a viewpoint of carcinogenic DNA damage and therapeutical modulation in cancer.

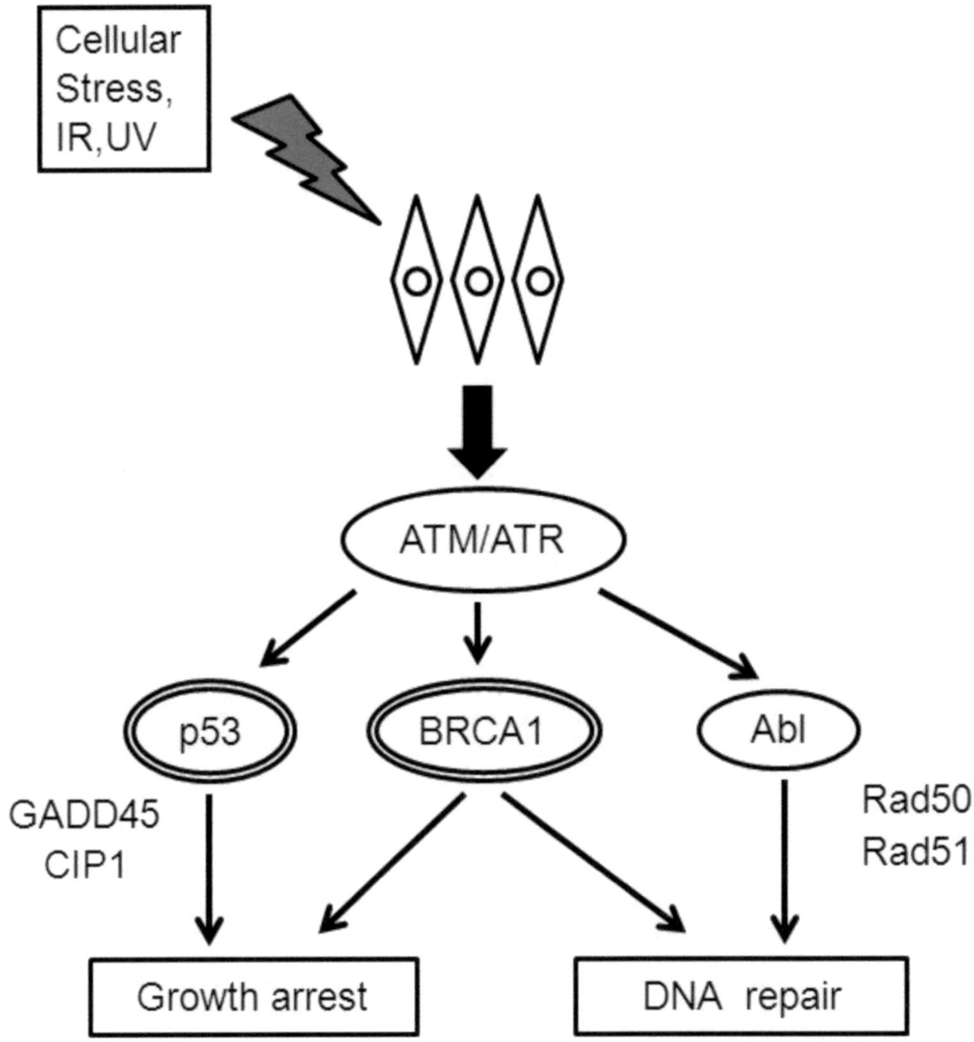

Figure 1. Schematic representation of the DNA repair and Growth arrest signaling pathways. Examples of the molecule known to act on the regulatory pathways are shown.

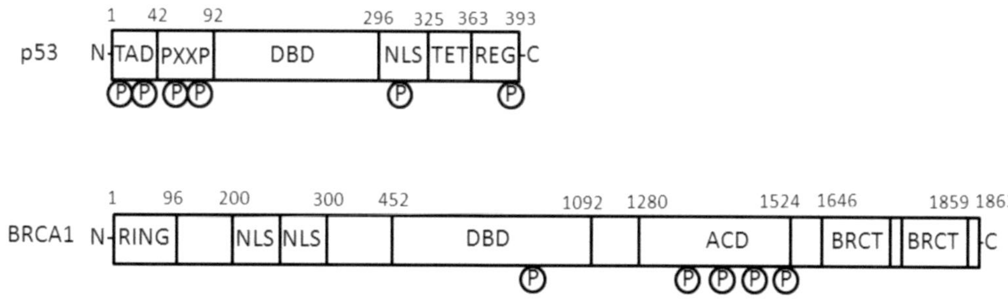

Figure 2. Schematic diagram indicating the domain structures of the p53 and BRCA1 proteins. The functionally important sites including the sites of protein phosphorylation are also shown.

2. Function and involvement of p53 in DNA repair pathway

The p53 is a transcription factor that regulates a number of genes and protects against genomic instability. It is inactive under normal physiological conditions and activated in response to various types of cellular stresses including DNA damage. Under the stress conditions, p53 functions to block cell cycle progression [10], and failure of the DNA repair mechanisms leads to p53 mediated induction of apoptotic cell death programs. The p53 protein is also induced and activated in the nucleus by a stress such as hypoxia and oxidative stress. In addition, p53 undergoes post-translational modifications such as acetylation of lysines, nitration of tyrosines, phosphorylation of serine/threonine residues in response to those stresses [11]. Activated p53 protein regulates its downstream genes and subsequently inhibits malignant transformation of normal cells. Because p53 plays an important role in the transcriptional regulation of genes encoding proteins involved in DNA repair and programmed cell death, the modification of p53 protein appears to be a pivotal determinant of cells fate in some conditions.

The p53 protein is involved in a lot of signaling pathways of cell growth regulation, and multiple mechanisms have been revealed to accomplish the regulation of p53 activity, which determines the selectivity of p53 for specific transcriptional targets, resulting in control of the p53 activity. A large number of molecules capable of activating p53 have been developed. Studies have documented the importance of Mdm2 in the control of the p53 activity [12]. MdmX is also recognized as the p53 negative regulators [13]. A p14 ARF controls the level of p53 by inhibiting the p53-specific ubiquitin ligase MDM2 [14]. The MdmX has been identified as a highly homologous gene that is closely related to Mdm2. Although MdmX possesses a p53 binding domain at its N-terminus, the MdmX does not have ubiquitin ligase activity like Mdm2. The 53BP1 protein also has a role in the cellular response to DNA damage. Convincing evidence exists for the 53BP1 affecting the outcome of DNA double strand break repair [15, 16]. Among a number of transcriptional targets of the p53, the p21WAF1 has been shown to play an important role in both p53-dependent and independent pathways [17]. The p21 WAF1 inhibits cell cycle progression through interaction with the cyclin and CDK complexes. CLCA2 has been reported as a p53 target gene that regulates the p53 induced apoptotic pathways. In addition, CLCA2 has been shown to be down-regulated in breast cancer tissues [18]. ABL1 includes nuclear localization signals and a DNA binding domain through which it mediates DNA damage repair functions. Several ABL targets including the p53 are primary regulators for the DNA damage induced apoptosis [19, 20]. Ciz1 is an estrogen-responsive gene (ER), whose product co-regulates ER by enhancing its transactivation activity. The Ciz1 protein induces hypersensitivity of breast cancer cells to estrogen and induces the expression of ER target gene such as cyclin D1 [21]. Moreover, Ciz1 promotes the proliferation, anchorage independent growth of breast cancer cells. The Ciz1 protein also interacts with a novel protein named PDRG1, which is regulated by the p53 and DNA damage [22].

The gene of the p53 is frequently mutated in multiple cancer tissues, suggesting that p53 plays a critical role in preventing cancers. Studies have shown that p53 is mutated or deleted in nearly half of all human cancers. During neoplastic progression, the p53 is often mutated and fails to perform its normal functions. Mutant p53 can be classified as a loss of function or a gain of function proteins depending on the type of mutation. The p53 activation by something cellular regulator including a gain of function-mutation may lead to regression of an early neoplastic lesion, and therefore may be important in developing cancer chemo-prevention.

3. Function and involvement of BRCA1 in DNA repair pathway

Mutations in the tumor suppressor gene BRCA1 confer an increased risk for the development of breast and ovarian cancers [23]. BRCA1 hereditary breast cancer is a type of cancer with defects in a DNA repair pathway. Actually, mutation of a single allele of the cancer susceptibility gene BRCA1 is associated with increased genomic instability in human breast epithelial cells [24], which accelerates the mutation rate of other critical genes. Several functions of BRCA1 may contribute to its tumor suppressor activity including roles in the DNA repair. Although BRCA1 gene mutations are rare in sporadic breast and/or ovarian cancers, BRCA1 protein expression is frequently reduced in the sporadic cases.

The BRCA1 has the important role in concert with BRCA2, Rad50 and Rad51 [25], in order to activate the checkpoints. For example, BRCA1 is colocalized with Rad51, a DNA recombinase related to the bacterial RecA protein. The BRCA1 protein becomes hyper-phosphorylated after exposure to the DNA damaging agents, and the function of BRCA1 seems to be regulated by the phosphorylation in response to DNA damage. Pharmacological inhibition of poly-ADP-ribose polymerase induces cell death in tumors with mutations in certain DNA repair pathways, when combined with DNA damaging chemotherapies. Then, poly-ADP-ribose polymerase inhibitors have been investigated for the treatment of patients with BRCA 1 mutation, as a strategy to potentiate the DNA damaging effects of chemotherapy and irradiation [26, 27].

The BRCA1 plays an important role in maintaining genomic integrity by protecting cells from double-strand breaks that arise after DNA damage. The BRCA1 cDNA encodes for 1863 amino acids protein with an amino terminal zinc ring finger motif and two putative nuclear localization signals (**Figure 2**). The amino-terminal domain possesses E3 ubiquitin ligase activity [28] and the carboxyl-terminal domain is involved in binding to specific phospho-proteins. The role of BRCA1 in cell cycle control has been understood by its ability to interact with various cyclins and cyclin-dependent kinases. The BRCA1 activates the CDK inhibitor p21 and the p53 tumor suppressor protein, which regulates several genes that control cell cycle checkpoints. BRCA1 also has binding domains for Rb, Rad50 and Rad51 [29, 30]. They may also be involved in DNA double strand break repair. Previous studies have suggested that the BRCA1 pathway dysfunction may also provide an opportunity for therapeutic intervention.

4. DNA repair and cancer therapy

DNA damaging strategies are frequently used as nonsurgical therapies against cancers. Among them, methylating agents such as cisplatin and ionizing radiation are important. DNA double strand breaks are induced following the exposure to the methylating agents [31]. Those also activate the DNA damage checkpoints, which induce cell cycle arrest in order to repair the DNA damage. However, down-regulation of DNA repair mechanism promotes genetic instability, which can lead to carcinogenesis. When defects in certain DNA repair molecules are present in immune system, for example, lymphocyte development can be compromised and the patients can consequently develop primary immune-deficiencies. Those patients often have a predisposition for cancer development. An additional consequence of defective DNA repair is cellular hypersensitivity to DNA damaging agents [32]. In another words, DNA damaging agents work well in cells with DNA repair defects. Mutations in BRCA1, for example, make cancer cells highly susceptible to inhibitors of a DNA repair pathway such as poly-ADP-ribose polymerase [33]. Inhibition of DNA repair pathway also seems to block the mechanisms that are required for survival in the presence of oncogenic mutations. As the consequence, selective elimination of the mutation bearing cells occurs, which can upregulate the DNA repair system. Epigenetic mechanisms such as histone modifications and DNA methylation have been evaluated with a view for enhancing the cancer therapy via the regulation of the expression of genes involved in DNA repair [34].

Treatment of cancers with DNA damaging therapy causes cytotoxicity through induction of high levels of the DNA damage. Cancer cells also respond to DNA damage by activation of the DNA repair and may counteract chemo and radiation efficacy. Actually, DNA repair have been shown to influence radiosensitivity, and the activation of DNA repair of cancer cells might be one of the most important factors in the therapeutical resistance. Inactivation of ATM give rise to cell cycle defects in response to irradiation and radiosensitise cancer cells [35]. In this way, Zebularine and 5-aza-2'-deoxycytidine are employed as radiosensitizing agents [36, 37]. Histone deacetylase inhibitors such as LBH589 and MS-275 have been shown to enhance radiosensitivity through the similar mechanisms [38]. Several histone deacetylase inhibitors exert direct cytotoxic effects and sensitize cancer cells to radiotherapy. For example, trichostatin A, which is the potent histone deacetylase inhibitor enhances radiosensitivity in a variety of human cancers [39]. A previous study has demonstrated that a histone deacetylase inhibitor downregulate the expression of Rad51, which participate in the DNA repair pathway. The marine product, psammaplin A, has been shown to have potent cytotoxicity against several cancer cells. As psammaplin A has been shown to exhibit histone deacetylase inhibitory activity, this may be a promising radiosensitizing agent [40]. Actually, the psammaplin A has the potential to increase radiosensitivity in lung cancer A549 and glioblastoma U373MG cells. Thus, it has been found that a variety of histone deacetylase inhibitors synergistically enhance the growth inhibition and apoptosis of DNA damaging drugs. As numerous parameters may influence cancer therapeutical sensitivity, the impairment of DNA repair may be one of the most crucial mechanisms underlying enhanced the therapeutical responses. So, detection of DNA damage and repair pathways is important component of the intrinsic therapy sensitivity (**Figure 3**).

Platinum compounds such as cisplatin and carboplatin are one of the most widely used and effective chemotherapeutic agents for several cancers including cerebellar tumor and medulloblastoma [41]. However, cancer cells often develop resistance to those genotoxic drugs. Improvements of the effectiveness to cancers are urgently needed. Some cell lines develop acute resistance to cisplatin in the presence of estrogen receptor antagonist. In the presence of it, cisplatin treated medulloblastoma cells show recruitment of Rad51 to the sites of damaged DNA lesions, and increase DNA repair activity. BRCA1 is required for subnuclear assembly of the Rad51 and survival following treatment with the cisplatin [42]. DNA damage in MCF7 cells in which estrogen receptor is activated, lead to the inhibition of cell cycle checkpoint, which results in less effective DNA repair [43]. DNA damage in the cancer cells in which estrogen receptor is inhibited, result in better DNA repair and improved cell survival, which attenuated cytotoxic action of cisplatin.

Proper intake of dietary nutrients including zinc has been considered crucial for preventing the initiation of events leading to the development of cancer. The zinc is an essential element that is integral to some transcription factors which regulate key cellular functions such as the response to oxidative stress and DNA damage repair. Zinc is involved in stabilization and activation of the p53 that appears to be an important component of the apoptotic process [44]. Thus, zinc provides an effective dietary chemopreventive approach to disease in a cancer, and zinc could be effective in the treatment of several cancers. However, it needs further exploration to investigate the genetic and epigenetic pathways of the effects by the zinc. There is interest in mechanisms of acquired resistance to epidermal growth factor receptor (EGFR) inhibitors that are being used in the treatment of a variety of cancers [45]. Acquired resistance to EGFR inhibitors is associated with the loss of p53 and cross resistance to irradiation. The p53 may enhance sensitivity to irradiation via induction of DNA damage repair at this point. The cytotoxic agents target stabilization of p53 through DNA damage. Thus, p53 represents an attractive target for therapeutic design and development of anticancer agents. Restoration of hypoxia induced p53-mediated signaling may well be effective in the targeting of hypoxic cells [46]. The DNA damage response is also induced in cells by the hypoxia.

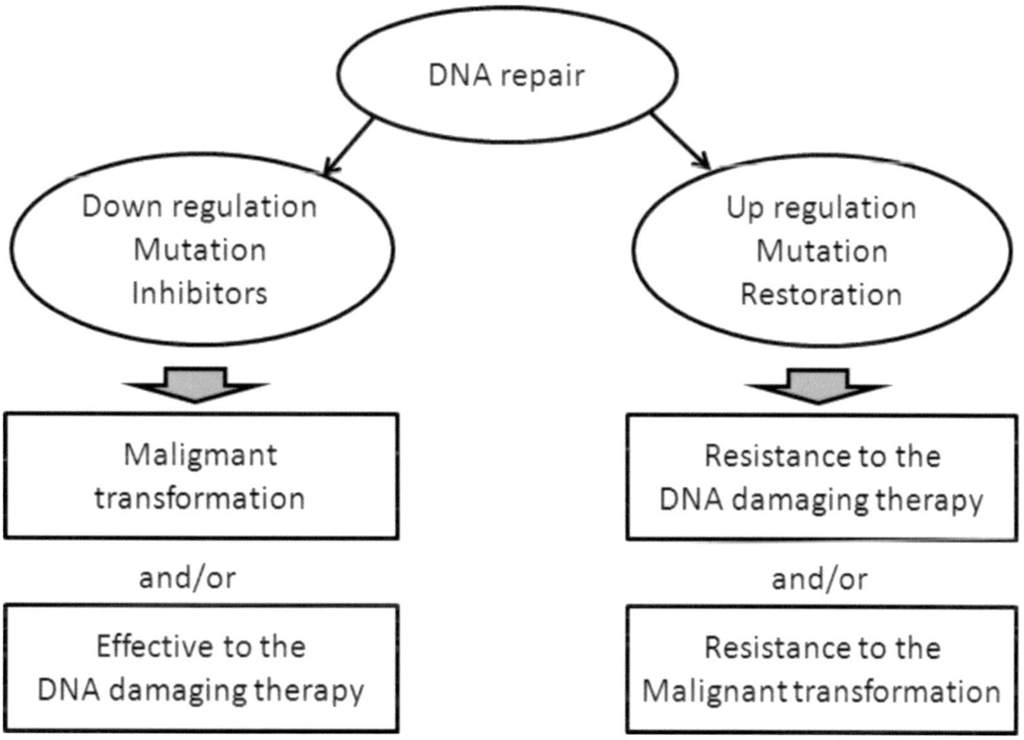

Figure 3. Implication of DNA repair modulations in cancer. DNA repair downregulation can contribute to genomic instability, which promotes malignant transformation of cells, and leads to cellular sensitivity to DNA damaging therapy. DNA repair upregulation can contribute to genomic stability, which lead to acquired resistance to the DNA damaging therapy.

5. Perspective

It has been paid more attention to the DNA repair as a therapeutic target, because DNA repair enzymes regulation and specific cytotoxic cancer therapy may be possible via the mechanism based on the appropriate DNA damaging approaches (**Figure 4**). The cancer cell genome is aberrant as a consequence of incomplete DNA repair. As many anticancer drugs further reduce the integrity of DNA, they may be able to cause more mutations and another cancer, if the lesions are not repaired. However, cancer cells, in which its DNA repair is down-regulated, have been shown to exhibit increased sensitivity to DNA damaging chemotherapy. A new therapeutic approach will be possibly developed, in which radiation therapy or cytotoxic anticancer agents are employed in conjunction with the DNA repair modulators. For example, cells exposing to hypoxia are sensitive to inhibition of components of the DNA damage response. The DNA damage response induced by hypoxia is distinct from the classical pathways induced by the DNA damaging agents due to the coincident repression of DNA repair in hypoxic conditions. The principle aims of the hypoxia induced DNA damage response seem to be the induction of p53 dependent apoptosis. Such combinations can cause severe genomic instability in cancer cells resulting

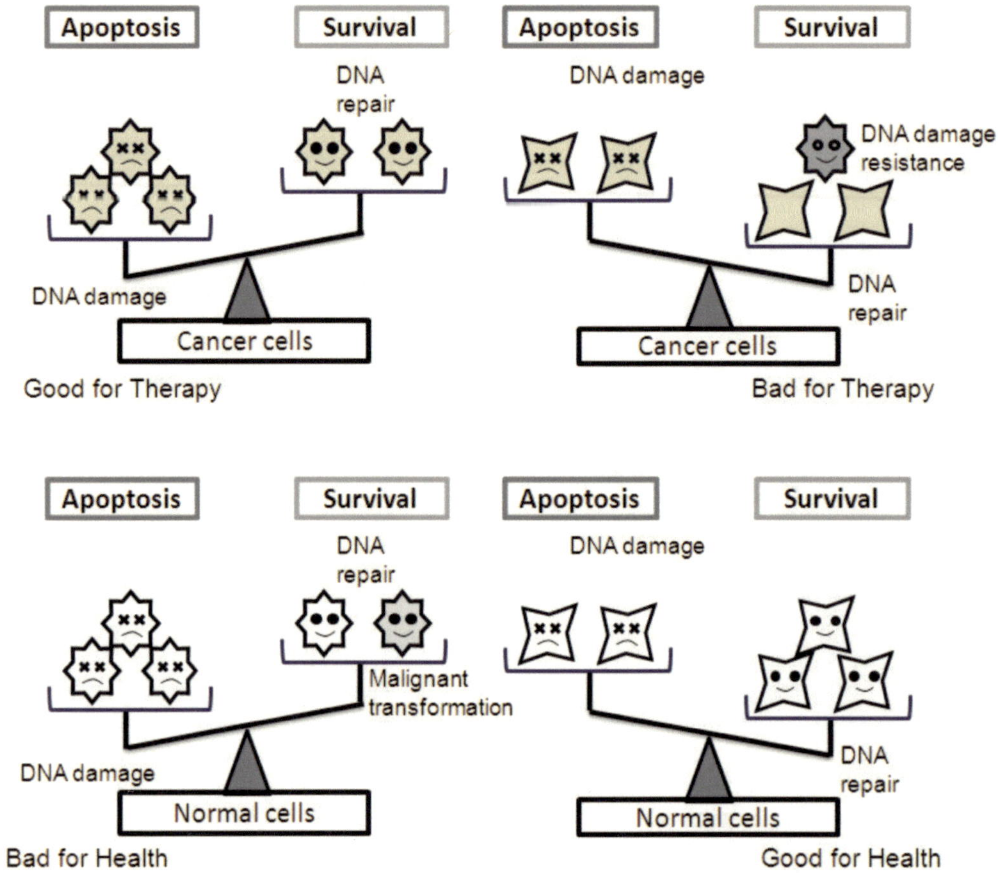

Figure 4. Survival or Apoptosis, that's the problem in cancer therapy and for individual health. The determination either survival or apoptosis is due to the balance between DNA damage and the DNA repair levels in cells.

in apoptotic cancer cell death. Tumor recurrence frequently occurs after genome damaging therapy, but the characteristics and the behavior of resistant cancer cells remain unknown. Recently, it has been reported that the peri-necrotic tumor cells after radiation therapy acquire hypoxia-inducible factor 1 (HIF-1) activity after surviving radiation, which triggers their translocation towards tumor blood vessels. So, the HIF-1 inhibitors suppress the incidence of post-irradiation tumor recurrence [47].

Understanding of the cellular aberrations of cancer cells has allowed the development of therapies to target biological pathways. Active inhibition of DNA repair enzyme in a tumor can lead to genomic instability and cell death by exploiting the paradigm of synthetic lethality, which potentiates anti-neoplastic effects of DNA damaging therapy including radiation. Several studies have evaluated the role of DNA repair enzyme inhibitors for treatment of cancer [48, 49]. In conclusion, the combination of DNA damaging agent and DNA repair enzyme inhibitor results in beneficial improved anticancer efficacy. However, side effects of the blocking of DNA repair system on the normal cell may overcome their benefit action. So it is important to precisely investigate the effects in both the target and normal cells. Optimizing treatment according to tumor status for DNA-repair biomarkers such as BRCA1 could predict response to DNA toxic cancer therapies and might improve the response of tumors to the therapies. Variation in DNA repair genes may also be informative. Further investigations will be required to identify other additional mechanisms associated with the therapeutic sensitivity and other epigenetic drugs such as the histone deacetylase inhibitors. Investigations are warranted to determine whether alterations in the methylation patterns of set of genes involved in DNA repair might be modulated by the inhibitors. Also, future studies should be conducted to determine whether the combination of DNA damaging agents and DNA repair modulator has potential for the treatment against cancer.

Competing interests statement

The authors declare that they have no competing financial interests.

Author details

Yasuko Kitagishi, Mayumi Kobayashi and Satoru Matsuda*
Department of Environmental Health Science, Nara Women's University Kita-Uoya, Nishimachi Nara, Japan

Acknowledgement

This work was supported by grants in-aid from the Ministry of Education, Culture, Sports, Science and Technology in Japan and Nara Women's University Intramural Grant for Project Research.

6. References

[1] Frame FM, Maitland NJ (2011) Cancer stem cells, models of study and implications of therapy resistance mechanisms. Adv Exp Med Biol. 720: 105-118.
[2] Athar M, Elmets CA, Kopelovich L (2011) Pharmacological activation of p53 in cancer cells. Curr Pharm Des. 17: 631-639.
[3] Pierce LJ, Haffty BG (2011) Radiotherapy in the treatment of hereditary breast cancer. Semin Radiat Oncol. 21: 43-50.
[4] Bolderson E, Richard DJ, Zhou BB, Khanna KK (2009) Recent advances in cancer therapy targeting proteins involved in DNA double-strand break repair. Clin Cancer Res. 15: 6314-6320.
[5] Bykov VJ, Lambert JM, Hainaut P, Wiman KG (2009) Mutant p53 rescue and modulation of p53 redox state. Cell Cycle. 8: 2509-2517.

* Corresponding Author

[6] Liu B, Chen Y, St Clair DK (2008) ROS and p53: a versatile partnership. Free Radic Biol Med. 44: 1529-1535.

[7] Gostissa M, Alt FW, Chiarle R (2011) Mechanisms that promote and suppress chromosomal translocations in lymphocytes. Annu Rev Immunol. 29: 319-350.

[8] Al-Ejeh F, Kumar R, Wiegmans A, Lakhani SR, Brown MP, Khanna KK (2010) Harnessing the complexity of DNA-damage response pathways to improve cancer treatment outcomes. Oncogene. 29: 6085-6098.

[9] Krystof V, Uldrijan S (2010) Cyclin-dependent kinase inhibitors as anticancer drugs. Curr Drug Targets. 11: 291-302.

[10] Kim E, Giese A, Deppert W (2009) Wild-type p53 in cancer cells: when a guardian turns into a blackguard. Biochem Pharmacol. 77: 11-20.

[11] Kim DH, Kundu JK, Surh YJ (2011) Redox modulation of p53: mechanisms and functional significance. Mol Carcinog. 50: 222-234.

[12] Chen H, Kolman K, Lanciloti N, Nerney M, Hays E, Robson C, Chandar N (2012) p53 and MDM2 are involved in the regulation of osteocalcin gene expression. Exp Cell Res. 318: 867-876.

[13] Biderman L, Poyurovsky MV, Assia Y, Manley JL, Prives C (2012) MdmX Is Required for p53 Interaction with and Full Induction of the Mdm2 Promoter after Cellular Stress. Mol Cell Biol. 32: 1214-1225.

[14] Gallagher SJ, Kefford RF, Rizos H (2006) The ARF tumour suppressor. Int J Biochem Cell Biol. 38: 1637-1641.

[15] Aly A, Ganesan S (2011) BRCA1, PARP, and 53BP1: conditional synthetic lethality and synthetic viability. J Mol Cell Biol. 3: 66-74.

[16] Kobayashi J, Iwabuchi K, Miyagawa K, Sonoda E, Suzuki K, Takata M, Tauchi H (2008) Current topics in DNA double-strand break repair. J Radiat Res. 49: 93-103.

[17] Lo PK, Lee JS, Sukumar S (2012) The p53-p21WAF1 checkpoint pathway plays a protective role in preventing DNA rereplication induced by abrogation of FOXF1 function. Cell Signal. 24: 316-324.

[18] Walia V, Ding M, Kumar S, Nie D, Premkumar LS, Elble RC (2009) hCLCA2 Is a p53-Inducible Inhibitor of Breast Cancer Cell Proliferation. Cancer Res. 69:6624-6632.

[19] Gonfloni S (2010) DNA damage stress response in germ cells: role of c-Abl and clinical implications. Oncogene. 29: 6193-6202.

[20] Yamaguchi T, Miki Y, Yoshida K (2010) The c-Abl tyrosine kinase stabilizes Pitx1 in the apoptotic response to DNA damage. Apoptosis. 15: 927-935.

[21] den Hollander P, Rayala SK, Coverley D, Kumar R (2006) Ciz1, a Novel DNA-binding coactivator of the estrogen receptor alpha, confers hypersensitivity to estrogen action. Cancer Res. 66: 11021-11029.

[22] Jiang L, Luo X, Shi J, Sun H, Sun Q, Sheikh MS, Huang Y (2011) PDRG1, a novel tumor marker for multiple malignancies that is selectively regulated by genotoxic stress. Cancer Biol Ther. 11: 567-573.

[23] Chionh F, Mitchell G, Lindeman GJ, Friedlander M, Scott CL (2011) The role of poly adenosine diphosphate ribose polymerase inhibitors in breast and ovarian cancer: current status and future directions. Asia Pac J Clin Oncol. 7: 197-211.

[24] Konishi H, Mohseni M, Tamaki A, Garay JP, Croessmann S, Karnan S, Ota A, Wong HY, Konishi Y, Karakas B, Tahir K, Abukhdeir AM, Gustin JP, Cidado J, Wang GM, Cosgrove D, Cochran R, Jelovac D, Higgins MJ, Arena S, Hawkins L, Lauring J, Gross AL, Heaphy CM, Hosokawa Y, Gabrielson E, Meeker AK, Visvanathan K, Argani P, Bachman KE, Park BH (2011) Mutation of a single allele of the cancer susceptibility gene BRCA1 leads to genomic instability in human breast epithelial cells. Proc Natl Acad Sci U S A. 108: 17773-17778.

[25] Rebbeck TR, Mitra N, Domchek SM, Wan F, Chuai S, Friebel TM, Panossian S, Spurdle A, Chenevix-Trench G; kConFab, Singer CF, Pfeiler G, Neuhausen SL, Lynch HT, Garber JE, Weitzel JN, Isaacs C, Couch F, Narod SA, Rubinstein WS, Tomlinson GE, Ganz PA, Olopade OI, Tung N, Blum JL, Greenberg R, Nathanson KL, Daly MB (2009) Modification of ovarian cancer risk by BRCA1/2-interacting genes in a multicenter cohort of BRCA1/2 mutation carriers. Cancer Res. 69: 5801-5810.

[26] Orlando L, Schiavone P, Fedele P, Calvani N, Nacci A, Cinefra M, D'Amico M, Mazzoni E, Marino A, Sponziello F, Morelli F, Lombardi L, Silvestris N, Cinieri S (2012) Poly (ADP-ribose) polymerase (PARP): rationale, preclinical and clinical evidences of its inhibition as breast cancer treatment. Expert Opin Ther Targets. 16:S83-S89.

[27] Banerjee S, Kaye S (2011) PARP inhibitors in BRCA gene-mutated ovarian cancer and beyond. Curr Oncol Rep. 13: 442-449.

[28] Shakya R, Reid LJ, Reczek CR, Cole F, Egli D, Lin CS, deRooij DG, Hirsch S, Ravi K, Hicks JB, Szabolcs M, Jasin M, Baer R, Ludwig T (2011) BRCA1 tumor suppression depends on BRCT phosphoprotein binding, but not its E3 ligase activity. Science. 334: 525-528.

[29] Maniccia AW, Lewis C, Begum N, Xu J, Cui J, Chipitsyna G, Aysola K, Reddy V, Bhat G, Fujimura Y, Henderson B, Reddy ES, Rao VN (2009) Mitochondrial localization, ELK-1 transcriptional regulation and growth inhibitory functions of BRCA1, BRCA1a, and BRCA1b proteins. J Cell Physiol. 219: 634-641.

[30] Deng CX, Brodie SG (2000) Roles of BRCA1 and its interacting proteins. Bioessays. 22: 728-737.

[31] Batista LF, Roos WP, Christmann M, Menck CF, Kaina B (2007) Differential sensitivity of malignant glioma cells to methylating and chloroethylating anticancer drugs: p53 determines the switch by regulating xpc, ddb2, and DNA double-strand breaks. Cancer Res. 67: 11886-11895.

[32] Damia G, D'Incalci M (2007) Targeting DNA repair as a promising approach in cancer therapy. Eur J Cancer. 43: 1791-1801.

[33] Nguyen D, Zajac-Kaye M, Rubinstein L, Voeller D, Tomaszewski JE, Kummar S, Chen AP, Pommier Y, Doroshow JH, Yang SX (2011) Poly(ADP ribose) polymerase inhibition enhances p53-dependent and -independent DNA damage responses induced by DNA damaging agent. Cell Cycle. 10: 4074-4082.

[34] Messner S, Hottiger MO (2011) Histone ADP-ribosylation in DNA repair, replication and transcription. Trends Cell Biol. 21: 534-542.

[35] Pugh TJ, Keyes M, Barclay L, Delaney A, Krzywinski M, Thomas D, Novik K, Yang C, Agranovich A, McKenzie M, Morris WJ, Olive PL, Marra MA, Moore RA (2009) Sequence variant discovery in DNA repair genes from radiosensitive and radiotolerant prostate brachytherapy patients. Clin Cancer Res. 15: 5008-5016.

[36] Champion C, Guianvarc'h D, Sénamaud-Beaufort C, Jurkowska RZ, Jeltsch A, Ponger L, Arimondo PB, Guieysse-Peugeot AL (2010) Mechanistic insights on the inhibition of c5 DNA methyltransferases by zebularine. PLoS One. 5: e12388.

[37] Chiam K, Centenera MM, Butler LM, Tilley WD, Bianco-Miotto T (2011) GSTP1 DNA methylation and expression status is indicative of 5-aza-2'-deoxycytidine efficacy in human prostate cancer cells. PLoS One. 6: e25634.

[38] Tan J, Cang S, Ma Y, Petrillo RL, Liu D (2010) Novel histone deacetylase inhibitors in clinical trials as anti-cancer agents. J Hematol Oncol. 3: 5.

[39] Karagiannis TC, Smith AJ, El' Osta A (2004) Radio- and chemo-sensitization of human erythroleukemic K562 cells by the histone deacetylase inhibitor Trichostatin A. Hell J Nucl Med. 7: 184-191.

[40] Ahn MY, Jung JH, Na YJ, Kim HS (2008) A natural histone deacetylase inhibitor, Psammaplin A, induces cell cycle arrest and apoptosis in human endometrial cancer cells. Gynecol Oncol. 108: 27-33.

[41] Paulino AC, Lobo M, Teh BS, Okcu MF, South M, Butler EB, Su J, Chintagumpala M (2010) Ototoxicity after intensity-modulated radiation therapy and cisplatin-based chemotherapy in children with medulloblastoma. Int J Radiat Oncol Biol Phys. 78: 1445-1450.

[42] Wagner JM, Karnitz LM (2009) Cisplatin-induced DNA damage activates replication checkpoint signaling components that differentially affect tumor cell survival. Mol Pharmacol. 76: 208-214.

[43] Cohen B, Shimizu M, Izrailit J, Ng NF, Buchman Y, Pan JG, Dering J, Reedijk M (2010) Cyclin D1 is a direct target of JAG1-mediated Notch signaling in breast cancer. Breast Cancer Res Treat. 123: 113-124.

[44] Song Y, Elias V, Loban A, Scrimgeour AG, Ho E (2010) Marginal zinc deficiency increases oxidative DNA damage in the prostate after chronic exercise. Free Radic Biol Med. 48: 82-88.

[45] Rosell R, Molina MA, Costa C, Simonetti S, Gimenez-Capitan A, Bertran-Alamillo J, Mayo C, Moran T, Mendez P, Cardenal F, Isla D, Provencio M, Cobo M, Insa A, Garcia-Campelo R, Reguart N, Majem M, Viteri S, Carcereny E, Porta R, Massuti B, Queralt C, de Aguirre I, Sanchez JM, Sanchez-Ronco M, Mate JL, Ariza A, Benlloch S, Sanchez JJ, Bivona TG, Sawyers CL, Taron M (2011) Pretreatment EGFR T790M mutation and BRCA1 mRNA expression in erlotinib-treated advanced non-small-cell lung cancer patients with EGFR mutations. Clin Cancer Res. 17: 1160-1168.

[46] Gopalani NK, Meena RN, Prasad DN, Ilavazhagan G, Sharma M (2012) Cooperativity between inhibition of cytosolic K+ efflux and AMPK activation during suppression of hypoxia-induced cellular apoptosis. Int J Biochem Cell Biol. 44: 211-223.

[47] Harada H, Inoue M, Itasaka S, Hirota K, Morinibu A, Shinomiya K, Zeng L, Ou G, Zhu Y, Yoshimura Y, McKenna WG, Muschel RJ, Hiraoka M (2012) Nature Communications 3, DOI: doi:10.1038/ncomms1786. in press.

[48] Davar D, Beumer JH, Hamieh L, Tawbi H (2012) Role of PARP Inhibitors in Cancer Biology and Therapy. Curr Med Chem. 19:3907-3921.

[49] Park Y, Moriyama A, Kitahara T, Yoshida Y, Urita T, Kato R (2012) Triple-negative breast cancer and poly(ADP-ribose) polymerase inhibitors. Anticancer Agents Med Chem. 12:672-677.

Section 3

A New Role of Oncogenes and Tumorsuppressorgenes

Chapter 6

Structure-Based Approaches Targeting Oncogene Promoter G-Quadruplexes

Dik-Lung Ma, Victor Pui-Yan Ma, Ka-Ho Leung, Hai-Jing Zhong, Hong-Zhang He, Daniel Shiu-Hin Chan and Chung-Hang Leung

Additional information is available at the end of the chapter

http://dx.doi.org/10.5772/54809

1. Introduction

The genetic information stored in DNA can be transcribed and translated into functional proteins with various biological roles, and the control of gene expression and cell division is tightly controlled under normal physiological conditions. However, genetic mutations arising during DNA replication can trigger uncontrolled cell growth, leading to the development of various types of cancers (Croce 2008). The cellular transformational events associated with cancer have been linked with mutations in particular genes, termed proto-oncogenes. These genes are necessary for the normal development and differentiation of cells, but when mutated into oncogenes they can lead to the overexpression of proteins involved in signal transduction and mitosis, ultimately resulting in cancer development. Blocking oncogenic translation using siRNAs has attracted intense attention in the literature (Heidenreich 2009; Ventura et al. 2009), but inhibiting oncogenic transcription through targeting DNA itself has been less explored.

While DNA is a well-established biomolecular target for anti-cancer therapy, most DNA-binding drugs such as cisplatin (Alderden et al. 2006) and its analogues interact with DNA non-selectively, resulting in adverse side effects (Jung et al. 2007). Consequently, this has driven interest in the targeting of unusual, non-canonical structures in DNA, in order to achieve selectivity for particular (onco)genes while potentially reducing adverse side effects. One such DNA structure that has attracted significant attention in the recent literature as an anti-cancer target is the G-quadruplex. While G-quadruplexes were initially regarded as somewhat of a structural curiosity when they were first discovered, accumulating evidence over the past decade have suggested that these non-canonical DNA structures may play important roles in modulating various biological processes (Lipps et al. 2009).

G-quadruplexes are four-stranded guanine-rich DNA structures that were first found at the ends of eukaryotic telomeres, and the role of telomeric G-quadruplexes for inhibiting telomerase activity has been intensely studied since the early 1990s (Blackburn 1991). Human telomeric DNA is usually 4–14 kilobases long, and is comprised of TTAGGG tandem repeats. Up-regulated telomerase activity in cancer cells maintains the length of telomeres after cell division, conferring immortality. Hurley and co-workers demonstrated that the activity of telomerase can be inhibited by small molecule-induced stabilization of telomeric G-quadruplex (Wheelhouse et al. 1998).

A few years later, Hurley and co-workers reported the seminal discovery of a potential G-quadruplex structure in the nuclease hypersensitive element III_1 ($NHEIII_1$) of the promoter region of the c-*myc* oncogene, and they further demonstrated that the transcriptional repression of c-*myc* can be achieved by induction of putative G-quadruplex formation by a small molecule (Siddiqui-Jain et al. 2002). Evidently, c-*myc* transcription was inhibited by the putative formation of the G-quadruplex structure in the promoter region, thus suppressing oncogenic expression. Later, other studies identified the presence of G-quadruplex-forming sequences in the promoter regions of other oncogenes such as c-*kit* (Rankin et al. 2005), KRAS (Cogoi et al. 2006), *bcl*-2 (Dai et al. 2006) and VEGF (Jiang et al. 1991). In 2007, Huppert and Balasubramanian conducted a large-scale bioinformatics analysis throughout the human genome, and found that G-quadruplex-forming sequences are enriched in the promoter regions of genes, and that >40% of annotated genes bears at least one potential G-quadruplex sequence within 1kb of the transcription start site (Huppert et al. 2007). Recent evidence has suggested that G-quadruplexes may exist *in vivo* and may play putative roles in various biological processes, such as the regulation of gene expression (Dexheimer et al. 2009; Gonzalez et al. 2009). Consequently, targeting the oncogenic G-quadruplexes using small molecules has emerged as an alternative strategy for the potential treatment of cancers (Balasubramanian et al. 2009).

Since the discovery of the first c-*myc* G-quadruplex stabilizer TMPyP4 and inhibitor of c-*myc* oncogenic expression by Hurley and co-workers, many other c-*myc* interactive small molecule ligands have been identified. For example, cationic porphyrins (Grand et al. 2002), quindoline and berberine derivatives (Ou et al. 2007; Lu et al. 2008; Ma et al. 2008), and trisubstituted isoalloxazines (Bejugam et al. 2007) have been demonstrated to interfere with the oncogenic transcription *in vitro*. Quarfloxin, developed by Cylene Pharmaceuticals, entered clinical trials due to its ability to interact with G-quadruplexes *in vivo* (Duan et al. 2001). Interestingly, quarfloxin concentrates in the nucleus and disrupts the G-quadruplex-nucleolin interaction, leading to the redistribution of nucleolin in the nucleoplasm which ultimately triggers the apoptosis and inhibition of cancer cell growth.

With advances in computer processing power and in the development of algorithms for molecular stimulation and docking, the use of high-throughput virtual screening for drug discovery has become increasingly popular (McInnes 2007). The rapid screening of a large chemical library using computational programs can efficiently weed out non-binding ligands *in silico*, thus dramatically reducing the number of compounds to be tested *in vitro*. While the use of computer-aided virtual screening for discovering enzyme antagonists has been widely employed, the use of computational analysis for identifying G-quadruplex ligands has been comparatively less explored (Ma et al. 2012). In this chapter, we first describe the general structure of G-quadruplexes and their involvement in transcriptional events, particularly those relevant to oncogenic expression. We then discuss the use of *in silico* methods to identify small molecule ligands of oncogenic promoter G-quadruplexes, and identify features or limitations of each method. Finally, we highlight recent, representative, examples of promoter G-quadruplex targeting by small molecules discovered using *in silico* methods.

2. General structure of the G-quadruplex and its involvement in transcriptional events

G-quadruplexes are constructed from stacks of G-tetrads, which consist of four guanine bases aligned in a co-planar arrangement stabilized by Hoogsteen hydrogen-bonding and monovalent cations (e.g. K^+ and Na^+) in the central cavity (Figure 1) (Mergny et al. 1998; Parkinson et al. 2002; Huppert et al. 2007). G-quadruplexes exhibit a high degree of structural polymorphism, contributing to the wide variety of distinct G-quadruplex topologies that differ in strand orientation, loop size, surface and groove dimensions (Burge et al. 2006). Consequently, G-quadruplexes formed from different DNA sequences may exhibit unique structural features that can be specifically targeted by small molecule ligands (Monchaud et al. 2008).

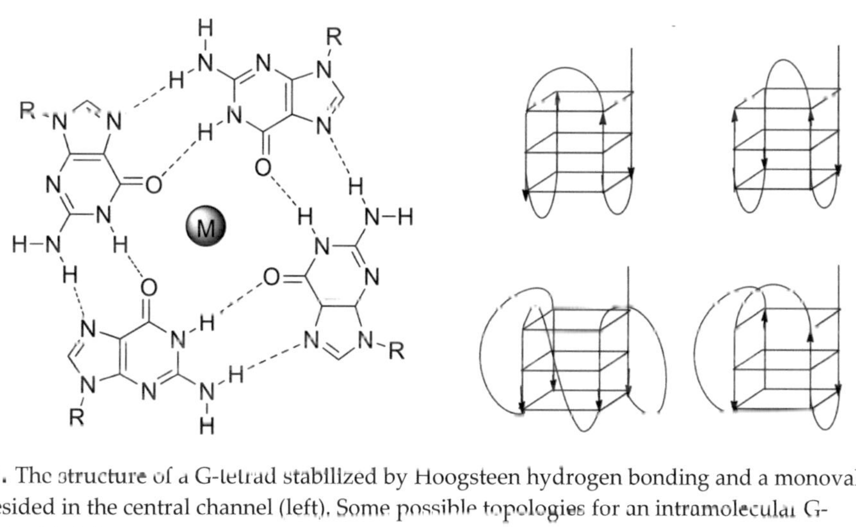

Figure 1. The structure of a G-tetrad stabilized by Hoogsteen hydrogen bonding and a monovalent cation resided in the central channel (left). Some possible topologies for an intramolecular G-quadruplex (right).

As previously mentioned, the occurrence of G-quadruplex-forming regions in the promoter region of oncogenes offers an alternative therapeutic avenue for the treatment of cancer. The induction of the G-quadruplex structure in the promoter region of the target gene could inhibit transcription of the oncogene, thus suppressing the production of the resultant oncoprotein. The potential to repress oncogenic expression by G-quadruplex formation can be illuminated by considering the history of the efforts targeted against well-studied oncogene c-*myc*.

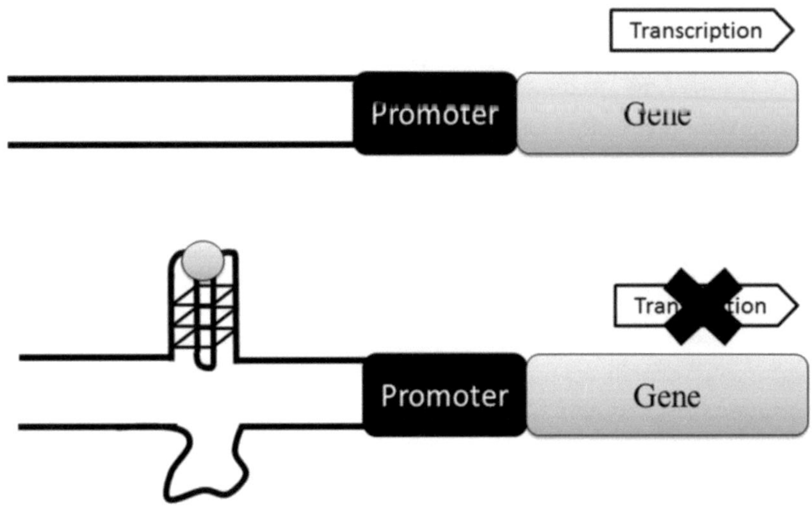

Figure 2. Transcription regulation of oncogenes by promoter G-quadruplex formation mediated by small molecules (circle).

MYC protein is a transcription factor that controls cell proliferation, differentiation and apoptosis (Marcu et al. 1992), and its cellular level is strictly regulated in normal cells. Mutation of c-*myc* and the overexpression of the MYC protein are observed in around 80% of solid tumors, including cervical carcinoma, myeloid leukemias and osteosarcomas (Lutz et al. 2002; Meyer et al. 2008; Wierstra et al. 2008). Accumulating evidence has revealed that the c-*myc* promoter region plays a pivotal role in the regulation of c-*myc* transcriptional activity. In particular, the nuclear hypersensitivity element III_1 (NHE III_1), a 27 bp guanine rich sequence located upstream of the c-*myc* protein, has been reported to control around 90% of c-*myc* transcription (Davis et al. 1989). *In vitro* experiments suggested that this sequence is able to fold into an intramolecular parallel G-quadruplex with predominant 1:2:1 and 2:1:1 loop topologies (Seenisamy et al. 2004). Hurley and co-workers showed the basal transcription activity of c-*myc* can be significantly enhanced by destabilizing the c-*myc* G-quadruplex through a guanine-to-thymine mutation in the quadruplex-forming sequence (Siddiqui-Jain et al. 2002). In the same report, they demonstrated the suppression of oncogenic c-*myc* transcription activity by a cationic porphyrin that can stabilize the G-quadruplex structure (Siddiqui-Jain et al. 2002). These results demonstrated that the c-*myc* promoter G-quadruplex may act as a regulator of oncogenic transcription, and that small molecule stabilizers of the G-quadruplex could potentially down-regulate the expression of oncogenes (Figure 2).

These promoter G-quadruplex-stabilizing ligands have potential advantages as alternative anti-cancer compounds compared to conventional protein or enzyme inhibitors (Balasubramanian et al. 2011). Firstly, since the availability of G-quadruplexes in cells is generally limited, a lower concentration of inhibitor could theoretically be used to achieve the desired biological effect. Secondly, due to the unique structural diversity of G-quadruplex motifs, superior selectivity towards a particular G-quadruplex may be potentially achieved by the rational design and modification of the lead compound. Thirdly, a number of oncogenes such as c-*kit*, BRAF and c-*myc*, which have been reported to contain G-quadruplex-forming motifs in their promoter regions, encode kinase or protein products that have been clinically validated as targets for the treatment of cancer. However, a number of issues remain for the development of effective promoter G-quadruplex ligands for the treatment of human diseases. These include acquiring more detailed and comprehensive structural information on the relevant topologies of G-quadruplexes in living systems, as well as developing ligands with sufficient G-quadruplex selectivity and affinity for potential *in vivo* application. Leading experts Balasubramanian, Hurley and Neidle have recently reviewed the targeting of oncogenic promoter G-quadruplexes as a potential anti-cancer strategy (Balasubramanian et al. 2011).

3. *In silico* methods in drug discovery

Virtual screening techniques have recently emerged as a complementary technique to traditional high-throughput screening technologies employed in the pharmaceutical industry (Shoichet 2004; Ghosh et al. 2006; Cavasotto et al. 2007). Using computer-aided methodologies, large numbers of compounds can be rapidly screened in order to efficiently eliminate non-binding compounds *in silico*, thus dramatically reducing the costs associated with preliminary testing in a drug discovery project. However, while the application of *in silico* techniques for discovering enzyme inhibitors has been well-established, the targeting of DNA structures using virtual screening has been comparatively less explored. Broadly speaking, virtual screening can be sub-divided into pharmacophore modelling and molecular docking. A representative list of commercially available molecular docking softwares for both pharmacophore modelling and molecular docking (receptor-ligand modelling) is given in Table 1.

Pharmacophore modelling can be further classified into structure-based and ligand-based methods. In structure-based pharmacophore modelling, the structure of receptor must be first determined using techniques such as X-ray crystallography and nuclear magnetic resonance (NMR). Alternatively, if the structure of particular target is not known, a model can be constructed by homology with closely-related structures. In general, a structure containing the biomolecular target complexed with its ligand is advantageous for virtual screening since the key features of the interaction between the ligand and the binding pocket can be directly examined. Some commercially available computational software programs such as LIGANDSCOUT (Wolber et al. 2004) and POCKET v.2 (Chen et al. 2006) are able to analyse the binding interaction and calculate the relevant contributions of each feature to the specificity and inhibitory potency of the ligand. Ligand–target interactions can include hydrogen bonding, ionic interactions and hydrophobic interactions, and this information can be harnessed to generate a three-dimensional (3D) pharmacophore model.

Company/Institution	Software	Uses
Accelrys	Discovery Studio, Insight II	Pharmacophore modelling, receptor-ligand docking, de novo drug design, molecular stimulation
MolSoft	ICM-Pro	Pharmacophore modelling, receptor-ligand docking, 3D QSAR model constructions
Tripos	Sybyl	Receptor-ligand docking, chemoinformatics, 3D QSAR model constructions
Scripps Research Institute	Autodock	Receptor-ligand docking
Schrodinger	Phase	Receptor-ligand docking, pharmacophore modelling

Table 1. Examples of commercially available drug discovery softwares.

In contrast, a prior knowledge of the biomolecular target is not needed in ligand based pharmacophore modelling, but instead a library of compounds with known potencies towards the biomolecular target is required for the construction of a training set. *In silico* techniques are then employed to generate a 3D pharmacophore that bears the representative electronic and steric features of the compounds from the training set. To obtain a reliable 3D pharmacophore, the training set should include structurally diverse compounds with *in vitro* potencies spanning a few orders of magnitude.

To confirm the validity of the 3D pharmacophore generated from either structure-based or ligand-based pharmacophore modelling, cost analysis techniques can be carried out based on statistical calculations in order to generate the "best" hypothetical structure. The validated pharmacophore is then subjected to virtual screening from chemical libraries to identify molecules that possess similar steric and electronic features with the pharmacophore. However, a drawback of pharmacophore modelling is that since the affinity calculation only involves the matching of geometry and functional groups of the potential ligand with the 3D pharmacophore, the screening process will tend to reveal ligands that structurally and electronically resemble the training set of compounds, rather than uncovering novel hit scaffolds.

On the other hand, molecular docking represents a totally different approach for virtual screening of bioactive compounds. Molecular docking involves stimulating the interactions between biomolecules and the ligands by computational algorithms. Molecular modelling has been gaining in popularity due to the increasing availability of biomolecular structures determined by either X-ray crystallography or NMR. In addition, advances in computational power and the continual development of more refined docking algorithms help to mitigate the relatively high computational strain demanded by molecular docking. In molecular docking, knowledge of the 3D biomolecular structure is essential, with or without the binding ligand. As previously described, the use of a biomolecular structure co-crystallized with a ligand is preferred as the binding pocket of the ligand can be easily identified and the subsequent docking analysis can then be restricted to the areas around the binding pocket in order to avoid wastage of computational resources and to eliminate false positives that interact outside of the binding site.

After completion of a virtual screening campaign, the resulting hit list of compounds can be subjected to experimental assays for hit validation (Figure 3). Alternatively, the hit structures can be used to construct analogues that can be screened *in silico* to potentially generate more potent ligands before chemical synthesis and biological testing.

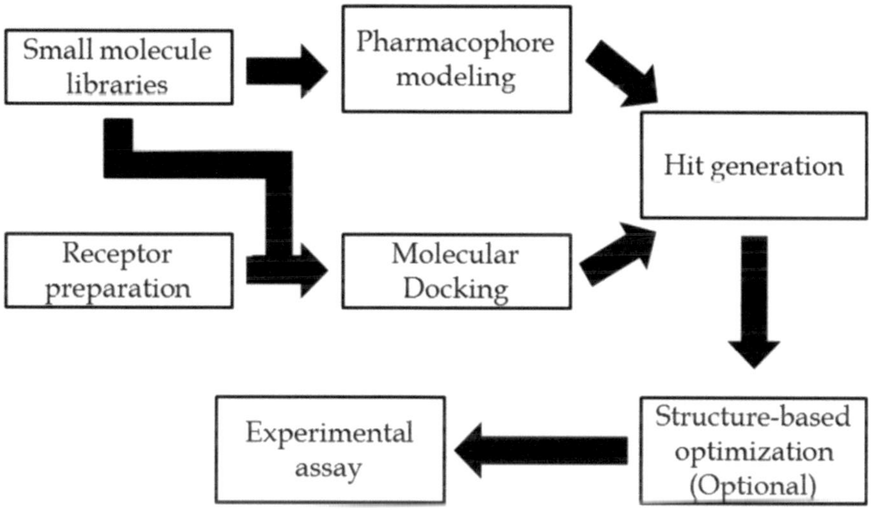

Figure 3. Pipeline of computer-aided drug discovery and lead optimization processes.

4. Molecular docking to discover promoter G-quadruplex stabilizing ligands

In order to drive the development of more potent and selective ligands targeting promoter G-quadruplexes, it is important to understand the detailed interactions between the G-quadruplex and the ligand at the molecular scale. Molecular modelling can provide a tool for visualizing the three-dimensional interactions of the G-quadruplex-ligand complex in order to better understand the structural or functional features required for effective binding. Compared to pharmacophore-based methods, molecular docking can potentially make more effective use of the structural information of the receptor for the discovery of novel G-quadruplex-targeting compounds. In particular, high-quality structural data on the distinctive features of different promoter G-quadruplexes may aid the design and optimization of bioactive ligands that are able to discriminate between related G-quadruplex topologies. In this section, we give a general overview for the *in silico* structure-based discovery of oncogenic promoter G-quadruplex stabilizing ligands.

Computer-aided high-throughput molecular docking and hit validation usually involves three stages (Tang et al. 2006). The first stage is the construction and preparation/selection of the chemical library, and the preparation of the biomolecular model for molecular docking. The second stage is the docking of the individual compounds of the chemical library against the biomolecule, followed by score calculation. In the third stage, the high-scoring compounds can be selected for *in vitro* biological assays to validate their activities towards the biomolecular target.

4.1. Selection of chemical library

A poorly-designed chemical library can result a high rate of false positives, or otherwise poor-quality hits. Therefore, the careful selection of a chemical library containing members possessing favourable pharmacokinetic properties (absorption, distribution, metabolism, excretion, and toxicity; ADMET) or structural diversity could improve the hit rate of a single docking campaign. Today, most chemical libraries are focused in some way by applying a manually selected pre-filter. For example, the Lipinski rule-of-five is a common filter that represents a collection of structural properties correlated with desirable solubility and bioavailability of small molecules (Lipinski et al. 2001). Screening compounds libraries with a pre-filter reduces the likelihood of identifying hit compounds with undesirable ADMET properties, therefore minimizing any loss of investment in chemical synthesis or biological assays. Two types of chemical libraries commonly chosen for virtual screening campaigns are drug/drug-like databases and natural product libraries.

Name	Company	Size of library	URL
ChEMBL	European Bioinformatics Institute (EBI)	>1.1 million	https://www.ebi.ac.uk/chembl/
ZINC	Bioinfomatics and Chemical Informatics Research Center (BCIRC)	>21 million	http://zinc.docking.org/
IBS Database	InterBioScreen Ltd	>45000	http://www.ibscreen.com/natural.shtml
NatDiverse	Analyticon Discovery	>20000	http://www.ac-discovery.com
Super Drug Database	Humboldt-University	~3000	http://bioinf.charite.de/superdrug/
DrugBank	University of Alberta	6711	http://www.drugbank.ca/

Table 2. Examples of commercially available chemical libraries used in computer-aided drug discovery.

Approved drugs usually have favourable or validated pharmacokinetic properties and toxicological profiles, which can improve the hit rate of the screening campaign, and could allow promising hit compounds to potentially bypass early-stage testing, thus streamlining the hit-to-lead optimization process. However, the use of an existing drug library for virtual screening cannot uncover novel bioactive compounds against the biological target. On the other hand, natural products represent the largest class of compounds in the chemical world. The interactions of natural products with biomolecules have been refined throughout evolutionary timescales, and these unique interactions can be harnessed by medicinal chemists to discover potential drugs. Since most natural products do not strictly adhere to Lipinski rule-of-fives, the virtual screening of natural product libraries can yield novel bioactive scaffolds that could not be obtained from drug-like or combinatorial libraries. Examples of commercially available drug databases and natural product libraries that can be used in high-throughput virtual screening are shown in Table 2.

4.2. Receptor preparation

To construct the receptor model for molecular docking, the atomic coordinates of G-quadruplex solved by the X-ray crystallography and NMR studies with or without bound ligand can usually be retrieved from the Protein Data Bank (Berman et al. 2000) or Nucleic Acid Database (Berman et al. 1996). Generally, structural data obtained from X-ray crystallography is considered more advantageous compared to those from solution NMR studies, as more detailed structural information can be obtained at the atomic scale. For G-quadruplexes lacking hard structural data, a model can be constructed by homology by modification of known, related G-quadruplex structures determined by X-ray crystallography. Commercially available software such as Discovery Studio (Accelrys Inc.) or ICM-Pro (Molsoft) can perform modification of the G-quadruplex conformation or topology through the addition or deletion of nucleobases, addition of monovalent cations in the central ion channel, or modification of the loop length and/or addition of nucleotides in the loop region (Lee et al. 2010).

4.3. G-quadruplex flexibility

The receptor model prepared can then be subjected to local energy minimization to generate the most suitable conformer for subsequent molecular docking analysis. While the small molecule ligands are usually assumed to be flexible so that the binding geometry of the ligand can be corrected predicted, the target is usually assumed to be mostly rigid, as the explicit treatment of receptor flexibility in the docking calculations would be too computationally expensive. Several approaches have been proposed to account for receptor flexibility in virtual screening campaigns. In the case of the G-quadruplex, the flexibility of the loop regions could be important especially for G-quadruplex groove-binding ligands.

An early approach tackling the problem of receptor flexibility was the "soft-docking" method (Jiang et al. 1991). In this approach, the compounds need not fit perfectly to the binding pocket of receptor and a certain degree of steric crash is allowed. During the docking process, the ligand and the receptor adjust their conformations continuously in order to achieve the most suitable conformation with maximum interaction. However, this method only utilizes a single receptor conformation, and thus the choice of receptor model for docking is of the utmost importance.

An alternative strategy that may be useful in G-quadruplex ligand discovery is the use of multiple receptor conformations (MRC) to probe the receptor flexibility (Totrov et al. 2008). This could involve a combination of multiple structures experimentally determined by X-ray crystallography or NMR, or could be generated by molecular stimulation (MD). By considering the different receptor features from multiple conformations, a more representative receptor conformation could be generated for virtual screening. Some modern docking algorithms are able to explicitly model receptor flexibility, but this is usually constrained to the ligand binding domain in order to conserve computing resources. A more thorough discussion of the common approaches used to model receptor flexibility can be found in review articles by Kavraki and co-worker (Teodoro et al. 2003), and Durrant and co-worker (Durrant et al. 2010).

4.4. Global energy optimization

The compounds from the chemical libraries are docked to the receptor structure individually. Generally, assigning the docking site across the entire G-quadruplex structure yields end-stacking compounds as the highest-scoring hits. For discovering groove-binders, which typically display weaker binding affinities, the search area for docking can be limited to the groove or loop regions of the G-quadruplex. Once the compound has been docked into the receptor, most computer algorithms will perform global energy optimization of the small molecule inside the binding pocket to find the most favourable orientation of the small molecule (Abagyan et al. 1994). For example, ICM-Pro (Molsoft) docking software (Abagyan et al. 1997) includes the following steps for global energy optimization:

1. A random conformational change of free variables according to a predefined continuous probability distribution.
2. A local energy minimization of analytical differentiable terms.
3. A calculation of the complete energy including non-differentiable terms such us entropy and solvation energy.
4. An acceptance or rejection of the total energy based on the Metropolis criterion and a return to the first step.

4.5. Score assignment

After the global energy optimization, score assignment is then performed to rank the compounds according to their predicted binding affinities. The score is a qualitative parameter that reflects the binding strength of the compound to the receptor and is composed a collection of factors such as hydrophobic interactions, van der Waal interactions, hydrogen bonding, and electrostatic interactions. However, the accuracy of the docking score will necessarily be limited by the assumptions and approximations of the scoring function. Other factors which may not be explicitly predicted by the computational algorithms, such as solvent environment and binding pocket availability, could also influence the actual binding affinity of the ligand.

Different docking programs may employ different scoring functions, which are generally classified into the following types: 1) force-field functions; 2) knowledge-based scoring functions; and 3) empirical scoring functions (Kitchen et al. 2004). These scoring functions perform calculations that involve different parameters such as statistical potential and weighted interaction terms to rank the apparent potency of the compounds. To improve the accuracy of the scoring assignment, the consensus scoring approach has been investigated. This strategy involves the combination of the weighted scores obtained for a single ligand from different score functions, to improve the hit rate of a docking campaign (Charifson et al. 1999; Clark et al. 2002; Baber et al. 2005; Yang et al. 2005).

5. Structure-based lead optimization

In the conventional drug discovery, validation of a screening hit by *in vitro* assays is usually followed by the synthesis of a range of structurally related analogues in order to optimize the binding and selectivity of the ligand towards the target. However, this approach necessarily entails a significant investment into manpower and materials, and can be very time-consuming. An alternative strategy utilizes the principles of computer-aided structure-based design in order to achieve the more efficient allocation of resources towards analogues with higher predicted binding affinities. By analysis of the receptor-ligand complex determined using X-ray crystallography or molecular modelling, a library of derivatives can be generated *in silico* that retain the important features of hit ligand that contribute to high binding affinity. This focused library can then undergo a second round of molecular docking procedure to identify the most promising derivatives for synthesis and evaluation.. The application of *in silico* structure-based optimization has also been applied for the development of oncogenic promoter G-quadruplex stabilizing ligands.

6. Discovery of oncogenic promoter G-quadruplex-stabilizing ligands using structure-based approaches

The use of *in silico* virtual screening to discover promoter G-quadruplex-stabilizing ligands has only been recently reported. Tang and co-workers utilized ligand-based pharmacophore modelling techniques to identify two non-planar alkaloids as groove binders of the parallel G-quadruplex (Li et al. 2009). In their report, the representative pharmacophore was constructed using the CATALYST software package (version 4.11, Accelrys Inc.) (Nicklaus et al. 1997). A total of 38 1,4-disubstituted anthraquinone derivatives comprised the training set, with IC_{50} values against rat glioma C6 cells spanning three orders of magnitudes (from 0.07 mM to 103 mM). Ten hypothetical models were constructed using the HypoGen hypothesis process, with the best pharmacophore containing one hydrogen bond receptor, one hydrogen bond donor, one positive ionizable group and two hydrophobic sites. The best pharmacophore model was selected for virtual screening and was mapped against a natural product database containing *ca.* 10,000 compounds derived from Chinese herbal medicines. A total of 176 hit compounds were identified with a diversity of scaffolds different to those of the training set, and 20 compounds were chosen for further evaluation based on compound availability. Intriguingly, the hit compounds included two neutral non-planar compounds, peimine (**1**) and peimimine (**2**). In UV melting experiments, peimine (**2**) and peimimine (**3**) were found to stabilize the tetramolecular G-quadruplex motif with significant increases in T_m. Further experiments indicated that both compounds were selective for parallel G-quadruplexes, and did not stabilize other G-quadruplex topologies or duplex DNA. Circular dichroism (CD) experiments found that compound **1** was able to enhance the characteristic parallel G-quadruplex CD signal at 262 nm of all the parallel G-quadruplexes examined, including c-*kit* oncogenic promoter G-quadruplex. The study from Tang and co-workers demonstrated the feasibility of employing ligand-based pharmacophore modelling to identity novel oncogenic promoter G-quadruplex-stabilizing compounds. However, further research would be required to fully characterize the possible biological effects of the compound in living cells.

In 2010, our group has employed high-throughput virtual screening techniques to identify fonsecin B (**3**) as a c-*myc* G-quadruplex stabilizer (Lee et al. 2010). Since no X-ray structure of the c-*myc* G-quadruplex was available, a molecular model of the predominant 1:2:1 loop isomer of c-*myc* G-quadruplex was constructed using the X-ray crystal structure of the related intramolecular human telomeric G-quadruplex. The model was built by the insertion or deletion of nucleobases and modification of the loop size to correspond to the 1:2:1 loop isomer of the c-*myc* G-quadruplex (Ou et al. 2007) using ICM-Pro (Molsoft). After the preparation of the receptor model, over 20,000 compounds from a natural product library were docked against the molecular model using the Molsoft ICM-Pro (3.6.1 d) docking protocol. Since most G-quadruplex stabilizing ligands possess a large polyaromatic scaffold for end-stacking, the docking area to the termini of the G-quadruplex was restricted to avoid the wastage of computational time. From the results of the virtual screening campaign, four hits were identified and tested in a preliminary *in vitro* PCR stop assay to assess their abilities to stabilize the c-*myc* G-quadruplex, and fonsecin B (**3**) emerged as the top candidate.

A variety of experiments were performed to analyze the interaction and selectivity of fonsecin B towards the c-*myc* G-quadruplex. UV-visible absorption spectroscopy revealed that compound **3** displayed 5.5-fold and 16.5-fold higher binding affinities for the c-*myc* G-quadruplex over duplex and single-stranded DNA, respectively. We then performed a detailed molecular modelling experiment in order to investigate the binding mode of the compound to the c-*myc* G-quadruplex. The modelling results revealed that **3** was stacked against the 3′-terminal of G-quadruplex with a binding energy of –48 kcal mol^{-1}. The phenolic and carbonyl oxygen atoms were predicted to orientate towards the central ionic channel, where the two oxygen atoms could possibly be stabilized by electrostatic interactions with the potassium ion. By comparison, intercalation of **3** into the G-quadruplex was calculated to be extremely unfavourable, with a binding energy of *ca.* 25 kcal mol^{-1}. PCR stop assays showed that **3** was able to stabilize the c-*myc* G-quadruplex with the similar potency to the well-known G-quadruplex ligand TmPyP4.

Apart from the high-throughput virtual screening of chemical libraries, structure-based optimization by *in silico* approaches have also been employed to improve the potency of the lead compounds to a particular oncogenic promoter G-quadruplex target. In 2009, Che and co-workers developed a series of Pt(II) complexes as c-*myc* G-quadruplex stabilizing ligands using an *in silico* structure-based optimization strategy (Wu et al. 2009). Among a series of Pt(II)-salphen complexes tested in preliminary *in vitro* assays, complex **4** was found to be most potent and was chosen for *in silico* structural modification. Over 60 derivatives of complex **4** were designed that contained side chains with various lengths and functional groups to interact with the grooves of the G-quadruplex, and these compounds were docked to the c-*myc* G-quadruplex using the ICM program. In the molecular docking analysis, the highest scoring compound **5** was found to bind more favorably to the c-*myc* G-quadruplex compared to the parent complex **4** due to the additional interactions between the side chains of **5** with the G-quadruplex grooves regions. Compound **5** was then synthesized for biological evaluation, and the PCR stop assay results showed **5** could stabilize the formation of the c-*myc* G-quadruplex with an IC_{50} value of 4.4 μM, which was an order lower than that of parent compound **4**. In this report, Che and co-workers successfully demonstrate the use of structure-based optimization of a Pt(II)-salphen complex to devise a more promising scaffold for stabilization of the c-*myc* oncogenic promoter G-quadruplex.

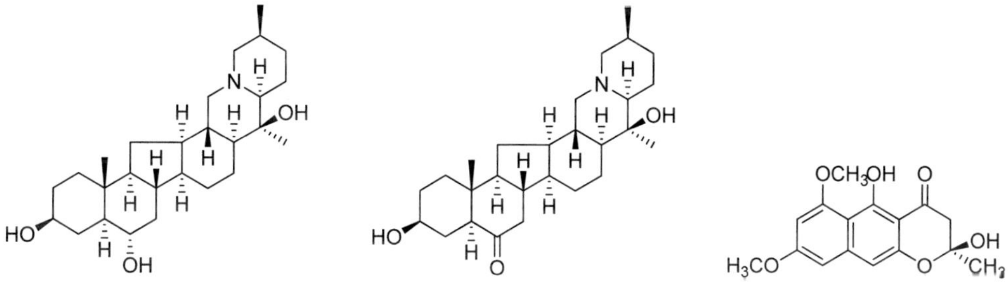

1 **2** **3**

Figure 4. Structures of promoter G-quadruplex-targeting compounds discovered via high-throughput virtual screening.

Later, the Che group reported another successful application of computer-based lead optimization of Pt(II) metal complexes to discover efficient c-*myc* G-quadruplex stabilizing ligands (Wang et al. 2010). Based on hit complex **6**, over 550 derivatives were designed by attaching side chains of various lengths and functionality to the parent scaffold, the library of compounds were rapidly screened *in silico*. Three of the highest scoring complexes **7–9** were then synthesized and subjected to comprehensive *in vitro* assays to evaluate their ability to stabilize the c-*myc* G-quadruplex. In the UV-Vis absorption experiments, all three complexes showed at least 10-fold higher binding affinities towards the c-*myc* G-quadruplex over duplex DNA. Furthermore, the complexes increased the T_m of the c-*myc* G-quadruplex by over 9 °C, and displayed improved potency at stabilizing the c-*myc* G-quadruplex in the PCR stop assay when compared to the parent compound. Subsequent reverse transcriptase PCR (RT-PCR) experiments showed that the mRNA level of the c-*myc* gene could be significantly diminished in the presence of complexes **7–9**, suggesting that these compounds could be used as suppressors of oncogenic expressing in living cells. This report by Che and co-workers again demonstrated the feasibility of *in silico* structure-based lead optimization of metal complexes, and suggested that the use of a larger chemical library of derivatives could generate a larger diversity of hits with potentially improved potencies.

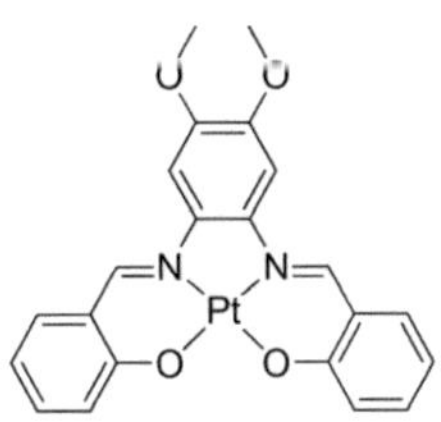

4

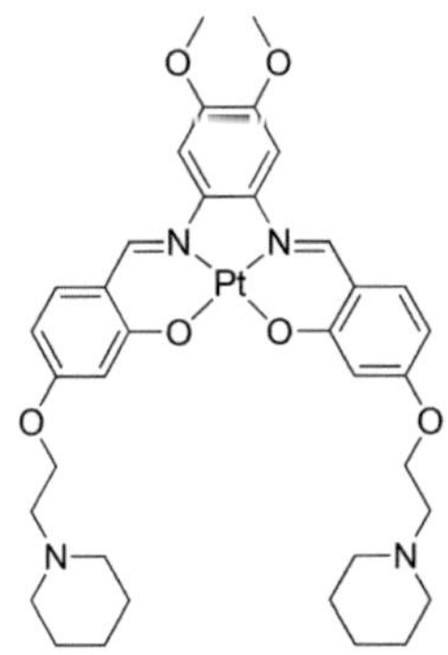

5

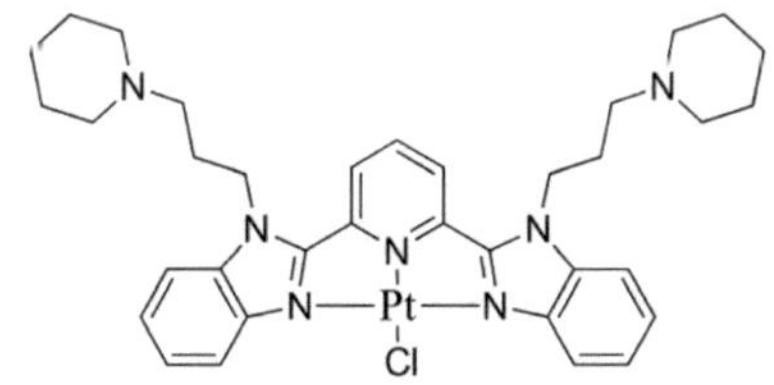

8

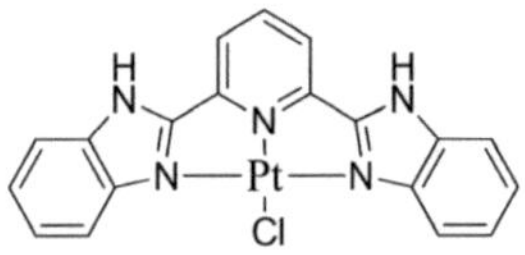

6

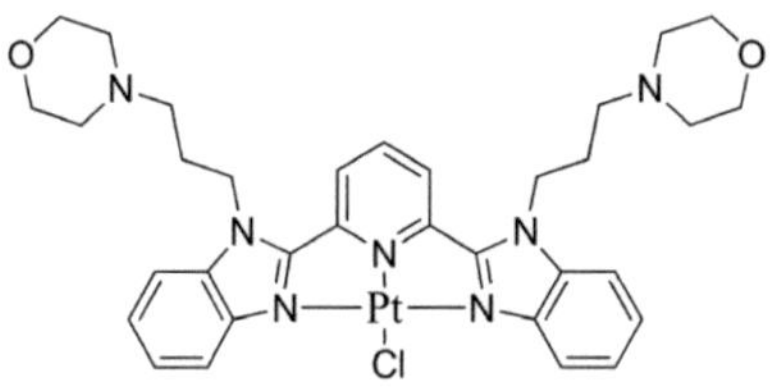

7

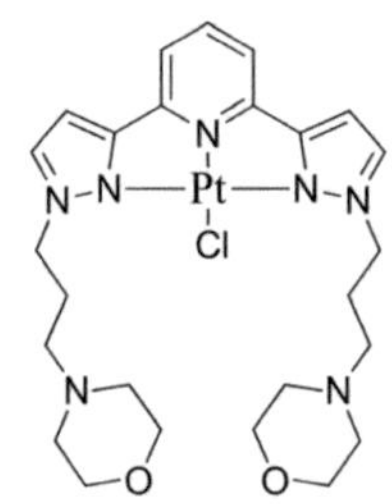

9

Figure 5. Chemical structures of the platinum(II) complexes discovered through *in silico* structure-based optimization as c-*myc* oncogenic G-quadruplex stabilizing ligands.

Our group has recently reported the structural-based optimization of FDA-approved drug methylene blue (MB) to generate more potent analogues as c-*myc* G-quadruplex stabilizers (Chan et al. 2011). Over 3,000 FDA-approved drugs were screened *in silico* against the 1:2:1 loop isomer model of the c-*myc* G-quadruplex developed by our group, and MB emerged as the top candidate. Although the MB is a well-known DNA intercalator and has been previously reported to bind the G-quadruplex, its application as a c-*myc* oncogenic promoter G-quadruplex stabilizer was first discovered by our group. 50 MB derivatives were designed *in silico* and were docked against the c-*myc* G-quadruplex using ICM-Pro software. Compounds **10a–c** bearing a bromophenyl pendant linked by an aliphatic side chain showed the greatest binding energy from the virtual screening, and they were synthesized for biological evaluation. In the fluorescence intercalator displacement (FID) assay, compound **10b** was found to effectively displace thiazole orange (TO) from the c-*myc* G-quadruplex with a DC_{50} value of 0.75 μM, while compounds **10a** and **10c** displayed higher DC_{50} values of *ca.* 6 and 2 μM, respectively. Furthermore, compound **10b** could inhibit *Taq* polymerase mediated-extension of the c-*myc* sequence through induction of the G-quadruplex structure in the PCR stop assay with superior potency compared to the parent compound MB. Detailed molecular docking analysis revealed that compound **10b** was predicted to form strong end-stacking interactions with the terminal of c-*myc* G-quadruplex with groove interactions, whereas the parent compound MB was predicted to interact with the G-quadruplex *via* a mostly intercalative mode. In living cells, compound **10b** was shown to be effectively down-regulate the c-*myc* promoter activity with an IC_{50} value of *ca.* 1 μM as revealed by a luciferase assay. The increased activity of the **10b** compared to MB against c-*myc* promoter activity could be potentially attributed, at least in part, to the stabilization of c-*myc* G-quadruplex structure. This report demonstrated the structure-based lead optimization approach effectively generate novel analogues of existing drug as oncogenic G-quadruplex stabilizing ligands.

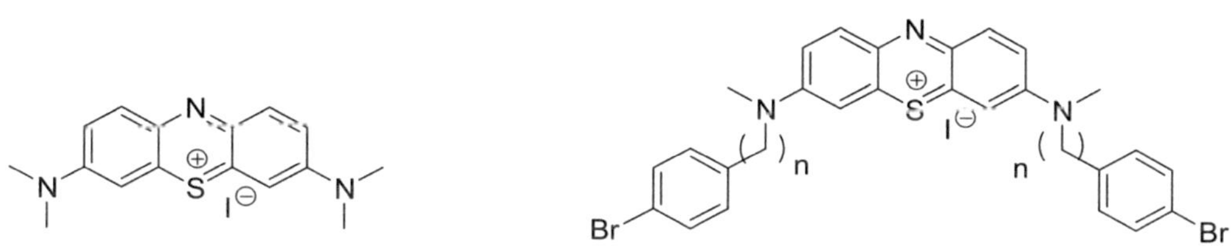

Methylene blue (MB)

10a: n = 0
10b: n = 2
10c: n = 3

Figure 6. Chemical structures of the FDA-approved drug methylene blue and its analogues designed by a structural-based optimization strategy as c-*myc* oncogenic G-quadruplex stabilizing ligands.

7. Conclusion

The identification of oncogenes involved in the progression of various types of tumours has stimulated the development of various anti-cancer strategies targeting oncogenic expression. The discovery of G-quadruplex motifs in the promoter regions of oncogenes and the elucidation of their putative roles in the regulation of oncogenic transcription has opened a new potential therapeutic avenue for the treatment of cancer. However, it should be noted that the application of G-quadruplex-stabilizing ligands for the modulation of oncogenic activity in living systems is still in its infancy. Most promoter quadruplex ligands discovered thus far have not yet progressed past pre-clinical investigation. To advance further, several important criteria have to be addressed. These include the bioavailability of G-quadruplex-binding compounds as well their conformational rigidity and promiscuity for other physiological targets. In particular, the action of the lead candidates against the large number of other gene promoters and G-quadruplex structures that are likely to be present in normal cells should be rigorously assessed. These factors would aid in the determination of the permissible dosage and therapeutic window of the G-quadruplex-targeting compounds for the potential treatment of cancer. With continual advances in computational technologies and modelling techniques, as well as the concurrent development of more focused yet diverse chemical libraries, we envisage that the discovery and investigation of novel promoter G-quadruplex-stabilizing ligands would continue to thrive in the near future. Furthermore, *in silico* hit-to-lead optimization allows the chemical space around hit compounds to be explored without necessitating the actual synthesis of analogue molecules, thus significantly reducing expenses associated with materials and manpower.

Author details

Dik-Lung Ma*, Victor Pui-Yan Ma, Ka-Ho Leung, Hong-Zhang He
and Daniel Shiu-Hin Chan
Department of Chemistry, Hong Kong Baptist University, Kowloon Tong, Hong Kong

Hai-Jing Zhong and Chung-Hang Leung*
State Key Laboratory of Quality Research in Chinese Medicine, Institute of Chinese, Medical Science, University of Macau, Macao, China

Acknowledgement

This work is supported by Hong Kong Baptist University (FRG2/11-12/009), Environment and Conservation Fund (ECF Project 3/2010), Centre for Cancer and Inflammation Research, School of Chinese Medicine (CCIR-SCM, HKBU), the Health and Medical Research Fund (HMRF/11101212), the Research Grants Council (HKBU/201811 and HKBU/204612), the Science and Technology Development Fund, Macao SAR (001/2012/A) and the University of Macau (SRG013-ICMS12-LCH, MYRG091(Y1-L2)-ICMS12-LCH and MYRG121(Y1-L2)-ICMS12-LCH).

8. References

Abagyan, R. and M. Totrov (1994). "Biased Probability Monte Carlo Conformational Searches and Electrostatic Calculations for Peptides and Proteins." *J Mol Biol* 235: 983-1002.

Abagyan, R. and M. Totrov (1997). "Flexible protein-ligand docking by global energy optimization in internal coordinates." *Proteins* 29: 215-220.

Alderden, R. A., M. D. Hall and T. W. Hambley (2006). "The Discovery and Development of Cisplatin." *J Chem Educ* 83: 728.

Baber, J. C., W. A. Shirley, Y. Gao and M. Feher (2005). "The Use of Consensus Scoring in Ligand-Based Virtual Screening." *J Chem Inf Model* 46: 277-288.

Balasubramanian, S., L. H. Hurley and S. Neidle (2011). "Targeting G-quadruplexes in gene promoters: a novel anticancer strategy?" *Nat Rev Drug Discov* 10: 261-275.

Balasubramanian, S. and S. Neidle (2009). "G-quadruplex nucleic acids as therapeutic targets." *Curr Opin Chem Biol* 13: 345-353.

* Corresponding Authors

Bejugam, M., S. Sewitz, P. S. Shirude, R. Rodriguez, R. Shahid and S. Balasubramanian (2007). "Trisubstituted Isoalloxazines as a New Class of G-Quadruplex Binding Ligands: Small Molecule Regulation of c-kit Oncogene Expression." *J Am Chem Soc* 129: 12926-12927.

Berman, H. M., A. Gelbin and J. Westbrook (1996). "Nucleic acid crystallography: A view from the nucleic acid database." *Prog Biophys Mol Biol* 66: 255-288.

Berman, H. M., J. Westbrook, Z. Feng, G. Gilliland, T. N. Bhat, H. Weissig, et al. (2000). "The Protein Data Bank." *Nucleic Acids Res* 28: 235-242.

Blackburn, E. H. (1991). "Structure and function of telomeres." *Nature* 350: 569-573.

Burge, S., G. N. Parkinson, P. Hazel, A. K. Todd and S. Neidle (2006). "Quadruplex DNA: sequence, topology and structure." *Nucleic Acids Res* 34: 5402-5415.

Cavasotto, C. and A. Orry (2007). "Ligand docking and structure-based virtual screening in drug discovery." *Curr Top Med Chem* 7: 1006-1014.

Chan, D. S.-H., H. Yang, M. H.-T. Kwan, Z. Cheng, P. Lee, L.-P. Bai, et al. (2011). "Structure-based optimization of FDA-approved drug methylene blue as a c-myc G-quadruplex DNA stabilizer." *Biochimie* 93: 1055-1064.

Charifson, P. S., J. J. Corkery, M. A. Murcko and W. P. Walters (1999). "Consensus Scoring: A Method for Obtaining Improved Hit Rates from Docking Databases of Three-Dimensional Structures into Proteins." *J Med Chem* 42: 5100-5109.

Chen, J. and L. Lai (2006). "Pocket v.2: Further Developments on Receptor-Based Pharmacophore Modeling." *J Chem Inf Model* 46: 2684-2691.

Clark, R. D., A. Strizhev, J. M. Leonard, J. F. Blake and J. B. Matthew (2002). "Consensus scoring for ligand/protein interactions." *J Mol Graph Model* 20: 281-295.

Cogoi, S. and L. E. Xodo (2006). "G-quadruplex formation within the promoter of the KRAS proto-oncogene and its effect on transcription." *Nucleic Acids Res* 34: 2536-2549.

Croce, C. M. (2008). "Oncogenes and Cancer." *New Engl J Med* 358: 502-511.

Dai, J., D. Chen, R. A. Jones, L. H. Hurley and D. Yang (2006). "NMR solution structure of the major G-quadruplex structure formed in the human BCL2 promoter region." *Nucleic Acids Res* 34: 5133-5144.

Davis, T. L., A. B. Firulli and A. J. Kinniburgh (1989). "Ribonucleoprotein and protein factors bind to an H-DNA-forming c-myc DNA element: possible regulators of the c-myc gene." *Proc Natl Acad Sci USA* 86: 9682-9686.

Dexheimer, T. S., S. S. Carey, S. Zuohe, V. M. Gokhale, X. Hu, L. B. Murata, et al. (2009). "NM23-H2 may play an indirect role in transcriptional activation of c-myc gene expression but does not cleave the nuclease hypersensitive element III1." *Mol Cancer Ther* 8: 1363-1377.

Duan, W., A. Rangan, H. Vankayalapati, M.-Y. Kim, Q. Zeng, D. Sun, et al. (2001). "Design and Synthesis of Fluoroquinophenoxazines That Interact with Human Telomeric G-Quadruplexes and Their Biological Effects1." *Mol Cancer Ther* 1: 103-120.

Durrant, J. D. and J. A. McCammon (2010). "Computer-aided drug-discovery techniques that account for receptor flexibility." *Curr Opin Pharmacol* 10: 770-774.

Ghosh, S., A. Nie, J. An and Z. Huang (2006). "Structure-based virtual screening of chemical libraries for drug discovery." *Curr Opin Chem Biol* 10: 194-202.

Gonzalez, V., K. Guo, L. Hurley and D. Sun (2009). "Identification and Characterization of Nucleolin as a c-myc G-quadruplex-binding Protein." *J Biol Chem* 284: 23622-23635.

Grand, C. L., H. Han, R. M. Muñoz, S. Weitman, D. D. Von Hoff, L. H. Hurley, et al. (2002). "The Cationic Porphyrin TMPyP4 Down-Regulates c-MYC and Human Telomerase Reverse Transcriptase Expression and Inhibits Tumor Growth in Vivo 1 This research was supported by grants from the NIH and the Arizona Disease Control Research Commission.1." *Mol Cancer Ther* 1: 565-573.

Heidenreich, O. (2009). Targeting Oncogenes with siRNAs. siRNA and miRNA Gene Silencing. M. Sioud, Humana Press. 487: 221-242.

Huppert, J. L. and S. Balasubramanian (2007). "G-quadruplexes in promoters throughout the human genome." *Nucleic Acids Res* 35: 406-413.

Jiang, F. and S.-H. Kim (1991). "“Soft docking”: Matching of molecular surface cubes." *J Mol Biol* 219: 79-102.

Jung, Y. and S. J. Lippard (2007). "Direct Cellular Responses to Platinum-Induced DNA Damage." *Chem Rev* 107: 1387-1407.

Kitchen, D. B., H. Decornez, J. R. Furr and J. Bajorath (2004). "Docking and scoring in virtual screening for drug discovery: methods and applications." *Nat Rev Drug Discov* 3: 935-949.

Lee, H.-M., D. S.-H. Chan, F. Yang, H.-Y. Lam, S.-C. Yan, C.-M. Che, et al. (2010). "Identification of natural product Fonsecin B as a stabilizing ligand of c-myc G-quadruplex DNA by high-throughput virtual screening." *Chem Commun* 46: 4680-4682.

Li, Q., J. Xiang, X. Li, L. Chen, X. Xu, Y. Tang, et al. (2009). "Stabilizing parallel G-quadruplex DNA by a new class of ligands: Two non-planar alkaloids through interaction in lateral grooves." *Biochimie* 91: 811-819.

Lipinski, C. A., F. Lombardo, B. W. Dominy and P. J. Feeney (2001). "Experimental and computational approaches to estimate solubility and permeability in drug discovery and development settings." *Adv Drug Deliver Rev* 46: 3-26.

Lipps, H. J. and D. Rhodes (2009). "G-quadruplex structures: in vivo evidence and function." *Trends Cell Biol* 19: 414-422.

Lu, Y.-J., T.-M. Ou, J.-H. Tan, J.-Q. Hou, W.-Y. Shao, D. Peng, et al. (2008). "5-N-Methylated Quindoline Derivatives as Telomeric G-Quadruplex Stabilizing Ligands: Effects of 5-N Positive Charge on Quadruplex Binding Affinity and Cell Proliferation." *J Med Chem* 51: 6381-6392.

Lutz, W., J. Leon and M. Eilers (2002). "Contributions of Myc to tumorigenesis." *BBA-Rev Cancer* 1602: 61-71.

Ma, D.-L., V. P.-Y. Ma, D. S.-H. Chan, K.-H. Leung, H.-J. Zhong and C.-H. Leung (2012). "In silico screening of quadruplex-binding ligands." *Methods* 57: 106-114.

Ma, Y., T.-M. Ou, J.-Q. Hou, Y.-J. Lu, J.-H. Tan, L.-Q. Gu, et al. (2008). "9-N-Substituted berberine derivatives: Stabilization of G-quadruplex DNA and down-regulation of oncogene c-myc." *Bioorg Med Chem* 16: 7582-7591.

Marcu, K. B., S. A. Bossone and A. J. Patel (1992). "myc Function and Regulation." *Annu Rev Biochem* 61: 809-858.

McInnes, C. (2007). "Virtual screening strategies in drug discovery." *Curr Opin Chem Biol* 11: 494-502.

Mergny, J.-L. and C. Helene (1998). "G-quadruplex DNA: A target for drug design." *Nat Med* 4: 1366-1367.

Meyer, N. and L. Z. Penn (2008). "Reflecting on 25 years with MYC." *Nat Rev Cancer* 8: 976-990.

Monchaud, D. and M.-P. Teulade-Fichou (2008). "A hitchhiker's guide to G-quadruplex ligands." *Org Biomol Chem* 6: 627-636.

Nicklaus, M. C., N. Neamati, H. Hong, A. Mazumder, S. Sunder, J. Chen, et al. (1997). "HIV-1 Integrase Pharmacophore: Discovery of Inhibitors through Three-Dimensional Database Searching†." *J Med Chem* 40: 920-929.

Ou, T.-M., Y.-J. Lu, C. Zhang, Z.-S. Huang, X.-D. Wang, J.-H. Tan, et al. (2007). "Stabilization of G-Quadruplex DNA and Down-Regulation of Oncogene c-myc by Quindoline Derivatives." *J Med Chem* 50: 1465-1474.

Parkinson, G. N., M. P. H. Lee and S. Neidle (2002). "Crystal structure of parallel quadruplexes from human telomeric DNA." *Nature* 417: 876-880.

Rankin, S., A. P. Reszka, J. Huppert, M. Zloh, G. N. Parkinson, A. K. Todd, et al. (2005). "Putative DNA Quadruplex Formation within the Human c-kit Oncogene." *J Am Chem Soc* 127: 10584-10589.

Seenisamy, J., E. M. Rezler, T. J. Powell, D. Tye, V. Gokhale, C. S. Joshi, et al. (2004). "The Dynamic Character of the G-Quadruplex Element in the c-MYC Promoter and Modification by TMPyP4." *J Am Chem Soc* 126: 8702-8709.

Shoichet, B. K. (2004). "Virtual screening of chemical libraries." *Nature* 432: 862-865.

Siddiqui-Jain, A., C. L. Grand, D. J. Bearss and L. H. Hurley (2002). "Direct evidence for a G-quadruplex in a promotor region and its targeting with a small molecule to repress c-MYC transcription." *Proc Natl Acad Sci USA* 99: 11593-11598.

Tang, Y., W. Zhu, K. Chen and H. Jiang (2006). "New technologies in computer-aided drug design: Toward target identification and new chemical entity discovery." *Drug Discov Today Technol* 3: 307-313.

Teodoro, M. L. and L. E. Kavraki (2003). "Conformational flexibility models for the receptor in structure based drug design." *Curr Pharm Des* 9: 1635-1648.

Totrov, M. and R. Abagyan (2008). "Flexible ligand docking to multiple receptor conformations: a practical alternative." *Curr Opin Struct Biol* 18: 178-184.

Ventura, A. and T. Jacks (2009). "MicroRNAs and Cancer: Short RNAs Go a Long Way." *Cell* 136: 586-591.

Wang, P., C.-H. Leung, D.-L. Ma, S.-C. Yan and C.-M. Che (2010). "Structure-Based Design of Platinum(II) Complexes as c-myc Oncogene Down-Regulators and Luminescent Probes for G-Quadruplex DNA." *Chem Eur J* 16: 6900-6911.

Wheelhouse, R. T., D. Sun, H. Han, F. X. Han and L. H. Hurley (1998). "Cationic Porphyrins as Telomerase Inhibitors: the Interaction of Tetra-(N-methyl-4-pyridyl)porphine with Quadruplex DNA." *J Am Chem Soc* 120: 3261-3262.

Wierstra, I. and J. Alves (2008). The c-myc Promoter: Still MysterY and Challenge. Advances in Cancer Research. F. V. W. George and K. George, Academic Press. Volume 99: 113-333.

Wolber, G. and T. Langer (2004). "LigandScout: 3-D Pharmacophores Derived from Protein-Bound Ligands and Their Use as Virtual Screening Filters." *J Chem Inf Model* 45: 160-169.

Wu, P., D.-L. Ma, C.-H. Leung, S.-C. Yan, N. Zhu, R. Abagyan, et al. (2009). "Stabilization of G-Quadruplex DNA with Platinum(II) Schiff Base Complexes: Luminescent Probe and Down-Regulation of c-myc Oncogene Expression." *Chem Eur J* 15: 13008-13021.

Yang, J.-M., Y.-F. Chen, T.-W. Shen, B. S. Kristal and D. F. Hsu (2005). "Consensus Scoring Criteria for Improving Enrichment in Virtual Screening." *J Chem Inf Model* 45: 1134-1146.

Chapter 7

Cancer Genes and Chromosome Instability

Alexey Stepanenko and Vadym Kavsan

Additional information is available at the end of the chapter

http://dx.doi.org/10.5772/54017

1. Introduction

The census of cancer genes (http://www.sanger.ac.uk/genetics/CGP/Census/) includes 487 mutated genes (data on September 2012) manually curated from the scientific literature, which are proved to induce or accelerate cancer development when appropriately changed (point mutations, deletions, translocations or amplifications) (see criteria for inclusion in the cancer gene census in [1]). Studies in mice have magnified the number of the potential cancer genes to more than 3000 [2] and the number of mutated genes revealed in tumor sequencing studies are gradually approaching this number (NCG 3.0, http://bio.ifom-ieo-campus.it/ncg) [3, 4]. Nevertheless, despite the impressive data accumulated from studies of gene mutations and pathway alterations, an overwhelming amount of diverse molecular information has offered limited understanding of the general mechanisms of cancer [5, 6].

For decades tumor development from precancerous lesions to obvious malignancy and metastases has been considered as a result of deterministic sequential accumulation of mutations in the handful of "driver" cancer genes, occurring in a continuous linear pattern of cancer progression, while genome/karyotype changes were judged as a by-product of transformation (see ref. in [5-10]). However, only a few genes have been shown to be commonly mutated in cancer sequencing studies, and they are neither highly prevalent nor in multiple tumor types [11-14]. Furthermore, the whole exome sequencing of multiple spatially separated samples obtained from the same tumor followed by phylogenetic reconstruction of tumor progression has revealed significant intratumoral heterogeneity with "no dominant clones in the cancer tissue" [15], "punctuated clonal evolution… without observable intermediate branching" [16] or "branched evolutionary tumor growth" with 63 to 69% of all somatic mutations not detectable across every tumor region and some genes undergoing multiple distinct and spatially separated inactivating mutations within a single tumor [17]. High-resolution SNP array of B-cell chronic lymphocytic leukemia (B-CLL) has demonsterated "clearly a nonlinear, branching sub-clonal hierarchy in B-CLL with multiple ancestral subclones" [18]. Similarly, it has been concluded that CLL progression can occur in "either a linear or branching manner, with multiple genetic subclones evolving either in succession or in parallel" [19]. Evaluation of the clonal relationships among pancreatic cancer metastases and primary tumor has led to conclusion that the genetic heterogeneity of metastases reflects heterogeneity already existing within the primary carcinoma, and that the primary carcinoma is a mixture of numerous subclones [20]. Thus, as Cahill et al [21] point out, "The tumor is clonal only in the sense that all cells within a tumor are derived from the same cell precursor. Genetic instability makes the tumor itself a population under change – a huge collection of coexisting subclones, each with the potential for future changes in the face of selective pressures". Altogether, these data seriously contradict to deterministic sequential accumulation of mutations in the handful of "driver" cancer genes occurring in a continuous linear pattern of cancer progression postulated by conventional gene mutation theory of cancer.

In contrast, chromosome instability (CIN) and the resulting magnitude of intratumor clonal/non-clonal heterogeneity are recognized to be the main driving forces of tumor evolution (immortalization, transformation, metastasis, acquisition of drug resistance) (reviewed in [5-10]). CIN results from persistent defects in mitotic fidelity and implies both whole chromosome instability and segmental chromosome instability (translocations, deletions, and amplifications). Although defects in telomere maintenance, sister chromatid cohesion, kinetochore-microtubule attachments, assembly of amphitelic bipolar mitotic spindles, as well as translocations containing breakpoints within fragile sites, instability of satellite repeats in heterochromatin, cell-in-cell formation by entosis (as a result, cytokinesis frequently fails, generating binucleate cells that produce aneuploid cell lineages) and random fragmentation of the entire chromosome (chromothripsis) in which chromosomes are broken into many pieces and then randomly stitched back together can contribute to CIN during tumor evolution, in established cancer cell lines mechanism of centrosome amplification and clustering is proposed to be the major contributor to CIN (discussed below). It is documented that extreme CIN relative to tumors with intermediate CIN is associated with improved survival outcome in cancer and experimental models have evidenced that extreme CIN has a negative impact on cellular fitness, generating nonneoplastic and nonviable cells, and constrains tumorigenesis. However, CIN represents early and causative event in cancer progression and significantly correlates with tumorigenic potential of cells and such clinical variables as tumor progression from precancerous lesions to malignant tumors and then to metastases, survival, treatment sensitivity, and the risk of acquired therapy resistance (reviewed in [22]).

In this review we provide evidence that tumorigenic action of cancer genes or mutagenic and non-mutagenic carcinogens is directly linked to centrosome deregulation and CIN. Any factors or stresses that contribute to CIN inevitably promote the evolution of cancer. CIN and clonal/non-clonal intratumor heterogeneity are the interconnected driving forces of immortalization and transformation and the reasons of oncogene addiction independence of tumors from any particular oncogene and general ineffectiveness of targeted therapy in clinic.

2. Immortalization and transformation: The central role of karyotype

Comparing gene expression in glioblastoma, the most aggressive form of human brain tumors, to the normal brain cells we have found *CHI3L1* among the genes with the highest expression level in glioblastomas [23, 24]. Addition of CHI3L1 to cell medium increased mitogenic and proliferative properties of 293 cells (human embryonic kidney 293 cells, also often referred to as HEK293) [25, 26]. 293 cells stably transfected with *CHI3L1* have an accelerated growth rate relatively to the parental cells and can undergo anchorage-independent growth in soft agar that is one of the consistent indicators of oncogenic transformation [25, 27]. Furthermore, 293_*CHI3L1* cells implanted in the rat brain of adult immunocompetent animals have given rise to the large intracerebral tumors with the newly ingrown blood vessels [27, 28].

Previously, similar data on transformation of immortalized 293 cells by one gene transfection was obtained for multiple diverse genes (see ref. in [29, 30]). However, 293 cells themselves (the same as many other cell lines) are already immortalized. In a given case, ectopic expression of CHI3L1 alone results in the tumorigenic conversion of previously immortalized 293 cells with shared adenovirus 5 DNA [31]. An immortalized cell (as well as a normal cell) must acquire a number of chromosome changes to become a fully malignant tumor cell. Karyotype analysis of 293_*CHI3L1* clones have shown that these cells differ from wild type [31, 32] and control cells (293_pcDNA3.1) in modal chromosome number and structure of chromosomes (manuscript in preparation). Other authors have also shown that overexpression, for example, of tripeptidyl-peptidase II [33], EBNA1 binding protein 2 [34], GLI1 transcripton factor [35] or Cut homeobox 1 trancription factor [36] have triggered centrosome and chromosomal abnormalities in 293 cells.

Transformation with one oncogene is not cell type-spesific. Analysis of literature has revealed that different oncogenes with diverse and nonoverlapping intracellular functions are characterized by the same ability: to trigger conversion of immortalized cells (e.g., 293, NIH3T3, HMEC, MCF10A, HCT116) or even primary cells into malignant tumor cells or aggravate tumorigenicity of tumor cells (reviewed in [30]). What is the basis for cell immortalization and how do different cancer genes trigger conversion of immortalized and even primary normal cells into malignant tumor cells *in vitro* and *in vivo*? Overcoming of senescence and acquisition of immortality is an essential rate-limiting step in the process of malignant transformation of mammalian somatic cells. *In vitro* immortalization of various cell types was successfully implemented by the introduction of viral genomes/oncogenes, ectopic expression of human telomerase reverse transcriptase (hTERT), some transcription factors (e.g. c-MYC, BMI1, ZNF217, or β-catenin), or carcinogen treatment, whereas spontaneously immortalized cells emerge at an extremely low frequency *in vitro* (about 10^{-7}) [30]. Multiple investigations have revealed that irrespectively of the nature of "immortalizing/transforming agent" for immortalization/transformation *in vitro* cells must overcome cellular senescence by inactivating/dysregulating p16^{INK4A}-pRB and/or ARF-p53 pathways and maintaining their telomeres by activation of *hTERT* expression (a predominant way) or by an alternative mechanism for lengthening telomeres (ALT) [30].

However, *in vivo* research has shown that telomerase-deficient primary mouse embryonic fibroblasts (MEFs) have generated tumors in nude mice following transformation [37]. Transformation of human primary fibroblasts and human primary mesodermal cells has resulted in cells capable to form colonies in soft agar and tumors in mice but they and the majority of the tumors derived from them have lacked telomerase activity, and telomere erosion has been observed [38]. To the point, human primary melanomas show telomere maintenance as a late event in tumor progression (metastatic melanoma); thus, telomere maintenance/immortalization is associated with progression rather than initiation of melanoma [39]. Moreover, approximately 40% of glioblastomas have no defined telomere maintenance mechanism (nither telomerase expression nor the alternative lengthening of telomeres mechanism) [40]. Numerous studies have proved that telomere dysfunction in the absence of telomerase activity drives chromosomal instability/karyotype evolution through telomere-telomere type rearrangements (breakage-fusion-bridge cycles) promoting the appearance of chromosomal rearrangements and numerical chromosome aberrations, contributing to genomic intratumor diversity and favoring cell immortalization, the acquisition of a tumor phenotype and increased metastasis [41-46]

Studing karyotype evolution in both individual cells and cell populations during various stages of cellular immortalization process in *in vitro* cell culture model it has been revealed that the karyotype evolution with the complex interplay between clonal and non-clonal chromosome abberations serves as the driving force for immortalization. By repeating the same experiments or analyzing the parallel clones derived from the same initial cell population, it has been found out that the immortalized cells display unique distinctive karyotypes, demonstrating the stochastic nature of karyotype evolution during cellular immortalization (reviewed in [5, 10]). Additional follow-up experiments have demonstrated that genome-based evolution can be detected in most of the major transition steps in cancer including immortalization, transformation, metastasis, and drug resistance [5]. Similarly, analyzing the karyotypes of clonal tumorigenic cell lines arising from the mass cultures of human cells within months after transfection with the same set of artificially activated oncogenes it has been found that different tumorigenic cell lines had individual clonal karyotypes and phenotypes and the phenotypes and karyotypes of different tumors induced by these lines in different mice have been karyotypic and phenotypic variants of the parental prototypes [47].

Thus, the process of immortalization/transformation is not simply a number of well defined events like inactivation of cell cycle negative regulators (p16^{INK4A}-pRB and/or ARF-p53) and activation of telomerase (hTERT) but, instead, is associated with karyotype/genome abnormalities (structural and numeral aneuploidy as well as abberant methylation and gene mutations) and, as a consequence, with global changes in gene expression and function. Analysis of 45 spontaneously transformed murine cell lines from normal epithelial cells has demonstrated that supernumerary centrosomes, aneuploidy and CIN precedes immortalization and transformation [48]. Also, CIN precedes chemical induced malignant transformation [7-9]. All immortalized and malignantly transformed cells have abnormal karyotypes irrespectively of "immortalizing/transforming agents", and karyotype evolution plays the central role in immortalization, transformation, metastasis, and drug resistance (reviewed in [5-10, 22, 30, 47, 49-52]).

3. Tumor genome profile output

In 2008 The International Cancer Genome Consortium (http://www.icgc.org/icgc) stated the primary goal to comprehensively characterize over 25,000 cancer genomes from 50 different cancer types and/or subtypes at the genomic, epigenomic, and transcriptomic levels to reveal the repertoire of oncogenic mutations and signaling networks, which can be exploited for the development of new cancer therapies [53]. Thus, "designed to identify the Achilles' heel of cancer" [54] and "driver universal cancer genes" [55] whole exome and genome sequencing studies (see ref. in [3, 4]) instead have revealed a large number of stochastic gene mutations in solid tumors for each individual with the same cancer type [11-14]. Searching for the "universal" cancer genes among deleted, amplified and sequence mutated genes across breast, colon, pancreatic cancers and glioblastoma has shown that only one gene, *TP53*, is commonly mutated in all four major cancer types [55, 56] and no single gene is commonly deleted or amplified [55]. Similarly, from more than 1,000 mutated genes identified across whole exome or genome sequencing of 10 tumor types, only 46 genes have been found mutated in two types, 7 (*TP53, CDKN2A, RB1, PIK3CA, KRAS, NF1*, and *KIAA0774*) in three types and only 1 (*TP53*) in four types (in 6 types) [3]. Ongoing Cancer Cell Line Project (http://www.sanger.ac.uk/genetics/CGP/CellLines/), which target is to sequence all known cancer genes in ~800 cell lines, has confirmed that *TP53, CDKN2A, RB1, PTEN, PIK3CA, KRAS*, and *BRAF* are the most frequenly mutated genes.

Interestingly, analysis of 70 tyrosine kinases with altered gene expression or located at a genomic site of copy number gain or loss in 95 chronic lymphocytic leukemias (CLLs) has revealed no somatic mutations [57]. Extension of this research, sequencing of 515 kinase genes in 23 CLLs, has revealed only six somatically acquired mutations (e.g., in *RAS* and *RAF*) across all kinase genes [58]. Further *B-RAF* sequencing in 250 CLLs has detected four *B-RAF* mutations, none involving B-RAF amino acid residue 600, which is the predominant B-RAF mutation found across human tumors. *N-RAS* mutations were found in 2 cases and none of *K-RAS* among 231 CLLs analyzed [58].

High-resolution analysis of somatic copy-number alterations (SCNAs) from 3,131 cancer specimens, belonging largely to 26 histological types, revealed a total of 75,700 gains and 55,101 losses across the cancers, for a mean of 24 gains and 18 losses per sample [59]. An average of 17% of the genome was amplified and 16% deleted in a typical cancer sample. From all SCNAs only 158 regions of focal SCNA were altered at significant frequency across several cancer types, of which 122 could not be explained by the presence of a known cancer target gene located within these regions [59]. High-resolution aCGH analysis of 598 human cancer cell lines derived from 29 different tissues revealed 2424 amplifications and 14010 deletions across the entire cell line panel [60]. SNP array screening of 746 cancer cell lines identified 2428 somatic homozygous deletions, which overlie 11% of protein-coding genes [61]. These cell lines have also been sequenced for mutations in the coding exons of 46 known cancer genes. In total, 1753 putative oncogenic mutations were identified [61]. Another research group identified 2576 somatic mutations across 1507 coding genes from 441 tumors comprising breast, lung, ovarian and prostate cancer types and subtypes [62].

Thus, the list of "non-universal" cancer genes and mutations within them is growing proportionally to seqencing studies stuffing databases. The Network of Cancer Genes (NCG 3.0, http://bio.ifom-ieo-campus.it/ncg) collects information on hundreds of cancer genes that have been found mutated in 16 different cancer types [4]. These genes were collected from the Cancer Gene Census as well as from 18 whole exome and 11 whole-genome screenings of cancer samples (see referenses in [3, 4]. COSMIC database (http://www.sanger.ac.uk/genetics/CGP/cosmic/) combines cancer mutation data manually curated from the scientific literature with the output from the Cancer Genome Project [63, 64]. COSMIC catalogues all somatic mutations in benign and malignant tumors as well as tumor cell lines [65]. Release v61 (September 2012) includes 22170 genes, 405271 mutations (224649 unique mutations), and 8931 gene fusions, described in 773098 tumor samples (2556 whole genomes).

It is worth noting that the total number of mutations in tumor samples are significantly underestimated, as the current methods of DNA sequencing detect a single base change only if it presents in >10% of the molecules, that is, therefore predominately clonal mutations [14]. Methodologies for studing patterns of genomic changes (e.g., aCGH and SNP) also detect only dominant clonal aberrations [10]. Estimate of all mutations including sub-clonal and random suggests that each cancer cell within most tumors contains >10,000 mutations and by the time a tumor is clinically detected (10^8–10^9 cells) it might harbour >10^{11} different mutations [14].

Importantly, genome profiling of a tumor bulk produces average profile of genetic changes in a tumor sample and does not mirror heterogeneity of genetic changes within tumor sample, i.e., changes restricted to the separate populations of tumor cells or single tumor cells [66]. However, there is a high level of genomic and (epi)genetic heterogeneity within individual lesions, as well as between primary tumors, metastatic cells, and relapses (see ref. in [22]).

4. Cancer genes induce, promote and licence CIN

CIN/random aneuploidy and intratumor heterogeneity drive tumor evolution. Which should surveillance mechanisms be disrupted to unleash CIN? As it follows from tumor sequencing studies, beyond the overwhelming "mutator phenotype", the most altered signaling pathways within and across different cancer types are p14^{ARF}-p53 pathway (*CDKN2A/ARF* and *TP53* genes), p16^{INK4A}-pRB pathway (*CDKN2A/INK4A* and *RB1* genes), MAPK pathway (*NF1, KRAS,* and *BRAF* genes) and PI3K-AKT pathway (*PTEN* and *PIK3CA* genes).

CIN results from persistent defects in mitotic fidelity and is strongly favored in cells with disrupted p14^{ARF}-p53 and/or p16^{INK4A}-pRB pathways explaining their highest deregulation frequency in immortalized and tumor cells [29]. Patients with Li-Fraumeni syndrome characterized by germline mutations of *TP53* develop a wide range of malignancies (reviewed in [67]). Mice expressing the *TP53* mutants have increased incidence of sarcomas and carcinomas (reviewed in [68, 69]). In contrast, "super *TP53*" mice, carrying *TP53* alleles in addition to the two endogenous alleles, exhibit an enhanced response to DNA damage and are significantly protected from cancer when compared with normal mice [70]. Cancer patients with missense mutations in *TP53* often have a poorer prognosis than those lacking *TP53* entirely, as the presence of dominantly mutated p53 not only confers loss of tumor suppressor activity but also provides a gain of oncogenic function [68, 71]. P53 gain of oncogenic function mutants have enhanced oncogenic potential and effectively induce CIN [68, 69, 72]. *In vitro* and *in vivo* data have established that loss of p53 activity and, to a greater degree, dominantly mutated p53 is the major event responsible for increased expression of cell-cycle and proliferation-associated genes (reviewed in [73]). The presence of disrupted *TP53*/dysregulated p53 pathway is significantly associated with intratumor genetic heterogeneity/clonal diversity [74], radio- and (multi)drug resistance [75-78]. Strikingly, high-grade serous ovarian cancer is characterized by *TP53* mutations in 96% of tumours (303 of 316 samples analysed) [79], and *TP53* is the most frequently known altered gene in acute myeloid leukemias with complex karyotype (CK-AML) [80]. Multivariable analysis of 234 CK-AMLs revealed that *TP53* alteration (70% of samples) was the most important prognostic factor in CK-AML, outweighing all other variables [80]. Evaluation of CIN in Barrett's esophagus tissue has revealed that CIN is highly correlated with *TP53* LOH [81]. In agreement, patients with LOH in *TP53* are 16 times more likely to progress from premalignant Barrett's esophagus to esophageal adenocarcinoma than patients without *TP53* LOH, supporting the hypothesis that expansion of CIN clones drive malignancy [82, 83]. Moreover, usage of integrated DNA sequence and copy number information to reconstruct the order of abnormalities in individual cutaneous squamous cell carcinomas and serous ovarian adenocarcinomas have allowed to reveal that loss of the second *TP53* allele appears to precede not only the development of CIN but also a vast expansion of simple mutations [84]. Mutation in *TP53* is the most common genetic alteration reported during metastasis to the brain in breast cancer [85]. Analysis of breast cancer cell line MCF-7 variant overexpressing a dominantly mutated *TP53* have showed that impaired p53 function drives breast cancer progression by CIN, which generates karyotypic variability, leading to transcriptome signatures that are responsible for cell proliferation, epithelial-to-mesenchymal transition, chemoresistance, and invasion [86]. Indeed, correlation of expression profiles with karyotypic parameters of the NCI-60 cancer cell line panel has revealed that CIN is associated with higher expression of genes implicated in epithelial-to-mesenchymal transition, cancer invasiveness, and metastasis and with lower expression of genes involved in cell cycle checkpoints, DNA repair, and chromatin maintenance [87]. P53-dependent pathways (as well as pRB1 pathways) alterations promote epithelial-to-mesenchymal transition in tumor cells through both CIN licencing and global aberrant transcription regulation (reviewed in [88, 89]). Furthermore, proliferation of aneuploid human cells is limited by p53 pathway [90]. In support, in genetically engineered mutant mice that are prone to aneuploidy *TP53* is a limiting factor in aneuploidy-induced tumorigenesis [91]. All together, these data justify reputation of mutant p53 as "the demon of the guardian of the genome" [92] and "a master regulator of human malignancies" [93].

Survivors of hereditary retinoblastoma, a childhood cancer of the eye caused by germline mutations of the *RB1* tumor suppressor gene, have an elevated risk of developing sarcomas, brain cancer, melanoma or some epithelial cancers [94, 95]. It was shown that inactivation of the pRB1 pathway in the developing mouse or human retina was accompanied by p19^{ARF}-p53 pathway activation and *RB1*-deficient retinoblasts underwent p53-mediated apoptosis and exited the cell cycle [96]. In contrast, *RB1*-deficient cell with inactivated p14^{ARF}-p53 pathway had growth advantage, clonally expanded, and formed retinoblastoma [96]. As it is expected, retinoblastoma is characterized by CIN, strengthening the view that the chromosomal changes contribute to the development and progression of malignancy [97, 98]. Also, analysis of hundreds of chronic lymphocytic leukemias (CLLs) has revealed a strong association between *RB1* deletion and aberrant p53 pathway with elevated genomic complexity, which is a strong independent predictor of rapid disease progression, disease aggressiveness, short remission duration, short survival, and therapy efficaciousness in CLL [99-101].

PRB1 plays a critical role in proper chromosome condensation and cohesion, centromeric function, and chromosome stability in mammalian cells (reviewed in [102, 103]). Inactivation of pRB1 not only allows inappropriate proliferation but also undermines mitotic fidelity leading to CIN and ploidy changes [102, 103]. pRB1 pathways deregulation correlates with (multi)drug and radioresistance [104, 105]. Screening of more than 25,000 compounds in human fibroblasts in which pRB1 activity was compromised by viral oncoproteins revealed that the only compounds selective for *RB1*-deficient cell death were topoisomerase II inhibitors (e.g., doxorubicin) [106]. Moreover, *RB1*-deficient cells displayed increased proliferation in the presence of the PI3K (LY294002) and MEK1/2 (U0126) inhibitors [107].

The *CDKN2A* locus comprises the *INK4A* and *ARF* genes encoding tumor suppressors p16INK4A and p14ARF (p19ARF in mice) that up-regulate the activities of pRB1 and p53 transcription factors, respectively [108]. Inactivation of *INK4A*, *ARF* or both genes strongly predisposes mice to tumor development (reviewed in [69]). Loss of p16^{INK4A} plays a causal role in centrosome dysfunction and the subsequent generation of CIN cells in multiple cell types [109]. Furthermore, both *CDKN2A* and TP53 are rate-limiting for reprogramming of somatic cells [110]. *CDKN2A* or TP53 inactivation has a profound positive effect on the efficiency of induced pluripotent stem (iPS) cell generation, increasing both the kinetics of reprogramming and the number of emerging iPS cell colonies [110, 111]. Reprogramming of somatic cells is accompanied by chromosome abnormalities, point mutations, epigenetic changes, and the drastic gene expression changes (reviewed in [112]). *CDKN2A* or TP53 inactivation leads to CIN and tumorigenicity of iPS cells (reviewed in [113]). In contrast, iPS cells containing an extra copy of the *TP53* or *CDKN2A* show reduced tumorigenic potential in various *in vitro* and *in vivo* assays and an improved response to anticancer drugs [114]. In addition to the reprogramming process itself the (epi)genomic stability of both iPS and human embrionic stem cells is affected by *in vitro* environmental conditions and the techniques used for cell derivation. Also, there is no passage number threshold ensuring safety of iPS. However, the risk of abnormalities increases with the time in culture [113].

PTEN can increase p53 stability and its DNA binding activity through physical association with p53 [115]. Germline mutations of *PTEN* have been found in cancer susceptibility Cowden and Bannayan–Riley–Ruvalcaba syndromes, which are now collectively referred to as the PTEN hamartoma tumor syndrome. Mice heterozygous for *PTEN* develop spontaneous tumors and conditional tissue-specific disruption of *PTEN* leads to different tumors in the affected tissues (reviewed in [116]). PTEN plays a fundamental role in the maintenance of chromosomal stability through the physical interaction with centromeres and control of DNA repair. *PTEN* null cells exhibit extensive centromere breakages and chromosomal translocations [117, 118]. Interestingly, comparison of spectra of *PTEN* and *TP53* somatic mutations across tumors has revealed that they are usually independent and even mutually exclusive [116].

Neurofibromatosis type 1 (NF1), a tumor predisposition syndrome, is characterised by the growth of benign and malignant tumors involving the peripheral and central nervous system and results from inactivating germline mutations of the *NF1* gene [119, 120]. *NF1* gene encodes a neurofibromin, which plays a role in MAPK, AKT-mTOR, adenylate cyclase, and PKC mediated pathways [121]. One of the main features of neurofibromatosis type 1 is benign neurofibromas, 10% of which become transformed into malignant peripheral nerve sheath tumors [119]. *TP53, CDKN2A,* and *RB1* mutations or deletions are detected in malignant peripheral nerve sheath tumors but not in benign neurofibromas [119, 120, 122]. In consistence with it, but in contrast to benign neurofibromas, malignant peripheral nerve sheath tumors are caracterized by CIN [119, 122].

Hyperactivation of the MAPK or PI3K-AKT pathway induces frequently cell cycle arrest and senescence *in vitro* and *in vivo*. Oncogene-induced senescence program, a state of stable cell-cycle arrest, together with oncogene induced apoptosis are recognized to represent an important barrier against tumor development *in vivo* [123]. Senescence cells are characterized by the inability to proliferate despite the presence of a steady supply of abundant nutrients, mitogens, ample room for expansion, and by maintenance of cell viability/resistance to apoptosis and metabolic activity for months. Expression of activated forms of RAS (N-RAS^{G12D}, H-RAS^{V12}, K-RAS^{G12V}), B-RAF^{E600} or MEK was shown to elicit cell cycle arrest and senescence in primary fibroblasts, Schwann cells, hepatocytes, T lymphocytes, keratinocytes, astrocytes, epithelial intestinal cells and other cell types, AKT overexpression induced senescence of primary and immortalized esophageal epithelial cells, primary MEFs, primary human aortic endothelial cells, human dermal microvascular endothelial cells, and human umbilical vein endothelial cells. Moreover, *in vitro* and/or *in vivo* inactivation of PTEN, VHL, RB1, NF1 or activation of RHEB, PKC, EGFR, TGFβ, INFβ, Cyclin E, Cyclin D, STAT5, c-MYC, β-Catenin, E2F, Rho small GTPases and many other proteins triggers senescence (reviewed in [30, 123-126]). Furthermore, mouse embrionic fibroblasts deficient in DNA damage response and DNA repair genes (*ATM, NBS1, TopBP1, BRCA1, BRCA2, Ku86, XRCC4, WRN* and *ERCC1*) undergo premature senescence (reviewed in [125]. Importantly, oncogene-induced senescence is frequently observed in premalignant lesions both in animal tumor models and in human patients but is essentially absent in advanced cancers, suggesting that malignant tumor cells have found ways to bypass or escape senescence [125, 126]. *In vitro* and *in vivo* models have shown that senescence and/or apoptosis evasion requires $p14^{ARF}/p19^{ARF}$-p53 and/or $p16^{INK4A}$-pRB pathway inactivation, which results in immortalization and malignant transformation *in vitro* and invasive tumor formation *in vivo* [30, 123-126].

The ability to induce CIN after inactivation/hyperactivation is not restricted to cancer genes the most frequently mutated across cancer types. BCR-ABL oncogene is mainly associated with Philadelphia chromosome positive chronic myeloid leukemia (>90% of patients) but is also found in acute lymphoblastic leukemia and occasionally in acute myelogenous leukemia. It results from a reciprocal translocation between chromosome 9 and 22. BCR-ABL is engaged in multiple signaling pathways and its expression in cells induces CIN (reviewed in [127, 128]). Heterozygous germline mutations in tumor supressors *BRCA1* or *BRCA2* are associated with hereditary cancers (e.g., breast and ovarian). BRCA1 and BRCA2 proteins have multiple functions including participating in a pathway that mediates repair of DNA double strand breaks by error-free methods. Inactivation of *BRCA1* or *BRCA2* results in centrosome amplification, cell-cycle checkpoint defects, DNA damage and CIN (reviewed in [129-131]). Von Hippel-Lindau disease is caused by germline mutations in the *VHL* tumour suppressor gene. *VHL* mutations predispose to the development of a variety of tumors (reviewed in [132]). Loss of VHL causes the mitotic spindle misorientation and CIN (reviewed in [133, 134]). Adenomatous polyposis coli (*APC*) was identified as a tumor suppressor gene mutated in familial colon cancer. Now it is well documented that loss of *APC* function plays an important role in CIN induction (reviewed in [135, 136]). Ataxia telangiectasia syndrome is characterized by extreme sensitivity to radiation, cell-cycle checkpoint defects, CIN, and predisposition to cancer. The disease is caused by germline mutations in the *ATM* gene involved in DNA double-strand break signaling and repair (reviewed in [137, 138]). Multiple endocrine neoplasia type 1 (MEN1) is an inherited cancer predisposition syndrome characterized by development of tumors in both endocrine and nonendocrine organs in patients and a mouse model of MEN1 [139]. *MEN1* encodes a tumor suppressor menin participating in regulation of cell proliferation, apoptosis, and DNA damage response/genome stability in part localizing to the promoters of thousands of human genes and regulating transcription mediated by interactions with chromatin modifying enzymes (reviewed in [140, 141]). Aberrant MYC activity is associated with the appearance of DNA damage-associated markers and CIN (reviewed in [142, 143]).

Furthermore, *in vitro* and *in vivo* research has proven that dozens of proteins involved in regulation of chromosome cohesion, centrosome amplification, spindle assembly checkpoint, kinetochore-microtubule attachment, cell cycle as well as homologous and non-homologous recombination can trigger centrosome amplifiction and CIN in primary or chromosomaly stable immortalized cells and induce tumors in genetically engineered mice (reviewed in [144-148] "offering proof of principle that CIN alone can be the root cause of spontaneous tumors in mammals" [71]. Moreover, diverse growth factors, transmembrane receptors, transcription factors when extopically overexpressed in cells also trigger centrosome amplification and CIN and are able to transform cells. Also, there is a significant association between global hypomethylation and CIN [149-153]. DNA methyltransferase deficient cells are chromosomally unstable [154, 155], and mice models have demonstrated that genomewide DNA hypomethylation can induce tumors [156-158]. Thus, a specific effect of oncoproteins is to cause aneuploidization [50] and the elevation of stochastic CIN [10].

5. All roads lead to centrosome

In cancer cells mechanism of centrosome amplification and clustering is proposed to be the major contributor to CIN [159, 160]. Centrosomes are microtubule-organizing structures that determine the organization of the mitotic spindle poles that segregate duplicated chromosomes between dividing cells. Mechanistically, CIN is driven by bipolar spindle formation through centrosomal clustering, which increases the formation of merotelic attachments (an error in which a single kinetochore is attached to microtubules emanating from both spindle poles [161]) producing chromosome missegregation [159, 160]. Chromosome missegregation was widely considered to occur due to anaphase lagging chromosomes. Nevertheless, recently it has been evidenced that most lagging chromosomes end up in the correct daughter cell, and the largest contribution to missegregation without obvious lagging in anaphase makes chromosomes with multimerotelic kinetochores, those with many microtubules oriented toward the wrong pole [162]. Centrosomal clustering allows successful completion of a cell division. In contrast, progeny of rarely and spontaneously arising multipolar cell divisions are often unviable undergoing mitotic cell death or cell-cycle arrest [159]. Whole-chromosome segregation errors frequently results in double-strand breaks, which can lead to unbalanced translocations in the daughter cells [163, 164] and chromosome pulverization/ chromothripsis defined by small-scale DNA copy number changes and extensive inter- and intrachromosomal rearrangements [165, 166]. Structural chromosomal aberrations lead to loss of heterozygosity for tumor suppressor genes [165, 167-170]. The transplantation of the generated *Drosophila* larval neural stem cells with extra centrosomes in normal hosts can induce the formation of metastatic tumors [171]. Centrosome abnormalities have been reported in most cancers.

Centrosome is made up of and regulated by more than 350 proteins (reviewed in [172-174] and numerous additional centrosome component candidates were revealed [175]. Genome-wide RNA interference screens have confirmed that about 200 genes contribute to spindle assembly [176], 32 genes are involved in centriole duplication and centrosome maturation [177], and 133 genes are engaged in centrosome clustering in drosophila cells [178]; silencing of 82 genes has resulted in the prevention of spindle multipolarity in human oral squamous cell carcinoma cells with supernumerary centrosomes [179]. Moreover, a system-wide two-hybrid screen on 94 proteins implicated in spindle function in *Saccharomyces cerevisiae* has uncovered 604 protein-protein interactions [180], and a cell cycle phosphoproteome of 18 yeast centrosome proteins has identified 297 phosphorylation sites [181]. Thus, accounting only these figures and that all these genes/proteins are regulated on multiple levels and changes of the abundance or activity of any one will affect the whole process, it is easy to understand why introduction of an oncogene into a cell directly or indirectly but inevitably will result in CIN. Indeed, monitoring phosphorylation of the histone variant H2AX, an early mark of DNA damage, it was identified hundreds of genes whose downregulation led to elevated levels of H2AX phosphorylation [182], and screening of 2,000 reduction-of-function alleles (1038 genes) for 90% of essential genes in *Saccharomyces cerevisiae* has generated a catalogue of 692 CIN genes whose disruption may lead to CIN [183]. Enriched gene ontology together with sequence orthologs created a list of human CIN candidate genes, which, when was cross-referenced to published somatic mutation databases, revealed hundreds of mutated CIN candidate genes [183].

Thus, irrespectively of their functions oncogenes and tumor suppressors directly or indirectly converge on centrosomes and mitotic checkpoints (reviewed in [144, 147, 148]). Deregulation of oncogenic and tumor suppressor pathways triggers and collaborates with CIN during tumorigenesis [184]. In contrast, supernumerary centrosome formation and CIN is reduced by overexpression of tumor suppressors in CIN cells [185-188]. Relationship between CIN and cancer genes explains well why such large number of cancer genes was identified (487 genes, data on September 2012) and why hundreds of oncogenes with diverse functions, when are ectopically overexpressed, are characterized by the same ability: to transform a cell or aggravate tumorigenicity.

6. CIN induction: Beyond cancer genes

CIN/aneuploidy induction is not restricted to cancer genes. Exposure of cells to drugs, chemical agents, and physical influences, as well as contacts with bacterial cells and infection with some viruses do induce centrosome amplification, CIN and can eventually result in transformation or aggravate transformed phenotype.

Metals in general are considered to be weak mutagens, if mutagenic at all, still many metals are carcinogenic (reviewed in [9, 189]). All of the carcinogenic metals are able to induce CIN. It was systematically shown that carcinogenic metals cause centrosome amplification, centriolar defects, spindle assembly checkpoint bypass, suppression of the dynamic instability of microtubules (reviewed in [189, 190]). Non-mutagenic carcinogen asbestos causes centrosome amplification and CIN [191] by binding to a subset of proteins that include regulators of the cell cycle, cytoskeleton, and mitotic process [192]. Non-mutagenic carcinogens polycyclic aromatic hydrocarbons including dioxins or benzo[a]pyrene also provoke CIN [9]. One of the possible mechanisms is through activation of a cytoplasmic aryl hydrocarbon receptor (reviewed in [193]), which itself when is ectopically overexpressed can induce centrosome amplification [194]. Nanomaterials give rise to aneuploidy mainly by interfering with microtubules (reviewed in [195]). Both intestinal commensal *Enterococcus faecalis* and pathogen *Helicobacter pylori* are potential important contributors to the etiology of sporadic colorectal cancers and can contribute to cellular transformation and tumorigenesis triggering DNA double breaks and CIN [196, 197]. Human papillomavirus oncoproteins E6 and E7 induce centrosome abnormalities and CIN (reviewed in [198]).

Thus, any factor, genetic or non-genetic, internal or external, producing stress-induced genome system instability and its mediated increase in the cell population heterogeneity will contribute to cancer evolution [5, 6].

7. Oncogene addiction concept

The term "oncogene addiction" was first coined by B. Weinstein to describe the dependency of certain tumor cells on a single activated oncogenic protein or pathway to maintain their malignant properties, despite the likely accumulation of multiple gain and loss-of-function mutations that contribute to tumorigenicity. Decoding oncogene addiction in cancer is believed to provide a key for effective molecular targeted therapy [199-204]. The concept of oncogene addiction has been obtained from various human tumor-derived cell lines and conditional transgenic animal models in which acute inactivation of the overexpressed wild type (e.g., *MYC* and *WNT1*) or mutated oncogenes (e.g., *EGFR*, *K-RAS*, *H-RAS*, *B-RAF*, *MET*, *FGFR3*, *ALK*, *AURK*, and *RET*) *via* switching off an inducible oncogene, siRNA, or small-molecule inhibitors typically has resulted in rapid apoptosis, or sometimes growth arrest and differentiation of tumor cells causing regression of the tumor [199-201, 206, 207]. However, many research groups monitoring long-term tumor response in diverse conditional mice models after oncoprotein withdrawal have repeatedly observed tumor relapses: H-RAS and p16^{INK4A}-/- (melanoma model), HER2/NEU (mammary carcinoma model), BCR-ABL (acute B-cell lymphoma model) (reviewed in [206]), MYC (lymphoma and mammary carcinoma models) [206, 208, 209], WNT1 (mammary carcinoma model) [206, 208, 210], MYC and K-RAS (mammary carcinoma model) [207], K-RAS and MAD2 (lung carcinoma model) [211], K-RAS (glioma model) [212] (see also [50] for additional examples), supporting the statement that "the nature of the initiating oncogene appears to be of little influence on the response of the resulting tumors to oncogene inactivation" [211]. In many cases tumor escape from oncogene dependence upon the primary oncogene inactivation was attributed to the acquired diverse novel genetic lesions [206, 211]. For example, MYC-induced lung cancers after oncogene inactivation failed to regress completely because of secondary activating events in K-RAS associated pathways [212] and the loss of *TP53* resulted in the absence of tumor regression [213], whereas loss of one *TP53* allele dramatically facilitated the progression of WNT1-induced mammary tumors to a oncogene independent state both by impairing the regression of primary tumors and by promoting the recurrence of fully regressed tumors following oncogene inactivation [214]. The acquisition of oncogene independence and tumor recurrence in K-RAS glioma model coincided with loss of *CDKN2A* [215]. Concurrent mutational inactivation of the *PTEN* and *RB1* tumor suppressors was determined as a mechanism for loss of B-RAF/MEK dependence in melanomas harboring B-RAF mutations [216]. Loss-of-function mutations in *PTEN* genes rendered T cell acute lymphoblastic leukemia independent of the MYC oncogene in conditional zebrafish model [209]. It is worth recalling that *TP53*, *RB1*, *CDKN2A*, *K-RAS*, and *PTEN* are among the most frequently mutated genes in human tumors [3]. It follows that advanced tumors already harbour "escape mechanisms"!

Importantly, acquisition of novel genetic lesions as primary oncogene dependence escape mechanisms is accompanied by CIN in tumor models. Analysis of relapsed lymphomas after MYC de-induction in conditional mice model showed that every relapsed tumor exhibited additional chromosomal rearrangements, both numerical and structural, compared with the primary tumor of origin [217] and high levels of aneuploidy in the primary tumor and in remaining cells survived after K-RAS and MAD2 oncoproteins withdrawal correlated with lung tumor relapses [218].

Observation of tumor relapses after oncogene inactivation and unsuccess of targeted therapies in multiple diverse clinical trials inclined many researchers to accept the pitfalls of oncogene addiction concept [6, 199, 200, 202, 211, 219-222]. Majority of tumors contain a heterogeneous cell population with a number of stochastic genome alterations, extensively rewired signaling networks and addicted to multiple oncogenes [6, 200, 220]. Furthermore, the addicted states can easily switch with each other during cancer progression and in particular during medical intervention [5, 202]. It is proposed that the concept of "network addiction", rather than "oncogene addiction", recapitulates more closely what is happening during tumor development and after exposure to therapeutic agents [219]. There is no particular pathway that would play a prominent role in maintaining cell viability [221]. For example, over 100 altered signaling pathways were identified in squamous cell lung carcinoma [222]. Illusion of oncogene dependence [199] and limited relevance of oncogene addiction concept for the majority of tumors [211] led to eradication of the hope of targeting the key addictive oncogene that maintains one's cancer [220]. Really, the obvious success of targeted therapy based on oncogene addiction concept is mainly restricted only to chronic myelogenous leukaemia (CML) in clinic [22, 223], which possesses in chronic phase, a major phase of drug response, a homogeneous population of tumor cells arisen from a single driver mutation, although still with high frequency of resistance development (35% of patients in chronic phase treated with imatinib) [224, 225].

Oncogene addiction concept and models, which it has been derived from, have obvious shortcomings and pitfalls. Cell lines display a genetic drift and low heterogeneity different from tumors *in vivo* as a consequence of selection and adaptation for cell culture conditions [226, 227]. Numerous tissue-specifc genetically engineered mouse cancer models have been developed that exhibit many biologic hallmarks of human cancer (reviewed in [69, 228]), however, they still poorly reproduce spontaneous tumors (reviewed in [229]). In transgenic mice models all the cells share the same genetic defects, which can not be the case in most sporadic cancers. Activated oncogenes form a dominant pathway through artificial selection favoring cancer progression and promoting cancer evolution much more strongly than what occurs in nature. It results in drastically reduced genome heterogeneity, which helps investigators illustrate the importance of favored genes [6]. Limited number of initiating genetic alterations, artificially activated oncogenes, benign levels of CIN, intratumor genetic homogeneity, and fostered evolution make mice tumors inappropriate models for the targeted treatment of cancers [6, 50, 218, 229]. Cancer therapy based on oncogene addiction concept is palliative rather than curative in clinic [22]. Also, the uniqueness and significance of oncogene addiction concept should be questioned by a growing list of non-oncogenes that are not inherently oncogenic themselves (not mutated or altered in any way) but required for tumor initiation and maintenance in a variety of cancer models [230-234]. This has led to establishment of non-oncogene addiction concept (reviewed in [233]).

Now it is supposed that insights into tumor evolution and the changes of tumor heterogeneity upon targeted therapy will allow identifying the non-responsive clones and targeting them [235-237]. However, underestimated intratumor heterogeneity can be a serious obstacle making this strategy hardly clinically implementable [15-20, 238].

8. Conclusion

Solid tumor evolution is cyclical and consists of two distinct phases: a punctuated phase (high CIN, frequent non-clonal chromosome aberrations) and a stepwise phase (low CIN, clonal evolution with dominant clonal chromosome aberrations). Shifts between phases are induced by stress and subsequent selection [5, 6, 10]. Thus, severity of CIN can be changed during tumour evolution and is affected by diverse genetic and non-genetic, internal and external stresses (modulation of expression of cancer genes, drugs, chemical agents/carcinogens, physical influences, and microenvironment changes). CIN results in genomic and (epi)genetic heterogeneity facilitating evolution of cancers and creating multiclonal tumour architecture, which increases the chance of pre-existance before or appearance during therapy of resistant sublones. There is a significant correlation in primary tumors between the degree of CIN and treatment sensitivity, the risk of acquired resistance and further tumor relapses. $p14^{ARF}$-p53 and $p16^{INK4A}$-pRB pathways are the main safeguards of mitotic fidelity. Once $p14^{ARF}$-p53 or/and $p16^{INK4A}$-pRB pathway is compromised, CIN is unleashed. Oncogene/stress induced senescence or apoptosis evasion requires $p14^{ARF}$/$p19^{ARF}$-p53 and/or $p16^{INK4A}$-pRB pathway inactivation, which results in successful immortalization and malignant transformation *in vitro* and invasive tumor formation *in vivo*. Consequently, increasing both the kinetics of reprogramming and the number of emerging iPS cell colonies by disrupting *CDKN2A* or *TP53* will inevitably result in transformation.

CIN and the resulting clonal/non-clonal intratumor heterogeneity elucidate why large scale tumor genome sequencing and high-resolution analysis of somatic copy-number alterations have failed to reveal "universal" cancer genes except well known for decades (*TP53, CDKN2A, RB1, PIK3CA, KRAS,* and *NF1*), and type- and stage-specific recurrent aberrations in solid tumors, whereas most recurrent chromosome abberations (deletions, amplifications, and translocations) ever ocurring genome-wide in tumors can be explained by 3D genome organization, spatial proximity among chromosome loci, and replication timing of sites producing rearrangements [239-241]. CIN explains how non-mutagenic chemical agents, physical influences, contacts with bacterial cells, and infection with some viruses induce or promote transformation of cells *in vitro* and tumor development *in vivo*, as well as spontaneous *in vitro* transformation of primary and immortalized cells and tumorigenicity of induced pluripotent stem (iPS) cells. CIN accounts for the acquisition of oncogene independence and tumor recurrence after inductor withdrawal in oncogene on/off conditional transgenic mice models. CIN and intratumor heterogeneity are the reasons of oncogene addiction independence of solid tumors from any particular oncogene and general ineffectiveness of targeted therapy in clinic. Any factors or stresses that contribute to CIN can potentially promote the evolution of cancer.

Author details

Alexey Stepanenko and Vadym Kavsan*
State Key Laboratory on Molecular and Cellular Biology,
Institute of Molecular Biology and Genetics, Kyiv, Ukraine

Acknowledgement

This work was supported in part by grant SFFR F46/457-2011 "State key laboratory of molecular and cellular biology" and by Informatization of Ukraine in frames of mutual Ukrainian-Russian program of fundamental research, project F40.4/018 "Search and characterization of oncogenes and tumor suppressor genes involved in the initiation and development of gliomas".

9. References

[1] Futreal PA, Coin L, Marshall M, Down T, Hubbard T, Wooster R, Rahman N, Stratton MR (2004) A census of human cancer genes. Nat. rev. cancer. 4: 177-183.
[2] Touw IP, Erkeland SJ (2007) Retroviral insertion mutagenesis in mice as a comparative oncogenomics tool to identify disease genes in human leukemia. Mol. ther. 15: 13-19.
[3] Ciccarelli FD (2010) The (r)evolution of cancer genetics. BMC biol. doi:10.1186/1741-7007-8-74.
[4] D'Antonio M, Pendino V, Sinha S, Ciccarelli FD (2012) Network of Cancer Genes (NCG 3.0): integration and analysis of genetic and network properties of cancer genes. Nucleic acids res. 40: 978-983.
[5] Heng HH, Stevens JB, Bremer SW, Ye KJ, Liu G, Ye CJ (2010) The evolutionary mechanism of cancer. J. cell biochem. 109: 1072-1084.
[6] Heng HH, Stevens JB, Bremer SW, Liu G, Abdallah BY, Ye CJ (2011) Evolutionary mechanisms and diversity in cancer. Adv. cancer res. 112: 217-53.
[7] Duesberg P, Rasnick D (2000) Aneuploidy, the somatic mutation that makes cancer a species of its own. Cell motil. cytoskeleton. 47: 81-107.
[8] Duesberg P, Fabarius A, Hehlmann R (2004) Aneuploidy, the primary cause of the multilateral genomic instability of neoplastic and preneoplastic cells. IUBMB life. 56: 65-81.
[9] Duesberg P, Li R, Fabarius A, Hehlmann R (2005) The chromosomal basis of cancer. Cell oncol. 27: 293-318.

* Corresponding Author

[10] Heng HH, Stevens JB, Liu G, Bremer SW, Ye KJ, Reddy PV, Wu GS, Wang YA, Tainsky MA, Ye CJ (2006) Stochastic cancer progression driven by non-clonal chromosome aberrations. J. cell physiol. 208: 461-472.

[11] Fox EJ, Salk JJ, Loeb LA (2009) Cancer genome sequencing - an interim analysis. Cancer res. 69: 4948-4950.

[12] Salk JJ, Fox EJ, Loeb LA (2010) Mutational heterogeneity in human cancers: origin and consequences. Annu. rev. pathol. 5: 51-75.

[13] Stratton MR, Campbell PJ, Futreal PA (2009) The cancer genome. Nature. 458: 719-724.

[14] Loeb LA (2011) Human cancers express mutator phenotypes: origin, consequences and targeting. Nat. rev. cancer. 11: 450-457.

[15] Xu X, Hou Y, Yin X, Bao L, Tang A, Song L, Li F, Tsang S, Wu K, Wu H, He W, Zeng L, Xing M, Wu R, Jiang H, Liu X, Cao D, Guo G, Hu X, Gui Y, Li Z, Xie W, Sun X, Shi M, Cai Z, Wang B, Zhong M, Li J, Lu Z, Gu N, Zhang X, Goodman L, Bolund L, Wang J, Yang H, Kristiansen K, Dean M, Li Y, Wang J (2012) Single-cell exome sequencing reveals single-nucleotide mutation characteristics of a kidney tumor. Cell. 148: 886-895.

[16] Navin N, Kendall J, Troge J, Andrews P, Rodgers L, McIndoo J, Cook K, Stepansky A, Levy D, Esposito D, Muthuswamy L, Krasnitz A, McCombie WR, Hicks J, Wigler M (2011) Tumour evolution inferred by single-cell sequencing. Nature. 472: 90-94.

[17] Gerlinger M, Rowan AJ, Horswell S, Larkin J, Endesfelder D, Gronroos E, Martinez P, Matthews N, Stewart A, Tarpey P, Varela I, Phillimore B, Begum S, McDonald NQ, Butler A, Jones D, Raine K, Latimer C, Santos CR, Nohadani M, Eklund AC, Spencer-Dene B, Clark G, Pickering L, Stamp G, Gore M, Szallasi Z, Downward J, Futreal PA, Swanton C (2012) Intratumor heterogeneity and branched evolution revealed by multiregion sequencing. N. engl. j. med. 366: 883-892.

[18] Knight SJ, Yau C, Clifford R, Timbs AT, Akha ES, Dréau HM, Burns A, Ciria C, Oscier DG, Pettitt AR, Dutton S, Holmes CC, Taylor J, Cazier JB, Schuh A (2012) Quantification of subclonal distributions of recurrent genomic aberrations in paired pre-treatment and relapse samples from patients with B-cell chronic lymphocytic leukemia. Leukemia. doi:10.1038/leu.2012.13.

[19] Braggio E, Kay NE, Vanwier S, Tschumper RC, Smoley S, Eckel-Passow JE, Sassoon T, Barrett M, Van Dyke DL, Byrd JC, Jelinek DF, Shanafelt TD, Fonseca R (2012) Longitudinal genome wide analysis of patients with chronic lymphocytic leukemia reveals complex evolution of clonal architecture at disease progression and at the time of relapse. Leukemia. doi. 10.1038/leu.2012.14.

[20] Yachida S, Jones S, Bozic I, Antal T, Leary R, Fu B, Kamiyama M, Hruban RH, Eshleman JR, Nowak MA, Velculescu VE, Kinzler KW, Vogelstein B, Iacobuzio-Donahue CA (2010) Distant metastasis occurs late during the genetic evolution of pancreatic cancer. Nature. 467: 1114-1117.

[21] Cahill DP, Kinzler KW, Vogelstein B, Lengauer C (1999) Genetic instability and darwinian selection in tumours. Trends cell biol. 9: 57-60.

[22] Stepanenko AA, Kavsan VM (2012) Evolutionary karyotypic cancer theory *versus* conventional cancer gene mutation theory. Biopol. cell. 28: in press.

[23] Garifulin OM, Shostak KO, Dmitrenko VV, Rozumenko VD, Khomenko OV, Zozulya Yu A, Zehetner G, Kavsan VM (2002) The genes SOX-2 and HC gp-39 are overexpressed in astrocytic gliomas. Biopol. cell. 18: 324-329.

[24] Shostak K., Labunskyy V., Dmitrenko V., Malisheva T., Shamayev M., Rozumenko V., Zozulya Y., Zehetner G., Kavsan V (2003) HC gp-39 gene is upregulated in glioblastomas. Cancer lett. 198: 203-210.

[25] Balynska OV, Baklaushev VP, Areshkov PO, Avdieiev S S, Boyko OI, Chekhonin VP, Kavsan VM (2011) Characterization of new cell line stably expressing CHI3L1 oncogene. Biopol. cell. 27: 285-290.

[26] Areshkov PO, Avdieiev SS, Balynska OV, Leroith D, Kavsan VM (2012) Two closely related human members of chitinase-like family, CHI3L1 and CHI3L2, activate ERK1/2 in 293 and U373 cells but have the different influence on cell proliferation. Int. j. biol. sci. 8: 39-48.

[27] Kavsan VM, Baklaushev VP, Balynska OV, Iershov AV, Areshkov PO, Yusubalieva GM, Grinenko NPh, Victorov IV, Rymar VI., Sanson M, Chekhonin VP (2011) Gene Encoding Chitinase 3-Like 1 Protein (CHI3L1) is a Putative Oncogene. Int. j. biomed. sci. 7: 230-237.

[28] Baklaushev VP, Kavsan VM, Balynska OV, Yusubalieva GM, Abakumov MA and Chekhonin VP (2012) New Experimental Model of Brain Tumors in Brains of Adult Immunocompetent Rats. Brit. j. med. med. res. 2: 206-215.

[29] Kavsan VM, Iershov AV, Balynska OV (2011) Immortalized cells and one oncogene in malignant transformation: old insights on new explanation. BMC cell biol. doi:10.1186/1471-2121-12-23

[30] Stepanenko AA and Kavsan VM (2012) Immortalization and malignant transformation of eukaryotic cells. Tsitol. genet. 2: 96-129.

[31] Graham FL, Smiley J, Russell WC, Nairn R (1977) Characteristics of a human cell line transformed by DNA from human adenovirus type 5. J. gen. virol. 36: 59-74.

[32] Bylund L, Kytölä S, Lui WO, Larsson C, Weber G (2004) Analysis of the cytogenetic stability of the human embryonal kidney cell line 293 by cytogenetic and STR profiling approaches. Cytogenet. genome res. 106: 28-32.

[33] Stavropoulou V, Xie J, Henriksson M, Tomkinson B, Imreh S, Masucci MG (2005) Mitotic infidelity and centrosome duplication errors in cells overexpressing tripeptidyl-peptidase II. Cancer res. 65: 1361-1368.

[34] Lee MC, Hsieh CH, Wei SC, Shen SC, Chen CN, Wu VC, Chuang LY, Hsieh FJ, Wu CH, Tsai-Wu JJ (2008) Ectopic EBP2 expression enhances cyclin E1 expression and induces chromosome instability in HEK293 stable clones. BMB rep. 41: 716-721.

[35] Leonard JM, Ye H, Wetmore C, Karnitz LM (2008) Sonic Hedgehog signaling impairs ionizing radiation-induced checkpoint activation and induces genomic instability. J. cell biol. 183: 385-391.

[36] Sansregret L, Vadnais C, Livingstone J, Kwiatkowski N, Awan A, Cadieux C, Leduy L, Hallett MT, Nepveu A (2011) Cut homeobox 1 causes chromosomal instability by promoting bipolar division after cytokinesis failure. Proc. natl. acad. sci. USA. 108: 1949-1954.

[37] Blasco MA, Lee HW, Hande MP, Samper E, Lansdorp PM, DePinho RA, Greider CW (1997) Telomere shortening and tumor formation by mouse cells lacking telomerase RNA. Cell. 91: 25-34.

[38] Seger YR, García-Cao M, Piccinin S, Cunsolo CL, Doglioni C, Blasco MA, Hannon GJ, Maestro R (2002) Transformation of normal human cells in the absence of telomerase activation. Cancer cell. 2: 401-413.

[39] Soo JK, Mackenzie Ross AD, Kallenberg DM, Milagre C, Heung Chong W, Chow J, Hill L, Hoare S, Collinson RS, Hossain M, Keith WN, Marais R, Bennett DC (2011) Malignancy without immortality? Cellular immortalization as a possible late event in melanoma progression. Pigment. cell melanoma res. 24: 490-503.

[40] Royds JA, Al Nadaf S, Wiles AK, Chen YJ, Ahn A, Shaw A, Bowie S, Lam F, Baguley BC, Braithwaite AW, MacFarlane MR, Hung NA, Slatter TL (2011) The CDKN2A G500 allele is more frequent in GBM patients with no defined telomere maintenance mechanism tumors and is associated with poorer survival. PLoS one. doi:10.1371/journal.pone.0026737.

[41] der-Sarkissian H, Bacchetti S, Cazes L, Londoño-Vallejo JA (2004) The shortest telomeres drive karyotype evolution in transformed cells. Oncogene. 23: 1221-1228.

[42] Soler D, Genescà A, Arnedo G, Egozcue J, Tusell L (2005) Telomere dysfunction drives chromosomal instability in human mammary epithelial cells. Genes chromosomes cancer. 44: 339-350.

[43] Pampalona J, Soler D, Genescà A, Tusell L (2010) Whole chromosome loss is promoted by telomere dysfunction in primary cells. Genes chromosomes cancer. 49: 368-378.

[44] Genescà A, Pampalona J, Frías C, Domínguez D, Tusell L (2011) Role of telomere dysfunction in genetic intratumor diversity. Adv. cancer res. 112: 11-41.

[45] Bojovic B, Crowe DL (2011) Dysfunctional telomeres promote genomic instability and metastasis in the absence of telomerase activity in oncogene induced mammary cancer. Mol carcinog. Available: http://onlinelibrary.wiley.com/doi/10.1002/mc.21834/abstract;jsessionid= 83C6173AF75E AF527A75BF7CE71606BE.d03t04. doi: 10.1002/mc.21834. Accessed 2011 Nov 15.

[46] Bojovic B, Crowe DL (2011) Telomere dysfunction promotes metastasis in a TERC null mouse model of head and neck cancer. Mol. cancer res. 9: 901-913.

[47] Nicholson JM, Duesberg P (2009) On the karyotypic origin and evolution of cancer cells. Cancer genet. cytogenet. 194: 96-110.

[48] Padilla-Nash HM, Hathcock K, McNeil NE, Mack D, Hoeppner D, Ravin R, Knutsen T, Yonescu R, Wangsa D, Dorritie K, Barenboim L, Hu Y, Ried T (2011) Spontaneous transformation of murine epithelial cells requires the early acquisition of specific chromosomal aneuploidies and genomic imbalances. Genes chromosomes cancer. 51: 353-374.

[49] Fabarius A, Li R, Yerganian G, Hehlmann R, Duesberg P (2008) Specific clones of spontaneously evolving karyotypes generate individuality of cancers. Cancer genet. cytogenet. 180: 89-99.

[50] Klein A, Li N, Nicholson JM, McCormack AA, Graessmann A, Duesberg P (2010) Transgenic oncogenes induce oncogene-independent cancers with individual karyotypes and phenotypes. Cancer Genet. Cytogenet. 200: 79-99.

[51] Duesberg P, Mandrioli D, McCormack A, Nicholson JM (2011) Is carcinogensis a form of speciation? Cell cycle. 10: 2100-2114.

[52] Duesberg P, Iacobuzio Donahue C, Brosnan JA, McCormack A, Mandrioli D, Chen L (2012) Origin of metastases: Subspecies of cancers generated by intrinsic karyotypic variations. Cell cycle. 11: 1151-1166.

[53] Ledford H (2010) Big science: The cancer genome challenge. Nature. 464: 972-974

[54] Heng HH (2007) Cancer genome sequencing: the challenges ahead. Bioessays. 29: 783-794.

[55] Bessarabova M, Pustovalova O, Shi W, Serebriyskaya T, Ishkin A, Polyak K, Velculescu VE, Nikolskaya T, Nikolsky Y (2011) Functional synergies yet distinct modulators affected by genetic alterations in common human cancers. Cancer res. 71: 3471-3481.

[56] Syed AS, D'Antonio M, Ciccarelli FD (2010) Network of Cancer Genes: a web resource to analyze duplicability, orthology and network properties of cancer genes. Nucleic acids res. 38: 670-675.

[57] Brown JR, Levine RL, Thompson C, Basile G, Gilliland DG, Freedman AS (2008) Systematic genomic screen for tyrosine kinase mutations in CLL. Leukemia. 22: 1966-1969.

[58] Zhang X, Reis M, Khoriaty R, Li Y, Ouillette P, Samayoa J, Carter H, Karchin R, Li M, Diaz LA Jr, Velculescu VE, Papadopoulos N, Kinzler KW, Vogelstein B, Malek SN (2011) Sequence analysis of 515 kinase genes in chronic lymphocytic leukemia. Leukemia. 25: 1908-1910.

[59] Beroukhim R, Mermel CH, Porter D, Wei G, Raychaudhuri S, Donovan J, Barretina J, Boehm JS, Dobson J, Urashima M, Mc Henry KT, Pinchback RM, Ligon AH, Cho YJ, Haery L, Greulich H, Reich M, Winckler W, Lawrence MS, Weir BA, Tanaka KE, Chiang DY, Bass AJ, Loo A, Hoffman C, Prensner J, Liefeld T, Gao Q, Yecies D, Signoretti S, Maher E, Kaye FJ, Sasaki H, Tepper JE, Fletcher JA, Tabernero J, Baselga J, Tsao MS, Demichelis F, Rubin MA, Janne PA, Daly MJ, Nucera C, Levine RL, Ebert BL, Gabriel S, Rustgi AK, Antonescu CR, Ladanyi M, Letai A, Garraway LA, Loda M, Beer DG, True LD, Okamoto A, Pomeroy SL, Singer S, Golub TR, Lander ES, Getz G, Sellers WR, Meyerson M (2010) The landscape of somatic copy-number alteration across human cancers. Nature. 463: 899-905.

[60] Mattison J, Kool J, Uren AG, de Ridder J, Wessels L, Jonkers J, Bignell GR, Butler A, Rust AG, Brosch M, Wilson CH, van der Weyden L, Largaespada DA, Stratton MR, Futreal PA, van Lohuizen M, Berns A, Collier LS, Hubbard T, Adams DJ (2010) Novel candidate cancer genes identified by a large-scale cross-species comparative oncogenomics approach. Cancer res. 70: 883-895.

[61] Bignell GR, Greenman CD, Davies H, Butler AP, Edkins S, Andrews JM, Buck G, Chen L, Beare D, Latimer C, Widaa S, Hinton J, Fahey C, Fu B, Swamy S, Dalgliesh GL, Teh BT, Deloukas P, Yang F, Campbell PJ, Futreal PA, Stratton MR (2010) Signatures of mutation and selection in the cancer genome. Nature. 463: 893-898.

[62] Kan Z, Jaiswal BS, Stinson J, Janakiraman V, Bhatt D, Stern HM, Yue P, Haverty PM, Bourgon R, Zheng J, Moorhead M, Chaudhuri S, Tomsho LP, Peters BA, Pujara K, Cordes S, Davis DP, Carlton VE, Yuan W, Li L, Wang W, Eigenbrot C, Kaminker JS, Eberhard DA, Waring P, Schuster SC, Modrusan Z, Zhang Z, Stokoe D, de Sauvage FJ, Faham M, Seshagiri S (2010) Diverse somatic mutation patterns and pathway alterations in human cancers. Nature. 466: 869-873.

[63] Shepherd R, Forbes SA, Beare D, Bamford S, Cole CG, Ward S, Bindal N, Gunasekaran P, Jia M, Kok CY, Leung K, Menzies A, Butler AP, Teague JW, Campbell PJ, Stratton MR, Futreal PA (2011) Data mining using the Catalogue of Somatic Mutations in Cancer BioMart. Database (Oxford). doi: 10.1093/database/bar018.

[64] Forbes SA, Bindal N, Bamford S, Cole C, Kok CY, Beare D, Jia M, Shepherd R, Leung K, Menzies A, Teague JW, Campbell PJ, Stratton MR, Futreal PA (2011) COSMIC: mining complete cancer genomes in the Catalogue of Somatic Mutations in Cancer. Nucleic acids res. 39: 945-950.

[65] Bell DW (2010) Our changing view of the genomic landscape of cancer. J. pathol. 220: 231-243.

[66] Heng HH, Liu G, Stevens JB, Bremer SW, Ye KJ, Abdallah BY, Horne SD, Ye CJ (2011) Decoding the genome beyond sequencing: the new phase of genomic research. Genomics. 98: 242-252.

[67] Varley JM (2003) Germline TP53 mutations and Li-Fraumeni syndrome. Hum. mutat. 21: 313-320.

[68] Kenzelmann Broz D, Attardi LD (2010) In vivo analysis of p53 tumor suppressor function using genetically engineered mouse models. Carcinogensis. 31: 1311-1318.

[69] Taneja P, Zhu S, Maglic D, Fry EA, Kendig RD, Inoue K (2011) Transgenic and knockout mice models to reveal the functions of tumor suppressor genes. Clin. med. insights oncol. 5: 235-257.

[70] García-Cao I, García-Cao M, Martín-Caballero J, Criado LM, Klatt P, Flores JM, Weill JC, Blasco MA, Serrano M (2002) "Super p53" mice exhibit enhanced DNA damage response, are tumor resistant and age normally. EMBO j. 21: 6225-6235.

[71] Coschi CH, Dick FA (2012) Chromosome instability and dysregulated proliferation: an unavoidable duo. Cell mol. life sci. doi: 10.1007/s00018-011-0910-4.

[72] Liu DP, Song H, Xu Y (2010) A common gain of function of p53 cancer mutants in inducing genetic instability. Oncogene. 29: 949-956.

[73] Brosh R, Rotter V (2010) Transcriptional control of the proliferation cluster by the tumor suppressor p53. Mol. biosyst. 6: 17-29.

[74] Allred DC, Wu Y, Mao S, Nagtegaal ID, Lee S, Perou CM, Mohsin SK, O'Connell P, Tsimelzon A, Medina D (2008) Ductal carcinoma in situ and the emergence of diversity during breast cancer evolution. Clin. cancer res. 14: 370-378.

[75] Zenz T, Mohr J, Edelmann J, Sarno A, Hoth P, Heuberger M, Helfrich H, Mertens D, Dohner H, Stilgenbauer S (2009) Treatment resistance in chronic lymphocytic leukemia: the role of the p53 pathway. Leuk. lymphoma. 50: 510-513.

[76] Michaelis M, Rothweiler F, Barth S, Cinatl J, van Rikxoort M, Löschmann N, Voges Y, Breitli76ng R, von Deimling A, Rödel F, Weber K, Fehse B, Mack E, Stiewe T, Doerr

HW, Speidel D, Cinatl J Jr (2011) Adaptation of cancer cells from different entities to the MDM2 inhibitor nutlin-3 results in the emergence of p53-mutated multi-drug-resistant cancer cells. Cell death dis. doi: 10.1038/cddis.2011.129.

[77] Knappskog S, Lønning PE (2012) P53 and its molecular basis to chemoresistance in breast cancer. Expert opin. ther. targets. 16: 23-30.

[78] Martinez-Rivera M, Siddik ZH (2012) Resistance and gain-of-resistance phenotypes in cancers harboring wild-type p53. Biochem. pharmacol. 83: 1049-1062.

[79] Cancer Genome Atlas Research Network (2011) Integrated genomic analyses of ovarian carcinoma. Nature. 474: 609-615.

[80] Rücker FG, Schlenk RF, Bullinger L, Kayser S, Teleanu V, Kett H, Habdank M, Kugler CM, Holzmann K, Gaidzik VI, Paschka P, Held G, von Lilienfeld-Toal M, Lübbert M, Fröhling S, Zenz T, Krauter J, Schlegelberger B, Ganser A, Lichter P, Döhner K, Döhner H (2011) TP53 alterations in acute myeloid leukemia with complex karyotype correlate with specific copy number alterations, monosomal karyotype, and dismal outcome. Blood. 119: 2114-2121.

[81] Lai LA, Paulson TG, Li X, Sanchez CA, Maley C, Odze RD, Reid BJ, Rabinovitch PS (2007) Increasing genomic instability during premalignant neoplastic progression revealed through high resolution array-CGH. Genes chromosomes cancer. 46: 532-542.

[82] Maley CC, Galipeau PC, Finley JC, Wongsurawat VJ, Li X, Sanchez CA, Paulson TG, Blount PL, Risques RA, Rabinovitch PS, Reid BJ (2006) Genetic clonal diversity predicts progression to esophageal adenocarcinoma. Nat. genet. 38: 468-473.

[83] Reid BJ, Kostadinov R, Maley CC (2011) New strategies in Barrett's esophagus: integrating clonal evolutionary theory with clinical management. Clin. cancer res. 17: 3512-3519.

[84] Durinck S, Ho C, Wang NJ, Liao W, Jakkula LR, Collisson EA, Pons J, Chan SW, Lam ET, Chu C, Park K, Hong SW, Hur JS, Huh N, Neuhaus IM, Yu SS, Grekin RT, Mauro TM, Cleaver JE, Kwok PY, Leboit PE, Getz G, Cibulskis K, Aster JC, Huang H, Purdom E, Li J, Bolund L, Arron ST, Gray JW, Spellman PT, Cho RJ (2011) Temporal dissection of tumorigenesis in primary cancers. Cancer discov. 1: 137-143.

[85] Lo Nigro C, Vivenza D, Monteverde M, Lattanzio L, Gojis O, Garrone O, Comino A, Merlano M, Quinlan PR, Syed N, Purdie CA, Thompson A, Palmieri C, Crook T (2012) High frequency of complex TP53 mutations in CNS metastases from breast cancer. Br. j. cancer. 106: 397-404.

[86] D'Assoro AB, Leontovich A, Amato A, Ayers-Ringler JR, Quatraro C, Hafner K, Jenkins RB, Libra M, Ingle J, Stivala F, Galanis E, Salisbury JL (2010) Abrogation of p53 function leads to metastatic transcriptome networks that typify tumor progression in human breast cancer xenografts. Int. j. oncol. 37: 1167-1176.

[87] Roschke AV, Glebov OK, Lababidi S, Gehlhaus KS, Weinstein JN, Kirsch IR (2008) Chromosomal instability is associated with higher expression of genes implicated in epithelial-mesenchymal transition, cancer invasiveness, and metastasis and with lower expression of genes involved in cell cycle checkpoints, DNA repair, and chromatin maintenance. Neoplasia. 10: 1222-1230.

[88] Jiang Z, Jones R, Liu JC, Deng T, Robinson T, Chung PE, Wang S, Herschkowitz JI, Egan SE, Perou CM, Zacksenhaus E (2011) RB1 and p53 at the crossroad of EMT and triple-negative breast cancer. Cell cycle. 10: 1563-1570.

[89] Ansieau S, Courtois-Cox S, Morel AP, Puisieux A (2011) Failsafe program escape and EMT: a deleterious partnership. Semin. cancer biol. 21: 392-396.

[90] Thompson SL, Compton DA (2010) Proliferation of aneuploid human cells is limited by a p53-dependent mechanism. J. cell biol. 188: 369-381.

[91] Li M, Fang X, Baker DJ, Guo L, Gao X, Wei Z, Han S, van Deursen JM, Zhang P (2010) The ATM-p53 pathway suppresses aneuploidy-induced tumorigenesis. Proc. natl acad sci. USA. 107: 14188-14193.

[92] Sigal A, Rotter V (2000) Oncogenic mutations of the p53 tumor suppressor: the demons of the guardian of the genome. Cancer res. 60: 6788-6793.

[93] Blandino G, Deppert W, Hainaut P, Levine A, Lozano G, Olivier M, Rotter V, Wiman K, Oren M (2012) Mutant p53 protein, master regulator of human malignancies: a report on the fifth Mutant p53 Workshop. Cell death differ. 19: 180-183.

[94] Kleinerman RA, Tucker MA, Tarone RE, Abramson DH, Seddon JM, Stovall M, Li FP, Fraumeni JF Jr (2005) Risk of new cancers after radiotherapy in long-term survivors of retinoblastoma: an extended follow-up. J. clin. oncol. 23: 2272-2279.

[95] Marees T, Moll AC, Imhof SM, de Boer MR, Ringens PJ, van Leeuwen FE (2008) Risk of second malignancies in survivors of retinoblastoma: more than 40 years of follow-up. J. natl. cancer inst. 100: 1771-1779.

[96] Laurie NA, Donovan SL, Shih CS, Zhang J, Mills N, Fuller C, Teunisse A, Lam S, Ramos Y, Mohan A, Johnson D, Wilson M, Rodriguez-Galindo C, Quarto M, Francoz S, Mendrysa SM, Guy RK, Marine JC, Jochemsen AG, Dyer MA (2006) Inactivation of the p53 pathway in retinoblastoma. Nature. 444. 61-66.

[97] Amare Kadam PS, Ghule P, Jose J, Bamne M, Kurkure P, Banavali S, Sarin R, Advani S (2004) Constitutional genomic instability, chromosome aberrations in tumor cells and retinoblastoma. Cancer genet. cytogenet. 150: 33-43.

[98] Choy KW, Pang CP, Fan DS, Lee TC, Wang JH, Abramson DH, Lo KW, To KF, Yu CB, Beaverson KL, Cheung KF, Lam DS (2004) Microsatellite instability and MLH1 promoter methylation in human retinoblastoma. Invest. ophthalmol. vis. sci. 45: 3404-3409.

[99] Kujawski L, Ouillette P, Erba H, Saddler C, Jakubowiak A, Kaminski M, Shedden K, Malek SN (2008) Genomic complexity identifies patients with aggressive chronic lymphocytic leukemia. Blood. 112: 1993-2003.

[100] Ouillette P, Fossum S, Parkin B, Ding L, Bockenstedt P, Al-Zoubi A, Shedden K, Malek SN (2010) Aggressive chronic lymphocytic leukemia with elevated genomic complexity is associated with multiple gene defects in the response to DNA double-strand breaks. Clin. cancer res. 16: 835-847.

[101] Ouillette P, Collins R, Shakhan S, Li J, Li C, Shedden K, Malek SN (2011) The prognostic significance of various 13q14 deletions in chronic lymphocytic leukemia. Clin. cancer res. 17: 6778-6790.

[102] Sage J, Straight AF (2010) RB's original CIN? Genes dev. 24: 1329-1333.

[103] Manning AL, Dyson NJ (2011) pRB, a tumor suppressor with a stabilizing presence. Trends cell biol. 21: 433-441.

[104] Knudsen ES, Wang JY (2010) Targeting the RB-pathway in cancer therapy. Clin cancer res. 16: 1094-1099.

[105] Lehn S, Fernö M, Jirström K, Rydén L, Landberg G (2011) A non-functional retinoblastoma tumor suppressor (RB) pathway in premenopausal breast cancer is associated with resistance to tamoxifen. Cell cycle. 10: 956-962.

[106] Dolma S, Lessnick SL, Hahn WC, Stockwell BR (2003) Identification of genotype-selective antitumor agents using synthetic lethal chemical screening in engineered human tumor cells. Cancer cell. 3: 285-296.

[107] Stengel KR, Dean JL, Seeley SL, Mayhew CN, Knudsen ES (2008) RB status governs differential sensitivity to cytotoxic and molecularly-targeted therapeutic agents. Cell cycle. 7: 1095-1103.

[108] Sherr CJ, McCormick F (2002) The RB and p53 pathways in cancer. Cancer Cell. 2: 103-112.

[109] McDermott KM, Zhang J, Holst CR, Kozakiewicz BK, Singla V, Tlsty TD (2006) p16(INK4a) prevents centrosome dysfunction and genomic instability in primary cells. PLoS biol. doi:10.1371/journal.pbio.0040051.

[110] Li H, Collado M, Villasante A, Strati K, Ortega S, Cañamero M, Blasco MA, Serrano M (2009) The Ink4/Arf locus is a barrier for iPS cell reprogramming. Nature. 460: 1136-1139.

[111] Pasi CE, Dereli-Öz A, Negrini S, Friedli M, Fragola G, Lombardo A, Van Houwe G, Naldini L, Casola S, Testa G, Trono D, Pelicci PG, Halazonetis TD (2011) Genomic instability in induced stem cells. Cell death. differ. 18: 745-753.

[112] Blasco MA, Serrano M, Fernandez-Capetillo O (2011) Genomic instability in iPS: time for a break. EMBO j. 30: 991-993.

[113] Lund RJ, Närvä E, Lahesmaa R (2012) Genetic and epigenetic stability of human pluripotent stem cells. Nat. rev. genet. 13: 732-744.

[114] Menendez S, Camus S, Herreria A, Paramonov I, Morera LB, Collado M, Pekarik V, Maceda I, Edel M, Consiglio A, Sanchez A, Li H, Serrano M, Belmonte JC (2012) Increased dosage of tumor suppressors limits the tumorigenicity of iPS cells without affecting their pluripotency. Aging cell. 11: 41-50.

[115] Freeman DJ, Li AG, Wei G, Li HH, Kertesz N, Lesche R et al. (2003). PTEN tumor suppressor regulates p53 protein levels and activity through phosphatase-dependent and -independent mechanisms. Cancer cell. 3: 117-130.

[116] Yin Y, Shen WH (2008) PTEN: a new guardian of the genome. Oncogene. 27: 5443-5453.

[117] Shen WH, Balajee AS, Wang J, Wu H, Eng C, Pandolfi PP, Yin Y (2007) Essential role for nuclear PTEN in maintaining chromosomal integrity. Cell. 128: 157-170.

[118] Mukherjee A, Karmakar P (2012) Attenuation of PTEN perturbs genomic stability via activation of Akt and down-regulation of Rad51 in human embryonic kidney cells. Mol. carcinog. doi: 10.1002/mc.21903.

[119] Upadhyaya M, Han S, Consoli C, Majounie E, Horan M, Thomas NS, Potts C, Griffiths S, Ruggieri M, von Deimling A, Cooper DN (2004) Characterization of the somatic mutational spectrum of the neurofibromatosis type 1 (NF1) gene in neurofibromatosis patients with benign and malignant tumors. Hum. mutat. 23: 134-146.

[120] Upadhyaya M, Kluwe L, Spurlock G, Monem B, Majounie E, Mantripragada K, Ruggieri M, Chuzhanova N, Evans DG, Ferner R, Thomas N, Guha A, Mautner V (2008) Germline and somatic NF1 gene mutation spectrum in NF1-associated malignant peripheral nerve sheath tumors (MPNSTs). Hum. mutat. 29: 74-82.

[121] Lee MJ, Stephenson DA (2007) Recent developments in neurofibromatosis type 1. Curr. opin. neurol. 20: 135-141.

[122] Spurlock G, Knight SJ, Thomas N, Kiehl TR, Guha A, Upadhyaya M (2010) Molecular evolution of a neurofibroma to malignant peripheral nerve sheath tumor (MPNST) in an NF1 patient: correlation between histopathological, clinical and molecular findings. J. cancer res. clin. oncol. 136: 1869-1880.

[123] Gorgoulis VG, Halazonetis TD (2010) Oncogene-induced senescence: the bright and dark side of the response. Curr. opin. cell biol. 22: 816-827.

[124] Caino MC, Meshki J, Kazanietz MG (2009) Hallmarks for senescence in carcinogensis: novel signaling players. Apoptosis. 14: 392-408.

[125] Larsson LG (2011) Oncogene- and tumor suppressor gene-mediated suppression of cellular senescence. Semin. cancer biol. 21: 367-376.

[126] Saab R (2011) Senescence and pre-malignancy: how do tumors progress? Semin. cancer biol. 21: 385-391.

[127] Burke BA, Carroll M (2010) BCR-ABL: a multi-faceted promoter of DNA mutation in chronic myelogeneous leukemia. Leukemia. 24: 1105-1112.

[128] Rumpold H, Webersinke G (2011) Molecular pathogenesis of Philadelphia-positive chronic myeloid leukemia - is it all BCR-ABL? Curr. cancer drug targets. 11: 3-19.

[129] Venkitaraman AR (2009) Linking the cellular functions of BRCA genes to cancer pathogenesis and treatment. Annu. rev. pathol. 4: 461-487.

[130] Vollebergh MA, Jonkers J, Linn SC. (2012) Genomic instability in breast and ovarian cancers: translation into clinical predictive biomarkers. Cell mol. life sci. 69: 223-245.

[131] Kais Z, Chiba N, Ishioka C, Parvin JD (2012) Functional differences among BRCA1 missense mutations in the control of centrosome duplication. Oncogene. 31: 799-804.

[132] Maher ER, Neumann HP, Richard S (2011) von Hippel-Lindau disease: a clinical and scientific review. Eur. j. hum. genet. 19: 617-623.

[133] Thoma CR, Toso A, Meraldi P, Krek W (2009) Double-trouble in mitosis caused by von Hippel-Lindau tumor-suppressor protein inactivation. Cell cycle. 8: 3619-3320.

[134] Thoma CR, Toso A, Meraldi P, Krek W (2011) Mechanisms of aneuploidy and its suppression by tumour suppressor proteins. Swiss med. wkly. doi: 10.4414/smw.2011.13170.

[135] Rusan NM, Peifer M (2008) Original CIN: reviewing roles for APC in chromosome instability. J. cell. biol. 181: 719-726.

[136] Bahmanyar S, Nelson WJ, Barth AI (2009) Role of APC and its binding partners in regulating microtubules in mitosis. Adv. exp. med. biol. 656: 65-74.

[137] Lavin MF, Birrell G, Chen P, Kozlov S, Scott S, Gueven N (2005) ATM signaling and genomic stability in response to DNA damage. Mutat res. 569: 123-132.

[138] Derheimer FA, Kastan MB (2010) Multiple roles of ATM in monitoring and maintaining DNA integrity. FEBS lett. 584: 3675-3681.

[139] Loffler KA, Biondi CA, Gartside M, Waring P, Stark M, Serewko-Auret MM, Muller HK, Hayward NK, Kay GF (2007) Broad tumor spectrum in a mouse model of multiple endocrine neoplasia type 1. Int. j. cancer. 120: 259-267.

[140] Wu T, Hua X (2011) Menin represses tumorigenesis via repressing cell proliferation. Am. j cancer res. 1: 726-739.

[141] Yang Y, Hua X (2007) In search of tumor suppressing functions of menin. Mol. cell. endocrinol. 265-266: 34-41.

[142] Wade M, Wahl GM (2006) c-Myc, genome instability, and tumorigenesis: the devil is in the details. Curr. top. microbiol. immunol. 302: 169-203.

[143] Prochownik EV (2008) c-Myc: linking transformation and genomic instability. Curr. mol. med. 8: 446-458.

[144] Fukasawa K (2007) Oncogenes and tumour suppressors take on centrosomes. Nat. rev. cancer. 7: 911-924.

[145] Rao CV, Yamada HY, Yao Y, Dai W (2009) Enhanced genomic instabilities caused by dysregulated microtubule dynamics and chromosome segregation: a perspective from genetic studies in mice. Carcinogensis. 30: 1469-1474.

[146] Schvartzman JM, Sotillo R, Benezra R (2010) Mitotic chromosomal instability and cancer: mouse modelling of the human disease. Nat. rev. cancer. 10: 102-115.

[147] Thompson SL, Bakhoum SF, Compton DA (2010) Mechanisms of chromosomal instability. Curr. biol. 20: 285-295.

[148] Harrison MK, Adon AM, Saavedra HI (2011) The G1 phase Cdks regulate the centrosome cycle and mediate oncogene-dependent centrosome amplification. Cell div. doi:10.1186/1747-1028-6-2.

[149] Watanabe Y, Maekawa M (2010) Methylation of DNA in cancer. Adv. clin. chem. 52: 145-167.

[150] Toyota M, Suzuki H (2010) Epigenetic drivers of genetic alterations. Adv. genet. 70: 309-323.

[151] Kanai Y (2008) Alterations of DNA methylation and clinicopathological diversity of human cancers. Pathol. int. 58: 544-558.

[152] Daniel FI, Cherubini K, Yurgel LS, de Figueiredo MA, Salum FG (2011) The role of epigenetic transcription repression and DNA methyltransferases in cancer. Cancer. 117: 677-687.

[153] Barra V, Schillaci T, Lentini L, Costa G, Di Leonardo A (2012) Bypass of cell cycle arrest induced by transient DNMT1 post-transcriptional silencing triggers aneuploidy in human cells. Cell div. doi:10.1186/1747-1028-7-2

[154] Karpf AR, Matsui S (2005) Genetic disruption of cytosine DNA methyltransferase enzymes induces chromosomal instability in human cancer cells. Cancer res. 65: 8635-8639.

[155] Dodge JE, Okano M, Dick F, Tsujimoto N, Chen T, Wang S, Ueda Y, Dyson N, Li E (2005) Inactivation of Dnmt3b in mouse embryonic fibroblasts results in DNA hypomethylation, chromosomal instability, and spontaneous immortalization. J. biol. chem. 280: 17986-17991.

[156] Gaudet F, Hodgson JG, Eden A, Jackson-Grusby L, Dausman J, Gray JW, Leonhardt H, Jaenisch R (2003) Induction of tumors in mice by genomic hypomethylation. Science. 300: 489-492.

[157] Eden A, Gaudet F, Waghmare A, Jaenisch R (2003) Chromosomal instability and tumors promoted by DNA hypomethylation. Science. doi: 10.1126/science.1083557.

[158] Howard G, Eiges R, Gaudet F, Jaenisch R, Eden A (2008) Activation and transposition of endogenous retroviral elements in hypomethylation induced tumors in mice. Oncogene. 27: 404-408.

[159] Ganem NJ, Godinho SA, Pellman D (2009) A mechanism linking extra centrosomes to chromosomal instability. Nature. 460: 278-282.

[160] Silkworth WT, Nardi IK, Scholl LM, Cimini D (2009) Multipolar spindle pole coalescence is a major source of kinetochore mis-attachment and chromosome mis-segregation in cancer cells. PLoS one. doi:10.1371/journal.pone.0006564.

[161] Gregan J, Polakova S, Zhang L, Tolić-Nørrelykke IM, Cimini D (2011) Merotelic kinetochore attachment: causes and effects. Trends cell. biol. 21: 374-381.

[162] Thompson SL, Compton DA (2011) Chromosome missegregation in human cells arises through specific types of kinetochore-microtubule attachment errors. Proc. natl. acad. sci. USA. 108: 17974-17978.

[163] Janssen A, Kops GJ, Medema RH (2009) Elevating the frequency of chromosome mis-segregation as a strategy to kill tumor cells. Proc. natl. acad. sci. USA. 106: 19108-19113.

[164] Guerrero AA, Martínez-A C, van Wely KH (2010) Merotelic attachments and non-homologous end joining are the basis of chromosomal instability. Cell div. doi:10.1186/1747-1028-5-13.

[165] Stephens PJ, Greenman CD, Fu B, Yang F, Bignell GR, Mudie LJ, Pleasance ED, Lau KW, Beare D, Stebbings LA, McLaren S, Lin ML, McBride DJ, Varela I, Nik-Zainal S, Leroy C, Jia M, Menzies A, Butler AP, Teague JW, Quail MA, Burton J, Swerdlow H, Carter NP, Morsberger LA, Iacobuzio-Donahue C, Follows GA, Green AR, Flanagan AM, Stratton MR, Futreal PA, Campbell PJ (2011) Massive genomic rearrangement acquired in a single catastrophic event during cancer development. Cell. 144: 27-40.

[166] Crasta K, Ganem NJ, Dagher R, Lantermann AB, Ivanova EV, Pan Y, Nezi L, Protopopov A, Chowdhury D, Pellman D (2012) DNA breaks and chromosome pulverization from errors in mitosis. Nature. 482: 53-58.

[167] Baker DJ, Jin F, Jeganathan KB, van Deursen JM (2009) Whole chromosome instability caused by Bub1 insufficiency drives tumorigenesis through tumor suppressor gene loss of heterozygosity. Cancer cell. 16: 475-486.

[168] Sotillo R, Schvartzman JM, Benezra R (2009) Very CIN-ful: whole chromosome instability promotes tumor suppressor loss of heterozygosity. Cancer cell. 16: 451-452.

[169] Baker DJ, van Deursen JM (2010) Chromosome missegregation causes colon cancer by APC loss of heterozygosity. Cell cycle. 9: 1711-1716.

[170] Kloosterman WP, Hoogstraat M, Paling O, Tavakoli-Yaraki M, Renkens I, Vermaat JS, van Roosmalen MJ, van Lieshout S, Nijman IJ, Roessingh W, van 't Slot R, van de Belt J, Guryev V, Koudijs M, Voest E, Cuppen E (2011) Chromothripsis is a common mechanism driving genomic rearrangements in primary and metastatic colorectal cancer. Genome biol. doi:10.1186/gb-2011-12-10-r103.

[171] Basto R, Brunk K, Vinadogrova T, Peel N, Franz A, Khodjakov A, Raff JW (2008) Centrosome amplification can initiate tumorigenesis in flies. Cell. 133: 1032-1042.

[172] Doxsey SJ (2005) Molecular links between centrosome and midbody. Mol. cell. 20: 170-172.

[173] Nogales-Cadenas R, Abascal F, Díez-Pérez J, Carazo JM, Pascual-Montano A (2009) CentrosomeDB: a human centrosomal proteins database. Nucleic acids res. 37: 175-180.

[174] Müller H, Schmidt D, Dreher F, Herwig R, Ploubidou A, Lange BM (2011) Gene ontology analysis of the centrosome proteomes of Drosophila and human. Commun. integr. biol. 4: 308-311.

[175] Jakobsen L, Vanselow K, Skogs M, Toyoda Y, Lundberg E, Poser I, Falkenby LG, Bennetzen M, Westendorf J, Nigg EA, Uhlen M, Hyman AA, Andersen JS (2011) Novel asymmetrically localizing components of human centrosomes identified by complementary proteomics methods. EMBO j. 30: 1520-1535.

[176] Goshima G, Wollman R, Goodwin SS, Zhang N, Scholey JM, Vale RD, Stuurman N (2007) Genes required for mitotic spindle assembly in Drosophila S2 cells. Science. 316: 417-421.

[177] Dobbelaere J, Josué F, Suijkerbuijk S, Baum B, Tapon N, Raff J (2008) A genome-wide RNAi screen to dissect centriole duplication and centrosome maturation in Drosophila. PLoS biol. doi:10.1371/journal.pbio.0060224.

[178] Kwon M, Godinho SA, Chandhok NS, Ganem NJ, Azioune A, Thery M, Pellman D (2008) Mechanisms to suppress multipolar divisions in cancer cells with extra centrosomes. Genes dev. 22: 2189-2203.

[179] Leber B, Maier B, Fuchs F, Chi J, Riffel P, Anderhub S, Wagner L, Ho AD, Salisbury JL, Boutros M, Krämer A (2010) Proteins required for centrosome clustering in cancer cells. Sci. transl. med. 2: 33-38.

[180] Keck JM, Jones MH, Wong CC, Binkley J, Chen D, Jaspersen SL, Holinger EP, Xu T, Niepel M, Rout MP, Vogel J, Sidow A, Yates JR 3rd, Winey M (2011) A cell cycle phosphoproteome of the yeast centrosome. Science. 332: 1557-1561.

[181] Paulsen RD, Soni DV, Wollman R, Hahn AT, Yee MC, Guan A, Hesley JA, Miller SC, Cromwell EF, Solow-Cordero DE, Meyer T, Cimprich KA (2009) A genome-wide siRNA screen reveals diverse cellular processes and pathways that mediate genome stability. Mol. cell. 35: 228-239.

[182] Wong J, Nakajima Y, Westermann S, Shang C, Kang JS, Goodner C, Houshmand P, Fields S, Chan CS, Drubin D, Barnes G, Hazbun T (2007) A protein interaction map of the mitotic spindle. Mol. biol. cell. 18: 3800-3809.

[183] Stirling PC, Bloom MS, Solanki-Patil T, Smith S, Sipahimalani P, Li Z, Kofoed M, Ben-Aroya S, Myung K, Hieter P (2011) The complete spectrum of yeast chromosome

instability genes identifies candidate CIN cancer genes and functional roles for ASTRA complex components. PLoS genet. doi:10.1371/journal.pgen.1002057.

[184] Woo RA, Poon RY (2004) Gene mutations and aneuploidy: the instability that causes cancer. Cell cycle. 3: 1101-1103.

[185] Moynahan ME, Cui TY, Jasin M (2001) Homology-directed dna repair, mitomycin-c resistance, and chromosome stability is restored with correction of a Brca1 mutation. Cancer res. 61: 4842-4850.

[186] Nam HJ, Chae S, Jang SH, Cho H, Lee JH (2010) The PI3K-Akt mediates oncogenic Met-induced centrosome amplification and chromosome instability. Carcinogensis. 31: 1531-1540.

[187] Solomon DA, Kim T, Diaz-Martinez LA, Fair J, Elkahloun AG, Harris BT, Toretsky JA, Rosenberg SA, Shukla N, Ladanyi M, Samuels Y, James CD, Yu H, Kim JS, Waldman T (2011) Mutational inactivation of STAG2 causes aneuploidy in human cancer. Science. 333: 1039-1043.

[188] Shinmura K, Tao H, Nagura K, Goto M, Matsuura S, Mochizuki T, Suzuki K, Tanahashi M, Niwa H, Ogawa H, Sugimura H (2011) Suppression of hydroxyurea-induced centrosome amplification by NORE1A and down-regulation of NORE1A mRNA expression in non-small cell lung carcinoma. Lung cancer. 71: 19-27.

[189] Wise SS, Wise JP (2010) Aneuploidy as an early mechanistic event in metal carcinogensis. Biochem. soc. trans. 38: 1650-1654.

[190] Holmes AL, Wise JP (2010) Mechanisms of metal-induced centrosome amplification. Biochem. soc. trans. 38: 1687-1690.

[191] MacCorkle RA, Slattery SD, Nash DR, Brinkley BR (2006) Intracellular protein binding to asbestos induces aneuploidy in human lung fibroblasts. Cell motil. cytoskeleton. 63: 646-657.

[192] Cortez Bde A, Quassollo G, Caceres A, Machado-Santelli GM (2011) The fate of chrysotile-induced multipolar mitosis and aneuploid population in cultured lung cancer cells. PLoS one. doi:10.1371/journal.pone.0018600.

[193] Marlowe JL, Puga A (2005) Aryl hydrocarbon receptor, cell cycle regulation, toxicity, and tumorigenesis. J. cell. biochem. 96: 1174-1184.

[194] Korzeniewski N, Wheeler S, Chatterjee P, Duensing A, Duensing S (2010) A novel role of the aryl hydrocarbon receptor (AhR) in centrosome amplification - implications for chemoprevention. Mol. cancer. doi:10.1186/1476-4598-9-153.

[195] Gonzalez L, Decordier I, Kirsch-Volders M (2010) Induction of chromosome malsegregation by nanomaterials. Biochem. soc. trans. 38: 1691-1697.

[196] Wang X, Allen TD, May RJ, Lightfoot S, Houchen CW, Huycke MM (2008) Enterococcus faecalis induces aneuploidy and tetraploidy in colonic epithelial cells through a bystander effect. Cancer res. 68: 9909-9917.

[197] Toller IM, Neelsen KJ, Steger M, Hartung ML, Hottiger MO, Stucki M, Kalali B, Gerhard M, Sartori AA, Lopes M, Müller A (2011) Carcinogenic bacterial pathogen Helicobacter pylori triggers DNA double-strand breaks and a DNA damage response in its host cells. Proc. natl. acad. sci. USA. 108: 14944-14949.

[198] Korzeniewski N, Spardy N, Duensing A, Duensing S (2011) Genomic instability and cancer: lessons learned from human papillomaviruses. Cancer lett. 305: 113-122.

[199] Sharma SV, Settleman J (2006) Oncogenic shock: turning an activated kinase against the tumor cell. Cell cycle. 5: 2878-2880.

[200] Sharma SV, Settleman J (2007) Oncogene addiction: setting the stage for molecularly targeted cancer therapy. Genes dev. 21: 3214-3231.

[201] Weinstein IB, Joe A (2008) Oncogene addiction. Cancer res. 68: 3077-3080

[202] Yan W, Zhang W, Jiang T (2011) Oncogene addiction in gliomas: implications for molecular targeted therapy. J. exp. clin. cancer res. doi:10.1186/1756-9966-30-58.

[203] McCormick F (2011) Cancer therapy based on oncogene addiction. J. surg. oncol. 103: 464-467.

[204] Settleman J (2012) Oncogene addiction. Curr. biol. 22: 43-44.

[205] Torti D, Trusolino L (2011) Oncogene addiction as a foundational rationale for targeted anti-cancer therapy: promises and perils. EMBO mol. med. 3: 623-636.

[206] Giuriato S, Felsher DW (2003) How cancers escape their oncogene habit. Cell cycle. 2: 329-332.

[207] Jechlinger M, Podsypanina K, Varmus H (2009) Regulation of transgenes in three-dimensional cultures of primary mouse mammary cells demonstrates oncogene dependence and identifies cells that survive deinduction. Genes dev. 23: 1677-1688.

[208] Jang JW, Boxer RB, Chodosh LA (2006) Isoform-specific ras activation and oncogene dependence during MYC- and Wnt-induced mammary tumorigenesis. Mol. cell biol. 26: 8109-8121.

[209] Gutierrez A, Grebliunaite R, Feng H, Kozakewich E, Zhu S, Guo F, Payne E, Mansour M, Dahlberg SE, Neuberg DS, den Hertog J, Prochownik EV, Testa JR, Harris M, Kanki JP, Look AT (2011) Pten mediates Myc oncogene dependence in a conditional zebrafish model of T cell acute lymphoblastic leukemia. J. exp. med. 208: 1595-1603.

[210] Debies MT, Gestl SA, Mathers JL, Mikse OR, Leonard TL, Moody SE, Chodosh LA, Cardiff RD, Gunther EJ (2008) Tumor escape in a Wnt1-dependent mouse breast cancer model is enabled by p19Arf/p53 pathway lesions but not p16 Ink4a loss. J. clin. invest. 118: 51-63.

[211] Jonkers J, Berns A (2004) Oncogene addiction: sometimes a temporary slavery. Cancer cell. 6: 535-538.

[212] Tran PT, Bendapudi PK, Lin HJ, Choi P, Koh S, Chen J, Horng G, Hughes NP, Schwartz LH, Miller VA, Kawashima T, Kitamura T, Paik D, Felsher DW (2011) Survival and death signals can predict tumor response to therapy after oncogene inactivation. Sci. transl. med. doi: 10.1126/scitranslmed.3002018.

[213] Tran PT, Fan AC, Bendapudi PK, Koh S, Komatsubara K, Chen J, Horng G, Bellovin DI, Giuriato S, Wang CS, Whitsett JA, Felsher DW (2008) Combined Inactivation of MYC and K-Ras oncogenes reverses tumorigenesis in lung adenocarcinomas and lymphomas. PLoS one. doi:10.1371/journal.pone.0002125.

[214] Gunther EJ, Moody SE, Belka GK, Hahn KT, Innocent N, Dugan KD, Cardiff RD, Chodosh LA (2003) Impact of p53 loss on reversal and recurrence of conditional Wnt-induced tumorigenesis. Genes dev. 17: 488-501.

[215] Vanbrocklin MW, Robinson JP, Lastwika KJ, McKinney AJ, Gach HM, Holmen SL (2012) Ink4a/Arf loss promotes tumor recurrence following Ras inhibition. Neuro oncol. 14: 34-42.

[216] Xing F, Persaud Y, Pratilas CA, Taylor BS, Janakiraman M, She QB, Gallardo H, Liu C, Merghoub T, Hefter B, Dolgalev I, Viale A, Heguy A, De Stanchina E, Cobrinik D, Bollag G, Wolchok J, Houghton A, Solit DB (2011) Concurrent loss of the PTEN and RB1 tumor suppressors attenuates RAF dependence in melanomas harboring (V600E)BRAF. Oncogene. doi: 10.1038/onc.2011.250.

[217] Karlsson A, Giuriato S, Tang F, Fung-Weier J, Levan G, Felsher DW (2003) Genomically complex lymphomas undergo sustained tumor regression upon MYC inactivation unless they acquire novel chromosomal translocations. Blood. 101: 2797-2803.

[218] Sotillo R, Schvartzman JM, Socci ND, Benezra R (2010) Mad2-induced chromosome instability leads to lung tumour relapse after oncogene withdrawal. Nature. 464: 436-440.

[219] Tonon G (2008) From oncogene to network addiction: the new frontier of cancer genomics and therapeutics. Future oncol. 4: 569-577.

[220] Mahoney DJ, Stojdl DF (2012) Fighting fire with fire: rewiring tumor cells for oncolytic virotherapy. Future oncol. 8: 219-221.

[221] Ng K, Chen CC (2011) Oncogene addiction and non-oncogene addiction in glioblastoma therapy. Chin. med. j. (Engl). 124: 2565-2568.

[222] Shi I, Hashemi Sadraei N, Duan ZH, Shi T (2011) Aberrant signaling pathways in squamous cell lung carcinoma. Cancer inform. 10: 273-285.

[223] Sawyers CL (2009) Shifting paradigms: the seeds of oncogene addiction. Nat. med. 15: 1158-1161.

[224] Santos FP, Kantarjian H, Quintás-Cardama A, Cortes J (2011) Evolution of therapies for chronic myelogenous leukemia. Cancer j. 17: 465-476.

[225] Shaffer BC, Gillet JP, Patel C, Baer MR, Bates SE, Gottesman MM (2012) Drug resistance: Still a daunting challenge to the successful treatment of AML. Drug resist. updat. doi: 10.1016/j.drup.2012.02.001.

[226] Bertotti A, Burbridge MF, Gastaldi S, Galimi F, Torti D, Medico E, Giordano S, Corso S, Rolland-Valognes G, Lockhart BP, Hickman JA, Comoglio PM, Trusolino L (2009) Only a subset of Met-activated pathways are required to sustain oncogene addiction. Sci. signal. doi: 10.1126/scisignal.2000643.

[227] Liedtke C, Wang J, Tordai A, Symmans WF, Hortobagyi GN, Kiesel L, Hess K, Baggerly KA, Coombes KR, Pusztai L (2010) Clinical evaluation of chemotherapy response predictors developed from breast cancer cell lines. Breast cancer res. treat. 121: 301-309.

[228] Politi K, Pao W (2011) How genetically engineered mouse tumor models provide insights into human cancers. J. clin. oncol. 29: 2273-2281.

[229] Cheon DJ, Orsulic S (2011) Mouse models of cancer. Annu rev pathol. 6: 95-119.

[230] Solimini NL, Luo J, Elledge SJ (2007) Non-oncogene addiction and the stress phenotype of cancer cells. Cell. 130: 986-988.

[231] Shaffer AL, Emre NC, Lamy L, Ngo VN, Wright G, Xiao W, Powell J, Dave S, Yu X, Zhao H, Zeng Y, Chen B, Epstein J, Staudt LM (2008) IRF4 addiction in multiple myeloma. Nature. 454: 226-231.

[232] Hussain S, Zhang Y, Galardy PJ (2009) DUBs and cancer: the role of deubiquitinating enzymes as oncogenes, non-oncogenes and tumor suppressors. Cell cycle. 8: 1688-1697

[233] Luo J, Solimini NL, Elledge SJ (2009) Principles of cancer therapy: oncogene and non-oncogene addiction. Cell. 136: 823-837.

[234] Chen DY, Liu H, Takeda S, Tu HC, Sasagawa S, Van Tine BA, Lu D, Cheng EH, Hsieh JJ (2010) Taspase1 functions as a non-oncogene addiction protease that coordinates cancer cell proliferation and apoptosis. Cancer res. 70: 5358-5367.

[235] Almendro V, Fuster G (2011) Heterogeneity of breast cancer: etiology and clinical relevance Clin. transl. oncol. 13: 767-773

[236] Aktipis CA, Kwan VS, Johnson KA, Neuberg SL, Maley CC (2011) Overlooking evolution: a systematic analysis of cancer relapse and therapeutic resistance research. PLoS one.; doi:10.1371/journal.pone.0026100.

[237] Navin N, Hicks J (2011) Future medical applications of single-cell sequencing in cancer. Genome med. doi:10.1186/gm247.

[238] Longo DL (2012) Tumor heterogeneity and personalized medicine. N. engl. j. med. 366: 956-957.

[239] De S, Michor F (2011) DNA replication timing and long-range DNA interactions predict mutational landscapes of cancer genomes. Nat. biotechnol. 29: 1103-1108.

[240] Fudenberg G, Getz G, Meyerson M, Mirny LA (2011) High order chromatin architecture shapes the landscape of chromosomal alterations in cancer. Nat. biotechnol. 29: 1109-1113.

[241] Zhang Y, McCord RP, Ho YJ, Lajoie BR, Hildebrand DG, Simon AC, Becker MS, Alt FW, Dekker J (2012) Spatial organization of the mouse genome and its role in recurrent chromosomal translocations. Cell. 148: 908-921.

Chapter 8

Human Papillomaviruses Oncoproteins

Gabriela Anton, Adriana Plesa, Coralia Bleotu, Anca Botezatu,
Mariana Anton, Lorelei Irina Brasoveanu and Mihai Stoian

Additional information is available at the end of the chapter

http://dx.doi.org/10.5772/55342

1. Introduction

One of the most common sexually transmitted diseases is human papillomavirus (HPV) infection that affects around 80% of sexually active women. Although most of the women clear HPV infection, individuals with inadequate immune responses develop persistent infections which lead to premalignant lesions such as high-grade cervical intraepithelial neoplasia (CIN-III), with high potential to progress to cervical carcinoma. Based on molecular and epidemiological data, high risk papillomaviruses (hrHPVs) are now recognized as etiologic agents of cervical carcinoma, although some additional events are required [1, 2].

From 200 HPV genotypes identified so far, nearly 40 can infect cervix and at least 15 hrHPVs (16, 18, 45, 31, 52, 33, 58, 35, 59, 51, 56, 39, 68, 73, and 82) are usually associated with the development of carcinomas. Although HPVs 26, 53, and 66 are probably high-risk types limited data link them to cervix cancer [3]. HPV16 accounts for near 60% of the cervical cancer cases in most countries, followed by HPV-18, -31 and -45.

HPVs are small non-enveloped double-stranded DNA viruses of about 8000-base pair long [4]. The viral genome codes for eight proteins and is divided in three functional regions: early (E1-E6), late (L1-L2) and long coding region (LCR). Early genes are synthesized in the infected basal cells and the late ones are expressed in differentiated cells [5], the replication of HPV cycle depending on complete squamous differentiation of the host epithelium. Except for E1 and E2 proteins (necessary for viral replication), papillomaviruses use the host cell machinery for viral DNA synthesis.

New data confirmed that papillomavirus genomes are organized in the form of chromatin-like structures composed by nucleoprotein complexes (nucleosomes) interconnected by a DNA filament. Treatment of CaSki human cervical carcinoma cell line with methidiumpropyl-EDTA-Fe (II) reveals nucleosomes in specific positions on the LCR and the E6 and E7 genes. First observed by electron microscopy for bovine papillomavirus (BPV) and HPV from human plantar warts, respectively [6], they were subsequently confirmed for CaSki cell line where the localization of nucleosomes was found at LCR, E6 and E7 genes level. The role of nucleosomes is to repress the activity of the E6 promoter. An open chromatin structure (transcriptionally active status) at early and late viral promoter regions was characterized by the presence of dimethylated forms of histone H3K4 as well as acetylated histones H3 and H4 [7]. These observations suggest the involvement of histone modification in HPV transcription regulation.

2. HPV oncogenesis

Most cervical cancers arise at the squamo-columnar junction, a site characterized by continuous metaplastic changes. The highest metaplastic activity occurs in young women who are reported to have the highest incidence of HPV infection. As cervical cancer is frequently detected in women over 35 years, it was suggested that the disease is a consequence of a slow progression of the viral infection acquired at younger age [8].

HPVs complete their life cycle only in fully differentiated squamous epithelium and the presence of viral genomes in the infected cells is essential both for papillomaviruses and their associated pathologies. HPV cervical infections result in three types of clinical manifestations: (a) productive infection which lead to virions production; viral genes expression is strictly associated with host cell differentiation; (b) latent (asymptomatic) infection (characterized by viral genome presence in basal layers) develops within the first three months or it can remain undetected for years [2]; (c) abortive infection, associated in particular with high risk HPV genotypes, arises especially in sites which are non-optimal for productive infection. Squamous and glandular carcinomas do not support the productive program.

Both *in vivo* and *in vitro* studies associated cervical cancer with three viral oncogenes (E5, E6 and E7) coded by hrHPVs [9]. HPV-induced carcinogenesis is a complex process characterized by alterations in tumour-suppressor genes. The aberrant function of these genes and the genomic instability determined by HPV viral genes, cumulated with the action of various cofactors, lead to progressive lesions and finally to cancer. Nevertheless, in the absence of persistent infection, the risk of cervical cancer is low [10].

The switch from productive to abortive infection is determined by a deregulated expression of E6 and E7 viral oncogenes in proliferating cells, thus leading to an extended lifespan [11]. The oncoproteins E6 and E7 interfere with tumor suppressors p53 and pRb respectively, and favour cells to overcome senescence barrier. Moreover, these proteins target a growing number of other cellular proteins/ factors. Epidemiologic and experimental data showed that also the E6 and E7 genes of low-risk types interfere with p53 and pRb and under certain circumstances are able to induce cervical neoplasia.

While in the normal viral life cycle, the genome replicates as episomal molecules, the up-regulation of viral oncogenes expression is associated with the HPV genome integration into the host cell chromosome [12]. As a result of integration, viral E1 and E2 genes are disrupted and their repressive action on E6 and E7 open reading frames is discontinued. Recent data point out that E2hrHPV proteins exhibit new oncogenic properties which rely on their ability to induce abnormal mitoses, leading to either loss or excess of DNA, together with DNA breaks during anaphase [13]. Although HPV integration plays an important role in the progression to cancer, the mechanisms are still unclear. Viral integration seems to confer selective advantage for oncogenes transcription and stability for transcripts encoding the E6 and E7 proteins which affect the key tumor suppressors p53 and pRB [14]. Cytogenetic mapping of multiple integration sites suggests that HPV integration occurrs preferentially in chromosomal fragile sites (CFS) [15] although it is under debate whether these sites present a greater susceptibility or accessibility to integration [16]. Sometimes, hrHPVs integration occurs within or adjacent to cellular oncogenes like myc, APM1, TP63, hTERT [17, 18]. Generally, coding regions are rarely targeted by HPV but gene expression and mRNA structure can be altered by insertion of the strong HPV promoter [14, 19].

Up-regulation of viral oncogenes expression together with loss of inhibitory effects of E2, result in cellular immortalization, deregulated proliferation and increased genomic instability [20]. The viral oncogenes are transcribed by a nucleoprotein complex (enhanceosome) that consists of transcriptional factors (JunB/Fra2) and a chromatin remodelling factor (HMG-I(Y) [21]. SMARCA2, a member of the SWI/SNF family of proteins, similar to the brahma (Brm) protein from *Drosophila,* is involved in transcriptional regulation of certain genes by altering the chromatin structure. When HPV is present as episome, SMARCA2 associates with E2 promoter and enhances E2 transcriptional activation [22]. SMARCA2 mRNA is a specific target for miR-199a-5p and miR-199a-3p in tumor cell lines, being often silenced in tumor cells at the post-transcriptional levels [23]. That might offer an alternative pathway for E2 gene silencing in HPV transforming infection.

The expression of the HPV oncogenes is necessary and sufficient for the initiation of cervical carcinogenesis, but host genome mutations are needed for malignant progression. In cervical cancer, cells accumulate a wide range of numerical and structural chromosomal abnormalities [24] including lagging chromosomal material, anaphase bridges, and multipolar mitoses [25]. As mentioned, *persistent infection* with HPV could lead, under certain conditions, to the insertion of viral genes into the host genome. As a consequence host defense mechanisms, including methylation machinery are activated [26]. Some viruses can find ways to regulate their gene expression (e.g. by modulating DNA methylation) in order to facilitate persistent infection and circumvent immune system [27]. Viral oncoproteins have the ability to modulate the methylation machinery in order to silent tumor suppressor genes. Studies on biological samples revealed an inverse correlation between the hypomethylation status of LCR region, E6 gene expression and the severity of lesion suggesting that hypomethylation accompanies progression to cancer [28, 29]. The studies of Badal et al. [30] revealed a clonal heterogeneity of methylation status in various regions of the viral genome, thus indicating that methylation of the viral oncogenes in cervical lesions is not an event that causes neoplastic progression but the result of transcriptional activity levels.

As mentioned, cellular transformation is a consequence of persistent infection by hrHPVs that leads to clonal progression of the persistently infected epithelium. Viral oncogenes are essential for carcinogenesis and their expression induces the tumorigenic state which ensures cell survival, essential for viral replication and the spread of progeny [31] Although the viral oncogenes were intensively studied, new data bring more information about their involvement in cervix carcinogenesis.

3. E6 HPV

High-risk E6 proteins are known for their ability to associate and degrade tumor suppressor p53. E6HPVs inactivate p53 in the infected cells, by inducing its degradation through the ubiquitin–proteasome pathway (Mdm2 E3, E6AP) [32]. This interaction prevents p53 from inducing growth arrest and apoptosis and promotes the perpetuation of damaged DNA during the host cell reproduction. Even both high and low risk E6HPV proteins interact with p53, only high risk oncogenes are capable of binding to the core region of p53. This step is mediated by recruitment of E6-AP (E3 ubiquitin ligase) which interacts with the viraloncogene and forms a complex with both E6 and target proteins [33].

E6 may inhibit p53 signalling pathways independent of protein degradation through p53 sequestration in the cytoplasm or by enhancing p53 nuclear export [34]. As a consequence, E6 oncoprotein precludes the growth-suppressive activities of p53 by transcriptional suppression of its target genes. It inhibits p53 activity by abrogation of the p53 transactivation *via* interaction with CBP/p300 [35, 36] or hADA3 histone acetyl-transferases, proteins involved in the regulation of transcription and DNA replication [37][38]. E6hrHPV proteins display a PDZ (*postsynaptic density protein, discs large tumor suppressor, and the epithelial tight junction protein, Z0-1*) motif designated as S/TXV at their C-terminus end which mediates E6 binding to proteins with these specific domains [39]. There are many studies focused on these interactions with proteins involved in proliferation control such as hDlg1 [40], hScrib [41], MAGI, PTPN3, MUPP1 [42, 43]. hScrib functions as a tumor suppressor that negatively regulates proliferation. hDlg and hScrib are proteins associated with cell junctions mediating the adhesion of basal cells to the ECM. Both are targeted for ubiquitination by high risk E6–E6AP complex, thus affecting epithelial cell growth [41]. MAGI proteins (membrane-associated guanylate kinase homologues –MAGUKs) are found at the tight junctions in epithelial cells and are thought to act in signalling pathways. Their degradation by E6 disrupts regulation of epithelial proliferation [42, 43]. Experimental evidence indicates that the interaction of E6 with PDZ proteins is necessary for the development of epithelial hyperplasia [44].

Several proteins involved in apoptosis and immune evasion (Bak, FADD,c-Myc, NFX1, procaspase 8, etc) [45, 46, 47, 48] are also targeted by E6 HPV. Bak, a member of the Bcl-2 family, is a proapoptotic protein whose interaction with the viral oncogene leads to the inhibition of apoptosis. This strategy by which the virus circumvents apoptosis might contribute to its oncogenic potential.

E6 oncoprotein is also able to modulate transcription from other cellular signaling pathways by interacton with three G-protein (E6TP, Gps2, Tuberin). E6 binds and degrades E6TP1 (*E6-*

targeted protein 1) in an E6AP dependent manner [49]. E6TP1 has homology to GAPs (*GTPase activating proteins*) for Rap [50] and its interaction with E6 was observed only in cancer-associated high-risk HPV but not in lesion-associated low-risk HPV. E6TP1 is involved in regulating cell proliferation and malignant cellular transformation, and its degradation by ubiquitination seems to be related to cellular immortalization suggesting a critical role of functional inactivation of E6TP1 in E6-induced cellular immortalization.

Tuberin is another protein with GAP activity which is degraded by E6. Tuberin functions in the harmatin–tuberin complex, which exhibits GAP activity toward Rheb proten. This complex is a negative regulator of mTOR signaling [51]. E6 also binds and degrades Gps2, that is involved in suppressing G-protein signaling pathway and c-Jun N-terminal kinase (JNK) activity [52].

E6 is involved in the blockage of apoptosis acting in both major apoptotic pathways:

a. the extrinsic pathway, which triggers extracellular signals that induce the activation of "death receptors" on the cell surface: 1) E6 binds to the death receptor TNFR-1, inhibiting TNFR-1 association with the TRADD (*TNFR1- associated death domain adapter molecule*) and blocking TNFR-1 death domain mediated apoptosis [47]; 2) E6 inhibits apoptosis by binding and degrading both the FADD adapter protein and caspase-8 [53].

b. the intrinsic pathway, which triggers sensing apoptotic signals that arise within the cell (DNA damage, oxidative stress) [54]. The lr/hrE6 oncoproteins block intrinsic apoptotic signaling interacting with Bak, inducing its proteasomal-dependent degradation [55], or using a mechanism depending or not on E6AP and E3 ubiquitin ligases [56].

Another biological activity of E6 oncoprotein consists in alteration of cell adhesion in order to allow proliferation of differentiated cells and inhibition of terminal differentiation: extracellular matrix adhesion, cell:cell contact and cytoskeletal organization. For example, Paxillin and zyxin are focal adhesion molecules involved in binding cellular cytoskeleton to the ECM and transmitting signals along the actin network from the ECM to nucleus. Focal adhesions form a structural link between the extracellular matrix and the actin cytoskeleton, and are important sites of signal transduction. Paxillin has been shown to bind to β-integrin, oncoproteins such as v-Src, v-Crk, p210BCR/ABL, p125FAK, vinculin, and talin, and is involved in changing the organization of the actin cytoskeleton. E6HPV interacts with paxillin [57], and the binding leads to the disruption of the actin cytoskeleton, a characteristic of many transformed cells.

E6 interacts with proteins involved in chromosomal stability within the HPV infected cell. Viral protein mediates MCM7 (*minichromosome maintenance* 7) degradation via E6AP and leads to chromosomal abnormalities in HPV infected cells [58]. Moreover, its interactions with XRCC1 and O(6)-methylguanine-DNA methyltransferase (MGMT) (proteins involved in single strand DNA break repair) induce DNA damage [59] or sensitize HPV infected cells to alkylating DNA damage [60]. These interactions increase genomic instability and accelerate the progression to carcinogenesis.

E6 hrHPV is also involved in immune evasion by interacting with IFR-3 (*Interferon regulatory factor-3*) [61], that is required for the expression of type I interferon. IFR-3 is activated by virus infection to form a complex with transcriptional regulators of the IFN-beta. Therefore IFR-3 inhibition affects its transactivation ability and results in the induction of IFN-β following viral infection [62]. Interferon induced growth arrest is dependent on p53 acetylation, a modification which affects p53 stability and increases its transcriptional activity. As E6 targets p53 directly or through p300/CBP, the virus induces proliferation of HPV infected cells in the presence of interferon [63]. Moreover, E6 inhibits TLR9 transcription, leading to a functional loss of TLR9 signaling pathways within the cell [61]. By activating telomerase, E6 promotes malignancy as the mutant cells continue to reproduce uncontrollably [64]

It was noticed that oncogenic E6HPV is able to modulate the expression of many cellular miRNAs *via* p53. For example, miR-34a gene is a direct transcriptional target of p53 and its expression is transactivated by p53 binding to a consensus p53 binding site in the miR-34a promoter region [65, 66, 67]. As E6 is a regulator of p53, viral oncoprotein leads to the reduction of miR-34a, and this affects the expression of cell cycle regulators, including cyclin E2, cyclin D1, CDK4, CDK6, Bcl-2, SIRT1, and p18Ink4c [68, 69]. The hypothesis that p53 modulates cellular miRNAs down-regulation mediated by E6HPV16 was sustained by the fact that the genes encoding miR-34a and miR-23b contain a promoter region with a p53 binding site [70].

4. E7HPV

The HPV life cycle is associated with the differentiation process of the infected epithelial cell. Interaction between E7 and pRB determines degradation and phosphorylation of pRB with the release of E2F and activation of genes that promote cellular proliferation. The actions of E7 induce cells to enter in the S phase of cell cycle (including suprabasal epithelial cells) which ensures all cellular factors necessary for viral replication. On the other hand, E7 can directly bind E2F1 and enhance E2F1-mediated transcription [71]. E2F transcription factors are critical regulators of G1 exit and S-phase progression. In addition, cellular differentiation, apoptosis and genomic instability are controlled by E2Fs [72]. E7 also interacts with pRb associated proteins (p107, p130) which are negative regulators of the cell cycle involved in G1/S and G2/M transition, via the LXCXE motif in CR2 [73].

E7hrHPV can associate and alter the activities of multiple cellular factors that normally contribute to the regulation of the cell cycle. In addition to targeting pRB for proteasomal degradation [74] E7 inhibits p21 functions by direct binding, thus contributing to sustained activity of CDK [73, 75, 76]. Cyclin dependent kinases (cdks) are the most important in cell division cycle. Expression of cyclins E and A, the regulatory subunits of cdk2, which drives S-phase entry and progression, is under E2F control and they are both expressed at higher levels in E7 expressing cells [77].

A cell infected by virus will usually respond by producing interferons (IFNs) that have an antiviral and antitumour effect. HPV16 E7 protein has been shown to block IFN-α activity and inhibit IFN-β promoter [78]. Besides its role in cell proliferation E7 also regulates apoptosis. Some studies underlined that the actions of E7 appear to be anti-apoptotic. On the other hand, overexpression of E7 in genital keratinocytes induces spontaneous cell death. However, its effect on cellular apoptotic pathways is pleiomorphic.

E7hrHPV increases genomic instability in primary human cells [79] and generates mitotic defects and aneuploidy as a consequence of gains or losses of entire chromosomes during mitosis, or by induction of supernumerary centrosomes and multipolar mitoses [25]. Supernumerary centrosomes and associated multipolar mitoses have been detected in cells that express low copy numbers of episomal E7HPV [80] and their incidence increases in cells with integrated HPV, presumably due to higher E7 expression. Induced aberrant centriole synthesis is dependent on cdk2 activity in E7 expressing cells [81, 82]. The ability of HPV16 E7 to induce supernumerary centrosomes is at least in part independent from the ability to target pRB family members. A possible pRB/p107/p130 independent mechanism involves the association of E7 with the centrosomal regulator γ-tubulin [83]. E7HPV expression also causes other types of mitotic abnormalities including lagging chromosomal material and anaphase bridges that may represent chromosomal fusions caused by double stand DNA breaks [84]. The presence of DNA repair foci indicates that E7 may induce double strand DNA breaks or interfere with break repair. This may facilitate viral genome integration.

High-risk E7 proteins are also able of direct the interaction with chromatin modifiers such as histone deacetylases HDACs 1, 2, 3 and 8, events independent of pRB inactivation. HDACs are involved in regulation of transcription of different genes, including those that present promoters activated by E2F transcriptional factor [84]. This interaction additionally affects the expression of S phase genes. Experimental studies showed that L67 mutation of HPV31 E7 protein determines the impossibility to bind HDACs, and affects the virus ability to remain in an episomal status or to complete the later stages of the viral life cycle [85]. Currently, there is no study to prove the connection between the viral replication and the binding of E7 to HDACs. E7hrHPV also interacts with c-myc, augments c-myc transactivation, contributing to an efficient immortalization.

As we mentioned before, HPV16 E7 oncoprotein interacts with complexes formed between E2F6 and polycomb transcriptional repressor (PRCs) [86]. PRCs associate with histone H3 lysine 27 trimethyl (H3K27me3) [87] and inactivate p14ARF tumor suppressor [88]. Highly HPV16E7 expression correlates with high levels of H3K27me3 [89] and an increased expression of p16INK4A through KDM6B induction. This process is not dependent of pRB inactivation by E7 oncogene, but several genes (Hox) regulated by KDM6A or KDM6B are highly expressed, promoting cell proliferation and escape from senescence. Gathering these data, HPV16E7 expression may cause epigenetic reprogramming in host cells, inducing alterations in H3K27me3 levels and transcriptional changes. On the other hand, KDM5 has been linked to oncogenesis process [86]: E2 protein recruits KDM5 in order to repress the transcription of the E6 and E7 oncoproteins through the HPV LCR [90, 91]. The interplay between histone methyl-transferases and demethylases in the context of viral oncogenes activity is shown in figure 1.

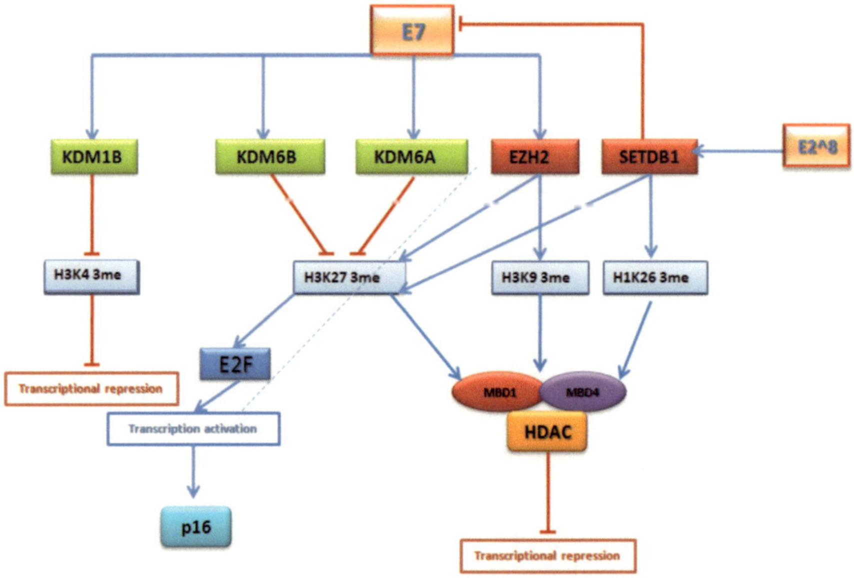

Figure 1. The interplay between histone methyl-trasferases and demethylases in the context of viral oncogenes activity

Expression of both early and late HPV genes seems to be subject to miRNA-mediated regulation at the post-transcriptional level in cervical cancer cell lines [68, 69].

E7 increases the expression of miR-15/16 cluster through pRB degradation and release of E2, a factor which promotes miR-15a/16-1 cluster expression [68, 69]. On the other hand, E7hrHPV down-regulates the expression of miR-203 [92], a micromolecule involved in the control of the keratinocytes differentiation by shift from a proliferative to a nonproliferative status [93, 94]. Another cause of miR-203 down-regulation is due to methylation of CpG islands in the promoter region. Hypermethylation of miR203 as well as miR-34b and miR-124 was correlated with CIN III and cervical cancer [95].

Beside the E6 and E7 oncogenes, recent studies emphasize the role of two other viral proteins in HPV induced oncogenesis: E5 and E2.

5. E5 HPV

E5 HPV16 is a hydrophobic protein (83 amino acid long), localized in the intracellular membranes (plasma membrane, endoplasmic reticulum, nuclear envelope and Golgi apparatus) [96]. Based on its interactions with cellular proteins, E5 seems to be a weak transforming protein. These interactions lead to alterations in normal biological activity and evasion of the immune response. E5 gene encodes short hydrophobic peptides, which have mitogenic activity, synergic with EGF (*epidermal growth factor*) [97]. In hrHPV infections, (*e.g.* HPV 16) EGF receptor increases 2-5 times in the human keratinocytes expressing E5, leading to cell proliferation. This suggests that HPV16 E5 plays a major role in expanding populations of HPV16-infected basal keratinocytes *in vivo* by augmenting extracellular growth signals in viral infected cells (enhancing ligand-dependent EGF-R activation). E5 oncoprotein binds and inhibits the activity of the 16 kDa subunit of vacuolar ATP-ase (V-ATPase), altering the endosomal acidification and degradation of EGF-R [98, 99]. The delay of EGF-R degradation can be reached by E5 interference with membrane trafficking and the fusion of early and late endosomes [100].

E5 activates EGF-R signaling pathway through either EGF-dependent or EGF-independent processes, but it is also capable of interacting with, enhancing/ altering the signaling of other different classes of growth factor receptors like:

- G protein-coupled endothelin receptor [96]; this interaction induces mitogenic activity of ET-1, leading to the chronic stimulation of keratinocyte proliferation;
- keratinocyte growth factor receptor/ fibroblast growth factor receptor 2b (KGF-R/FGF-R2b); these receptors are down-modulated by E5, through reduction of transcripts and protein [101, 102].
- connexin 43 interferes with E5, in order to inhibit gap junction-mediated communication between epithelial cells in monolayer [103] and in raft cultures [104]; this makes the transformed cells more insensitive to homeostatic growth control signals from adjacent normal cells. Moreover, E5 seems to be involved in induction of cell fusion [105, 106, 107] a critical event in the early stage of HPV-associated cervical cancer. There are experimental data which support E5 role in cervical cancer. It seems this viral protein increases the efficiency of keratinocytes immortalization induced by E6 and E7 oncogenes [108] and affects cell-cell communications [109]

In early infection, E5 appears to inhibit programmed cell death [110] using different mechanisms like: (a) down regulation of the total amount of Fas receptor and reduction of Fas surface location; and (b) alteration of the formation of *Death-Inducing Signalling Complex* (DISC) triggered by TRAIL [111]. While E5 did not down-regulate TRAIL receptor expression, it was found to inhibit TRAIL signaling by interfering with the formation of the TRAIL DISC and thereby inhibiting the cleavage of procaspases-3 and -8, as well as of PARP [111]. Therefore, it is possible that E5 interferes with the ability of the immune system to eliminate infected cells by impairing death receptor signaling. Together, the results of these studies provide strong evidence that E5 contributes to the evasion of immune surveillance during the early stages of HPV infection.

In contrast, HPV16E5 sensitizes human keratinocytes to apoptosis induced by osmotic stress, perhaps due to cell membrane modifications caused by this strong hydrophobic molecule [111]. On the other hand, E5 can inhibit the ER stress pathway, cyclooxygenase-2 (COX-2), XBP-1 and IRE1a, but this seems to be limited to the high risk genotypes, favoring viral replication and persistence [112].

The role of E5 in HPV transformation might be due to alteration of innate and adaptive immune responses. E5 protein seems to down-regulate MHC/HLA class I, through alkalinisation of the endomembrane compartments [113] and the direct interaction of E5 with the heavy chain of the MHC class I complex [114, 115]. E5 gene is often deleted during viral DNA integration into the host cell genome. This might suggest a dispensable role of this gene in oncogenesis but the fact that E5 mRNA is the most abundant viral transcript prior integration sustains its role in early phases of tumorigenesis.

6. E2 HPV

The E2HPV protein exhibits complex functions independent of transcription; it can modulate the host cells in concert with the viral vegetative cycle. Recent data point out that E2HPV could be involved in early carcinogenesis [13]. E2 is a repressor of E6 and E7 transcription in the HPV context. E2HPV is involved in viral transcription and replication [116, 117], forming together with E1 a complex with viral origin of replication and recruiting cellular DNA replication machinery (DNA polymerases, replication protein A, replication protein C, topoisomerase I/II and proliferating-cell nuclear antigen) in order to facilitate viral DNA replication [116]. It was noted that E2 protein is expressed at relatively high levels in differentiated cells of the intermediate layers of CIN lesions; on the other hand, its expression is decreased with progression of the lesions and is absent in most of the cancers *in situ*, being inversely correlated with expression of E7 [13, 118]. E2 is an unstable protein expressed in both the nuclei and cytoplasm of infected cells, and is degraded through the proteasome [119, 120]. In most cases, HPV integration occurs by breaking the E2 gene region. Re-expression of E2 in cervical carcinoma cell lines appears to be detrimental to cell proliferation due to the induction of G1 cell cycle arrest through repression of the endogenous E6/E7 expression, as well as due to induction of cellular senescence and apoptosis [121, 122]. The fact that E2 can regulate the activities of E6 and E7 via transcriptional control or by direct interaction [28], suggests that HPV genome integration may result from a strong selective pressure on the virus to avoid E2-induced apoptosis while modulating the survival of infected cells through the activities of E6 and E7.

E2 could enhance cellular DNA replication through abrogation of a mitotic checkpoint [123] and blocking the cell cycle in G2/M [124]; E2 activates the spindle assembly checkpoint and induces abnormal chromosome segregation after anaphase, leading to aneuploidy or DNA breaks [13]. The potential role of E2 to induce abnormal mitoses links E2 to HPV-associated carcinogenesis. This hypothesis is sustained by the fact that only E2 proteins from high-risk HPVs could induce abnormal mitotic phenotypes, in contrast to the E2 proteins from the low-risk HPV11 and 6 which are inactive [124].

7. Prevention of cervical carcinoma

The high risk human papillomaviruses are associated with cervical cancers and play an essential role in the pathogenesis of the disease. Although commercial prophylactic HPV vaccines are now available, they do not have therapeutic effect against established HPV infections and HPV-associated lesions which account for high morbidity and mortality worldwide. Advanced cervical cancer remains a public health issue despite the availability of preventive vaccines and population-based screening because they target a very young teenage population with a delayed impact on cervical cancer due to the peak of cervical cancer incidence at ages 45–55 [125]. Viral oncoproteins are critical for the induction and maintenance of cellular transformation in HPV-infected cells. Therefore, E6 and E7 are considered the ideal targets for therapeutic HPV vaccines. By contrast with the commercial preventive HPV vaccines (Gardasil and Cervarix) which use HPV virus-like particles to generate neutralizing antibodies, therapeutic vaccines can eliminate preexisting lesions and infections by generating cellular immunity against HPV-infected cells. Consequently, many therapeutic vaccine strategies have focused primarily on stimulating the production and activation of T cells that can recognize infected cells expressing the target antigens (E6 and E7).

A variety of vaccine strategies have been employed to target immune responses to these proteins. Various therapeutic HPV vaccines for cervical cancer, including live vector-, peptide-, protein-, nucleic acid-, or cell-based vaccines targeting the E6HPV and/or E7 antigens were developed.

Live vector-based vaccines (bacterial and viral vectors) are attractive due to their high immunogenicity and efficiency in delivering antigens or DNA encoding antigens of interest. Among them, ADXS11-001 (Listeria-based vaccine) targets E7 and is well tolerated by patients in end-stage of cervical cancer, who had failed prior chemotherapy, radiotherapy and/or surgery (phase I trial in patients with stage IVb cervical cancer) [126]. On the other hand, TA-HPV (a recombinant vaccinia virus expressing HPV-16/18 E6/E7 fusion protein), induces HPV antigen-specific T cell-mediated immune response (phase I/II trial in patients with Ib or IIa cervical cancer) [127]. MVA-E2 and MVA-HPV-IL2 (Modified Vaccinia Ankara-based vaccines expressing HPV16 E6/E7 and IL-2) showed some promises as 50% of the treated patients presented complete healing of lesions and E6 and E7 antigen levels below the detection limit of 6 months post vaccination (phase II trial in patients with CIN III) [128].

Cell-based vaccines (dendritic cells-DCs, modified tumor cells) are highly immunogenic and useful in expressing the relevant tumor antigens. Vaccination with E7-presenting DCs transfected with siRNA targeting Bim (Bcl-2-interacting mediator) was capable of generating a strong E7-specific CTL response and a marked therapeutic effect in vaccinated mice [129]. The vaccine was in clinical pilot study in patients with late stage cervical cancer [130] or phase I trial in patients with stage Ib or IIa cervical cancer [131], or with recurrent cervical cancer [132].

Peptide-based vaccines can combine multiple epitopes and enhance peptides for MHC binding. The peptide-based vaccine potency is increased by using adjuvants such as GM-CSF, 4-1BB ligand, and Montanide ISA 51) [133, 134]. Several vaccines from this category are in different phase trials: Lipopeptide lipidated E7 (HLA-A* 0201 - restricted epitope, a.a. 86– 93 lipopeptide) in phase I trial in patients with refractory cervical or vaginal cancer; Peptide & Montanide ISA -51 (HLA-A * 0201- HPV16 E7 epitopes restricted, a.a. 12 to 20 ± a.a. 86 -93) ligated to PADRE, adjuvant Montanide ISA 51, in phase I/II trial in patients with recurrent or residual cervical cancer. TriVax- HPV16-E7 epitope (E7 49-57 with CD40 mAb) in tumor-bearing mice [135] has not yet been tested in clinical trials.

The protein-based vaccines take the advantage of using fully purified proteins which are able to induce humoral and cellular immune response. Conformational epitopes of injected proteins are recognized by B cell receptors, triggering specific immunoglobulin synthesis row. Proteins are retrieved and processed by antigen presenting cells (dendritic cells, macrophages, etc.) in cooperation with T helper lymphocytes (by presenting peptides conjugated with MHC class II molecules) and cytotoxic T lymphocytes (by presenting peptides conjugated with MHC class I molecules). Adjuvants (Iscomatrix, AS02B, Poly ICLC) [136, 137] and fusion immunostimulatory proteins (heat shock protein derived from *Mycobacterium bovis*) improve CTL responses of HPV protein-based vaccines [138].

Nucleic acid-based vaccines are based on the direct introduction into the host cell of information encoding the antigen of interest, synthesized *in situ*. Recombinant DNA is introduced into tissues by intramuscular inoculation. Dendritic cells serves as central players for DNA vaccine development. pNGVL4a encodes the signal sequence *Sig* linked to a weakened form of HPV16 E7 fused to HSP70. It is used in phase I trial in patients with CIN II/III [139]. VGX-3100 vaccine expressing E6 and E7 HPV16/18 proteins was used in Phase I trial in patients with CIN II/III post-surgical or ablative treatment [140]. Regarding to the potential of E5 to contribute to HPV-associated carcinogenic process, it was suggested its role during the early tumorigenesis stage. Taking into account a limited immune response in malignat stage as a result in down-regulation of MHC class I and II molecules, a therapeutic vaccine targeting E5-expressing cells might be a good strategy to prevent the progression of premalignant lesions toward invasive cervical cancers [141]. Using a recombinant adenovirus which expresses E5HPV16 (AdV-based E5) in syngenic animals, it was observed a reduction of tumor growth correlated with tumor protection through CD8 T cells [142], but HPV16E5 25-33 peptide plus CpG oligodeoxynucleotides (ODN) proved to be more effective as vaccine [143]. The construction of different DNA vectors based on epitopes of E5 HPV oncogene (now under evaluation in animal models) was also described [144]. The immune effector cells in premalignanant lesions may eradicate tumor cells more efficiently than in the invasive cervical cancers.

8. Conclusions

The studies of HPV E6 and E7 oncogenes and the proteins coded will continue in order to discover new diagnostic and prognostic tools for cervical cancer. On the other hand, scientific studies will probably decipher new pathways of HPV oncogenesis molecular network and these will enrich the knowledge in this field.

Abbreviations

ABL Abelson murine leukemia
APM adipose most abundant gene transcript
Bcl-2 B cell leukemia/lymphoma 2
BCR breakpoint cluster region
Brm brahma
CREB cyclic AMP response element-binding protein
CBP CREB-binding protein

CDK cyclin-dependent kinases
CKI and II casein kinase I and II
COX-2 cyclooxygenase 2
E6-AP E6-associated protein
E6-BP E6-binding protein
ET1 etched1
FADD Fas-associated protein with death domain
FAK focal adhesion kinase
Fra2 Fos related antigen
GAP GTPase activating proteins
GM-CSF granulocyte-macrophage colony-stimulating-factor
Gps2 G-protein pathway suppressor 2
hADA3 transcriptional adaptor 3
HDAC histone deacetylase
hDlg human Drosophila discs large protein
hDlg1 discs large homolog 1
hE6TP1 human E6-targeted protein 1
HLA human leukocyte antigen
HMG high mobility group
HPV human papilloma virus
hScrib human Scribble tumor suppressor protein
hScrib scribbled homolog Drosophila
hTERT human telomerase reverse transcriptase
IFN interferon
IFNAR1 interferon-alpha receptor 1
IRE1a endoribonuclease/protein kinase IRE1-like protein
IRF-1 and -3 interferon regulatory factor 1 and 3
ISGF3 interferon-stimulated gene factor 3
KDM1 lysine (K)-specific demethylase 1A
M2-PK M2 pyruvate kinase
MAGI membrane-associated guanylate kinases
Mdm2 murine double minute 2
MHC major histocompatibility complex
MMP-7 multicopy maintenance protein 7
mTOR mechanistic/mammalian target of rapamycin (serine/threonine kinase)
MUPP1 multi-PDZ-domain protein 1
NFX1 nuclear factor (X can be any amino acids)
p18Ink4c Cyclin-dependent kinase 4 inhibitor C
PTPN3 protein tyrosine phosphatase, non-receptor type 3
Rb retinoblastoma protein
Rheb Ras homolog enriched in brain
S4 subunit 4
SIRT sirtuin (silent mating type information regulation 2 homologue) 1

SMARC SWI/SNF-related, matrix-associated, actin-dependent regulators of chromatin
SWI/SNF Switch/Sucrose nonfermentable
TBP TATA box-binding protein
TLR9 toll-like receptor 9
TNFR1 tumor necrosis factor receptor, member 1
TP63 tumor protein p63
TRADD TNFRSF1A-associated via death domain
TRAIL tumor necrosis factor-related apoptosis-inducing ligand
v- Src sarcoma viral oncogene
v-Crk sarcoma virus CT10 oncogene homolog (avian)-like
XBP-1 X-box binding protein 1
XRCC1 X-ray repair complementing defective repair in Chinese hamster cells 1

Author details

Gabriela Anton, Adriana Plesa, Coralia Bleotu, Anca Botezatu and Mihai Stoian
Viral Genetics Dept, Stefan S Nicolau Institute of Virology, Bucharest-Romania

Mariana Anton
Genetics Dept, Carol Davila University of Medicine and Pharmacy, Bucharest-Romania

Lorelei Irina Brasoveanu
Center of Immunology, Stefan S Nicolau Institute of Virology, Bucharest-Romania

Acknowledgement

PN2 -41030, PN2-41081 and VIASAN 223 Romanian National Grants.

9. References

[1] Walboomers JM, Jacobs MV, Manos MM, Bosch FX, Kummer JA, Shah KV, Snijders PJ, Peto J, Meijer CJ, Muñoz N. Human Papillomavirus is a Necessary Cause of Invasive Cervical Cancer Worldwide. Journal of Pathology 1999;189: 12-19.

[2] Muñoz N, Bosch FX, de Sanjose S, Herrero R, Castellsague X, Shah KV, Snijders PJ, Meijer CJ. Epidemiologic Classification of Human Papillomavirus Types Associated with Cervical Cancer. New England Journal of Medicine 2003;348: 518-527.

[3] Bosch FX, Lorincz A, Munoz N, Meijer CJ, Shah KV. The Causal Relation between Human Papillomavirus and Cervical Cancer. Journal of Clinical Pathology 2002;55: 244-65.

[4] Sinal SH, Woods CR. Human Papillomavirus Infections of the Genital and Respiratory Tracts in Young Children. Seminars in Pediatric Infectious Diseases 2005;16: 306-16.

[5] Molijn A, Kleter B, Quint W, van Doorn LJ. Molecular Diagnosis of Human Papillomavirus (HPV) Infections. Journal of Clinical Virology, 2005;32S: S43-S51.

[6] del Mar Pena L, Laimins LA. Differentiation-Dependent Chromatin Rearrangement Coincides with Activation of Human Papillomavirus Type 31 Late Gene Expression. Journal of Virology 2001;75: 10005-10013.
[7] Wooldridge TR, Laimins LA, Regulation of Human Papillomavirus Type 31 Gene Expression During the Differentiation-Dependent Life Cycle Through Histone Modifications and Transcription Factor Binding. Virology 2008;374: 371-380
[8] Burd EM. Human Papillomavirus and Cervical Cancer. Clinical Microbiology Reviews 2003;16: 1-17.
[9] Narisawa-Saito M, Kiyono T. Basic Mechanisms of High-Risk Human Papillomavirus Induced Carcinogenesis. Cancer Science. 2007;98: 1505-1511.
[10] Schiffman M, Wentzensen N, Wacholder S, Kinney W, Gage JC, Castle PE. Human Papillomavirus Testing in the Prevention of Cervical Cancer. Journal of the National Cancer Institute. 2011;103(5): 368-383.
[11] Clifford GM, Smith JS, Plummer M, Muñoz N, Franceschi S. Human Papillomavirus Types in Invasive Cervical Cancer Worldwide: a Meta-Analysis. British Journal of Cancer 2003;88: 63 73.
[12] Alazawi W, Pett M, Arch B, Scott L, Freeman T, Stanley MA, Coleman N. Changes in Cervical Keratinocyte Gene Expression Associated with Integration of Human Papillomavirus 16. Cancer Research 2002;62: 6959-6965.
[13] Bellanger S, Tan CL, Xue YZ, Teissier S, Thierry F. Tumor Suppressor or Oncogene? A Critical Role of the Human Papillomavirus (HPV) E2 Protein in Cervical Cancer Progression. American Journal of Cancer Research 2011;1(3): 373-389.
[14] Ziegert C, Wentzensen N, Vinokurova S, Kisseljov F, Einenkel J, Hoeckel M, von Knebel Doeberitz M. A Comprehensive Analysis of HPV Integration Loci in Anogenital Lesions Combining Transcript and Genome Based Amplification Techniques. Oncogene 2003;22: 3977-3984.
[15] Yu T, Ferber MJ, Cheung TH, Chung TK, Wong YF, Smith DI. The Role of Viral Integration in the Development of Cervical Cancer. Cancer Genetics and Cytogenetics 2005;158(1): 27-34.
[16] Woodman CBJ, Collins SI, Young LS. The Natural History of Cervical HPV Infection: Unresolved Issues. Nature Reviews Cancer 2007;7: 11-22.
[17] Ferber MJ, Thorland EC, Brink AA, Rapp AK, Phillips LA, McGovern R, Gostout BS, Cheung TH, Chung TK, Fu WY, Smith DI. Preferential Integration of Human Papillomavirus Type 18 near the c-myc Locus in Cervical Carcinoma. Oncogene 2003;22: 7233-7242.
[18] Ferber MJ, Montoya DP, Yu C, Aderca I, McGee A, Thorland EC, Nagorney DM, Gostout BS, Burgart LJ, Boix L, Bruix J, McMahon BJ, Cheung TH, Chung TK, Wong YF, Smith DI, Roberts LR. Integrations of the Hepatitis B Virus (HBV) and Human Papillomavirus (HPV) into the Human Telomerase Reverse Transcriptase (hTERT) Gene in Liver and Cervical Cancers. Oncogene 2003;22: 3813–3820.
[19] Wentzensen N, Vinokurova S, von Knebel Doeberitz. Systematic Review of Genomic Integration Sites of Human Papillomavirus Genomes in Epithelial Dysplasia and Invasive Cancer of the Female Lower Genital Tract. Cancer Research 2004;64: 3878-3884.

[20] Pett M, Coleman N. Integration of High-Risk Human Papillomavirus: a Key Event in Cervical Carcinogenesis? Journal of Pathology 2007;212(4): 356-367.

[21] Bouallaga I, Teissier S, Yaniv M, Thierry F. HMG-I(Y) and the CBP/p300 Coactivator are Essential for Human Papillomavirus Type 18 Enhanceosome Transcriptional Activity. Molecular and Cellular Biology 2003;23: 2329-2340.

[22] Kumar RA, Naidu SR, Wang X, Imbalzano AN, Androphy EJ. Interaction of Papillomavirus E2 Protein with the Brm Chromatin Remodeling Complex Leads to Enhanced Transcriptional Activation. Journal of Virology 2007;81: 2213-2220.

[23] Sakurai K, Furukawa C, Haraguchi T, Inada K, Shiogama K, Tagawa T, Fujita S, Ueno Y, Ogata A, Ito M, Tsutsumi Y, Iba H. MicroRNAs miR-199a-5p and -3p Target the Brm Subunit of SWI/SNF to Generate a Double-Negative Feedback Loop in a Variety of Human Cancers. Cancer Research 2011;71(5): 1680-9.

[24] Mitelman F, Johansson B, Mertens F (2007) Mitelman Database of Chromosome Aberrations in Cancer. http://cgap.nci.nih.gov/Chromosomes/Mitelman.

[25] Duensing S, Munger K. The Human Papillomavirus type 16 E6 and E7 Oncoproteins Independently Induce Numerical and Structural Chromosome Instability. Cancer Research 2002;62(23): 7075-7082

[26] Tao Q, Huang H, Geiman TM, Lim CY, Fu L, Qiu GH, Robertson KD. (2002) Defective *de novo* Methylation of Viral and Cellular DNA Sequences in ICF Syndrome Cells. Human Molecular Genetics 2002;11: 2091-2102.

[27] Tsai CN, Tsai CL, Tse KP, Chang HY, Chang YS. The Epstein-Barr Virus Oncogene Product, Latent Membrane Protein 1, Induces the Downregulation of E-Cadherin Gene Expression via Activation of DNA Methyltransferases. Proceedings of the National Academy of Sciences of the USA. 2002;99: 10084-10089.

[28] Badal V, Chuang LS, Tan EH, Badal S, Villa LL, Wheeler CM, Li BF, Bernard HU. CpG Methylation of Human Papillomavirus Type 16 DNA in Cervical Cancer Cell Lines and in Clinical Specimens: Genomic Hypomethylation Correlates with Carcinogenic Progression. Virology 2003;77: 6227-6234.

[29] Kalantari M, Calleja-Macías IE, Tewari D, Hagmar B, Lie K, Barrera-Saldaña HA, Wiley DJ, Bernard HU. Conserved Methylation Patterns of Human Papillomavirus Type 16 DNA in Asymptomatic Infection and Cervical Neoplasia. Journal of Virology 2004;78: 12762-12772.

[30] Badal S, Badal V, Calleja-Macías IE, Kalantari M, Chuang LS, Li BF, Bernard HU. The Human Papillomavirus-18 Genome is Efficiently Targeted by Cellular DNA Methylation. Virology 2004;324: 483-492.

[31] Garnett TO, Duerksen-Hughes PJ. Modulation of Apoptosis by Human Papillomavirus (HPV) Oncoproteins. Archives of Virology 2006;151: 2321-2335.

[32] Scheffner M, Werness BA, Huibregtse JM, Levine AJ, Howley PM. The E6 Oncoprotein Encoded by Human Papillomavirus Types 16 and 18 Promotes the Degradation of p53. Cell 1990;63(6): 1129–1136.

[33] Schwarz SE, Rosa JL, Scheffner M. Characterization of Human hect Domain Family Members and Their Interaction with UbcH5 and UbcH7. Journal of Biological Chemistry 1998;273(20): 12148-12154.

[34] Mantovani F, Banks L. The Human Papillomavirus E6 Protein and its Contribution to Malignant Progression. Oncogene 2001;20(54): 7874-7887.

[35] Patel D, Huang SM, Baglia LA, McCance DJ. The E6 Protein of Human Papillomavirus Type 16 Binds to and Inhibits Co-activation by CBP and p300. EMBO Journal 1999;18(18): 5061-5072.

[36] Zimmermann H, Koh CH, Degenkolbe R, O'Connor MJ, Muller A, Steger G, Chen JJ, Lui Y, Androphy E, Bernard HU. Interaction with CBP/p300 Enables the Bovine Papillomavirus Type 1 E6 Oncoprotein to Downregulate CBP/p300-Mediated Transactivation by p53. Journal of General Virology 2000;81(11): 11-23.

[37] Kumar A, Zhao Y, Meng G, Zeng M, Srinivasan S, Delmolino LM, Gao Q, Dimri G, Weber GF, Wazer DE, Band H, Band V. Human Papillomavirus Oncoprotein E6 Inactivates the Transcriptional Coactivator Human ADA3. Molecular and Cellular Biology 2002;22 (16): 5801-5812.

[38] Chen JJ, Hong Y, Rustamzadeh E, Baleja JD, Androphy EJ. Identification of an Alpha Helical Motif Sufficient for Association with Papillomavirus E6. Journal of Biological Chemistry 1998;273(22): 13537-13544.

[39] Tong X, Howley PM. The Bovine Papillomavirus E6 Oncoprotein Interacts with Paxillin and Disrupts the Actin Cytoskeleton. Proceedings of the National Academy of Sciences of the USA 1997;94(9): 4412-4417.

[40] Kiyono T, Hiraiwa A, Fujita M, Hayashi Y, Akiyama T, Ishibashi M. Binding of High Risk Human Papillomavirus E6 Oncoproteins to the Human Homologue of the Drosophila Discs Large Tumor Supressor Protein. Proceedings of the National Academy of Sciences of the USA 1997;94(21): 11612-11616.

[41] Nakagawa S, Huibregtse JM. Human Scribble (Vartul) is Targeted for Ubiquitin-Mediated Degradation by the High Risk Papillomavirus E6 Proteins and the E6AP Ubiquitin–Protein Ligase. Molecular and Cellular Biology 2000;20(21): 8244-8253.

[42] Jing M, Bohl J, Brimer N, Kinter M, Vande Pol SB. Degradation of Tyrosine Phosphatase PTPN3 (PTPH1) by Association with Oncogenic Human Papillomavirus E6 Proteins. Journal of Virology 2007;1(5): 2231-2239.

[43] Spanos WC, Geiger J, Anderson ME, Harris GF, Bossler AD, Smith RB, Klingelhutz AJ, Lee JH. Deletion of the PDZ Motif of HPV16 E6 Preventing Immortalization and Anchorage-Independent Growth in Human Tonsil Epithelial Cells. Head Neck 2008;30 (2): 139-147.

[44] Nguyen ML, Nguyen MM, Lee D, Griep AE, Lambert PF. The PDZ Ligand Domain of the Human Papillomavirus Type 16 E6 Protein is Required for E6's Induction of Epithelial Hyperplasia in vivo. Journal of Virology 2003;77(12): 6957-64.

[45] Spanos WC, Hoover A, Harris GF, Wu S, Strand GL, Anderson ME, Klingelhutz AJ, Hendriks W, Bossler AD, Lee JH. The PDZ Binding Motif of Human Papillomavirus Type 16 E6 Induces PTPN13 Loss, which Allows Anchorage Independent Growth and Synergizes with ras for Invasive Growth. Journal of Virology 2008;82(5): 2493–2500.

[46] Degenhardt YY, Silverstein S. Interaction of Zyxin, a Focal Adhesion Protein, with the e6 Protein from Human Papillomavirus Type 6 Results in its Nuclear Translocation. Journal of Virology 2001;75(23): 11791-11802.

[47] Filippova M, Song H, Connolly JL, Dermody TS, Duerksen-Hughes PJ. The Human Papillomavirus 16 E6 Protein Binds to Tumor Necrosis Factor (TNF) R1 and Protects Cells from TNF-Induced Apoptosis. Journal of Biological Chemistry 2002;277(24): 21730-21739.
[48] Filippova M, Johnson MM, Bautista M, Filippov V, Fodor N, Tungteakkhun SS,Williams K, Duerksen-Hughes PJ. The Large and Small Isoforms of Human Papillomavirus Type 16 E6 Bind to and Differentially Affect Procaspase 8 Stability and Activity. Journal of Virology 2007;81(8): 4116-4129.
[49] Lee C, Wooldridge TR, Laimins LA. Analysis of the Roles of E6 Binding to E6TP1 and Nuclear Localization in the Human Papillomavirus Type 31 Life Cycle. Virology 2007;358(1): 201–210.
[50] Gao Q, Srinivasan S, Boyer SN, Wazer DE, Band V. The E6 Oncoproteins of High-Risk Papillomaviruses Bind to a Novel Putative GAP Protein, E6TP1, and Target it for Degradation. Molecular and Cellular Biology 1999;19(1): 733-744.
[51] Huang J, Manning BD. The TSC1–TSC2 Complex: a Molecular Switchboard Controlling Cell Growth. Biochemical Journal 2008;412 (2): 179-190.
[52] Degenhardt YY, Silverstein SJ. Gps2, a Protein Partner for Human Papillomavirus E6 Proteins. Journal of Virology 2001;75(1): 151-160.
[53] Garnett TO, Filippova M, Duerksen-Hughes PJ. Accelerated Degradation of FADD and Procaspase 8 in Cells Expressing Human Papilloma Virus 16 E6 Impairs TRAIL-Mediated Apoptosis. Cell Death and Differentiation 2006;13(11): 1915-1926.
[54] Wang X. The Expanding Role of Mitochondria in Apoptosis. Genes and Development 2001;15(22): 2922-2933.
[55] Underbrink MP, Howie HL, Bedard KM, Koop JI, Galloway DA. The E6 Proteins from Multiple Beta HPV Types Degrade Bak and Protect Keratinocytes from Apoptosis after UVB Irradiation. Journal of Virology 2008;82(21): 10408-10417.
[56] Simmonds M, Storey A. Identification of the Regions of the HPV 5 E6 Protein Involved in Bak Degradation and Inhibition of Apoptosis. International Journal of Cancer 2008;123(10): 2260-2266.
[57] Tong X, Howley PM. The Bovine Papillomavirus E6 Oncoprotein Interacts with Paxillin and Disrupts the Actin Cytoskeleton. Proceedings of the National Academy of Sciences of the USA 1997;94(9): 4412-4417.
[58] Kuhne C, Banks L. E3-Ubiquitin Ligase/E6-AP Links Multicopy Maintenance Protein 7 to the Ubiquitination Pathway by a Novel Motif, the L2G Box. Journal of Biological Chemistry 1998;273(51): 34302-34309.
[59] Iftner T, Elbel M, Schopp B, Hiller T, Loizou JI, Caldecott KW, Stubenrauch F. Interference of Papillomavirus E6 Protein with Single-Strand Break Repair by Interaction with XRCC1. EMBO Journal 2002;21(17): 4741-4748.
[60] Srivenugopal KS, Ali-Osman F. The DNA Repair Protein, O(6)-Methylguanine-DNA Methyltransferase is a Proteolytic Target for the E6 Human Papillomavirus Oncoprotein. Oncogene 2002;21(38): 5940-5945.
[61] Hasan UA, Bates E, Takeshita F, Biliato A, Accardi R, Bouvard V, Mansour M, Vincent I, Gissmann L, Iftner T, Sideri M, Stubenrauch F, Tommasino M. TLR9 Expression and

Function is Abolished by the Cervical Cancer-Associated Human Papillomavirus Type 16. Journal of Immunology 2007;178 (5): 3186-3197.

[62] Ronco LV, Karpova AY, Vidal M, Howley PM. Human Papillomavirus 16 E6 Oncoprotein Binds to Interferon Regulatory Factor-3 and Inhibits its Transcriptional Activity. Genes and Development 1998;12: 2061-2072.

[63] Beglin M, Melar-New M, Laimins L. Human Papillomaviruses and the Interferon Response. Journal of Interferon and Cytokine Research. 2009;29(9): 629-35.

[64] Riley RR, Duensing S, Brake T, Münger K, Lambert PF, Arbeit JM. Dissection of Human Papillomavirus E6 and E7 Function in Transgenic Mouse Models of Cervical Carcinogenesis. Cancer Research 2003;63: 4862-71.

[65] He L, He X, Lim LP, de Stanchina E, Xuan Z, Liang Y, Xue W, Zender L, Magnus J, Ridzon D, Jackson AL, Linsley PS, Chen C, Lowe SW, Cleary MA, G.J. Hannon GJ. A MicroRNA Component of the p53 Tumour Suppressor Network. Nature 2007;447: 1130-1134.

[66] Chang TC, Wentzel EA, Kent OA, Ramachandran K, Mullendore M, Lee KH, Feldmann G,Yamakuchi M, Ferlito M, Lowenstein CJ, Arking DE, Beer MA, Maitra A, Mendell JT. Transactivation of miR-34a by p53 Broadly Influences Gene Expression and Promotes Apoptosis. Molecular Cell 2007;26: 745-752.

[67] Raver-Shapira N, Marciano E, Meiri E, Spector Y, Rosenfeld N, Moskovits N, Bentwich Z, Oren M. Transcriptional Activation of miR-34a Contributes to p53-Mediated Apoptosis. Molecular Cell. 2007;26: 731-743.

[68] Zheng ZM. Regulation of Cellular miRNA Expression by Human Papillomaviruses. Biochimica et Biophysica Acta. 2011;1809: 668-677

[69] Wang X, Tang S, Le SY, Lu R, Rader JS, Meyers C, Zheng ZM. Aberrant Expression of Oncogenic and Tumor-Suppressive MicroRNAs in Cervical Cancer is Required for Cancer Cell Growth. PLoS One. 2008;3(7): e2557

[70] Au Yeung CL, Tsang TY, Yau PL, Kwok TT. Human Papillomavirus Type 16 E6 Induces Cervical Cancer Cell Migration Through the p53/MicroRNA-23b/Urokinase-Type Plasminogen Activator Pathway. Oncogene 2011;30: 2401-2410.

[71] Hwang SG, Lee D, Kim J, Seo T, Choe J. Human Papillomavirus Type 16 E7 Binds to E2F1 and Activates E2F1-Driven Transcription in a Retinoblastoma Protein Independent Manner. Journal of Biological Chemistry 2002;277(4): 2923-2930.

[72] Dyson N. The Regulation of E2F by pRB-Family Proteins. Genes and Development 1998;12(15): 2245-2262.

[73] Dyson N, Guida P, Munger K, Harlow E. Homologous Sequences in Adenovirus E1A and Human Papillomavirus E7 Proteins Mediate Interaction with the Same Set of Cellular Proteins. Journal of Virology 1992;66(12): 6893-6902.

[74] Jones DL, Münger K. Analysis of the p53-Mediated G1 Growth Arrest Pathway in Cells Expressing the Human Papillomavirus Type 16 E7 Oncoprotein. Journal of Virology 1997;71: 2905-12.

[75] Tommasino M, Adamczewski JP, Carlotti F., Barth CF, Manetti R, Contorni M, Cavalieri F, Hunt T, Crawford L. HPV16 E7 Protein Associates with the Protein Kinase p33CDK2 and Cyclin A. Oncogene 1993;8(1): 195-202.

[76] McIntyre M.C, Frattini MG, Grossman SR, Laimins LA. Human Papillomavirus Type 18 E7 Protein Requires Intact Cys-X-X-Cys Motifs for Zinc Binding, Dimerization, and Transformation but not for Rb Binding. Journal of Virology 1993;67: 3142-3150.

[77] Zerfass K, Schulze A, Spitkovsky D, Friedman V, Henglein B, Jansen-Durr P. Sequential Activation of Cyclin E and Cyclin A Gene Expression by Human Papillomavirus Type 16 E7 Through Sequences Necessary for Transformation. Journal of Virology 1995;69(10): 6389-6399.

[78] Park JS, Kim EJ, Kwon HJ, Hwang ES, Namkoong SE, Um SJ. Inactivation of Interferon Regulatory Factor-1 Tumor Suppressor Protein by HPV E7 Oncoprotein. Implication for the E7-Mediated Immune Evasion Mechanism in Cervical Carcinogenesis. Journal of Biological Chemistry. 2000;275: 6764-6769.

[79] White AE, Livanos EM, Tlsty TD. Differential Disruption of Genomic Integrity and Cell Cycle Regulation in Normal Human Fibroblasts by the HPV Oncoproteins. Genes and Development 1994;8(6): 666–677.

[80] Duensing S, Duensing A, Flores ER, Do A, Lambert PF, Munger K. Centrosome Abnormalities and Genomic Instability by Episomal Expression of Human Papillomavirus Type 16 in Raft Cultures of Human Keratinocytes. Journal of Virology 2001;75(16): 7712-7716.

[81] Duensing S, Duensing A, Lee DC, Edwards KM, Piboonniyom SO, Manuel E, Skaltsounis L, Meijer L, Munger K. Cyclin-Dependent Kinase Inhibitor Indirubin-3'-Oxime Selectively Inhibits Human Papillomavirus Type 16 E7-Induced Numerical Centrosome Anomalies. Oncogene 2004;23(50): 8206-8215.

[82] Duensing A, Liu Y, Tseng M, Malumbres M, Barbacid M, Duensing S. Cyclin Dependent K2 is Dispensable for Normal Centrosome Duplication but Required for Oncogene-Induced Centrosome Overduplication. Oncogene 2006;25(20): 2943-2949.

[83] Nguyen CL, Eichwald C, Nibert ML, Munger K. Human Papillomavirus Type 16 E7 Oncoprotein Associates with the Centrosomal Component Gamma-tubulin. Journal of Virology 2007;81(24): 13533-13543.

[84] de Ruijter AJ, van Gennip AH, Caron HN, Kemp S, van Kuilenburg AB. Histone Deacetylases (HDACs): Characterization of the Classical HDAC Family. Biochemical Journal 2003;370: 737-749.

[85] Longworth MS, Laimins LA. The Binding of Histone Deacetylases and the Integrity of Zinc Finger-Like Motifs of the E7 Protein are Essential for the Life Cycle of Human Papillomavirus Type 31. Journal of Virology 2004;78: 3533-3541.

[86] McLaughlin-Drubin ME, Huh KW, Münger K. Human Papillomavirus Type 16 E7 Oncoprotein Associates with E2F6. Journal of Virology 2008;82: 8695-8705

[87] Schwartz YB, Pirrotta V. Polycomb Silencing Mechanisms and the Management of Genomic Programmes. Nature Reviews Genetics 2007;8: 9-22.

[88] Serrano M, Lin AW, McCurrach ME, Beach D, Lowe SW. Oncogenic ras Provokes Premature Cell Senescence Associated with Accumulation of p53 and p16INK4a. Cell 1997;88: 593-602.

[89] Agger K. The H3K27me3 Demethylase JMJD3 Contributes to the Activation of the INK4A-ARF Locus in Response to Oncogene- and Stress-Induced Senescence. Genes and Development 2009;23: 1171-1176.

[90] Hayami S, Yoshimatsu M, Veerakumarasivam A, Unoki M, Iwai Y, Tsunoda T, Field HI, Kelly JD, Neal DE, Yamaue H, Ponder BA, Nakamura Y, Hamamoto R. Overexpression of the JmjC Histone Demethylase KDM5B in Human Carcinogenesis: Involvement in the Proliferation of Cancer Cells Through the E2F/RB Pathway. Molecular Cancer. 2010;9: 59-72.

[91] Smith JA, White EA, Sowa ME Powell ML, Ottinger M, Harper JW, Howley PM. Genome-Wide siRNA Screen Identifies SMCX, EP400, and Brd4 as E2-Dependent Regulators of Human Papillomavirus Oncogene Expression. Proceedings of the National Academy of Sciences of the USA 2010;107, 3752-3757.

[92] Melar-New M, Laimins LA. Human Papillomaviruses Modulate Expression of MicroRNA 203 upon Epithelial Differentiation to Control Levels of p63 Proteins. Journal of Virology 2010;84: 5212-5221.

[93] Yi R, Poy MN, Stoffel M, Fuchs E. A Skin MicroRNA Promotes Differentiation by Repressing 'Stemness'. Nature 2008;452: 225-229

[94] Lena AM, Shalom-Feuerstein R, Rivetti D, Aberdam VD, Knight RA, Melino G, Candi E. miR-203 Represses 'Stemness' by Repressing DeltaNp63. Cell Death and Differentiation 2008;15: 1187-1195.

[95] Botezatu A, Goia-Rusanu CD, Iancu IV, Huica I, Plesa A, Socolov D, Ungureanu C, Anton G. Quantitative Analysis of the Relationship between MicroRNA-124a, -34b and -203 Gene Methylation and Cervical Oncogenesis. Molecular Medicine Reports 2011;4(1): 121-128.

[96] Venuti A, Salani D, Poggiali F, Manni V, Bagnato A. The E5 Oncoprotein of Human Papillomavirus Type 16 Enhances Endothelin-1-Induced Keratinocyte Growth. Virology 1998;248: 1-5.

[97] Bouvard V, Matlashewski G, Gu ZM, Storey A, Banks L. The Human Papillomavirus Type 16 Gene Cooperates with the E7 Gene to Stimulate Proliferation of Primary Cells and Increases Viral Gene Expression. Virology 1994;203: 73-80.

[98] Straight SW, Hinkle PM, Jewers RJ, McCance DJ. The E5 Oncoprotein of Human Papillomavirus Type 16 Transforms Fibroblasts and Effects the Down-regulation of the Epidermal Growth Factor Receptor in Keratinocytes. Journal of Virology 1993;67: 4521-4532.

[99] DiMaio D, Mattoon D. Mechanisms of Cell Transformation by Papillomavirus E5 Proteins. Oncogene 2001;20: 7866-7873

[100] Thomsen P, van Deurs B, Norrild B, Kayser L. The HPV16 E5 Oncogene Inhibits Endocytic Trafficking. Oncogene 2000;19: 6023-6032.

[101] Belleudi F, Leone L, Purpura V, Cannella F, Scrofani C, Torrisi MR. HPV16 E5 Affects the KGFR/FGFR2b-Mediated Epithelial Growth Through Alteration of the Receptor Expression, Signalling and Endocytic Traffic. Oncogene 2011;30(50): 4963-4976.

[102] Krawczyk E, Suprynowicz FA, Liu X, Dai Y, Hartmann DP, Hanover J, Schlegel R. Koilocytosis: a Cooperative Interaction between the Human Papillomavirus E5 and E6 Oncoproteins. American Journal of Pathology 2008;173: 682-688.

[103] Oelze I, Kartenbeck J, Crusius K, Alonso A. Human Papillomavirus Type 16 E5 Protein Affects Cell-Cell Communication in an Epithelial Cell Line. Journal of Virology 1995;69: 4489-4494.

[104] Tomakidi P, Cheng H, Kohl A, Komposch G, Alonso A. Connexin 43 Expression is Downregulated in Raft Cultures of Human Keratinocytes Expressing the Human Papillomavirus Type 16 E5 Protein. Cell and Tissue Research. 2000;301: 323-327.

[105] Hu L, Ceresa B. Characterization of the Plasma Membrane Localization and Orientation of HPV16 E5 for Cell-Cell Fusion. Virology 2009;393: 135-143.

[106] Hu L, Plafker K, Vorozhko V, Zuna RE, Hanigan MH, Gorbsky GJ, Plafker SM, Angeletti PC, Ceresa BP. Human Papillomavirus E5 Induces Bi-Nucleated Cell Formation by Cell-Cell fusion. Virology 2009;384: 125-134.

[107] Hu L, Potapova TA, Li S, Rankin S, Gorbsky GJ, Angeletti PC, Ceresa BP. Expression of HPV16 E5 Produces Enlarged Nuclei and Polyploidy through Endoreplication. Virology 2010;405: 342-351.

[108] Stoppler MC, StraightSW, Tsao G, Schlegel R, McCance DJ. The E5 Gene of HPV-16 Enhances Keratinocyte Immortalization by Full-Length DNA. Virology 1996;223: 251-254.

[109] Oelze I, Kartenbeck J, Crusius K, Alonso A. Human Papillomavirus Type 16 E5 Protein Affects Cell-Cell Communication in an Epithelial Cell Line. Journal of Virology 1995;69: 4489-4494.

[110] Zhang B, Spandau DF, Roman A. E5 Protein of Human Papillomavirus Type 16 Protects Human Foreskin Keratinocytes from UV B-Irradiation-Induced Apoptosis. Journal of Virology 2002;76: 220-231.

[111] Kabsch K, Alonso A. The Human Papillomavirus Type 16 (HPV-16) E5 Protein Sensitizes Human Keratinocytes to Apoptosis Induced by Osmotic Stress. Oncogene 2002;21: 947-953.

[112] Sudarshan SR, Schlegel R, Liu X. The HPV-16 E5 Protein Represses Expression of Stress Pathway Genes XBP-1 and COX-2 in Genital Keratinocytes. Biochemical and Biophysical Research Communications. 2010;399: 617-622.

[113] Schapiro F, Sparkowski J, Adduci A, Schlegel R, Grinstein S. Golgi Alkalinization by the Papillomavirus E5 Oncoprotein. Journal of Cellular Biology 2000;148: 305-315.

[114] Cortese MS, Ashrafi GH, Campo MS. All Four Di-Leucine Motifs in the First Hydrophobic Domain of the E5 Oncoprotein of Human Papillomavirus Type 16 are Essential for Surface MHC Class I Downregulation Activity and E5 Endomembrane Localization. International Journal of Cancer 2010;126(7): 1675-1682.

[115] Ashrafi GH, Haghshenas M, Marchetti B, Campo MS. E5 Protein of Human Papillomavirus 16 Downregulates HLA Class I and Interacts with the Heavy Chain via its First Hydrophobic Domain. International Journal of Cancer 2006;119: 2105-2112.

[116] Melendy T, Sedman J, Stenlund A. Cellular Factors Required for Papillomavirus DNA Replication. Journal of Virology 1995;69: 7857-7867.

[117] Thierry F. Transcriptional Regulation of the Papillomavirus Oncogenes by Cellular and Viral Transcription Factors in Cervical Carcinoma. Virology 2009;384: 375-379.

[118] Xue Y, Bellanger S, Zhang W, Lim D, Low J, Lunny D, Thierry F. HPV16 E2 is an Immediate Early Marker of Viral Infection, Preceding E7 Expression in Precursor Structures of Cervical Carcinoma. Cancer Research 2010;70: 5316-5325.

[119] Blachon S, Bellanger S, Demeret C, Thierry F. Nucleo-Cytoplasmic Shuttling of High Risk Human Papillomavirus E2 Proteins Induces Apoptosis. Journal of Biological Chemistry 2005;280: 36088-36098.

[120] Bellanger S, Demeret C, Goyat S, Thierry F. Stability of the Human Papillomavirus Type18 E2 Protein is Regulated by a Proteasome Degradation Pathway through its Amino-Terminal Transactivation Domain. Journal of Virology 2001;75: 7244-7251.

[121] Goodwin EC, DiMaio D. Repression of Human Papillomavirus Oncogenes in HeLa Cervical Carcinoma Cells Causes the Orderly Reactivation of Dormant Tumor Suppressor Pathways. Proceedings of the National Academy of Sciences of the USA 2000;97: 12513-12518.

[122] Dowhanick JJ, McBride AA, Howley PM. Suppression of Cellular Proliferation by the Papillomavirus E2 Protein. Journal of Virology 1995;69: 7791-7799.

[123] Frattini MG, Hurst SD, Lim HB, Swaminathan S, Laimins LA. Abrogation of a Mitotic Checkpoint by E2 Proteins from Oncogenic Human Papillomaviruses Correlates with Increased Turnover of the p53 Tumor Suppressor Protein. EMBO Journal 1997;16: 318-331.

[124] Bellanger S, Blachon S, Mechali F, Bonne-Andrea C, Thierry F. High-Risk but not Low-Risk HPV E2 Proteins Bind to the APC Activators Cdh1 and Cdc20 and Cause Genomic Instability. Cell Cycle 2005;4: 1608-1615.

[125] Scholl SM, Kenter G, Kurzeder C, Beuzeboc P. Pathway Profiling and Rational Trial Design for Studies in Advanced Stage Cervical Carcinoma: a Review and a Perspective. ISRN Oncol. 2011:403098.

[126] Maciag PC, Radulovic S, Rothman J. The First Clinical Use of a Live-Attenuated Listeria Monocytogenes Vaccine: a Phase I Safety Study of Lm-LLO-E7 in Patients with Advanced Carcinoma of the Cervix. Vaccine 2009;27(30). 3975-3983.

[127] Kaufmann AM, Stern PL, Rankin EM, Sommer H, Nuessler V, Schneider A. Safety and Immunogenicity of TA-HPV, a Recombinant Vaccinia Virus Expressing Modified Human Papillomavirus (HPV)-16 and HPV-18 E6 and E7 Genes, in Women with Progressive Cervical Cancer. Clinical Cancer Research 2002;8(12): 3676-3685.

[128] Garcia-Hernandez E, Gonzalez, Sanchez J L, Andrade-Manzano A, Contreras M L, Padilla S, Guzman CC. Regression of Papilloma High-Grade Lesions (CIN 2 and CIN 3) is Stimulated by Therapeutic Vaccination with MVA E2 Recombinant Vaccine. Cancer Gene Therapy 2006;13(6): 592-597.

[129] Kim JH, Kang TH, Noh KH, Bae HC, Kim SH, Yoo YD. Enhancement of Dendritic Cell-Based Vaccine Potency by Anti-Apoptotic siRNAs Targeting Key Pro-apoptotic Proteins in Cytotoxic CD8(+) T Cell-Mediated Cell Death. Immunological Letters. 2009;122(1): 58-67.

[130] Ferrara A, Nonn M, Sehr P, Schreckenberger C, Pawlita M, Durst M. Dendritic Cell-Based Tumor Vaccine for Cervical Cancer II: Results of a Clinical Pilot Study in 15 Individual Patients. Journal of Cancer Research and Clinical Oncology 2003;129(9): 521-530.

[131] Santin AD, Bellone S, Palmieri M, Zanolini A, Ravaggi A, Siegel ER. Human Papillomavirus Type 16 and 18 E7-Pulsed Dendritic Cell Vaccination of Stage IB or IIA

Cervical Cancer Patients: a Phase I Escalating-Dose Trial. Journal of Virology 2008;82(4): 1968-1979.

[132] National Taiwan University Hospital. Immunotherapy of Recurrent Cervical Cancers Using Dendritic Cells (DCs). 2009. Available from URL: http://www.clinicaltrials.gov.

[133] Steller MA, Gurski KJ, Murakami M, Daniel RW, Shah KV, Celis E. Cell-Mediated Immunological Responses in Cervical and Vaginal Cancer Patients Immunized with a Lipidated Epitope of Human Papillomavirus Type 16 E7. Clinical Cancer Research 1998;4(9): 2103-2109.

[134] Sharma RK, Elpek KG, Yolcu ES, Schabowsky RH, Zhao H, Bandura-Morgan L, Shirwan H. Costimulation as a Platform for the Development of Vaccines: a Peptide-Based Vaccine Containing a Novel Form of 4-1BB Ligand Eradicates Established Tumors. Cancer Research 2009;69(10): 4319-4326.

[135] Barrios K, Celis E. TriVax-HPV: an Improved Peptide-Based Therapeutic Vaccination Strategy against Human Papillomavirus-Induced Cancers. Cancer Immunology and Immunotherapy 2012;61(8): 1307-1317.

[136] Hallez S, Simon P, Maudoux F, Doyen J, Noel JC, Beliard A. Phase I/II Trial of Immunogenicity of a Human Papillomavirus (HPV) Type 16 E7 Protein-Based Vaccine in Women with Oncogenic HPV-Positive Cervical Intraepithelial Neoplasia. Cancer Immunology and Immunotherapy 2004;53(7): 642-650.

[137] Frazer IH, Quinn M, Nicklin JL, Tan J, Perrin LC, Ng P. Phase 1 Study of HPV16-Specific Immunotherapy with E6E7 Fusion Protein and ISCOMATRIX Adjuvant in Women with Cervical Intraepithelial Neoplasia. Vaccine 2004;23(2): 172-181.

[138] Einstein MH, Kadish AS, Burk RD, Kim MY, Wadler S, Streicher H. Heat Shock Fusion Protein-Based Immunotherapy for Treatment of Cervical Intraepithelial Neoplasia III. Gynecologic Oncology. 2007;106(3): 453-460.

[139] Trimble CL, Peng S, Kos F, Gravitt P, Viscidi R, Sugar E. A Phase I Trial of a Human Papillomavirus DNA Vaccine for HPV16+ Cervical Intraepithelial Neoplasia 2/3. Clinical Cancer Research 2009;15(1): 361-367.

[140] VGX Pharmaceuticals, Inc. Phase I of Human Papillomavirus (HPV) DNA Plasmid (VGX-3100)+ Electroporation for CIN 2 or 3, 2009. Available from URL: http://www.clinicaltrials.gov

[141] Kim SW, Yang JS. Human Papillomavirus type 16 E5 Protein as a Therapeutic Target. Yonsei Medical Journal 2006;47(1): 1-14.

[142] Liu DW, Tsao YP, Hsieh CH, Hsieh JT, Kung JT, Chiang CL, Huang SJ, Chen SL. Induction of CD8 T Cells by Vaccination with Recombinant Adenovirus Expressing Human Papillomavirus Type 16 E5 Gene Reduces Tumor Growth. Journal of Virology 2000;74(19): 9083-9089.

[143] Chen YF, Lin CW, Tsao YP, Chen SL. Cytotoxic-T Lymphocyte human Papillomavirus type 16 E5 Peptide with CpG-Oligodeoxynucleotide Can Eliminate Tumor Growth in C57BL/6 Mice. Journal of Virology 2004;78: 1333-1343.

[144] Mariz FC. Development of new biotechnology platforms for production of HPV vaccines: Approaches in the context of developing countries. J Vaccines Vaccin 2012;3:4.

Section 4

A New Approach on Cancer Mechanism

Chapter 9

Model Systems Facilitating an Understanding of Mechanisms for Oncogene Amplification

Takaaki Watanabe

Additional information is available at the end of the chapter

http://dx.doi.org/10.5772/55119

1. Introduction

Gene amplification is a copy number increase of a restricted region of a chromosome arm. Amplified chromosomal regions are present in acentric mini extra-chromosome (double minutes, DMs) or within a chromosome as repetitive arrays (homogeneously staining regions, HSRs); or distributed at various locations in the genome (scattered-type) (Fig. 1).

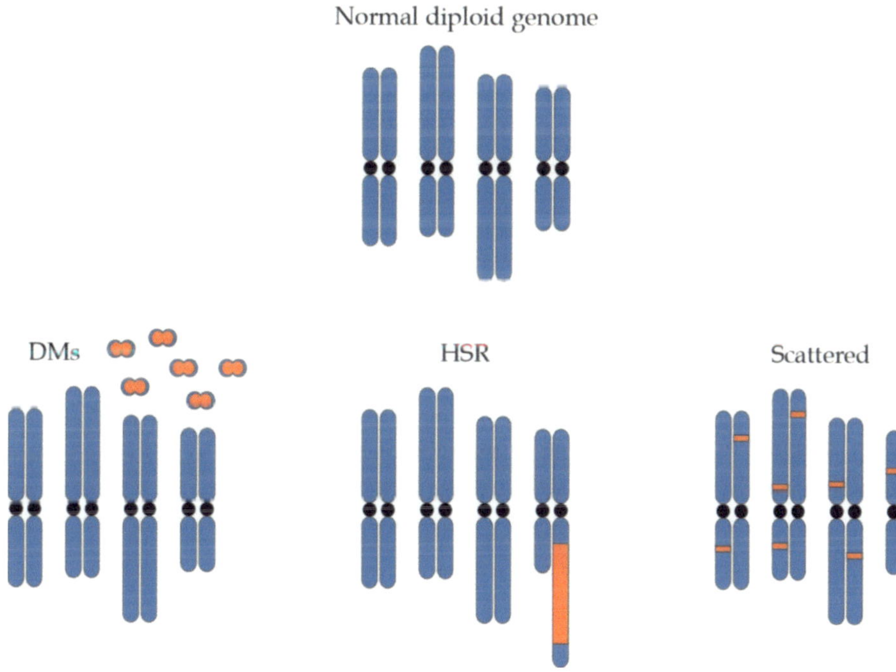

Figure 1. Typical amplification products in mammalian cells.

A schematic illustration of four-chromosome genome (above) and three types of amplification products (below) are depicted. Amplified regions are indicated in red, and black circles represent centromeres. See text for details.

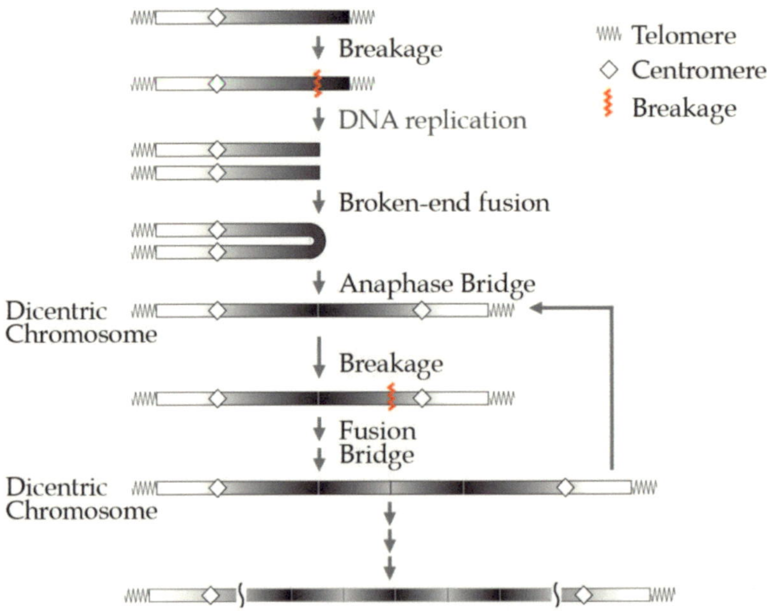

Figure 2. Breakage-fusion-bridge (BFB) cycles

The BFB cycle can be initiated by a DNA double-strand break. After DNA replication, the ends of the sister chromatids can fuse, giving rise to a dicentric chromosome. At anaphase, if the two centromeres go to the two opposite poles of the mitotic spindle, the dicentric chromosome can be broken. An asymmetric break will lead to a formation partially deleted or duplicated broken chromosomes. Subsequent cycles involving the chromosome with the duplication cause the increase in the copy number of the region of interest as inverted repeats. BFB cycles end when the broken chromosome ends are stabilized.

Oncogene amplification is common in human cancers and contributes to tumor progression and therapeutic resistance (Albertson, 2006; Tanaka and Yao, 2009). For example, ERBB2 amplification is often detected in advanced breast cancers, and overproduction of ERBB2 can accelerate tumor progression (Di Fiore et al., 1987; Muller et al., 1988; Slamon et al., 1987). Amplifications of MYC, CCND1, EGFR, MDM2, MYCN, JUN, TNK2, or ESR1 are also associated with aggressive phenotypes of tumors. BCR-ABL fusion gene is amplified in patients showing therapeutic resistance to Imatinib mesylate (Gorre et al., 2001). Amplifications of DHFR, TYMS, or MET are also associated with therapeutic resistance.

A variety of models are proposed to explain the amplification process, including unequal sister-chromatid exchange, localized over replication, fold-back priming, rolling-circle replication, and breakage-fusion-bridge (BFB) cycle (Kobayashi et al., 2004; McClintock, 1941; Rattray et al., 2005; Tower, 2004; Watanabe and Horiuchi, 2005). Cytogenetic features of BFB cycle have been repeatedly observed in tumor cells (Fig.2). BFB cycle is the most popular model to explain intra-chromosomal amplification (Mondello et al., 2010; Tanaka and Yao, 2009), especially in the early stage of the amplification. In cancer cells, HSRs are often organized as an inverted ladder associated with a deletion that spans from the amplicon toward a telomere (Debatisse and Malfor, 2005). According to the BFB model, such a complex rearrangement results from the following repeating cycle: an initial DSB; replication of the broken molecule; fusion of sister chromatids; formation of a bridge during anaphase; and asymmetrical breakage due to mechanical tension, which generates one chromatid with an inverted repeat at the broken end.

In extra-chromosomal amplification, replication-based models are often proposed. Breakage at stalled replication forks is proposed to cause DMs formation including EGFR gene (Vogt et al., 2004). Extra-rounds of replication are thought to lead to DMs containing N-myc gene. In N-myc amplification, extra-round of replication is expected to form an extra-chromosomal element leading to integration followed by intra-chromosomal amplification (Savelyeva and Schwab, 2001). However, only by these amplification models themselves, it is difficult to explain the entire processes of the amplification.

2. Barrier to efficient analyses

Despite their biological and clinical importance, mechanisms for amplifying oncogenes remain largely unknown. This is because the whole process of gene amplification has been difficult to analyze because of additional kinds of amplification processes and secondary chromosome rearrangements (Haber and Debatisse, 2006). There are at least three reasons for this difficulty: (1) previous approaches to understand mechanisms for amplification were based on the structural analysis of complex end products; (2) few model systems for gene amplification are available that allow chromosomal engineering, as is possible in yeast (Lengauer et al., 1998); (3) spontaneous gene amplification occurs at very low frequency.

The use of genome-wide scanning techniques, such as array comparative genomic hybridization (array CGH) and next-generation DNA sequencing, has recently demonstrated that most solid tumors contain amplified portions of their genomes (Albertson, 2006). However, even these recent genomic technologies cannot unambiguously assign sequences in amplified regions and accurately resolve their chromosomal structure. Thus, amplified regions have been largely refractory to standard human genetic analyses.

3. Model systems for understanding common features of gene amplification

3.1. DSB and inverted repeats

Long series of studies have shown that DNA double-strand break (DSB) and inverted repeats play an important role in gene amplification. DNA double-strand break (DSB) is one of the harmful forms of DNA damage, and can induce several types of chromosomal aberrations, including gene amplification, when not correctly repaired. Amplification is triggered by DNA-damaging agents, which can directly or indirectly cause DSBs (Kuo et al., 1994; Paulson et al., 1998; Poupon et al., 1996; Yunis et al., 1987). In mammalian genomes, there are regions prone to breakage known as common fragile sites (CFSs) (Debatisse et al., 2012; Glover et al., 2005). CFSs are involved in chromosomal aberrations, including gene amplification, and have been shown to play a major role in the early steps in gene amplification (Ciullo et al., 2002; Coquelle et al., 1997; Hellman et al., 2002; Kuo et al., 1998). In cooperation with DSBs, short inverted repeats could generate a palindromic dicentric chromosome, leading to gene amplification.

Model systems that use site-specific endonucleases, such as I-SceI or HO endonucleases, have been constructed in yeast and in mammalian cells. Yao's group first constructed a plasmid-based system in yeast containing an HO endonuclease cutting site and an adjacent inverted repeat (Butler et al., 1996). This system efficiently formed a palindromic mini-chromosome after induction of the endonuclease. They next used Chinese hamster ovary (CHO) cells and inserted a DHFR transgene into a chromosome of the cells with an I-SceI cutting site and an adjacent inverted repeat (Tanaka et al., 2002). This system formed a palindromic dimer after I-SceI cutting and consequently caused intra-chromosomal amplification, suggesting the formation of a dicentric chromosome and the involvement of subsequent BFB cycles.

We developed a new approach in which we design amplification processes and test whether the processes can produce the amplification seen in nature. Previously, in yeast, we constructed a system designed to induce a rapid amplification mode, double rolling-circle replication (DRCR) via chromosomal breaks induced by HO endonuclease (Watanabe and Horiuchi, 2005) (Fig.3). DRCR is a continuous process in which two replication forks chase each other (Fig.3A), and was first confirmed by Volkert and Broach for amplification of yeast 2μ plasmid (Volkert and Broach, 1986). To induce DRCR, we used break-induced replication (BIR), a nonreciprocal recombination-dependent replication process that is an effective mechanism to repair a broken chromosome (Fig.3B). The DRCR amplification is selected with an amplification marker, *leu2d*, which has a slight transcription activity and complements leucine auxotrophy if amplified (Erhart and Hollenberg, 1983). This system produced intra-/extra-chromosomal products resembling HSR and DMs seen in mammalian cells (Fig.3C). The HSR-type products contain up to ~100 copies of *leu2d* gene, which occupies 730kb (the rest of chromosome VI comprises 275 kb). Interestingly, HSR/DMs products were generated at low frequency without deliberate DNA cleavage, depending on the chromosome structure with the inverted repeats. These features strongly suggest that the processes described here may contribute to natural gene amplification in higher eukaryotes and natural amplification involves DRCR.

Lobachev et al constructed a yeast strain having an inverted repeat of Alu sequences, and showed that the repeat are fragile sites (Lobachev et al., 2002). The Alu inverted repeats can be cleaved and subsequently generate hairpin ends, which can be opened up by the Mre11/Rad50/Xrs2 complex in concert with the Sae2 protein. His group next demonstrated that Alu inverted repeats can trigger intra- and extra-chromosomal amplification in yeast (Narayanan et al., 2006).

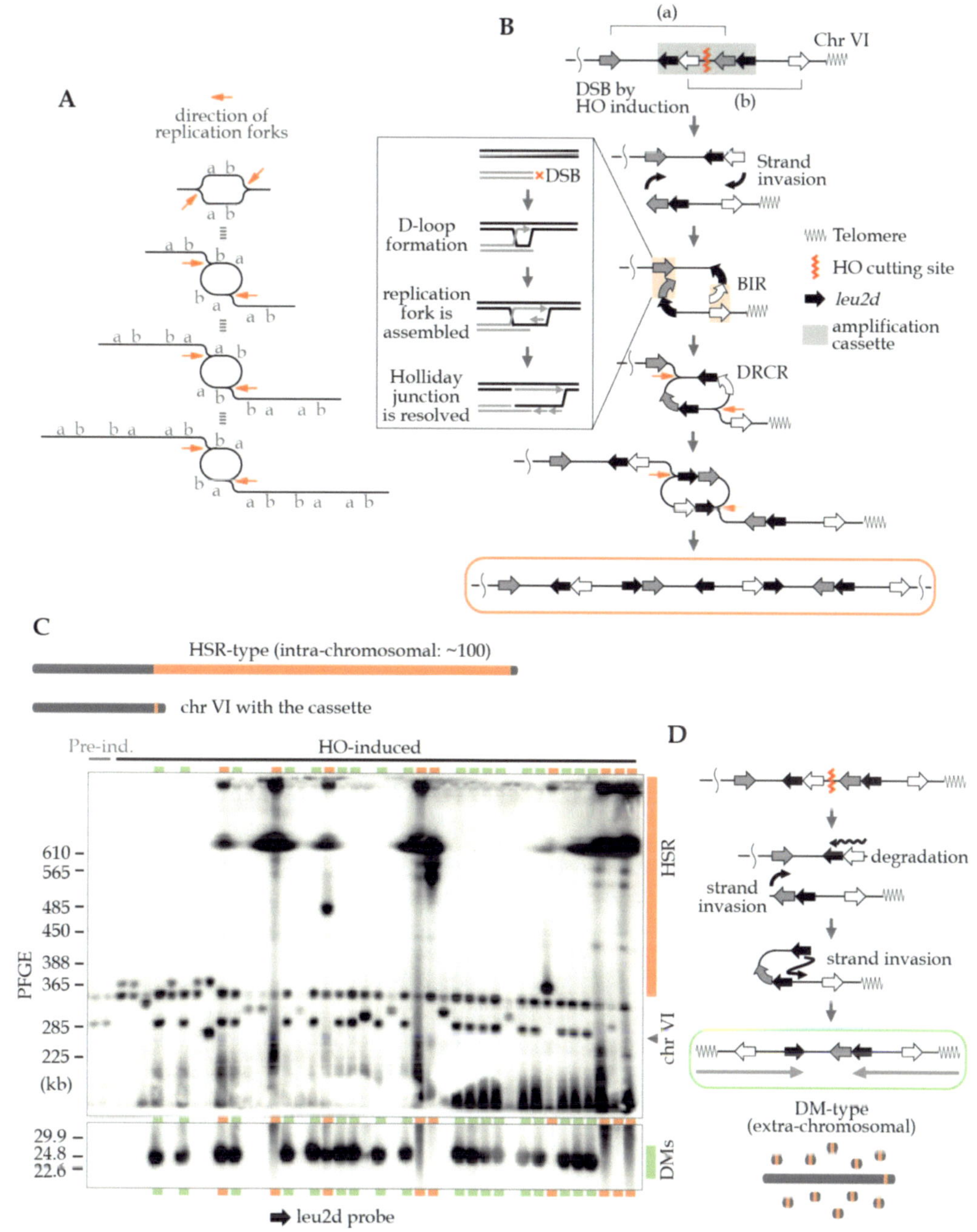

Figure 3. Gene amplification system based on DRCR utilizing break-induced replication (BIR).

(A) Double rolling-circle replication (DRCR). Two replication forks chase each other. One replication fork can replicate a template for the other fork and so amplification proceeds. (B) Structure of the amplification cassette and a model for DRCR amplification. This cassette contains two PCR-amplified sequences (white and gray arrows) derived from the nearby genomic region, forming two inverted pairs (a) and (b). The amplification marker, *leu2d*, has a slight transcription activity, and it will complement leucine auxotrophy if amplified. This yeast strain has galactose-inducible HO endonuclease gene. Following HO cutting, two chromosomal ends can invade each other, initiating two break-induced replication (BIR) events as in the insert box and subsequent DRCR. The DRCR process would terminate by recombination between bidirectionally elongated arms. (C) Southern analysis of uncut chromosomal DNA from Leu^+ survivors with the *leu2d* probe. The expression of HO endonuclease was induced on galactose medium without leucine (HO-induced). PFGE was performed with higher and lower size ranges. The lanes marked in red and green indicate intra- and extra-chromosomal amplification, respectively. Pre-ind.: preinduction conditions (cultured on glucose plates containing leucine). (D) Model for the production of extra-chromosomal products. These products are proposed to result from degradation of one broken end and the subsequent intramolecular BIR.

3.2. Replication stress within repeated sequences

Recently, DNA replication stress within repeated sequences is reported to contribute importantly to genome instability. Two recent yeast papers have shown that nearby inverted repeats recombine spontaneously to fuse, leading to the formation of dicentric and acentric chromosomes (Branzei and Foiani, 2010a; Mizuno et al., 2009; Paek et al., 2009). This fusion process does not appear to require DSB formation, and is likely caused by DNA replication-based mechanism involving an aberrant switch of replication templates.

Another example involves the re-replication event, the inappropriate firing of replication origins. Green et al. developed an elegant system in yeast that enables a locus-specific and transient re-replication by conditionally deregulating the replication origin (Green et al., 2010). They demonstrate that re-replication can generate duplication in cooperation with Ty repetitive elements, suggesting that this process is a potent inducer of gene amplification.

We have examined whether gene amplification can be induced when recombinational processes between inverted sequences are coupled with DNA replication. To efficiently induce the recombinational processes, Cre-lox site-specific recombination was used to design amplification system based on DRCR (Watanabe et al., 2011). This system successfully yielded HSR/DM-type products in yeast (Fig.4) and Chinese hamster ovary (CHO) cells (Fig.5). We first predicted that, if recombination occurs between un-replicated and recently replicated regions during replication (Fig.4A), the replication fork would make an additional copy of the replicated region. To induce DRCR, two sets of the recombinational process were utilized (Fig.4B and 4C). In yeast, the Cre induction caused a >7000-fold increase in the frequency of survivors and, surprisingly, over 10% of the Cre recombination-induced cells undergo gene amplification (Fig.4D). The HSR-type products appear to contain approximately 90-140 copies of the *leu2d* gene, corresponding to a 3.6~5.6-fold increase in the length of the original (275 kb) chromosome VI (Fig.4E).

For DRCR system in CHO cells, we constructed an amplification cassette on a rat genomic bacterial artificial chromosome (BAC), and integrated it into a specific site on a CHO cell chromosome using the Flp-FRT (Flp recombination target site) system (Fig.5A). An amplification marker, a mouse dihydrofolate reductase (DHFR) gene, provides methotrexate (MTX) resistance when amplified. This system successfully produced HSR/DM/Scattered-type amplification (Fig.5B-K).

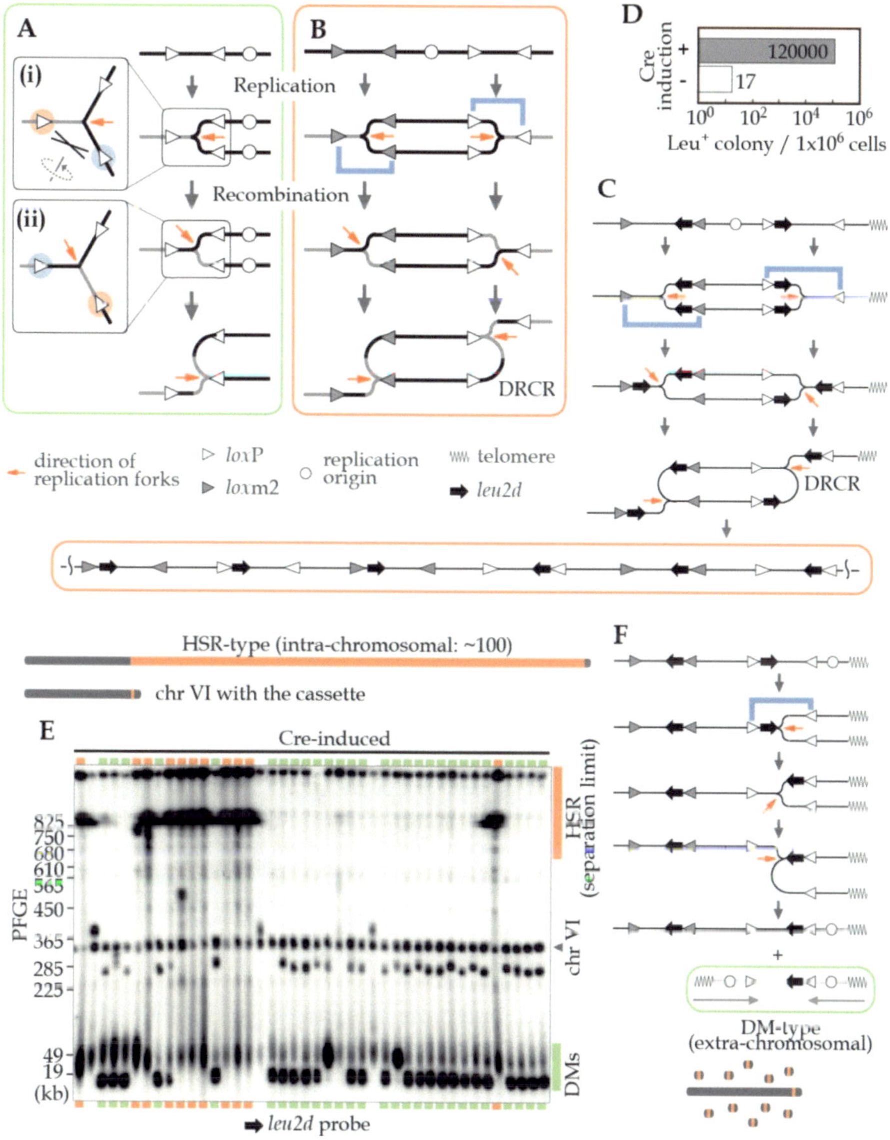

Figure 4. Gene amplification in yeast induced by Cre recombination.

(A) Recombinational process coupled with replication. The gray and black lines indicate the un-replicated and recently-replicated regions at the time of recombination, respectively. If recombination occurs between *lox*P sites marked red and blue (i), the replication template is switched and thereafter the replicated region is replicated again (ii). (B) DRCR induction. If both bidirectional DNA replications undergo the processes as described in (A), DRCR can be induced. Two different types of *lox* sequence, the wild-type *lox*P (lox for short) and a mutant-type *lox*m2 (m2 for short) were used. Cre recombination occurs between identical sites (*lox*-*lox* or m2-m2) but not between different sites (*lox*-m2). (C) Structure of the amplification cassette and a model for DRCR amplification. (D) Frequency of Leu+ colony formation. (E) Southern analysis of uncut chromosomal DNA from Leu$^+$ survivors with the *leu2d* probe. The expression of Cre recombinase was induced in galactose medium for 90 min (Cre-induced). PFGE was performed with a wide-size range. The lanes marked in red and green indicate intra- and extra-chromosomal amplification, respectively. (D) Model for the production of extra-chromosomal products. These products are proposed to result from a single recombinational process coupled with DNA replication.

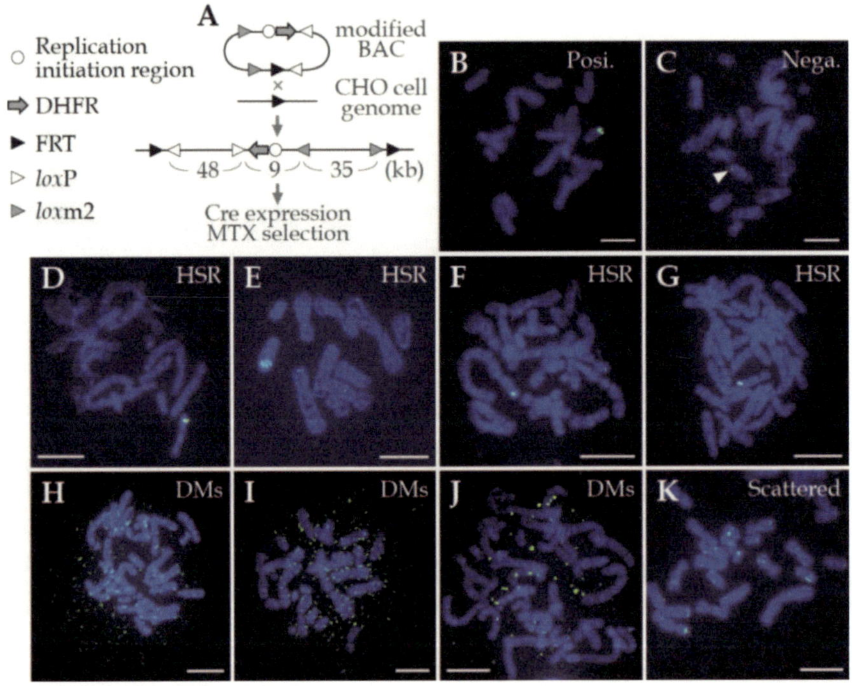

Figure 5. Gene amplification in CHO cells induced by Cre recombination.

(A) Structure of the modified BAC and construction of the CHO strain for gene amplification. The sizes (kb) of the three regions in the structure are indicated below. (B) to (K) Metaphase FISH analysis with FITC-labeled probes (green). As a positive control (B), the CHO DR1000L-4N strain that contains ~170 copies of DHFR was probed with a pSV2-dhfr plasmid. The BAC-CHO strain (C; negative control) without Cre induction and MTX selection and MTX-resistant clones (D-K) were probed with the BAC in (A). DNA is counterstained with DAPI (blue). The scale bars represent 10 μm. These amplified products would be derived from the integrated BAC construct.

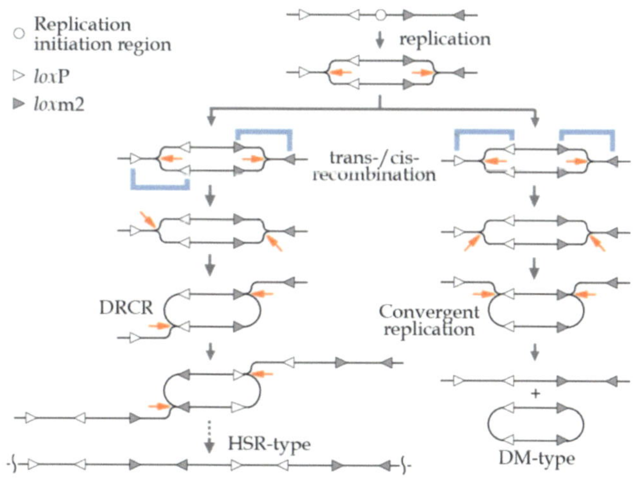

Figure 6. Model for HSR/DM production in the CHO system.

A model for the HSR and DMs production by Cre recombination coupled with replication. See in the text.

Our Cre-*lox* system can induce tissue-specific amplification, and therefore may allow a direct approach to examine which genetic elements contribute to oncogenesis or malignant potential in each tissue when amplified. In addition, our CHO system showed scattered-type amplification products resembling those seen in cancer cells, although in non-cancerous cell line. From these results, we reasoned that DRCR are centrally involved in amplification of drug-resistance genes and oncogene. This system can serve as a good model for amplification in mammalian cells and contribute to a better understanding of oncogene amplification and development of anticancer strategies in the future.

The formation of HSR/DM-type products can be explained by Cre recombination coupled with replication in two alternative ways, by trans- or cis-recombination, which can induce either DRCR or convergent replication, respectively (Fig.6). The scattered-type amplification may be generated by reintegration of DM-type products into ectopic chromosomes through interspersed repetitive elements. In gene amplification in mammalian cells, BFB cycles would form megabase-sized inverted repeats, which may induce DRCR if homology-based recombination is coupled with DNA replication. Recently, a similar process, replication template exchange, was reported to lead to acentric or dicentric chromosome formation in yeast, indicating an important contribution to genome instability (Branzei and Foiani, 2010a; Mizuno et al., 2009; Paek et al., 2009). We propose that such processes can occur in cultured cells and tumor cells through genome instability associated with deregulated replication (Aguilera and Gomez-Gonzalez, 2008; Branzei and Foiani, 2010b).

3.3. Rearrangements in amplified regions

In amplified chromosomal regions, intensive chromosome rearrangements are frequently observed, leading to the increase in the gene copy number and to the decrease in size of the amplification unit (Debatisse and Malfor, 2005; Mondello et al., 2010). Nuclear blebs and micronuclei are frequently observed in cells with gene amplification and found to contain amplified sequences and thus may be a location for rearrangement of amplified region. However, how the rearrangements proceed is a long-standing question. In oncogene amplification, the complex patterns of amplification generated by the rearrangements are closely associated with poor prognosis in cancer (Chin et al., 2006; Hicks et al., 2006). Interestingly, we have observed the rearrangement in all our DRCR systems (Fig.7A and 7B). Sequences flanked by inverted repeats, which are formed by DRCR amplification, were subject to frequent inversion. We call this phenomenon DRCR-dependent inversion. To explore the link between the rearrangements and the DRCR process, we constructed a system that can turn on or off the occurrence of DRCR, using yeast 2μ plasmid (Okamoto et al., 2011). This system demonstrated that inversions, deletions, or duplications could be intensively induced in a DRCR-dependent manner. This result suggests that DRCR may cause the rearrangements in amplification in nature.

DRCR-dependent inversion is an interesting phenomenon, but the mechanism remains unknown. DRCR is expected to form an unstable structure, a palindromic structure. We propose that DRCR-dependent inversion may disrupt the palindromic structure and substantially stabilize the highly repetitive array (Fig.7B). We also proposed a model in which DRCR markedly stimulates recombinational events (Fig.7C). In eukaryotes, a protein complex, cohesin, bundles newly replicated sister chromatids until anaphase and regulates the separation of sister chromatids during cell division (Nasmyth, 1999). In DRCR process, however, one of newly replicated sister chromatids is used as a template for another replication fork, and therefore cohesin would fail to bundle the sister chromatids together. These cohesion-free regions are expected to be recombinogenic based on some data indicating activated recombination under cohesion-deficient conditions (Grossenbacher-Grunder & Thuriaux, 1981; Kobayashi et al. 2004).

Recently, a chromosome catastrophe phenomenon termed chromothripsis, in which numerous rearrangements are apparently acquired in one single catastrophic event, was observed in multiple cancers (Liu et al., 2011). The formation of intensive rearrangements has been proposed to involve a replication-based mechanism, the fork stalling and template switching (FoSTeS) model (Lee et al., 2007). The FoSTeS process may be engaged also in the intensive rearrangements in amplified chromosomal regions.

In cancer and drug-resistant cells, BFB cycles form large regular inverted repeats in the early stages of amplification, and thereafter these repeats rapidly change into shorter highly amplified units. However, it remains largely unknown how complex end products can be rapidly generated after BFB cycles. We expect that DRCR process play a key role in linking BFB cycles to complex end products. DRCR process may be initiated by DSBs or DNA replication stress within inverted chromosome regions formed through BFB cycles. This involvement of DRCR is supported by a recent data that HSR was lengthened more rapidly than expected from BFB cycle model (Harada et al., 2011).

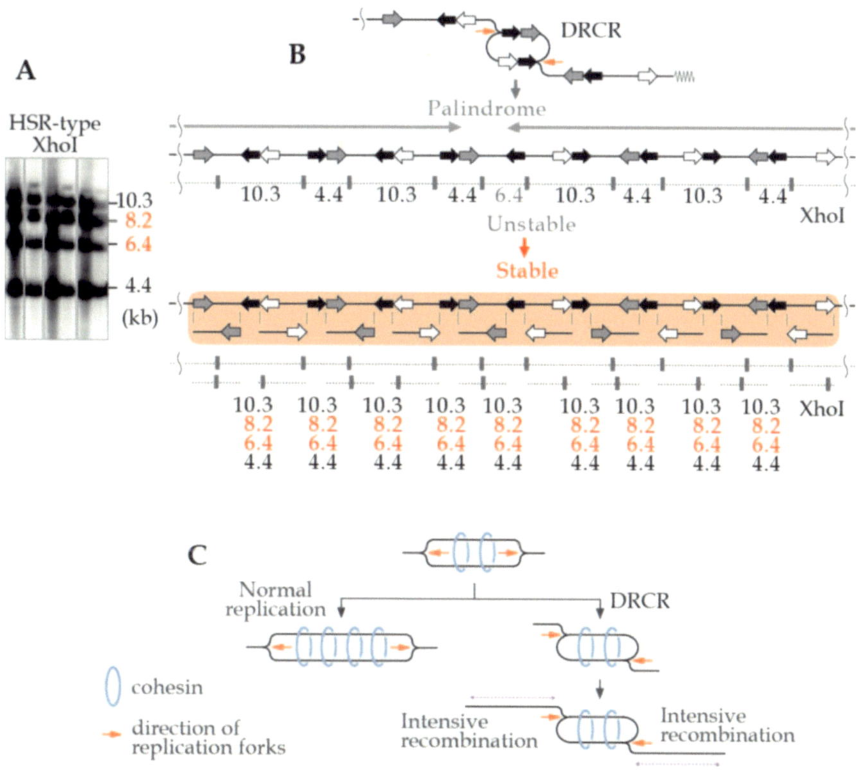

Figure 7. DRCR-dependent rearrangements

(A) Southern analysis of *Xho*I-digested DNA of some HSR-type samples in our BIR based DRCR system with the *leu2d* probe. The fragment sizes in black and red indicate the expected and unexpected band. (B) Schematic representation of the expected structure derived through the DRCR process and *Xho*I-restriction maps of the representative HSR-type structure. (C) Model of the recombinogenic feature of DRCR. While cohesin complexes bundle newly replicated sister chromatids in normal DNA replication, in DRCR, cohesin would fail to bundle the sister chromatids together, leading to the exposure of recombinogenic region.

4. Concluding remarks

The processes of oncogene amplification are difficult to analyze because of the infrequency of amplification and the plasticity of amplified products. The development of model systems is one of the best approaches to overcome the difficulties in elucidating the molecular mechanisms. The model systems can serve as a good model for a better understanding of oncogene amplification and contribute to development of anticancer strategies in future.

Gene amplification is a hallmark of most advanced solid tumors and amplified genes are useful therapeutic targets. Immortalized cells can undergo amplification when selected with appropriate drugs (10^{-4} to 10^{-7}), whereas gene amplification has never been detected in normal cells (<10^{-9}) (Tlsty et al., 1989; Wright et al., 1990). This observation strongly suggests the defect in control of genome integrity in cancer cells.

Furthermore, cancer cells are often dependent on (addicted to) only one or a few genes conferring malignancy and growth advantage, although the cells involve multiple genetic and epigenetic abnormalities (Weinstein and Joe, 2006). This phenomenon, called 'oncogene addiction', is frequently observed with oncogenes associated with amplification, such as MYC, ERBB2, CCND1, and BCR-ABL, indicating that the enhanced expression of amplified genes would become a meaningful therapeutic targets.

The direct involvement of DRCR-related processes in oncogene amplification has yet to be demonstrated. Amplified oncogenes manifest a structural diversity. MYC gene is thought to amplify first as DMs, and thereafter integration into a chromosome can lead to HSR amplification consisting of direct or inverted repeats. Although many tumor cells would undergo BFB cycles, which form inverted array, amplification of MYCN and ERBB2 can be found as HSR with direct tandem repeats (Albertson, 2006). Amplified EGFR genes are present on DMs (Albertson, 2006), and BCR-ABL amplification was found on a chromosome (Gorre et al., 2001). These amplifications could not be explained by only one versatile process, but DRCR-related process may contribute to a variety of oncogene amplification. HSR and DMs in MYC amplification might be produced via DRCR and its related process like convergent replication, respectively (Fig.6). Furthermore, Our system can be adapted to simple rolling-circle replication (RCR) by replacing inverted sequences in our amplification cassettes to direct ones. This RCR forms direct tandem array as seen in amplification of MYCN and ERBB2. The DRCR-related processes can be initiated by any important triggers, such as DSB, inverted repeats, and replication stress, which genome instability in tumor or cancer cells could provide. These trigger reactions may occur via interspersed repetitive elements, including Alus, and short or long interspersed nucleotide element (SINE/LINE). The DRCR-related processes can generate intensive chromosome rearrangement, a common feature of oncogene amplification. Thus, we propose that DRCR-related processes can provide broad contributions to oncogene amplification at multiple phases.

We also believe that optimization and improvement of the model amplification systems could provide benefits for the production of therapeutic proteins. Thus, works that utilize the model systems will have great impact not only on scientific understanding but also in the medical, industrial and economic fields.

Author details

Takaaki Watanabe
Department of Molecular Genetics, Cleveland Clinic Lerner Research Institute, USA

Acknowledgement

I am grateful to Prof. Takashi Horiuchi for his supervision in National Institute for Basic Biology (NIBB). I would like to thank all students, technicians, technologist, and faculty who have been supporting and guiding me. I appreciate Dr. Hisashi Tanaka giving me helpful discussion in Cleveland Clinic Lerner Research Institute. This was supported by Grant-in-Aid for Young Scientists (Japan Society for the Promotion of Science); Adaptable and Seamless Technology Transfer Program (Japan Science and Technology Agency); Research Project of the Center for the Promotion of Integrated Sciences of Sokendai.

5. References

Aguilera, A and Gomez-Gonzalez, B. 2008. Genome instability: a mechanistic view of its causes and consequences. *Nat Rev Genet* 9: 204-217.

Albertson, DG. 2006. Gene amplification in cancer. *Trends Genet* 22: 447-455.

Branzei, D and Foiani, M. 2010a. Leaping forks at inverted repeats. *Genes Dev* 24: 5-9.

Branzei, D and Foiani, M. 2010b. Maintaining genome stability at the replication fork. *Nat Rev Mol Cell Biol* 11: 208-219.

Butler, DK, Yasuda, LE, and Yao, MC. 1996. Induction of large DNA palindrome formation in yeast: implications for gene amplification and genome stability in eukaryotes. *Cell* 87: 1115-1122.

Chin, K, DeVries, S, Fridlyand, J, Spellman, PT, Roydasgupta, R, Kuo, WL, Lapuk, A, Neve, RM, Qian, Z, Ryder, T et al. 2006. Genomic and transcriptional aberrations linked to breast cancer pathophysiologies. *Cancer Cell* 10: 529-541.

Ciullo, M, Debily, MA, Rozier, L, Autiero, M, Billault, A, Mayau, V, El Marhomy, S, Guardiola, J, Bernheim, A, Coullin, P et al. 2002. Initiation of the breakage-fusion-bridge mechanism through common fragile site activation in human breast cancer cells: the model of PIP gene duplication from a break at FRA7I. *Hum Mol Genet* 11: 2887-2894.

Coquelle, A, Pipiras, E, Toledo, F, Buttin, G, and Debatisse, M. 1997. Expression of fragile sites triggers intrachromosomal mammalian gene amplification and sets boundaries to early amplicons. *Cell* 89: 215-225.

Debatisse, M, Le Tallec, B, Letessier, A, Dutrillaux, B, and Brison, O. 2012. Common fragile sites: mechanisms of instability revisited. *Trends Genet* 28: 22-32.

Debatisse, M and Malfor, B. 2005. Gene amplification mechanisms. in *Genome Instability in Cancer Development* (ed. E.A. Nigg), pp. 343-361. Springer, Netherlands.

Di Fiore, PP, Pierce, JH, Kraus, MH, Segatto, O, King, CR, and Aaronson, SA. 1987. erbB-2 is a potent oncogene when overexpressed in NIH/3T3 cells. *Science* 237: 178-182.

Erhart, E and Hollenberg, CP. 1983. The presence of a defective LEU2 gene on 2 mu DNA recombinant plasmids of Saccharomyces cerevisiae is responsible for curing and high copy number. *J Bacteriol* 156: 625-635.

Glover, TW, Arlt, MF, Casper, AM, and Durkin, SG. 2005. Mechanisms of common fragile site instability. *Hum Mol Genet* 14 Spec No. 2: R197-205.

Gorre, ME, Mohammed, M, Ellwood, K, Hsu, N, Paquette, R, Rao, PN, and Sawyers, CL. 2001. Clinical resistance to STI-571 cancer therapy caused by BCR-ABL gene mutation or amplification. *Science* 293: 876-880.

Green, BM, Finn, KJ, and Li, JJ. 2010. Loss of DNA replication control is a potent inducer of gene amplification. *Science* 329: 943-946.

Grossenbacher-Grunder, AM, and Thyriaux, P. 1981. Spontaneous and UV-induced recombination in radiation-sensitive mutants of *Schizosaccharomyces pombe*. *Mutat Res* 81: 37-48.

Haber, JE and Debatisse, M. 2006. Gene amplification: yeast takes a turn. *Cell* 125: 1237-1240.

Harada, S, Sekiguchi, N, and Shimizu, N. 2011. Amplification of a plasmid bearing a mammalian replication initiation region in chromosomal and extrachromosomal contexts. *Nucleic Acids Res* 39: 958-969.

Hellman, A, Zlotorynski, E, Scherer, SW, Cheung, J, Vincent, JB, Smith, DI, Trakhtenbrot, L, and Kerem, B. 2002. A role for common fragile site induction in amplification of human oncogenes. *Cancer Cell* 1: 89-97.

Hicks, J, Krasnitz, A, Lakshmi, B, Navin, NE, Riggs, M, Leibu, E, Esposito, D, Alexander, J, Troge, J, Grubor, V et al. 2006. Novel patterns of genome rearrangement and their association with survival in breast cancer. *Genome research* 16: 1465-1479.

Kobayashi, T, Horiuchi, T, Tongaonkar, P, Vu, L, and Nomura, M. 2004. *SIR2* regulates recombination between different rDNA repeats, but not recombination within individual rRNA genes in yeast. *Cell* 117: 441-453.

Kuo, MT, Sen, S, Hittelman, WN, and Hsu, TC. 1998. Chromosomal fragile sites and DNA amplification in drug-resistant cells. *Biochem Pharmacol* 56: 7-13.

Kuo, MT, Vyas, RC, Jiang, LX, and Hittelman, WN. 1994. Chromosome breakage at a major fragile site associated with P-glycoprotein gene amplification in multidrug-resistant CHO cells. *Mol Cell Biol* 14: 5202-5211.

Lee, JA, Carvalho, CM, and Lupski, JR. 2007. A DNA replication mechanism for generating nonrecurrent rearrangements associated with genomic disorders. *Cell* 131: 1235-1247.

Lengauer, C, Kinzler, KW, and Vogelstein, B. 1998. Genetic instabilities in human cancers. *Nature* 396: 643-649.

Liu, P, Erez, A, Nagamani, SC, Dhar, SU, Kolodziejska, KE, Dharmadhikari, AV, Cooper, ML, Wiszniewska, J, Zhang, F, Withers, MA et al. 2011. Chromosome catastrophes involve replication mechanisms generating complex genomic rearrangements. *Cell* 146: 889-903.

Lobachev, KS, Gordenin, DA, and Resnick, MA. 2002. The Mre11 complex is required for repair of hairpin-capped double-strand breaks and prevention of chromosome rearrangements. *Cell* 108: 183-193.

McClintock, B. 1941. The Stability of Broken Ends of Chromosomes in Zea Mays. *Genetics* 26: 234-282.

Mizuno, K, Lambert, S, Baldacci, G, Murray, JM, and Carr, AM. 2009. Nearby inverted repeats fuse to generate acentric and dicentric palindromic chromosomes by a replication template exchange mechanism. *Genes Dev* 23: 2876-2886.

Mondello, C, Smirnova, A, and Giulotto, E. 2010. Gene amplification, radiation sensitivity and DNA double-strand breaks. *Mutat Res* 704: 29-37.

Muller, WJ, Sinn, E, Pattengale, PK, Wallace, R, and Leder, P. 1988. Single-step induction of mammary adenocarcinoma in transgenic mice bearing the activated c-neu oncogene. *Cell* 54: 105-115.

Narayanan, V, Mieczkowski, PA, Kim, HM, Petes, TD, and Lobachev, KS. 2006. The pattern of gene amplification is determined by the chromosomal location of hairpin-capped breaks. *Cell* 125: 1283-1296.

Nasmyth, K. 1999. Separating sister chromatids. *Trends Biochem Sci* 24: 98-104.

Okamoto, H, Watanabe, TA, and Horiuchi, T. 2011. Double rolling circle replication (DRCR) is recombinogenic. *Genes to cells* 16: 503-513.

Paek, AL, Kaochar, S, Jones, H, Elezaby, A, Shanks, L, and Weinert, T. 2009. Fusion of nearby inverted repeats by a replication-based mechanism leads to formation of dicentric and acentric chromosomes that cause genome instability in budding yeast. *Genes Dev* 23: 2861-2875.

Paulson, TG, Almasan, A, Brody, LL, and Wahl, GM. 1998. Gene amplification in a p53-deficient cell line requires cell cycle progression under conditions that generate DNA breakage. *Mol Cell Biol* 18: 3089-3100.

Poupon, MF, Smith, KA, Chernova, OB, Gilbert, C, and Stark, GR. 1996. Inefficient growth arrest in response to dNTP starvation stimulates gene amplification through bridge-breakage-fusion cycles. *Mol Biol Cell* 7: 345-354.

Rattray, AJ, Shafer, BK, Neelam, B, and Strathern, JN. 2005. A mechanism of palindromic gene amplification in *Saccharomyces cerevisiae*. *Genes Dev* 19: 1390-1399.

Savelyeva, L, and Schwab, M. 2001. Amplification of oncogenes revisited: from expression profiling to clinical application. *Cancer Lett* 167: 115-123.

Slamon, DJ, Clark, GM, Wong, SG, Levin, WJ, Ullrich, A, and McGuire, WL. 1987. Human breast cancer: correlation of relapse and survival with amplification of the HER-2/neu oncogene. *Science* 235: 177-182.

Tanaka, H, Tapscott, SJ, Trask, BJ, and Yao, MC. 2002. Short inverted repeats initiate gene amplification through the formation of a large DNA palindrome in mammalian cells. *Proc Natl Acad Sci U S A* 99: 8772-8777.

Tanaka, H and Yao, MC. 2009. Palindromic gene amplification--an evolutionarily conserved role for DNA inverted repeats in the genome. *Nat Rev Cancer* 9: 216-224.

Tlsty, TD, Margolin, BH, and Lum, K. 1989. Differences in the rates of gene amplification in nontumorigenic and tumorigenic cell lines as measured by Luria-Delbruck fluctuation analysis. *Proc Natl Acad Sci U S A* 86: 9441-9445.

Tower, J. 2004. Developmental gene amplification and origin regulation. *Annu Rev Genet* 38: 273-304.

Vogt, N, Lefevre, SH, Apiou, F, Dutrillaux, AM, Cor, A, Leuraud, P, Poupon, MF, Dutrillaux, B, Debatisse, M, and Malfoy, B. 2004. Molecular structure of double-minute chromosomes bearing amplified copies of the epidermal growth factor receptor gene in gliomas. *Proc Natl Acad Sci U S A* 101: 11368-11373.

Volkert, FC and Broach, JR. 1986. Site-specific recombination promotes plasmid amplification in yeast. *Cell* 46: 541-550.

Watanabe, T and Horiuchi, T. 2005. A novel gene amplification system in yeast based on double rolling-circle replication. *EMBO J* 24: 190-198.

Watanabe, T, Tanabe, H, and Horiuchi, T. 2011. Gene amplification system based on double rolling-circle replication as a model for oncogene-type amplification. *Nucleic acids research* 39: e106.

Weinstein, IB and Joe, AK. 2006. Mechanisms of Disease: oncogene addiction—a rationale for molecular targeting in cancer therapy. *Nature Clinical Practice Oncology* 3: 448-457.

Wright, JA, Smith, HS, Watt, FM, Hancock, MC, Hudson, DL, and Stark, GR. 1990. DNA amplification is rare in normal human cells. *Proc Natl Acad Sci U S A* 87: 1791-1795.

Yunis, JJ, Soreng, AL, and Bowe, AE. 1987. Fragile sites are targets of diverse mutagens and carcinogens. *Oncogene* 1: 59-69.

Chapter 10

MLL Gene Alterations in Acute Myeloid Leukaemia (11q23/*MLL*+ AML)

Denisa Ilencikova and Alexandra Kolenova

Additional information is available at the end of the chapter

http://dx.doi.org/10.5772/55141

1. Introduction

Acute myeloid leukemia (AML) is characterized by the malignant transformation of myeloid cells from myeloblasts to a pathological cell clone. These pathological cell clones lose their ability to differentiate and mature, are no longer subject to regulatory mechanisms and suppress other components of normal hemopoiesis. AML does not fall under a single nosological entity. The heterogeneity of AML is reflected by differences in morphology and immunophenotype, as well as cytogenetic and molecular genetic abnormalities. It includes a number of subtypes, which can be further classified according to the FAB and World Health Organization (WHO) criteria.

Acute myeloid leukemia represents 15% to 20% of all childhood leukemias, approximately 33% of adolescent leukemias, and approximately 50% of adult leukemias. After a peak during the first 2 years of life, the subsequent annual incidence of AML slowly increases after 9 years of age (incidence rate 5/1 million in 5 to 9-year-olds, 9/1 million in 15 to 19-year-olds). In general, the biological features, other than age, of pediatric and adult AML appear to be similar, but the differences have not been reviewed systematically [1].

The rate of *therapy-related AML* (that is, AML caused by previous chemotherapy) is rising; therapy-related disease currently accounts for approximately10–20% of all cases of AML [2]. The incidence of secondary leukemias is increasing because of aging of the population (MDS is more frequent in elderly people) and widespread of successful use of chemoradiotherapy in cancer patients (solid tumors or hematological malignancies). The majority of secondary leukemias resulting from the use of cytotoxic drugs. Therapy – related AML is heterogeneous collection of diseases characterised by distinct chromosomal abnormalities. One subset of therapy related AMLs is associated with exposure to alkylating agents. The chromosomal abnormalities 5q- and monosomy 7 are commonly observed in leukemic cells in this groups. The other major subset of therapy-induced leukemia is associated with exposure to epipodophyloltoxin drugs teniposid and etoposid. A high proportion of epipodophyllotoxin - associated AMLs are of the M4 (monocytic) or M5 (myelomonocytic) subtype and have abnormalities at chromosome band 11q23 involving rearrangement of the MLL gene. The same genetic abnormality is also found in some secondary AMLs associated with exposure to antracyclines. These two classes of chemotherapeutic agents share a common mechanism of action that involves binding to and inhibition of DNA topoisomerase II.

Acute myeloid leukemia is a curable disease; the chance of cure for a specific patient depends on a number of prognostic factors. The current five-year survival rates of adult patients under age 60 range from 30% - 40%; for pediatric patients, five-year survival rates are up to 65% [3, 4].

The cure rates in pediatric AML have been achieved not only by the more effective use of anti-leukemic agents but also by improvements in supportive care and better risk-group stratification. Recurrent cytogenetic and genetic aberrations and early responses to treatment are important prognostic factors in AML and therefore are used for risk group stratification.

The prognostic value of cytogenetics is well established in all age groups. The biologic data differ considerably between infants and older age groups but only slightly between children, adolescents, and young adults. The distribution of cytogenetic aberrations in infants is different from that in older patients. Infants have almost no favorable aberrations but have frequent 11q23 aberrations and complex karyotypes, which is similar to older AML patients (>60 years)[1]. Schochet et al. [5] analyzed the effect of age and cytogenetics on clinical outcome in adult patients (>16 years). They found that both age and cytogenetics were independent prognostic parameters in AML; however, up to the age of 49 years, age had no major impact on prognosis, whereas the karyotype did. Therapy today consists of a limited number of intensive courses of chemotherapy based on cytarabine and an anthracycline. An important problem in the treatment of AML remains the high frequency of treatment-related deaths and long-term side effects [6,7].

This problem hampers further therapy-intensification, and most investigators therefore feel that we have reached a plateau in the number of patients that can be cured with current chemotherapy regimens. Our efforts should therefore focus on clarifying the biology of pediatric AML. This knowledge can be used for novel classification and risk-group stratification. In addition, it creates the potential for targeted, i.e., more leukemia-specific, therapy. It is anticipated that such therapies will increase the cure-rate and decrease the toxicity of treatment of patients with AML [4].

Leukemias bearing translocations involving chromosome 11q23 are of particular interest due to unique clinical and biological characteristics. The development of acute leukemias is associated with *MLL* gene alterations in about 10% of all leukemia cases of acute lymphoblastic leukemia and acute myeloid leukemia) [8].

***MLL* alterations** correlate with specific disease subtypes (acute myeloid and acute lymphocytic leukemias), a specific gene expression profile [9, 10], and outcomes (favorable or poor), depending on the particular *MLL* alteration [11]. Certain *MLL* alterations are independent unfavorable prognostic factors, and patients are usually treated according to high-risk protocols. For this reason, identifying *MLL* alterations has relevant implications for therapy decision-making. In pediatric AML, optimized intensive regimens for AML have also improved outcomes for *MLL*-rearranged AML. Patients have an intermediate outcome, with a 5 y OS (probability of overall survival at 5 years from diagnosis) ranging from 42-62% [12]. Therefore, further insights into the biology of *MLL*-rearranged AML, the development of reliable methods for screening in laboratory settings, and safe testing of new potential *MLL*-targeted therapies could have a significant impact on the overall outcomes for adult and pediatric patients.

The ***MLL* gene** was identified in 1991; a year later, it was completely characterized and cloned. The origin of the previous *ALL1* designation dates back to 1970, when van den Bergh described the reconstruction of the gene area for the first time in a patient with lymphoblastic leukemia [13]. Scientists later completed the characterization of the gene, and the gene was named *MLL* (mixed-lineage leukemia) based on the 11q23 translocation, which is observed in myelogenous and lymphoblastic types of leukemia. *MLL* has other synonyms as well, such as *HRX* (human trithorax) and *Htrx1*, which express its homology with the trithorax (*trx*) gene in *Drosophila melanogaster*. The ***MLL (ALL1, HRX, Htrx1)* gene** is located on the long arm of chromosome 11 (11q23), telomerically to the *PLFZ* gene and centromerically from the *RCK* gene (Figure 1).

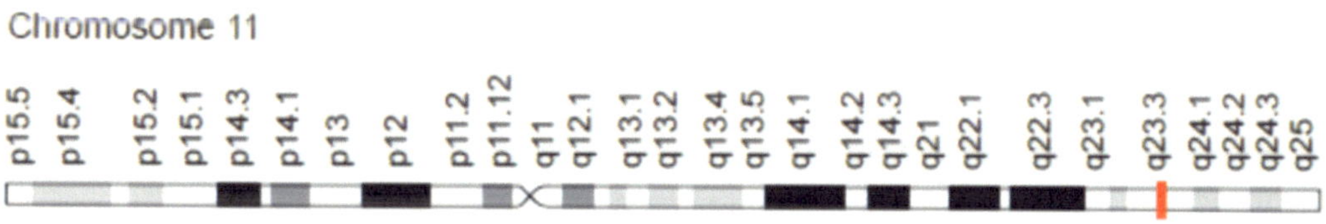

Figure 1. Chromosome 11. The red mark indicates the position of the *MLL* gene.

The *MLL* gene consists of 36 exons over 100 kb. The product of the resulting 12 kb mRNA is a protein with 3968 amino acids and a molecular mass of approximately 430 kD. It is transcribed from centromere to telomere. Most, but not all, breaks in the *MLL* gene are localized in the 8.3 kb breakpoint region (bcr – breakpoint cluster region). The bcr region can be divided into a centromeric portion and a telomeric portion. Breaks in the *MLL* gene in infant leukemia and t-AML occur primarily in the telomeric part, while breaks in patients with *de novo* AML are closer to the centromere [1] (Figure 2).

Several translocation partners of *MLL* were found recently to coexist in a super elongation complex (SEC) that includes known transcription elongation factors such as eleven-nineteen lysine-rich leukemia (ELL) and positive transcription elongation factor b (P-TEFb). The SEC is required for *HOX* (homeobox domain gene) gene expression in leukemic cells, suggesting that chromosomal translocations involving *MLL* could lead to the overexpression of *HOX* and other genes through the involvement of the SEC [14].

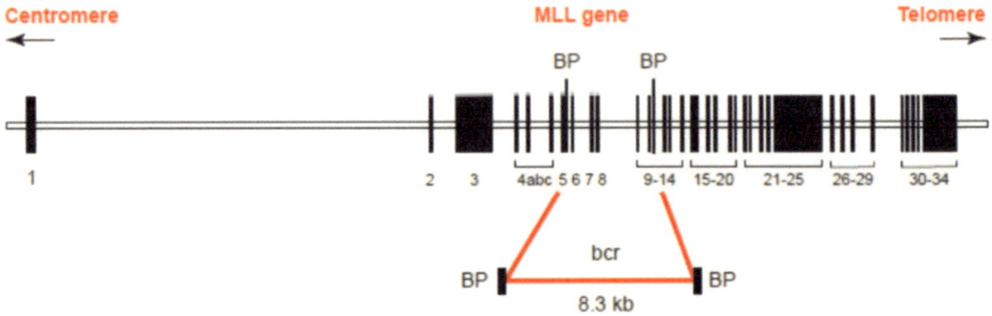

Figure 2. The structure of the *MLL* gene. Structure of the MLL gene: exon 1-34. Bcr (breakage region) region: exons 5-11, BP – break point.

The **MLL protein** is expressed in different tissues, such as the brain, colon, liver, spleen, thymus, kidneys, tonsils, heart, lungs, testes and thyroid. Genetic mutations of the *MLL* gene seem to occur preferentially in hematopoietic cells, suggesting that this system enables special permissivity, allowing for the survival and development of leukemic clones of different MLL fusion proteins. Specific signals are derived from stromal cells during fetal liver and definitive hematopoiesis. This enables the activation of anti-apoptotic pathways and stem cell maintenance necessary to receive survival signals caused by the presence of oncogenic MLL fusion proteins [15, 16].

The MLL protein is involved in chromatin regulation. It is specifically hydrolyzed by the endopeptidase Taspase1 and methylates histone core particles at histone H3 lysine 4 residues [17-19]. Therefore, MLL is part of an epigenetic system that co-regulates mitotic gene-expression signatures during embryonic development and tissue differentiation in mammalian organisms. The MLL complex binds to different promoters in various tissues. Recently, a genome-wide array study revealed that MLL was bound to more than 2000 different promoter regions [20]. This protein belongs to the group of Trithorax (trx-G) proteins, which are responsible for maintaining gene expression during growth. It is assumed that the MLL protein controls the expression of *HOX* genes. Several *HOX* genes are involved in the regulation of normal and leukemic hemopoiesis. The products of *HOX* genes are localized in the nucleus and represent a major class of transcription factors controlling cell proliferation/differentiation during early embryonic development [21].

2. Etiology and pathogenesis of causative *MLL* gene abnormalities in AML

The cause of 11q23/ *MLL*+ AML is unknown, but important factors include ionizing radiation (the highest incidence was observed five to seven years after radiation exposure), chemicals (such as benzene and various organic solvents), drugs (cytostatic drugs in particular), physical agents (such as electromagnetic fields), and environmental factors to which the fetus is exposed in utero. In infant AML, a prenatal origin has been suggested by data from neonatal bloodspots on Guthrie cards [22, 23]. The 11q23 locus is particularly sensitive to cleavage after treatment with topoisomerase-II inhibitors. Because DNA topoisomerase II seems to be highly expressed in the developing fetus, exposure to inhibitors of DNA topoisomerase II could induce *MLL* AML in utero. A large case-control study of maternal diet and infant leukemia showed that the amount of maternal consumption of food containing DNA topoisomerase II inhibitors was correlated with the risk of developing MLL-rearranged AML [24].

The pathogenesis of AML is related to oncogenic fusion proteins, the formation of which results from chromosomal translocations or inversions [25] (Table 1).

Chromosomal aberation	FAB subtype AML	Frequency	Fusion gene
t(8;21) (q22;q22)	AML- M2	18% (30%)	*AML1- ETO*
t(15;17) (q21-q11-22)	AML- M3	10% (98%)	*PML- RARα*
t(11;17) (q23;q21)	AML- M3	rare	*PLZF- RARα*
Inv(16) or t(16;16)	AML- M4Eo	8% (~100%)	*CBFβ- MYH11*
t(9;11) (p22;q23)	AML- M4	11% (30%)	*MLL- AF9*
t(6;11)	AML- M5	~ 35% AML	*MLL-AF6/AF6q21*
t(10;11)			*MLL-AF10;CALM-AF10*
t(11;17)			*MLL-AF17/AF17q25*
t(11;19)			*MLL-ENL/ENL/EEN*
t(4;11)			*MLL-AF4*
t(6;9) (p23;q34)	AML- M1,M2,M4,M5	1%	*DEK- KAN*
t(16;21) (p11;q22)	AML	< 1%	*TLS(FUS)- ERG*
t(16;21) (q24;q22)	t-AML, MDS	< 1%	*AML1- MTG16*
t(3;21)	AML	< 1%	*AML1- EVI1, EAP, MDS1*
t(7;11) (p15;p15)	AML- M2, M4	< 1%	*NUP98- HOX49*
t(1;11) (q23;p15)	AML- M2	< 1%	*NUP98- PMX1*
t(8;16) (p11;p13)	AML- M4, M5	< 1%	*MOZ- CBP*
Inv(8) (p11;q13)	AML- M0, M1, M5	< 1%	*MOZ- TIF2*
t(8;22) (p11;p13)	AML- M5	< 1%	*MOZ- p300*
t(12;22) (p13;q23)	AML- M4, CML	< 1%	*TEL- MN1*
t(5;12) (q33;p12)	CMMol	2-5%	*TEL- PDGFRβ*
t(1;19) (q23;p13)	AML- M7	< 1%	*OTT- MAL*

* The percentage of translocation in AML subtypes. Values in brackets indicate the frequency within the morphological or immunological disease subtype.

** Percentage refers to the frequency of reciprocal translocation chromosome products resulting. AML - acute myelogenous leukemia, t-AML (therapy-related AML) - AML associated with therapy, MDS - myelodysplastic syndrome; CMMoL - chronic myelomonocytic leukemia

Table 1. Common gene fusions caused by chromosomal abnormalities and associated with acute myeloid leukemia.

The WHO suggested characterizing 11q23/*MLL*+ AML within ALL as a separate entity with recurrent cytogenetic translocations in 1999. This hypothesis was supported by microarray analyses, which proved that 11q23/*MLL*+ AML has a unique profile of gene expression and that *MLL*+ leukemic blasts resemble very immature progenitor cells [9]. AML with *MLL* gene alterations is characterized by a high degree of clinical and immunological heterogeneity, resulting in immunophenotype variability. This variability originates in myeloid cells/monocytes [26]. The prognosis of AML is unfavorable and varies depending on the type of translocation and the phenotype and age of the patient. The prognostic effect of 11q23 aberrations may depend on *MLL* partner genes. Many studies have shown that the translocations of t(6;11)(q27;q23) and t(10;11)(p12;q23) are associated with an unfavorable prognosis; however, the t(9;11)(p22;q23) translocation is associated with a significantly longer patient survival rate [27, 28]. However, none of the 11q23 aberrations has a favorable prognosis. When different MLL fusion protein complexes were characterized, a novel cancer mechanism was uncovered. It has been known since 1999 that direct MLL fusion proteins are able to deregulate *HOX* genes, except when reciprocal MLL fusion proteins are present [29-31]. The leukemogenesis concept suggests that all MLL fusion proteins increase and maintain a high level of transcription of *MEIS1* (myeloid ecotropic viral integration site 1 homolog) and *HOXA* (homeobox A cluster) gene family members. The functional importance became the association of MEN1, LEDGF and MYB proteins at the N-terminal location of the MLL fusion [32-35]. Changes in the regulation of *HOXA* gene expression influence the function of the hematopoietic system during its development and therefore contribute to the initiation of leukemogenesis. *HOXA* genes are not deactivated, but a high expression of the *MEIS1* gene was observed [36]. Stam et al. [37] described low *HOXA* gene expression in pediatric leukemia patients with chromosomal translocation t(4;11), which is associated with a worse prognosis. Stumpel et al. [38] studied the methylation of promoter regions in samples with t(4;11), t(11;19) and t(9;11). His data indicated that different epigenetic mechanisms accompany the development of leukemia. Recent studies identified two mechanisms for leukemia development. One is the changing of epigenetic imprints, initiated by the presence of *MLL-MLLT3, MLL-MLLT10, MLL-MLLT1* or the reciprocal *AFF1-MLL* fusion protein through activation of P-TEFb kinase. The second function of the *MLL–AFF1 (*ALL1-*fused gene from chromosome 4 (*AF4*))* fusion protein is the ability to block apoptosis and to transcriptionally activate *HOXA* genes and *TERT* (telomerase reverse transcriptase) [39]. There is evidence that for all MLL-rearranged leukemias, this is the typical activation pattern of *HOXA* and *MEIS1* genes. Faber et al. [40] documented that overexpression of *HOXA9* (homeobox A9) in complex with *MEIS1* is able to drive the myeloid phenotype in mice.

3. Distribution of *MLL* gene alterations

AML with *MLL* gene alterations (11q23/*MLL*+AML) represents 3-4% of all AML cases and occurs most frequently in young people with *"de novo"* AML (5-7%) and in treatment-induced AML (t-AML) patients (10-15%). It is rarely seen in older patients (aged 60 and up) [5]. AML with *MLL* gene conversions occurs more frequently in infants than in adults and is usually manifested through the AML M4/M5 phenotype [41] Overall, the incidence of *MLL* gene conversions in children with AML varies within the range of 35-50% [42]. The percentages of representation are slightly different between individual studies because the sensitivity of 11q23/ *MLL*+ AML detection depends on the method of testing. The *MLL* gene is also a relatively frequent target of cryptic alterations, which were not always identified in the past using conventional karyotyping [8]. According to a report by Marschalek, more than 70 different fusion partner genes have been characterized at the molecular level. The analyzed *MLL* fusion alleles were classified according to their occurrence in ALL and AML patients. Of all *MLL* rearrangements, 80% are caused by *AF4* (80%), *AF9* (16%), *ENL* (11%), *AF10* (7%) and *ELL* (4%). The remaining 20% of MLL-rearranged leukemia patients displayed 59 different fusion partners, most of which were identified in single patients [8]. Approximately 50% of pediatric AML cases with an MLL consist of t(9,11)(p22,q23). The other 50% primarily include t(6,11)(q27,q23), t(10,11)(p12,q23), t(11,19)(q23,p13.1) and t(1,11)(q21,q23) [43]. This distribution is almost identical with adult AML, with the exception of t(6,11)(q27,q23), which has a greater distribution in adult *MLL*-rearranged AML [5]. Although *MLL* rearrangements are predominantly found in AML, they are also detected in 6% of pediatric ALL cases.

4. Conversion mechanism from an *MLL* proto-oncogene to an oncogene

Extensive cytogenetic and molecular studies have revealed that 11q23/MLL is a highly promiscuous locus. Based on the results of research from the past 19 years, 71 different *MLL* translocation partner genes and their specific breakpoint regions have been characterized (published and unpublished data [8]). Of these, 43 (60.5%) are reciprocal chromosomal translocations, 4 (5.7%) are 11q23ter deletions and 8 (11.3%) are 11q inversions. In 13 (18.3%) *MLL* fusion partners, more than two DNA strand breaks and the insertion of 11q23 material into another chromosome were identified. A very rare situation of three different *MLL* fusion partners has been described in 4.2% of all cases [44]. The *MLL* "recombinome" currently consists of 104 different areas of fusion [45]. The question remains: How many of them do we not yet know?

The *MLL* proto-oncogene can be transformed into an oncogene via several mechanisms, such as:

- chromosomal translocations
- complex chromosomal alterations, such as deletions, inversions in the area of 11q, MLL gene insertions into other chromosomes or the insertion of chromatin material into the MLL gene
- partial tandem duplications
- amplifications and gains

A. Translocations

The *MLL* gene is frequently involved in chromosomal translocations with other genes, leading to a break within the *MLL* locus and a partner gene, resulting in the emergence of a new fusion gene. *MLL* fusion proteins (the products of fusion genes) are often associated with the development of acute myelogenous types of leukemia, and their oncogenic characteristics have been extensively studied in vitro and *in vivo* in mouse models [28]. The *MLL* gene represents more complex rearrangements, with at least three or more DNA double-strand breaks. The reciprocal *MLL* fusion is cryptic in these cases; an *MLL* fusion gene cannot be detected. Complex rearrangements can be divided into three subgroups. The first group represents the participation of three independent chromosomes in complex translocation and results in three different fusion genes [45]. The most frequently fused genes are *AFF1/AF4, MLLT3/AF9, MLLT1/ENL, MLLT1/AF1Q* and *ELL*. The second group is built from reciprocal chromosomal translocations containing deletions on either of the involved chromosomes. The third group consists of chromosomal fragment insertions. In this type, a portion of chromosome 11 (including part of the *MLL* gene) is inserted into another chromosome. Translocations with transcription oriented toward the centromere belong to this subgroup. In these cases, three independent fusion genes are generated. There is also spliced fusion, generated by fusing the 5′- location of the *MLL* gene to the upstream region of a TPG (translocation partner gene). Approximately 50% of all recombination events are spliced fusions [44]. The final group of 3′*MLL* fusion represents head-to-head fusion. The transcriptional orientation of the fused transcriptional genes is opposite of the orientation of the *MLL* gene. This genetic situation often results in LOH. All known translocation participating genes (TPGs) were classified according to their cellular function. They can build membrane proteins and nuclear proteins. As membrane proteins, these TPGs function as extracellular proteins, cell adhesion proteins with functions in the organization of focal adhesion plaques, endocytotic proteins (EPS15 (epidermal growth factor receptor substrate 15) and PICALM (phosphatidylinositol binding clathrin assembly *protein)* proteins)), proteins involved in diverse signaling pathways (AF6 (actin-filament-binding*),* ABI1(abl-interactor 1) , GPHN (gephyrin), KIAA0284 (centrosomal protein 170kDa) and MYO1F (myosin IF) proteins), the organization and regulation of the cytoskeleton, metabolic functions and pre-apoptotic proteins (MLLT11/AF1Q (myeloid/lymphoid or mixed-lineage leukemia fused to ALL1 fused gene from chromosome 1q) protein). As nuclear proteins, they can control the cell cycle and take part in the organization of the nuclear cytoskeleton during cytokinesis (SEPTINS (cytoskeletal GTP-binding) protein), nucleic acid binding (TNRC18- trinucleotide repeat containing 18), chromosome association (CASC5- cancer susceptibility candidate 5), chromatin regulation (CREBBP- CREB binding *protein*), transcription factors (AF17 (*ALL1*-fused gene from chromosome 17), FOXO3 forkhead box O3)., FOXO4 forkhead box O3 , FRYL (furry homolog-like), MAML2 (mastermind-like 2) and TET1 (tet methylcytosine dioxygenase 1)) and regulation factors. Recurrence of *MLL* rearrangements was observed in approximately 44% of all TPGs. The most frequent translocations within *11q23/MLL+ AML* are illustrated in Figure 3 and Figure 4.

B. Partial tandem duplication (PTD) and MLL gene amplification

Approximately 7.5% of AML patients with a normal karyotype are hiding a PTD of the *MLL* gene. An *MLL* gene PTD is uniquely distinguished from other *MLL* gene alterations that result in chimeric gene fusions. In the PTD of the *MLL* gene, all of the protein domains encoded by the *MLL* gene are retained [46]. *MLL* PTD is common in adult AML patients but not in pediatric AML patients. It has also been identified at a low level in healthy humans [47]. The frequency of *MLL* gene PTD in infants with AML, as well as in older children with AML, is not well established. In adult patients with the *de novo* form of AML and a normal karyotype, the presence of an *MLL* gene PTD versus its absence is associated with poor prognosis (shorter remission time) [48, 38] (Figures 5 and 6).

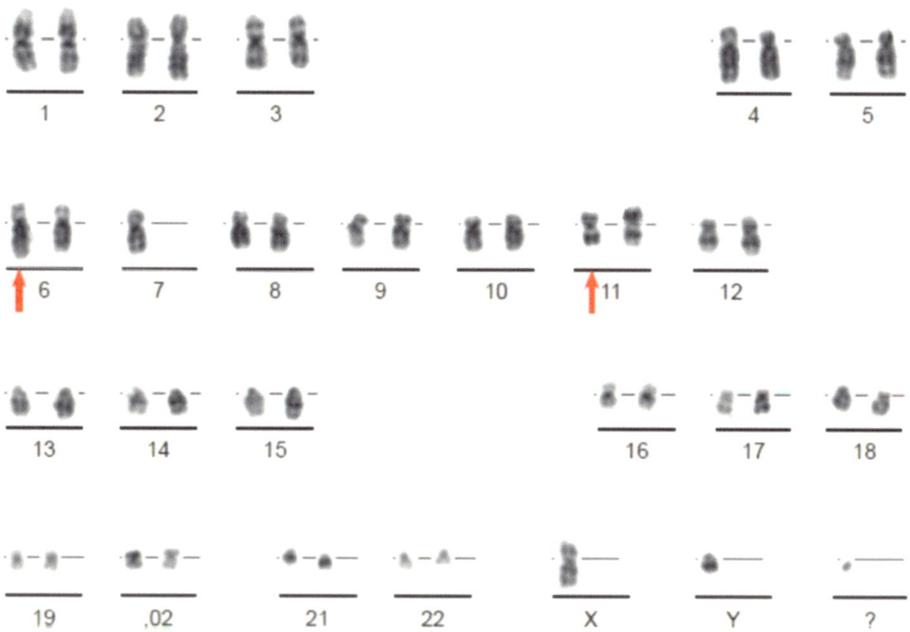

Figure 3. Complex karyotype with translocation *MLL/AF6*. Complex karyotype: 45,XY,-4,der(7)t(4;7)(q?12;q?11),+dimin/45,XY,idem,t(6;11)(q27;q23).

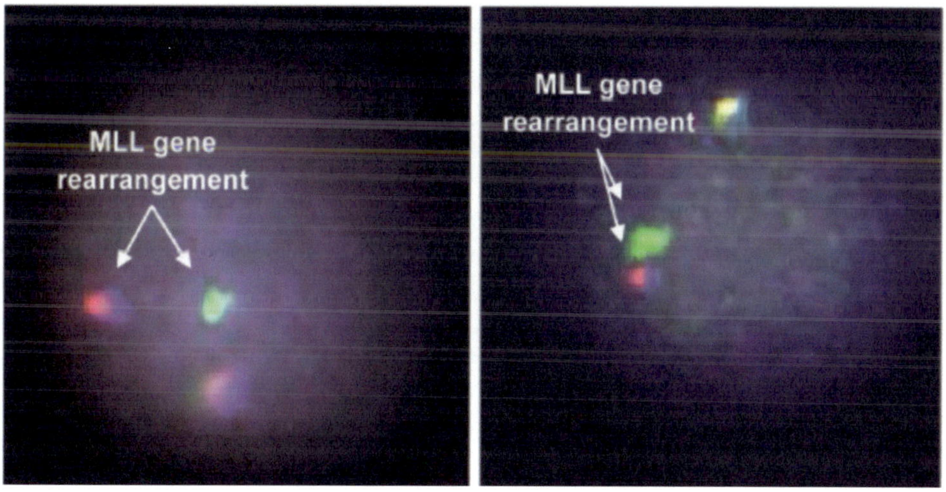

Figure 4. The results of fluorescence analysis of interphase nuclei obtained by taking a photograph with the CCD camera in a fluorescent microscope.

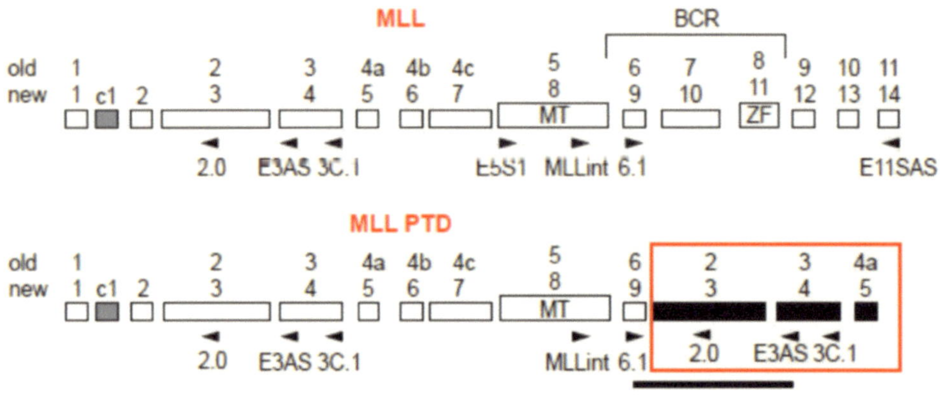

Figure 5. The *MLL* gene and *MLL* PTD. Above: the old nomenclature exon. Below: the new numbering.

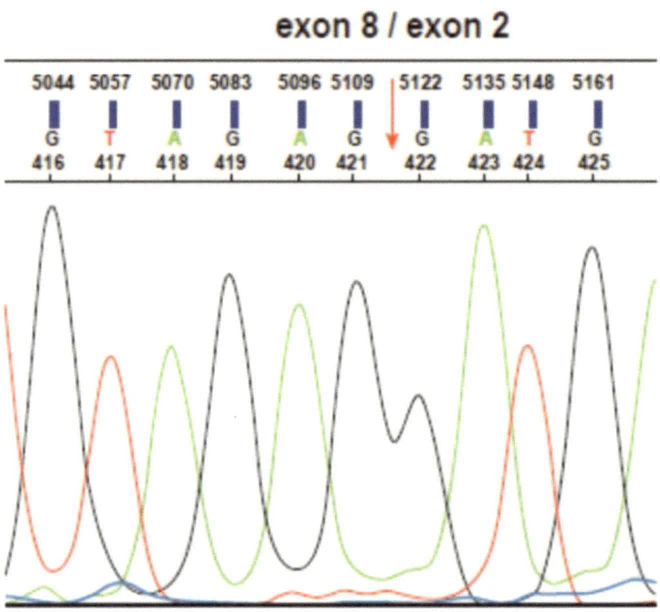

Figure 6. Sequence of *MLL* PTD from sequencing, showing a break in exon8/exon2 (exon3/exon11).

Previous studies have associated an *MLL* gene PTD with AML subtypes M1 and M2. Presently, according to FAB (the most widely used classification of AML, derived from the French-American-British group in 1976), the association of an *MLL* gene PTD with any specific FAB subtype of AML has not been confirmed. On the contrary, *MLL* translocations occur predominantly in the myelomonocytic (M4) and monocyte (M5) AML subtypes [49].

Some AML patients have an increased number of *MLL* gene copies in the form of double minute chromosomes, also called homogeneously staining regions. *MLL* gene amplification may occur through skipping translocations, in which the amplicon of chromosome 11 is integrated into one or more other chromosomes, creating multiple copies of the *MLL* gene.

In general, the amplification of the gene leads to an overgrowth of structurally normal copies of the gene, resulting in overproduction of the oncogene-stimulating protein. These extra proto-oncogene copies increase the amount of the gene product in a cell, thereby inducing unlimited cell proliferation. Gene amplification is usually manifested cytogenetically, either in an intra-chromosomal manner as a homogeneously staining region (HSR – homogeneously staining region) or in an extrachromosomal manner as double minute chromosomes (dmin). Identification of genes in the amplified region allows us to perform fluorescent in situ hybridization (Figure 7).

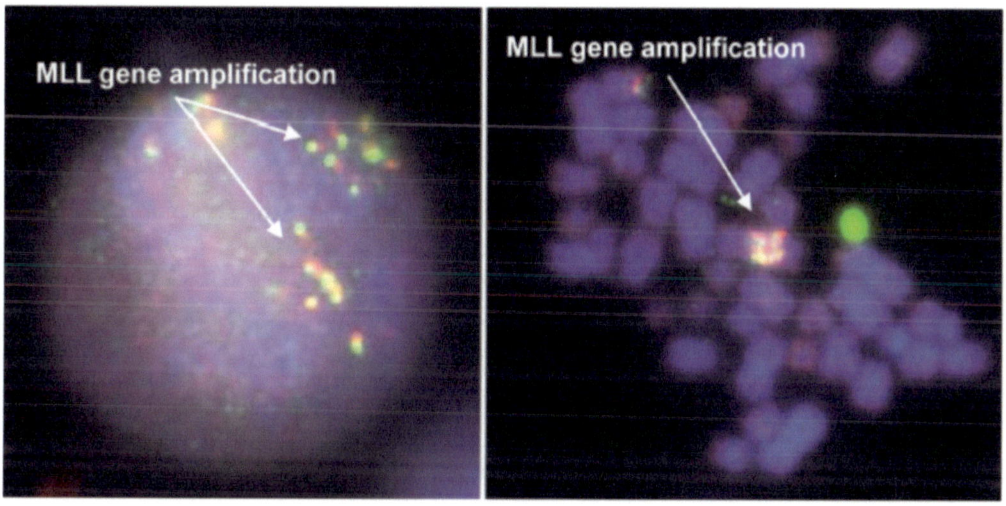

Figure 7. The results obtained from the analysis of a fluorescent CCD camera. Left: interphase nucleus. Right: mitosis. Amplification of MLL (9 copies) in a patient with karyotype 44, XY, -5, hsr (11) (q23), -18, +21, + mar (C).

The amplification of genes, a common occurrence in a wide range of tumors, is rarely observed in acute leukemia. Gene amplification is identified in approximately 1% of patients with AML by conducting a cytogenetic analysis in the form of dmin (the area of the *MLL* gene) [50].

It was found that patients with the *MLL* gene amplification share several common characteristics: they are older than 60 and have a *de novo* form of AML, a complex karyotype, and a short survival rate; 90% of them also have a 5q deletion.

5. Detection methods for *MLL* gene conversions

In diagnostic procedures, methods such as cytogenetic analysis, fluorescent in situ hybridization (FISH), and reverse transcriptase-polymerase chain reaction (RT-PCR) are routinely used for the identification of various regroupings within the *MLL* gene. Genomic molecular methods are also used, such as array comparative genomic hybridization (aCGH). Recently, the spectrum of diagnostics methods was expanded by long-distance inverse PCR (LDI-PCR), which detects rearrangements within the *MLL* gene at the molecular level [45].

Classical cytogenetics is used to determine a completed karyotype picture of the disease and to monitor the progress of the disease. It provides a full overview of qualitative and quantitative karyotype abnormalities and reveals primary and secondary clonal changes. Classical cytogenetics can reveal five most frequent *MLL* rearrangements include t(4;11)(q21;q23), *AFF1(AF4)/MLL;* t(6;11)(q27;q23), *MLLT4(AF6)/MLL;* t(9;11)(p22;q23), *MLLT3(AF9)/MLL;* t(11;19)(q23,p13.1), *MLL/ELL;* and t(11;19)(q23;p13.3), *MLL/MLLT1(ENL)*.Typically, conventional cytogenetics has been used to detect rearrangements involving the *MLL* gene. However, conventional cytogenetics may fail to detect nearly one-third of *MLL* rearrangements; therefore, fluorescence in situ hybridization (FISH) has emerged as the modality of choice for detection of such rearrangements. **Fluorescent in situ hybridization (FISH)** is a method of molecular cytogenetics that enables the detection of specific nucleotide sequences ranging from one to several hundred kilobases. The principle of this method lies in the ability of a single-strand DNA probe to bind with a complementary segment of single-stranded patient DNA. Using specific probes enables us to identify chromosome numbers and to identify specific chromosomal regions (loci). By running FISH on metaphase as well as interphase cells, one of the biggest problems of classical cytogenetic analysis has been overcome. The **LSI® MLL Dual Color, Break Apart Rearrangement Probe** (Vysis) is used for the detection of alterations, amplifications and deletions within the *MLL* gene.

Reverse transcriptase PCR (RT-PCR) is particularly useful if the internal organization of exons and introns within the gene is not known. The first step is isolating the mRNA of the respective gene from the tissue. Using a reverse transcriptase enzyme and an oligo dT primer, complementary DNA (cDNA) is created from an mRNA molecule, which then serves as a template for PCR. Using the appropriate primers allows for further amplification of a specific cDNA sequence. The resulting product is then visualized on an agarose gel.

Multiplexed reverse transcription PCR (MRT-PCR) Anderson et al., 2001, developed this quick and accurate method to identify the six most common *MLL* gene translocations: *MLL/AF4* (acute lymphoblastic leukemia), *MLL/AF6, MLL/AF9, MLL/AF10, MLL/ENL,* and *MLL/ELL.* MRT-PCR is based on two individual steps. The first step uses a mix of external (out) primers, and the second step uses a mix of internal (in) primers, which allows for the detection of six fusion genes in two multiplex PCR reactions. Thus, each sample is tested for the presence of the fusion gene twice. Primers are designed so that in the first step, there is a significantly greater amount of the product formed than in the second step, which increases the specificity of this method. If necessary, the MRT-PCR analysis can be extended by investigating other fusion genes [51].

5.1. Long-distance inverse PCR (LDI-PCR)

The different *MLL* translocation partner genes are identified by cytogenetic analyses, and only the most common *MLL* translocations are investigated by RT-PCR or by MRT-PCR analyses. However, the infrequent or unknown *MLL* translocations were excluded from further analyses. Therefore, it was a goal to establish a universal method that enables the detection of *MLL* rearrangements with genomic DNA. Mayer et al. [52] designed a universal long-distance inverse-PCR approach for clinical use and verified it as a very suitable method for the identification of known and unknown translocation partner genes (TPGs) and the establishment of patient-specific *MLL* fusion sequences (Figure 8).

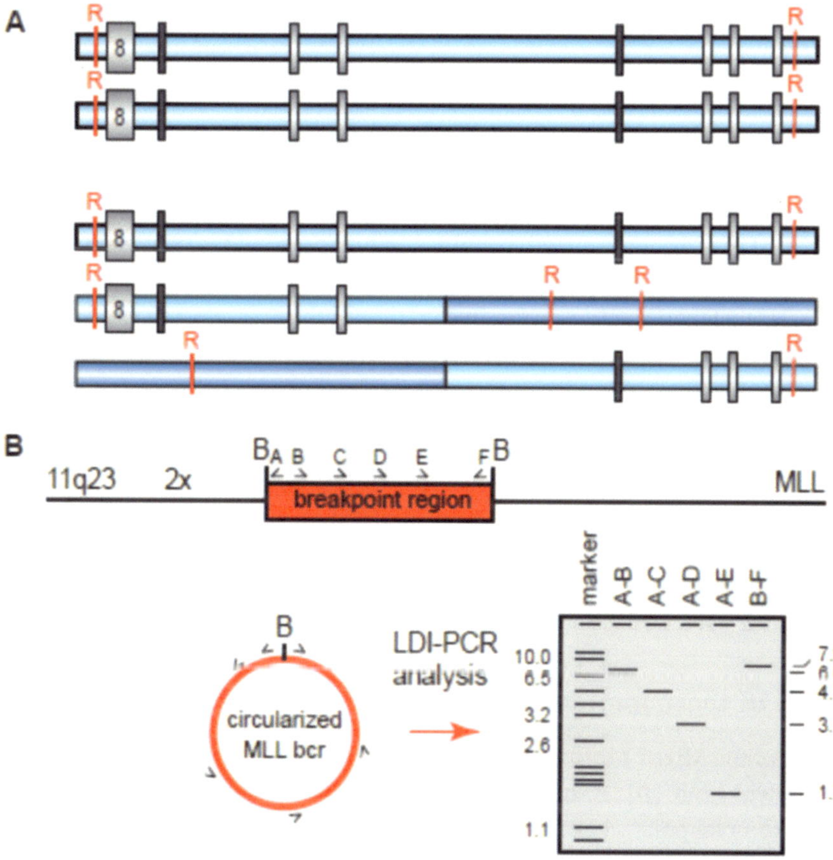

Figure 8. Principles of the LDI-PCR method. **A.** The schema summarizes how the genomic DNA is first restricted using distinct combinations of restriction enzymes (R: restriction site), then re-ligated to form two DNA circles that can be amplified with a specific set of oligonucleotides (A-B, A-C, A-D, and A-E). The primer combination B-F serves as internal control. **B.** *Bam*HI restriction recognition site. Translocation-bearing cells yield both wild-type and derivative templates, differing in size and detectible on the gel. PCR amplimers can be analyzed by sequence analysis using oligonucleotides.

LDI-PCR allows for the identification of a new class of *MLL* recombinations and for the discovery of new fusion genes, providing new insight into the origination mechanisms of *MLL* rearrangements. In this method, 1 µg of genomic DNA from the patient is isolated and digested with the restriction enzyme *BamHI.* The residual enzymatic activity is removed by phenol extraction and ethanol precipitation. After digestion, the DNA samples are re-ligated to form DNA circles (at 16ºC overnight in the presence of T4 DNA ligase). All ligation reactions are terminated at 65ºC for 10 minutes. *MLL* gene-specific oligonucleotides are designed according to GenBank accession no. AJ235379 DNA sequences. For digestion and re-ligation of DNA, the five oligonucleotides (A-E) are used in four combinations (A-B, A-C, A-D and A-E). A positive control containing the oligonucleotides B and F is included in each analysis to amplify a 7.9 kb DNA fragment of the *MLL* breakpoint cluster region. All LDI-PCR reactions are performed using the TripleMaster PCR system. PCR amplimers are separated on 0.8% agarose gels. Non-germline PCR amplimers are isolated from the gel and subjected to DNA sequence analyses to obtain the patient-specific fusion sequences. Annotation of fused *MLL* sequences is carried out by blasting the human genome database (Genomic BLAST, www.ncbi.nlm.nih.gov/genome/seq/Blast). The presence of a rearranged *MLL* allele can be identified by digestion and re-ligation of the two *MLL* alleles. Three different DNA circles are formed (der(11) and der(TP), TP presets translocation partner) that can be amplified by the designated primer combinations A-L. The DNA sequences of oligonucleotides A-L are available at www.biozentrum.unifrankfurt.de/PharmBiol/ Mitarbeiter/Marschalek/ download.html. In some cases, is necessary to analyze the cDNA to validate an *MLL* spliced fusion or to investigate alternative splice products from an *MLL* fusion gene. Because these identified fusion gene sequences are patient-specific and exist in only one copy per leukemic cell, they can be used as reliable markers for minimal residual disease studies and for minimal residual disease monitoring by quantitative PCR techniques.

Analyses of novel identified *MLL* fusion genes provide a rich source for future analyses of oncogenic MLL protein variants. These MRD markers contribute to stratification and improved treatment and outcomes of leukemia patients.

6. Outcomes of these methods

Translocations of the Mixed Lineage Leukemia (MLL) gene at 11q23 are found in both acute lymphoblastic leukemia (ALL) and acute myeloblastic leukemia (AML). The *MLL* gene contains an 8 kb breakpoint cluster region in which virtually all rearrangements occur. To date, more than 70 different fusion partners have been identified, although some of them have been observed only as a single case. The majority of *MLL* gene rearrangements are associated with infant ALL. Acute lymphoblastic leukemia (ALL) diagnosed within the first 12 months of life accounts for 2.5% to 5% of pediatric ALL cases and displays unique biologic, clinical, and prognostic features that are different from those of older children with ALL. Approximately 80% of infant cases harbor rearrangements of the *MLL* (chromosome band 11q23) [53]. Infants with ALL are treated with an intensive regimen of ALL- and AML-like chemotherapy, with the proportion of *MLL*-rearranged cases being responsible for the poor outcome in this age group [54].In contrast, in 75% of the *MLL*-rearranged pediatric AML cases, 4 partners are involved: *AF9/MLLT3* on chromosome 9p21, *AF10/MLLT10* on 10p12, *ELL* on 19p13.1, and *AF6/MLLT4* on 6q27 [55]. In infant AML, *AF9* and *AF10* are among the most frequent *MLL* fusion partners [9]. New translocation partners are still being reported, adding to the diversity of *MLL*-rearranged leukemia. Recently, *ABI2* on chromosome 2q33.2 has been identified as a new *MLL* translocation partner in an infant with

AML-M5 leukemia refractory to standard induction chemotherapy. This important c-Abl regulator is a functional homologue of *ABI1*, a recurrent *MLL*-translocation partner located on chromosome 10p11.2, and is implicated as a tumor suppressor by its inhibitory function in c-Abl signaling [56, 57].

Rearrangements of the *MLL* gene are found in most cases of infant AML and, regardless of age, confer an intermediate risk. The treatment of *MLL*-rearranged ALL in children includes intensified chemotherapy. *MLL*-rearranged AML is a heterogeneous disease in both biology and outcome. In addition to translocation partners, other variables such as hyperleucocytosis, age (older than 10), additional cytogenetic aberrations and early response to treatment have prognostic relevance and are independent prognostic factors. In general, certain *MLL* rearrangements are associated with poor outcomes in pediatric and adult acute myeloid leukemia. However, patients with *MLL*-rearranged AML have intermediate outcomes when treated with the optimized treatment regimens, with a 5-year event-free survival probability (5y-EFS) ranging from 32-54%. Currently, hematopoietic stem cell transplantation is no longer advised during the first remission for favorable MLL rearrangements. Recently, there have been new prognostic subgroups identified within 11q23. A favorable example is t(1,11)(q21,q23). It has an excellent clinical outcome (5y-EFS of 92% and 5y-OS of 100%) [58]. In contrast, subgroups t(10,11)(p12,q23) and t(6,11)(q27,q23) have poor prognoses, with 5y-EFS rates of 31 and 11%, and 5y-OS rates of 45 and 22% [12]. Adults with t(6,11)(q27,q23) also have poor outcomes [59]. Within the most common subgroup t(9,11)(p22,q23), the prognosis appears to be related to morphology, as a group with acute monoblastic leukemia (AML FAB M5) had a significantly better outcome than groups with other FAB subtypes [12].

As with other types of leukemia, the cause of MLL-rearranged AML is unknown. The pathogenesis of AML requires both type-I and type-II mutations. *MLL* rearrangements belong to type-II mutations [60] and lead to the impaired differentiation of hematopoietic cells. Type-I mutations mainly reflect molecular mutation hotspots in specific genes (*FLT3, KIT, NRAS, KRAS, PTPN11*), which are involved in the proliferation of hematopoietic cells [12]. Although *MLL*-rearranged AML harbored one of the lowest frequencies of type-I aberrations (43%), mutations in the RAS-signaling pathway interestingly represented the vast majority in *MLL*-rearranged AML. Cases are routinely screened for *MLL* rearrangements by conventional cytogenetics and FISH; however, these techniques do not guarantee 100% sensitivity. Thus, GEP (gene expression profiling) and LDI-PCR (long-distance inverse PCR) could be used to identify cases not detected with FISH, although these techniques are currently used only in research settings. As the outcome of AML is also dependent on translocation partners, Balgobind et al. [12] suggest that for the next risk group stratification, all *MLL*-rearranged cases should be screened for the favorable prognostic subgroups t(1,11)(q21,q23) and t(9,11)(p22,q23) with FAB5 and the poor prognostic subgroups t(10,11)(p12,q23) and t(6,11)(q27,q23). It can be assumed that a systematic analysis of the *MLL* recombinome will allow conclusions on certain aspects of the mechanisms of leukemogenesis to be drawn by identifying the MLL fusion proteins. This points to the translocation partner as having a role in the disease phenotype and functional heterogeneity of MLL fusions, but the molecular details of these associations are unclear.

The monitoring of MRD by RT-PCR detection of leukemia-specific targets (e.g., gene fusions, gene mutations, overexpressed genes) or by multi-parameter flow cytometry identifying leukemia-associated aberrant phenotypes remains an active field of investigation. Despite technical developments, there is still a paucity of large prospective trials demonstrating its clinical utility, except for APL (acute promyelocytic leukemia). Potentially useful applications of MRD monitoring include early assessment of response to therapy to improve risk stratification and guide post-remission therapy and post-treatment monitoring to detect impending relapse and to guide preemptive therapy. Real-time quantitative (RQ)–PCR assays have been developed for other fusion gene targets such as MLLT3-MLL and DEK-NUP214, but the data are very scarce due to the low frequencies of these leukemias [61]. In AML, there is a need for new agents that target specific biological markers with crucial roles in the development of leukemia and that are related to outcome. Benefits from specific treatments have been shown for specific AML FAB 3 - APL with ATRA and for CML and Ph+ ALL, imatinib mesylate.

There are several recently developed agents that may target the *MLL* complex or downstream targets, such as *FLT3*, tyrosine kinase, which is highly expressed in MLL-rearranged AML. FLT3 inhibitors such as PKC412 showed potential in phase I/II trials of adult AML. Other targets include Glycogen synthase kinase 3–*GSK3* inhibitors, *RAS* pathways, and inhibitors of *MEK*. Some of these new agents likely will not fully block leukemic transformation, but may have an additive effect with current treatment strategies by targeting the proliferative advantages of these leukemic cells [62]. Another possibility is to directly target the *MLL* complex or proteins recruited by the *MLL* complex. However, further safety studies are warranted because genetic disruptions in mice resulted in embryonic lethality [63]. Another possibility could be downstream targets of *MLL*-rearranged AML, such as the upregulation of *HOX* genes. Recent studies suggest that MLL-rearranged leukemias are largely driven by epigenetic dysregulation. Several epigenetic regulators that modify DNA or histones have been implicated in *MLL*-fusion driven leukemogenesis, including DNA methylation, histone acetylation, and histone methylation. The histone methyltransferase DOT1L has emerged as an important mediator of MLL-fusion–mediated leukemic transformation. The clinical development of targeted inhibitors of these epigenetic regulators may therefore hold promise for the treatment of MLL-rearranged leukemia [64].

7. Conclusion

Acute myeloid leukemia is a heterogeneous group of leukemias that result from the clonal transformation of hematopoietic precursors through the acquisition of many chromosomal rearrangements and multiple gene mutations. The cytogenetic aberrations are commonly used as diagnostic and prognostic markers for specific subgroups; in addition, they also have important impacts on achieving complete remission, risk of relapse and overall survival of patients.

Among these aberrations is a subgroup of *MLL* aberrations that have a heterogeneous impact on prognosis, predicting good, intermediate or poor outcomes. This outcome is dependent on different factors, such as translocation partner, age, WBC, and additional cytogenetic aberrations. For this reason, identifying the translocation partner with the methods discussed above has a crucial significance for the stratification of clinical risk groups, tailoring the intensity of treatment strategy and the overall outcome. Cases with favorable prognosis (t(1,11)(q21,q23)) may benefit from less intensive treatment, and cases with poor prognosis (t(6,11)(q27,q23) and t(10,11)(p21,q23)) need adjustment and alternative treatment approaches to improve outcome. It is commonly accepted that the AML phenotype results from multiple genetic/epigenetic lesions affecting differentiation, proliferation, and apoptosis. Distinguishing a particular gene signature for *MLL*-rearranged leukemias sheds light on the molecular mechanisms and potential therapeutic targets of these leukemias. It may also prove to have a useful role in both diagnosis and prognosis. Further investigation into the genetic aberrations of AML cells may provide the knowledge needed to develop new compounds directed against leukemia-specific targets. Consequently, the targeting of a single aberrant protein is unlikely to eradicate the leukemic clone. Although several molecularly-targeted therapies have been shown to be active in AML, it is clear from early clinical studies that most of these novel agents will need to be used in combination with conventional cytotoxic therapy.

However, although subgroup-directed and rationally targeted therapy offers possibilities for the improved care of patients with AML, it will also have implications for the design of clinical trials. In the long term, this may require large randomized trials with international subgroup-specific protocols.

The relationship of outcome with specific translocation partners requires that partners be searched for in the diagnostic work-up of AML and followed-up during treatment. However, to achieve further improvements in survival, unraveling the biology of AML is warranted.

Author details

Denisa Ilencikova
2nd. Department of Pediatrics Comenius University - Medical School University Children´s Hospital Bratislava, Slovakia

Alexandra Kolenova
Department of Pediatric Oncology, Faculty of Medicine, Comenius University – Medical School and University Children´s Hospital, Bratislava, Slovakia

8. References

[1] Creutzig U, Büchner T, Sauerland MC, Zimmermann M, Reinhardt D, Döhner H, Schlenk RF (2008) Significance of age in acute myeloid leukemia patients younger than 30 years: a common analysis of the pediatric trials AML-BFM 93/98 and the adult trials AMLCG 92/99 and AMLSG HD93/98A. Cancer. 112(3):562-71.

[2] Leone G, Mele L, Pulsoni A, Equitani F, Pagano, L (1999) The incidence of secondary leukemias. Haematologica. 84(10):937-45.

[3] Kolitz JE, George SL, Marcucci G, et al. (2010) P-glycoprotein inhibition using valspodar (PSC-833) does not improve outcomes for patients under age 60 years with newly diagnosed acute myeloid leukemia: Cancer and Leukemia Group B study 19808. Blood.116:1413 1421.

[4] Kaspers GJL, Zwaan, CHM (2007) Pediatric acute myeloid leukemia: towards high-quality cure of all patients. Haematologica 92: (11) 1519-1532.

[5] Schoch C, Schnittger S, Klaus M, et al. (2003) AML with 11q23/MLL abnormalities as defined by the WHO classification: incidence, partner chromosomes, FAB subtype, age distribution, and prognostic impact in an unselected series of 1897 cytogenetically analyzed AML cases. Blood, 102: 2395-2402.

[6] Slats AM, Egeler RM, Van Der Does-Van Den Berg A, Korbijn C, Hählen K, Kamps WA, et al. (2005) Causes of death – other than progressive leukemia – in childhood acute lymphoblastic (ALL) and myeloid leukemia (AML): the Dutch Childhood Oncology Group experience. Leukemia. 19:537- 44.

[7] Rubnitz JE, Lensing S, Zhou Y, Sandlund JT, Razzouk BI, Ribeiro RC, et al. (2004) Death during induction therapy and first remission of acute leukemia in childhood: the St. Jude experience. Cancer. 101:1677-84.

[8] Marshalek R. (2010) Mechanisms of leukemogenesis by MLL fusion proteins. British Journal of Haematology, 152: 141-154.

[9] Armstrong SA, Staunton JE, Silverman LB, Pieters R, den Boer ML, Minden MD., Sallan SE., Lander ES, Golub TR and Korsmeyer, SJ et al (2002) MLL translocations specify a distinct gene expression profile that distinguishes a unique leukemia. Nat Genet. 30: 41-47.

[10] Yoeh EJ, Ross ME, Shurleff SA, Williams WK, Patel D, Mafouz R, Behm FG, Raimondi SC, Relling MV, Patel A et al. (2002) Classification, subtype discovery, and prediction of outcome in pediatric acute lymphoblastic leukemia by gene expression profiling. Cancer Cell. 1: 133-143.

[11] Mrózek K, Heinonen K, Lawrence D, Carroll AJ, Koduru PR, Rao KW, Strout MP, Hutchison RE, Moore JO, Mayer RJ, et al. (1997) Adult patients with de novo acute myeloid leukemia and t(9; 11)(p22; q23) have a superior outcome to patients with other translocations involving band 11q23: a cancer and leukemia group B study. Blood 90: 4532-4538.

[12] Balgobind BV, Zwaan CM, Pieters R, van der Heuvel-Eibrink MM (2011) The heterogeneity of pediatric MLL-rearranged acute myeloid leukemia. Leukemia. 25: 1239-1248

[13] Cimino G, Rapanotti MC, Sprovieri T, Elia L (1998) All1 gene alternations in Acute leukemia: biological and clinical aspects. Haematologica. 83: 350-357.

[14] Lin C, Smith ER, Takahashi H, Lai KC, Martin-Brown S et al. (2010) AFF4, a komponent of the ELL/P-TEFb elongation complex and a shared subunit of MLL chimeras, can link transkription elongation to leukemia. Mol Cell. 37: 429-437.

[15] Arai F, Hirao A and Suda T (2005) Regulation of hematopoietic stem cells by the niche. Trends Cardiovasc. Med. 15: 75-79.

[16] De Toni F, Racaud-Sultan C, Chicanne G, Mas VM, Careven C, Mesange F et al. (2006) A crosstalk between the Wnt and the adhesion-dependent signaling pathways governs the chemosensitivity of acute myeloid leukemia. Oncogene. 25: 3113-3122.

[17] Hsieh JJD, Cheby EF and Korsmeyer SJ (2003) Taspasel: a threonine aspartase required for cleavage of MLL and proper HOX gene expression. Cell.115: 293-303.

[18] Nakamura T, Mori T, Tada S, Krajewski W, Rozovskaia T. et al. (2002) ALL-1 is a histone methyltransferase that assembler a supercomplex of proteins involved in transcriptional regulation. Mol Cell 10: 1119-1128.

[19] Yokohama A, Wang Z, Wysocka J, Sanyal M, Aufiero DJ et al. (2004) Leukemia proto-oncoprotein MLL forms a SET1-like histone methyltransferase complex with menin to regulace *Hox* gene expression. Mole Cell Biol. 24: 5639-5649.

[20] Guenter MG, Jenner RG, Chevalier B, Nakamura T, Croce CM et al. (2005) Global and Hox-specific roles for the MLL1 methyltransferase. Proc Natl Acad Sci USA. 102: 8603-8608.

[21] Giampaolo A, Felli N, Diverio D, Morsilli O, Samoggia P, Breccia M, Lo Coco F, Peschle, C, Testa, U. (2002) Expression pattern of HOXB6 homeobox gene in myelomonocytic differentiation and acute myeloid leukemia. Leukemia. 16: 1293-1301.

[22] Burjanivova T, Madzo J, Muzikova K, Meyer C, Schneider B, Votava F, Marschalek R, Stary J, Trka J, Zuna J. (2006) Prenatal origin of childhood AML occurs less frequently than in childhood ALL. BMC Cancer. 21(6): 100

[23] Jones LK, Neat MJ, van Delft FW, Mitchell MP, Adamaki M, Stoneham SJ, Patel N, Saha V. (2003) Cryptic rearrangement involving MLL and AF10 occurring in utero.Leukemia.17(8):1667-9.

[24] Spector LG, Davies SM, Robison LL, Hilden JM, Roesler M, Ross JA. Cancer Epidemiol Biomarkers Prev. (2007) Birth characteristics, maternal reproductive history, and the risk of infant leukemia: a report from the Children's Oncology Group.16(1):128-34.

[25] Alcalay M, Meani N, Gelmetti V, Fantozzi A, Fagioli M, Orleth A, Riganelli D, Sebastiani C, Cappelli E, Casciari C, Sciurpi et al. (2003) Acute myeloid leukemia fusion proteins deregulate genes involved in stem cell maintenance and DNA repair. JCI. 112: 1751–1761.

[26] Mikulasova Z, Ilencikova D, Slamka T, Durovcikova D. (2010) Acute Myeloblastic Leukaemia with Alterations of MLL Proto-Oncogene Protein (11q23/MLL+AML). Klin Onkol. 23(6): 401-407.

[27] Cox MCH, Panetta P, Lo-Coco F, Del Poeta G, Venditti A, Maurillo L, Del Principe MI, Mauriello A, Anemona L, Bruno A, Mazzone C, Palombo P, Amadori S. (2004) Chromosomal Aberration of the 11q23 Locus in Acute Leukemia and Frequency of MLL Gene Translocation. Am J Clin Pathol. 122: 298-306.

[28] Ayton PM, Cleary ML (2001) Molecular mechanisms of leukemogenesis mediated by MLL fusion proteins. Oncogene. 20: 5695-5707.

[29] Kawagoe H, Humphries RK, Blair A, Sutherland HJ and Hogge DE (1999) Expression of HOX genes, HoX cofactors, and MLL in phenotypically and functionally defined

subpopulations of leukemic and normal human hematopoietic cells. Leukemia. 13: 687-698.

[30] Imamura T, Morimoto A, Takanashi M, Hibi S, Sugimoto T, Ishii E and Imashuku, S. (2002) Frequent co-expression of HoXA9 and Meis1 genes in infant acute lymphoblastic leukaemia with MLL rearrangement. British Journal of Haematology. 119: 119-121.

[31] Ayton PM. and Cleary ML (2003) Transformation of myeloid progenitors by MLL oncoproteins is dependent on Hoxa7 and Hoxa9? Genes and Development. 17: 2298-2307.

[32] Milne TA, Dou Y, Martin ME, Brock HW, Roeder RG, and Hess JL (2005) MLL associates specifically with a subset of transcriptionally active target genes. Proceedings of the National Academy of Science of the USA. 102: 14765-14770.

[33] Caslini C, Yang Z, El-Osta M, Milne TA, Slany RK and Hess JL (2007) Interaction of Mll amino terminal sequences with menin is required information. Cancer Research. 67: 7275-7283.

[34] Yokoyama A and Cleary ML (2008) Menin critically links MLL proteins with LEDGF on cancer-associated target genes. Cancer Cell. 14: 36-46.

[35] Jin S, Zhao H, Yi Y, Nakata Y, Kalota A, and Gewirtz AM. (2010) c-Myb binds Mll through menin in human leukemia cells and is an important driver of MLL-asociated leukemogenesis. The Journal of Clinical Investigation. 120: 593-606.

[36] Trentin L, Giordan M, Dingermann T, Basso G, Te Kronnie G and Marschalek R (2009) Two independent gene signatures in pediatric t(4;11)-positive human leukemic cells. Blood. 106: 1559-3566.

[37] Stam RW, Schneider P, Hagelstein JA, van der Linden MH, Stumpel DJ, de Menezes, RX, de Lorenzo P, Valsecchi MG and Pieters R (2010) Gene expression profiling-based dissection of MLL translocated and MLL germline acute lymphoblastic leukemia in infants. Blood. 115: 2835-2844.

[38] Stumpel DJ, Schneider P, van Roon EH, Boer JM, de Lorenzo P, Valsecchi MG, de Menezes RX, Pieters R, and Stam RW (2009) Specific promoter methylation identifies different subgroups of MLL-rearranged infant acute lymphoblastic leukemia, influences clinical outcome, and provides therapeutic options. Blood. 114: 5490-5498.

[39] Gessner A, Thomas M, Garrido Castro P, Büchler L, Scholz A, Brümmendorf TH, Martinez Soria N, Vormoor J, Greil J and Heidenreich O (2010) Leukemic fusion genes MLL/AF4 and AML1/MTG8 support leukemic self-renewal by controlling expression of the telomerase sbunit TERT. Leukemi. 24: 1751-1759.

[40] Faber J, Krivtsov AV, Stubbs MC, Wright R, Davis TN, van den Heuvel-Eibrink M, Zwaan CM, Kung AL and Armstrong SA (2009) HOXA9 is required for survival in human MLL-rearranged acute leukemias. Blood. 113: 2375-2385.

[41] Haferlach T, Schoch C, Schnittger S, Kern W, Löffler H, Hiddemann W (2002) Distinct genetic patterns can be identified in acute monoblastic and acute monocytic leukaemia (FAB AML M5a and M5b): a study of 124 patients. Br J Haematol. 118: 426-431.

[42] Arnaud B, Douet-Guilbert N, Morel F, Le Bris MJ, Herry A et al. (2005): Screening by fluorescent in situ hybridization for MLL status at diagnosis in 239 unselected patients with acute myeloblastic leukemia. Cancer Genet Cytogenet. 161: 110-115.

[43] Raimondi SC, Chang MN, Ravindranath Y, Behm FG, Gresik MV, Steuber CP, Weinstein HJ, Carroll AJ (1999) Chromosomal abnormalities in 478 children with acute myeloid leukemia: clinical characteristics and treatment outcome in a cooperative pediatric oncology group study-POG 8821. Blood. 11:3707-16.

[44] Mayer C, Burmeister T, Strehl S, Schneider B, Hubert D, Zach O et al. (2007) Spliced MLL fusions: a novel mechanism to generate functional chimeric MLL-MLLT1 transcripts in t(11;19)(q23;p13.3) leukemia. Leukemia. 21:588-590.

[45] Meyer C, Kowarz E, Hofmann J, Renneville A, Zuna J, Trka J, Ben Abdelali R, Macintyre E, De Braekeleer E, De Braekeleer M, Delabesse E, et.al. (2009) New insights to the MLL recombinome of acute leukemias. Leukemia. 23(8):1490-1499.

[46] Whitman SP, Liu S, Vukosavljevic T, Rush LJ, Yu L, Liu CH, Klisovic MI, Maharry, K, Guimond M, Strout MP, Becknell B, Dorrance A, Klisovic RB, Plass CH, Bloomfield CD, Marcucci G, Caligiuri MA (2005) The MLL partial tandem duplication: evidence for recessive gain-of-function in acute myeloid leukemia identifies a novel patient subgroup for molecular-targeted therapy. Blood. 106: 345-352.

[47] Libura M, Asnafi V, Tu A, Delabesse E, Tigaud I, Cymbalista F, Bennaceur-Griscelli A, Villarese P, Solbu G, Hagemeijer A, Beldjord K, Hermine O, Macintyre E (2003) FLT3 and MLL intragenic abnormalities in AMLreflect a common category of genotoxic stress. Blood. 102: 2198-2204.

[48] Caligiuri MA, Strout M, Lawrence D, Arthur DC, Baer MR, Yu F, Knuutila S, Mrózek K, Oberkircher AR, Marcucci G, de la Chapelle A, Elonen E, Block AW, Rao PN, Herzig GP, Powell BL, Ruutu T, Schiffer CA, Bloomfield CD (1998) Rearrangement of *ALL1* (*MLL*) in acute myeloid leukemia with normal cytogenetics. Cancer Res. 58: 55-59.

[49] Schnittger S, Kinkelin U, Schoch C, Heinecke A, Haase D, Haferlach T, BÜchner T, WÖrmann B, Hiddemann W, Griesinger F (2000): Screening for MLL tandem duplication in 387 unselected patients with AML identify a prognostically unfavorable subset of AML. Leukemia. 14: 796-804.

[50] Wakui M, Kuriyama K, Miyazaki Y, Hata T, Taniwaki M, Ohtake S, Sakamaki H, Miyawaki S, Naoe T, Ohno R, Tomonaga M (2008) Diagnosis of acute myeloid leukemia according to the WHO classification in the Japan Adult Leukemia Study Group AML-97 protocol. Int J Hematol. 87: 144-151.

[51] Andersson A, Höglund M, Johansson B, Lassen C, Billström R, Garwicz S, Nilsson P, G., Mitelman F, Fioretos T (2001) Paired multiplex reverse-transcriptase polymerase chain reaction (PMRT-PCR) analysis as a rapid and accurate diagnostic tool for the detection of *MLL* fusion genes in hematologic malignancies. Leukemia. 15: 1293-1300.

[52] Mayer C, Schneider B, Reichel M, Angermueller S, Strehl S, Schnittger S et al. (2005) Diagnostic tool for the identification of MLL rearrangements including unknown partner genes. Proc Natl Acad Sci USA, 102:449-454.

[53] Mann G, Attarbaschi A, Schrappe M, De Lorenzo P, Peters C, Hann I, De Rossi G, Felice M, Lausen B, Leblanc T, Szczepanski T, Ferster A, Janka-Schaub G, Rubnitz J, Silverman LB, Stary J, Campbell M, Li CK, Suppiah R, Biondi A, Vora A, Valsecchi MG, Pieters R (2010) Interfant-99 Study Group. Blood. 116(15):2644-50.

[54] Chowdhury T, Brady HJ. (2008) Insights from clinical studies into the role of the MLL gene in infant and childhood leukemia. Blood Cells Mol Dis. 40(2):192-9.

[55] Balgobind BV, Zwaan CM, Meyer C, Marschalek R, Pieters R, Beverloo HB, et al. (2009) NRIP3: a novel translocation partner of MLL detected in a pediatric acute myeloid leukemia with complex chromosome 11 rearrangements. Haematologica. 94(7):1033.

[56] Coenen EA, Zwaan CM, Meyer C, Marschalek R, Pieters R, van der Veken LT, et al. (2011) KIAA1524: A novel MLL translocation partner in acute myeloid leukemia. Leuk Res.35(1):133–5.

[57] Coenen EA, Zwaan CM, Meyer C, Marschalek R, Creutzig U, Pieters R, Bradtke J, van den Heuvel-Eibrink MM. (2012) Abl-interactor 2 (ABI2): A novel MLL translocation partner in acute myeloid leukemia. Leuk Res. 6 (5):e113-5. Epub 2012 Feb 1.

[58] *Balgobind BV, Raimondi SC, Harbott J, Zimmermann M, Alonzo TA, Auvrignon A, Beverloo HB, Chang M, Creutzig U, Dworzak MN, et al. (2009)* Novel prognostic subgroups in childhood 11q23/MLL-rearranged acute myeloid leukemia: results of an international retrospective study. *Blood. 114(12):2489-96.*

[59] Blum W, Mrózek K, Ruppert AS, Carroll AJ, Rao KW, Pettenati MJ, Anastasi J, Larson RA, Bloomfield CD (2004) Adult de novo acute myeloid leukemia with t(6;11)(q27;q23): results from Cancer and Leukemia Group B Study 8461 and review of the literature. Cancer. 101(6):1420-7.

[60] Gilliand DG, Griffin, JD (2002) The roles of FLT3 in hematopoesis and leukemia. Blood. 100: 1532-1542.

[61] Döhner H, Estey EH, Amadori S, Appelbaum FR, Büchner T, Burnett AK, Dombret H, Fenaux P, Grimwade D, Larson RA, Lo-Coco F, Naoe T, Niederwieser D, Ossenkoppele GJ, Sanz MA, Sierra J, Tallman MS, Löwenberg B, Bloomfield CD European LeukemiaNet (2010) Diagnosis and management of acute myeloid leukemia in adults: recommendations from an international expert panel, on behalf of the European LeukemiaNet. Blood. 115(3):453-74.

[62] Sebolt-Leopold JS (2008) Advances in the development of cancer therapeutics directed against the RAS-mitogen-activated protein kinase pathway Clin Cancer Res. 14(12):3651-6.

[63] Ayton PM, Chen EH (2004) Cleary MLBinding to nonmethylated CpG DNA is essential for target recognition, transactivation, and myeloid transformation by an MLL oncoprotein. Mol Cell Biol. 24(23):10470-8.

[64] Bernt KM, Armstrong SA (2011) Targeting epigenetic programs in MLL-rearranged leukemias. Hematology Am Soc Hematol Educ Program. 2011:354-60.

Chapter 11

Dual Role of TLR3 in Inflammation and Cancer Cell Apoptosis

Yann Estornes, Olivier Micheau, Toufic Renno and Serge Lebecque

Additional information is available at the end of the chapter

http://dx.doi.org/10.5772/54772

1. Introduction

1.1. The concepts of recognition of non-self by innate immune receptors

Immunity may be regarded as the most sophisticated part of the tissue repair process. In order to reach the *"restitutio ad integrum"* of tissues while minimizing the general consequences of external aggression, multicellular organisms have evolved mechanisms that allow rapid detection of non-self or injured self. Early recognition represents the first stage of protection against pathogens that enables any cell to elicit promptly various forms of protective responses that altogether represent the so-called "innate immune response". In addition, the innate immune response turns on two types of specialized effector immune cells responsible for the adaptive immune response, the T and the B lymphocytes

During the last two decades, two concepts have emerged in an effort to elucidate the basis of the key-initiating step, i.e., the molecular recognition of non-self. On one side, it was first reasoned, and later amply demonstrated, that the structures that are recognized early by the so-called innate immunity must share some important features that allows their recognition as non-self. This led to the model of "Pathogen Associated Molecular Patterns" (or PAMPs), which implies that distinction relies on differences in shape of molecules shared by pathogens, as they have been conserved during the evolution to fulfill important functions. On the other side, the concept of Pathogen Recognition Receptors (PRRs) was built on the assumption that a limited number of germline-encoded receptors should have the capacity to detect the differences in shape displayed by the PAMPs. In agreement with the model, each of the main categories of PRRs displays features that are well suited for discriminating non-self.

The lectins are either soluble or membrane-bound proteins that recognize saccharides through single or multiple Carbohydrate Recognition Domains (CRD). Given the differences in enzymatic equipment for polysaccharide synthesis, and therefore in the nature (and the shape) of saccharides expressed at the surface of pathogens when compared to eukaryotic cells, those structures represent ideal targets for pathogen detection.

The cytoplasmic nucleotide-binding oligomerization domain (NOD)-like receptors (NLR) share domain architecture comprising a nucleotide-binding domain (NBD) and a leucine-rich repeat (LRR) domain. NOD1 and NOD2 recognize distinct building blocks of peptidoglycan (PGN) found in bacterial walls.

The RIG-I (retinoic acid inducible gene-I, DDX58) and MDA5 (melanoma-differentiation-associated gene-5, RH116) represent the RIG-I-like helicases (RLH) family of cytosolic sensors that specifically recognizes double stranded RNA (dsRNA), while AIM2 (absent in melanoma 2) appears to be essential for mediating inflammatory reactions triggered by cytoplasmic DNA that signs the presence of pathogens. Recently, a complex formed of three helicases DDX1-DDX21-DHX36 [1] and a fourth helicase DHX9 [2] have been shown to detect dsRNA in the cytosol of myeloid dendritic cells (mDCs).

Last but not least, the membrane-bound Toll-like receptors constitute a family of 10 members in human (11 in mouse) that share a LRR extracellular domain involved in the binding of PAMPs. TLR1, 2, 4, 5 and 6 are expressed at the cell surface membrane and recognize pathogens-derived lipids, lipopolysaccharides, PGN or proteins. In contrast, TLR3, 7, 8 and 9 recognize (poly)nucleotides in endolysosomes.

2. Toll-like receptor 3: a PRR that activates various types of cells in response to dsRNA

TLR3 is a highly glycosylated type I membrane receptor that appears to be dedicated to the recognition of dsRNA [3] that represents a replication intermediate for many viruses. TLR3 is thus involved in the innate immune response against various viruses [4], and plays a non-redundant role in HSV-1 infection of the CNS [5]. Like all TLRs, TLR3 possesses an extracellular domain made of (23) LRRs and a cytoplasmic toll/IL-1 receptor (TIR) domain required for downstream signaling. Compared with other PRRs also responsive to RNA, the specificity of TLR3 resides in its location at the membrane of endolysosomes and in its affinity for a large range of dsRNA sizes (form > 50 bp to over 2000 bp). In contrast, RIG-I and MDA5 are activated by the presence in the cytoplasm of short or long dsRNA, respectively, while the membrane-bound TLR7 detects the presence of single stranded RNA (i.e. bacterial mRNA).

The trachea, the pancreas and the placenta are the three organs that show the highest expression of TLR3 mRNA (http://www.ncbi.nlm.nih.gov/geoprofiles). However, TLR3 can also be detected by immunohistochemistry in many tissues, including the skin [6], the muscles [7], and the kidneys [8]. At the cellular level, myeloid dendritic cells and macrophages, but not other leukocytes, including monocyte precursors have been found to express TLR3. TLR3 is also present in non-immune cells such as epithelial cells of various origins (lung [9], intestine [10], breast [11], kidney [12], pancreas [13]) but also in mesenchymal cells [14] and in endothelial cells [15]. Of interest, TLR3 is the TLR that is expressed most strongly in the brain, especially in astrocytes, glia, and neurons[16].

External dsRNA appears to be first internalized by cells through the binding on surface scavenger receptors [17]. In endolysosomes, dsRNA binding leads to TLR3 dimerization and to recruitment through TIR domains homotypic interaction of a single adaptor, TRIF (TIR domain-containing adapter protein inducing interferon beta). TRIF in turns recruits several signaling kinases that activate different transcription factors: 1) through the activation of tumor necrosis factor receptor (TNFR)-associated factor (TRAF6) E3 ubiquitin ligase, TRIF recruits the transforming growth factor-β-activated kinase 1 (TAK1) which mediates downstream NF-kB activation[18]. 2) Protein kinase R (PKR) is associated with TAK1 and contributes to the activation of the p38 mitogen-activated protein kinase pathway by interaction with MKK6 [19]. 3) TRIF also recruits TBK1 and IKKε through TRAF3, which phosphorylates IRF3 [20, 21] Activated IRF3 translocates into the nucleus and induces expression of Type I IFN [22]. 4) The receptor interacting protein 1 kinase (RIP1K) is also essential for NF-kB activation but not for IRF3 activation by TRIF [23, 24].

3. Activities of TLR3 ligands on cancer cells

3.1. Inflammatory and proliferative responses of cancer cells

Many types of cancer cells express TLR3. This was established by immunohistochemistry on tumor tissue sections of breast carcinoma [25], oral squamous cell carcinoma [26], cervical carcinoma [27], ovarian carcinoma [28], prostate carcinoma, head and neck carcinoma [29]. Furthermore, the level of TLR3 expression by prostate cancer cells was shown to be significantly associated with higher probability of biochemical recurrence [30]. We have also observed TLR3 staining on lung squamous cell carcinoma and on a portion of HCC (our unpublished data). Furthermore, overexpression of TLR3 has been detected by flow cytometry, by western blot and/or by qPCR in melanoma cells [31, 32], esophageal squamous cell carcinoma[33], head and neck carcinoma cells [34] and multiple myeloma cells [35].

Like normal cells, human cancer cell lines will respond to TLR3 ligand by secreting inflammatory cytokines, IFN-I and chemokines. As an example, we found that NSCLC, OSCC and HCC cell lines could secrete IL-6, IL-8, RANTES, IP-10, and IFN-I, although at different levels depending on the line under consideration (our unpublished data). Likewise, prostate cancer cells secrete IL-8, chemokine (C C motif) ligand 3, CCL3, CCL5 and IP-10 in response to Poly(I:C) [36], and head and neck cancer cells secrete IL-1β, IL-6 and IL-8 [29].

Few data have been published regarding the changes of surface membrane protein expression by cancer cells after TLR3 activation. Nevertheless, two reports have shown that CD54 is upregulated, while MHC-I expression remained constant [29, 37].

Regarding cancer cells migration in response to TLR3 stimulation, divergent results have been reported. Studying nasopharyngeal carcinoma (NPC), Zhang et *al*. observed that TLR3 agonist downregulated the expression of chemokine receptor CXCR4 and inhibited cell migration in response to CXCR4 ligand stromal cell-derived factor-1alpha (SDF-1alpha) in chemotaxis assays [38]. Moreover, TLR3 activation reduced the capacity of NPC cells to form metastasis in draining lymph nodes when injected in athymic mice. In contrast, stimulation of TLR3-expressing head and neck OC2 cells with Poly(I:C) was found to induce the secretion of CCL5 and to promote CCL5-mediated migration in OC2 cells [26]. Similarly, Goto et *al*. showed that Poly(I:C) enhanced the migration of melanoma cells in vitro [32]. Related to those observations, we regularly observe significant changes in the morphology of cultured cancer cells in the presence of Poly(I:C), but little is known yet on the effects of TLR3 activation on the cytoskeleton.

Lastly, rare examples of cancer cells proliferating in response to TLR3 activation have been published. For example, one multiple myeloma cancer cell lines showed an NF-kB-dependent proliferation in response to Poly(I:C) [39]. Moreover, indirect evidences led to the conclusion that TLR3 might support the proliferation of some head and neck cancer cell lines proliferation through c-Myc upregulation [40], and of papillary thyroid carcinoma [41].

3.2. Anti-proliferative effects on cancer cell

Direct inhibition of tumor growth by TLR3 agonists has been reported in vitro for human breast, melanoma, prostate, head and neck, multiple myeloma, clear renal carcinoma, colon, lung, and cervical cancer cells [11, 31, 42-51]. Two mechanisms contribute to the inhibition of tumor growth upon TLR3 activation; (i) decrease of proliferation and (ii) induction of apoptotic cell death.

3.2.1. TLR3 decreases proliferation of cancer cells by blocking progression through the cell cycle

Decrease of tumor cell proliferation in response to TLR3 activation by Poly(I:C) dsRNA has been demonstrated by BrDu incorporation experiments for breast and prostate cancer cells [11, 46], and by Ki-67 staining in prostate cell lines [51], and likely participates to the dsRNA anti-tumoral effect in the other types of cancers listed above. The blockade of cell cycle appears to result form the combined downregulation of cyclin D1 and upregulation of cyclin-dependent kinase inhibitor p27 [11, 46, 52] and/or the inhibition of the Akt signaling pathway [51].

3.2.2. TLR3 triggers the apoptosis of cancer cells

a. General considerations on apoptosis

Apoptosis is an evolutionarily programmed cell death that was first described by Kerr and colleagues in 1972 [53]. It is crucial for successful embryonic development and for the maintenance of normal cellular homeostasis in adult organisms. Deregulation of apoptosis is involved in an extensive variety of diseases such as cancer and autoimmunity, but also in immunodeficiency, degenerative diseases, or infertility.

Apoptotic cell death results from the dismantlement of the cell by the sequential activation of cysteine proteases, called caspases, that cleaves numerous proteins in the cell. Two major pathways of apoptosis have been identified: the "extrinsic pathway" and the "intrinsic pathway". The first one is typically triggered by ligation of cell surface Death Receptors of the TNFRI superfamilly (such as TRAIL-R or FAS) which allows the formation of a supramolecular complex called DISC (for Death Inducing Signaling Complex) in which FADD plays a key role in the recruitment and the activation of the initiator caspase-8 (and also caspase-10) inside this platform. Inactive caspase-8 monomers are forced to dimerize when in close proximity inside the DISC, which triggers their catalytic activity leading to autocleavage and stabilization of caspase-8 in its active form. The "intrinsic pathway", also called the "mitochondrial pathway" is typically initiated by a diverse range of stress condition such as DNA damage, ER stress, or withdrawal, and leading to mitochondria alterations and cytochrome C release, and activation of the initiator caspase-9 in a molecular platform called Apoptosome. The "extrinsic" and "intrinsic" pathways are tightly regulated by FLIP and BCL-2 family proteins, respectively, and converge to the activation of the executioner caspase-3 and -7 that cleave essential proteins required for cellular homeostasis.

In "Type I cells", such as lymphocytes, activation of caspase-8 directly catalyzes the maturation of caspase-3 and triggers cell death. In other cells, such as hepatocytes, caspase-8 activation cleaves the BH3-only protein BID, generating a mitochondrion-permeabilizing fragment (t-BID for truncated BID) which creates an amplification loop of the death signal that is required for cell death to occur. These cells are called "Type II cells".

b. TLR3 activates the extrinsic pathway of apoptosis in cancer cells

The first demonstration that TLR3 activation by dsRNA Poly(I:C) can directly induce apoptotic death of cancer cells *in vitro* was recently achieved by our group in 2006, in a model of breast carcinoma cell lines [11]. Since this first observation, an increasing number of studies has been started, and to date, the direct inhibitory effect of TLR3 ligands on tumor cell survival has been reported on melanoma, head and neck, prostate, clear renal carcinoma, multiple myeloma, colon, cervical, and lung cancer cells. Moreover, the relevance of TLR3 expression in cancer cells for dsRNA antitumor effects has now been demonstrated in immunodeficient mouse models and has been validated as a biomarker for the therapeutic efficacy of dsRNA on metastatic relapse [25].This indicates that TLR3 targeting could represent an opportunity for the development of novel cancer therapy strategies.

Several studies have clearly demonstrated that TLR3-induced apoptosis in cancer cells is dependent on caspase-8 activation [44, 50, 54, 55], suggesting that TLR3 activation triggers the "extrinsic pathway" of apoptosis. Interestingly, caspase-8 activation and apoptosis triggering in response to TLR3 activation is independent of the classical Death Receptors since invalidation of these receptors by siRNA or by neutralizing antibodies do not block TLR3-mediated caspase-8-dependent apoptosis [54, 55].

The canonical activation of caspase-8 by Death Receptor relies on a particular domain shared by these receptors at their C-terminal side, and called Death Domain (DD). This DD is crucial for the assembling of the DISC through its association with the DD of the adapter FADD which in turn recruits caspase-8 through homotypic interaction between their respective Death Effector Domain (DED). However, TLR3 does not contain such a DD, and the mechanism by which TLR3 activates caspase-8 remained unexplained until recently.

c. TLR3 behaves like a Death Receptor in cancer cells

Clues to understand how TLR3 activates caspase-8 came from cell death models of ectopic TRIF transfection [56, 57]. Genetic modifications of TRIF allowed to conclude that the RHIM (RIP Homotypic Interaction Motif) C-terminal domain of TRIF is crucial for TRIF-induced caspase-8 activation. This domain was previously shown to be required for homotypic association with the RHIM domain of RIP1 kinase and for NF-kB signaling triggering [23]. Interestingly, RIP1 contains also a DD, and the hypothesis of a molecular platform containing TRIF/RIP1/FADD/caspase-8 and mediating apoptosis was born. However, evidences of the molecular assembly of this platform to TLR3 in physiologic conditions were lacking.

Our group and that of Martin Leverkus recently highlighted the molecular mechanism of TLR3-mediated cell death [54, 55]. In these two independent studies, TLR3 activation by dsRNA Poly(I:C) lead to the formation of a DISC-like complex containing caspase-8/FADD/FLIP/RIP1 and TRIF - RIP1 playing a crucial role in the formation of this complex - confirming at a physiologic level the previous studies. Generation of new anti-TLR3 monoclonal antibodies allowed us to establish that TLR3 was also present in the complex [55], indicating that even in absence of a DD in its C-terminal side, TLR3 is able to directly engage the "extrinsic pathway" of apoptosis by recruiting the initiator caspase-8 to itself, a characteristic initially observed for the death receptors TRAIL-R or FAS. We propose that dsRNA-mediated TLR3 dimerization allows the recruitment of TRIF through TIR homotypic interaction which in turn allows the recruitment of the DD-containing RIP1, the adapter FADD, and caspase-8 to trigger apoptosis (Figure 1a).

However, when we investigated the role of FADD in TLR3-mediated caspase-8 activation we were struck by the fact that invalidation of FADD by siRNA transfection did not prevent TLR3-induced caspase-8 activation and apoptosis whereas FAS- or TRAIL-R-dependent apoptosis were prevented [55]. FADD possesses both a DD and a DED, and was therefore expected to provide the molecular link between RIP1 and caspase-8. Additional works are required to elucidate the role of FADD in the TLR3-dependent caspase-8-containing complex, but we can hypothesize that another adapter (such as FAF1 [58]) might exert a redundant function, or that RIP1-caspase-8 association is direct and does not require an adaptor molecule (which was previously observed *in vitro* with purified proteins [59])

d. Several molecular checkpoints negatively regulates TLR3-induced apoptosis

When screening the effect of dsRNA on lung tumor cell lines, we observed that not all the cells were sensitive to dsRNA-induced apoptosis, even when they express a functional

TLR3. Moreover, normal lung epithelial cells were also resistant to apoptosis, indicating that physiologic negative regulators of the TLR3 apoptotic pathway exist in the cells. Two major and complementary checkpoints can be inferred from the literature.

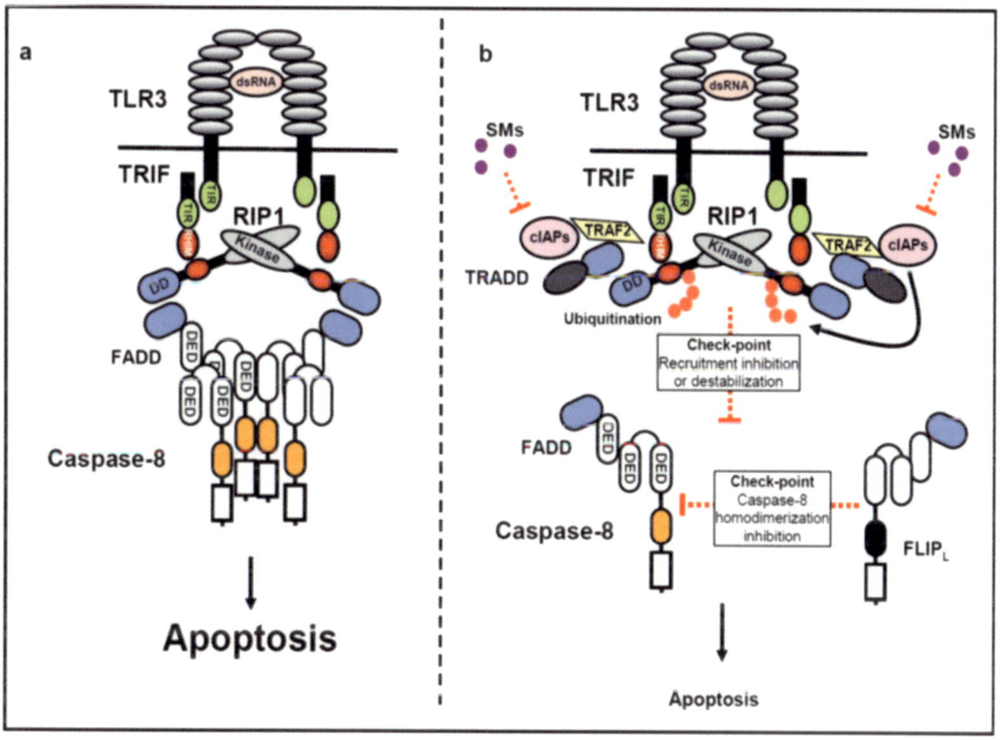

Figure 1. Hypothetical model of TLR3-triggered apoptosis: mechanisms. **a**, TLR3 activation by dsRNA induces the formation of an atypical caspase-8-activating complexe containing caspase-8/FADD/RIP1/TRIF and TLR3. Successive homotypic interactions are required for TLR3 to recruit caspase-8. TLR3 possesses a TIR domain that binds to the adaptor TRIF through homotypic TIR domain interaction, while TRIF possesses a RHIM (RIP Homotypic Interaction Motif) domain in its C-terminal side allowing its association with the RHIM domain of RIP1. Then, RIP1 can recruit FADD through homotypic interaction between their Death Domain (DD), and FADD recruits caspase-8 through theur respective Death Effector Domain (DED). **b**, Regulatory mechanisms of caspase-8 recruitment and activation by TLR3. In addition to RIP1, the adaptor TRIF recruits an ubiquitin ligase complexe containing the adaptor TRADD and the ubiquitin ligases TRAF2 and cIAPs which drives ubiquitination of RIP1, a post-translational modification required for NF kB activation, that limits its association with caspase-8 by directly preventing and/or destabilizing the binding. In absence of cIAPs, which can be achieved by smac mimetics (SMs) treatments that triggers cIAPs auto-ubiquitination and degradation by the proteasome, RIP1 is not ubiquitinated which favours the recruitment of caspase-8. In presence of FLIP at sufficient level, the affinity of FLIP for caspase-8 favours the formation of FLIP-caspase-8 heterodimers, hence preventing the formation of apoptotic caspase-8 homodimers. cIAPs and FLIP may constitute two different molecular checkpoints acting at two different levels for the negative regulation of caspase-8 recruitment by TLR3.

d.1. The upstream antiapoptotic IAPs-dependent checkpoint

The mammalian Inhibitor of APoptosis (IAP) proteins, c-IAP1, c-IAP2, and XIAP, are critical regulators of cell death through their direct activity towards caspases. IAPs are also well known modulators of inflammatory signaling and immunity. These proteins consist of three N-terminal Baculovirus IAP Repeat (BIR) domains, a C-terminal Really Interesting New Gene (RING) domain that confers E3 ubiquitin ligase activity, and a CAspase-Recruitment Domain (CARD) – in c-IAP1 and c-IAP2 – required for autoinhibition of their ligase activity at steady state. Notably, c-IAP1 and c-IAP2 regulate ubiquitin-dependent innate immune signaling in aval of TLRs or TNF-R, such as the activation of nuclear factors NF-kB, through their ubiquitin ligase activity toward key molecules of the signaling pathways. Based on the contribution of IAPs in cancer cell survival, small pharmacological inhibitors have recently been developed. These antagonist molecules, dubbed Smac-mimetics (SMs), mimic the N-terminal IAP-binding motif of SMAC (an endogenous mitochondrial IAP inhibitor), and selectively bind the BIR2 and BIR3 domains of IAPs. In particular, interaction of SMs with c-IAP1and c-IAP2 results in auto-ubiquitination activity and rapid proteasomal degradation [60-62].

The use of SMs shed new light on cIAPs functions. Notably, it has been demonstrated that non-degradative K63-linked ubiquitination of RIP1 by cIAPs is required for efficient NF-kB activation and prosurviving signaling in response to TNFR-I activation [61, 63, 64]. Moreover, RIP1 ubiquitination by cIAPs prevents RIP1 from binding caspase-8 and blocks apoptosis after TNF stimulation [63, 65, 66]. Hence, cIAPs dependent RIP1 ubiquitination functions as an early checkpoint to protect from TNF-RI-induced cell death until a later checkpoint take place via the expression of pro-survival genes through the NF-kB pathway (reviewed in [67]). Ubiquitination of RIP1 is also important for TLR3-induced NF-kB activation, and like for TNF signalling, the adaptor TRADD and the ubiquitin ligase TRAF2 are required for efficient RIP1 ubiquitination [68, 69].

Recently, two groups described a new RIP1-mediated death platform, termed the ripoptosome, which is formed upon downregulation of cIAPs and XIAP by SMs treatment or genotoxic stress [54, 70]. They showed that invalidation of IAPs allows the self-assembling of a cytosolic molecular complex containing RIP1, FADD and caspase-8, independently of Death Receptor signaling, and mediating apoptotic cell death.

Interestingly, IAPs inhibition by SMs treatment sensitizes a variety of cancer cells (melanoma, nasopharyngeal carcinoma, cervix, NSCLC…) to TLR3-mediated apoptosis [44, 49, 50, 54, 55]. cIAP1 and cIAP2 play non-redundant roles in this apoptotic process since specific invalidation of cIAP1 or cIAP2 can potentiate the deleterious effect of dsRNA. Two non-mutually exclusive models can be proposed to explain the sensitizing effect of cIAP invalidation. In the first one, cIAP elimination by SMs allows the formation of the ripoptosome which can bind to TRIF following TLR3 stimulation by dsRNA treatment, and favouring induction of apoptosis. In the second one, TLR3 ligation allows the recruitment of the adapter TRIF that functions as a platform to recruit signaling molecules such as RIP1, TRAF2, cIAPs, and TRADD for activation of the NF-kB pathway. In absence of cIAP, ubiquitination of RIP1 is defective which favours (or stabilizes) its association with caspase-8 and induces apoptosis (Figure 1b). This second model is supported by the fact that TLR3-induced apoptosis can occur without a prior invalidation of cIAPs in some tumor cells, and that ripoptosome formation may not be a prerequisite for caspase-8 activation.

d.2. The downstream antiapoptotic FLIP-dependent checkpoint

Two FLIP isoforms exist in the cell: FLIPs (short form) et FLIPL (long form). FLIPL is similar to caspase-8 but lacks the catalytic site. FLIPs contains the two DED and is structurally related to the FLIP inhibitor from viruses. FLIPs and FLIPL bind FADD and block caspase-8-mediated apoptosis in response to death receptor ligation [71, 72]. FLIP represents one of the most important anti-apoptotic proteins whose expression is tightly regulated by the NF-kB pathway for blocking TNF-mediated caspase-8-dependent apoptosis [73]. Moreover, heterodimers FLIP-caspase-8 assemble preferentially in the cell because of a greater affinity and/or stability than caspase-8 homodimers [74].

Like classical death receptors of the TNFR family, TLR3-induced caspase-8-mediated apoptosis is negatively regulated by FLIP. Indeed, FLIP invalidation by specific shRNA potentiates TLR3-dependent caspase-8 activation and apoptosis in different tumor cell lines ([54] and unpublished data). At the contrary, FLIPL overexpression blocks the apoptotic effect of dsRNA poly(I:C) treatment [54, 55]. In contrast to TNF-RI pathway, for which the role and the regulation of FLIP have been extensively studied, TLR3-mediated FLIP regulation as well as the mechanism of FLIP-dependent blockade of pro-apoptotic activation of caspase-8 are not clear and require further investigations. However, we can hypothesis (from death receptor signalling literature) that FLIP inhibit TLR3-induced apoptosis through associating with caspase-8 to form FLIP caspase-8 heterodimers, and hence, preventing the formation of apoptotic caspase-8 homodimers (Figure 1b)

Although both IAPs- and FLIP-dependent checkpoints are likely to protect cells form TLR3-triggered apoptosis, it remains unknown to which extent they each contribute to the resistance of normal cells and of different tumor cells. For example, it would be interesting to determine whether the higher sensitivity to TLR3-induced apoptosis of metastatic head and neck cancer cells relative to primary tumors [75] could be explained by differences in the efficacy of either or both of those two molecular barriers.

3.2.3. TLR3 and necroptosis

It is important to note that although FLIPL prevents apoptotic activation of caspase-8, FLIPL-caspase-8 heterodimers are proteolytically active, which is not true for FLIPs-caspase-8 heterodimers [74, 76, 77]. This non-apoptotic protease activity of FLIPL-caspase-8 heterodimers is required to protect from lethality of mouse embryos during development, indicating that caspase-8 plays a survival role [78]. Indeed, caspase-8 knock-out is lethal at around embryonic day 10.5 due to alteration in the development of yolk sac vasculature [79, 80]. A molecular mechanism of caspase-8-induced survival has been recently highlighted, and indicates that FLIPL-caspase-8 heterodimers confers protection from necroptosis [78, 81], a form of programmed necrotic cell death, which is regulated by RIP1 and RIP3 [82, 83]. To prevent necroptosis, caspase-8 protease activity is required to cleave and inactivate RIP1 and RIP3, but also CYLD, a deubiquitinating enzyme that removes Lys 63-linked polyubiquitin chains on RIP1 and regulates the interaction between RIP1 and caspase-8 [66, 84]. Necroptosis can be triggered by death receptor ligation in condition of caspase-8 inhibition, and is inhibited by necrostatin-1, a specific inhibitor of RIP1 kinase activity [85]. Necroptotic cell death is currently under intensive investigations (for review see [86-88])

Since TLR3 behaves like a death receptor and activates caspase-8 through the recruitment of RIP1, it is reasonable to assume that TLR3 could also induce necroptotic cell death in condition of caspase-8 inhibition. Indeed, it has been reported that Poly(I:C)-induced TLR3 activation can trigger necroptosis in presence of the pan-caspases inhibitor Z-VAD [54], this cell death is inhibited by necrostatin-1 treatment. FLIP isoforms play differential roles in this type of cell death, $FLIP_L$ preventing both apoptosis and necroptosis while $FLIP_S$ is an inhibitor of only apoptosis [54]. However, TLR3-mediated necroptosis seems to be cell specific and probably depends on the expression of RIP3 [54, 55], which is also true for other inductors of necroptosis. Nevertheless, these data indicate that TLR3 activation can trigger the formation of a "necroptosome" containing at least RIP1 and RIP3 which could have relevant function in virus-infected cell death and in immune responses. Further studies are required to address the role of necroptosis in virus-induced diseases and in TLR3-mediated tumor growth inhibition.

3.3. dsRNA in clinical trials

It is known for long time that in human and primate, Poly(I:C) has a short half-life(~6min) because of rapid hydrolysis by RNase from serum, and its capacity to induce IFN production is weak compare to what is observed in mouse models [89, 90]. Moreover, no GMP preparation are currently available and poly(I:C) has too much toxicity by causing fever, renal failure, coagulopathies and hypersensitivity reactions [90], indicating that Poly(I:C) can't be used in clinic. However, two type of Poly(I:C) analogues are currently evaluated in several clinical trials: Poly-ICLC that correspond to Poly(I:C) complexed with polylysine and carboxymethylcellulose, and Poly(I:C_{12}U) or Ampligen (Hemispherx Biopharma of Philadelphia) which is a Poly(I:C) modified by introduction of unpaired bases (uracil). Poly-ICLC is 4- to 10-fold more resistant to hydrolysis than Poly(I:C), with a longer half-life in serums of primate, and a great inducer of IFN [91]. Poly(I:C_{12}U) is a GMP-grade molecule that, in contrast to Poly-ICLC, undergoes accelerated hydrolysis because of regular regions of mismatching. However, Poly(I:C_{12}U) maintains pharmacological activity [92]. Poly-ICLC remains toxic – notably with doses greater than 12 mg/m2 – whereas Poly(I:C_{12}U) showed no evidence of dose-limiting organ toxicity. Indeed, Poly(I:C_{12}U) has been previously tested in the treatment for chronic fatigue syndrome and AIDS without apparent toxicity [92]. Moreover, Poly(I:C_{12}U) is shown to specifically target TLR3 [93].

Owing to its strong capacity to activate the adaptive immunity notably through its action on dendritic cells, dsRNA ligands are currently tested in several clinical trials mainly as adjuvant for antigen peptide vaccinations against various types of cancer [94]. The antigen peptide will be mainly taken up by the dendritic cells that play a major role in the innate immune response as professional Antigen-Presenting Cells (APCs). The peptide is then processed by APCs, and epitopes presented at the cell surface through MHC class I molecules for antigen cross-presentation to CD8+ T-cells. The adjuvant (here the dsRNA ligands) plays an important role for the up-regulation of co-stimulatory molecules by dendritic cells and their maturation, leading to direct activation of CD8+ and CD4+ T-cells through MHC class II and I molecules respectively, and indirectly to NK cells. Several phase 0/I/II clinical trials - http://www.clinicaltrials.gov/ - are in progress in which Poly-ICLC is used in ~ 80% of the studies as adjuvant for antigen-peptide vaccination such as TARP for prostate cancer, MUC1 for triple negative breast cancer or prostate cancer, or NY-ESO1 for ovarian cancer or melanoma. Poly-ICLC is also used in combination with radiotherapy for low-grade recurrent B and T cell lymphoma, and for brain and central nervous system tumors in phase I and II clinical phase. Interestingly, a phase II clinical trial from the North American Brain Tumor Consortium for 30 patients with newly diagnosed supratentorial glioblastoma showed that treatment with radiotherapy in combination with Poly-ICLC followed by Poly-ICLC as a single agent was relatively well-tolerated and enhanced the survival of patients compared to historical studies using radiotherapy alone [95]. Then, the New Approaches to Brain Tumor Therapy (NABTT) consortium assigned 365 patients with newly diagnosed glioblastoma in phase II clinical trial for testing novel agents in combination with radiation + temozolomide and compared the results with the data from the European Organization for Research and Treatment of Cancer (EORTC) phase II study [96, 97]. It is interesting to note that patients treated with radiation + temozolomide + Poly-ICLC had significantly longer survival than patients treated with only radiation + temozolomide between 2000 and 2002 [96]. However, these encouraging data have to be interpreted with circumspection because of the changing patterns of care. Concerning Ampligen product, only two clinical trials (phase I/II) are in progress (recruiting status) in which the dsRNA Ampligen is used as adjuvant for oxidized tumor cell lysate vaccination for patients with ovarian, fallopian tube, or primary peritoneal cancer, or as adjuvant for HER2 protein vaccination for patients with HER2-positive breast cancers.

4. Integrated view of the activities of TLR3 ligand in cancer

TLR3 agonist would have multiple cellular targets that could all contribute to the efficacy of their use in cancer.

As described above, targeting TLR3 expressed by tumor cells could trigger apoptosis and/or block cell cycle progression. It can also elicit the secretion of chemokines, which may recruit immune effectors at the site of the tumor and thereby enhance anticancer immune responses [36], or reduce the sensitivity of cancer cells to immuno-chemotherapy [98].Furthermore, many of the cytokines secreted by TLR3-stimulated cancer cells, and particularly the type I IFNs will enhance the intratumoral innate immune responses, while the upregulation of CD54 on cancer cells may also enhance the cytotoxic activity T cells, as it has been observed *in vitro* [37].

Among the human immune cells, TLR3 is mostly expressed by myeloid Dendritic Cells (mDC) [99], which represent the major Antigen-Presenting Cells, and by macrophages. However, TLR3 is only one of the dsRNA receptor present in mDC, altogether with RIG-I, MDA-5 and the two helicases complexes DDX1-DDX21-DHX36 and DHX9. In the presence of Poly(I:C), human mDC undergo phenotypic maturation and produce high amounts of IL-12 p70 [100, 101]. Moreover, TLR3 activation had been shown to enhance the antigen cross-presentation capability of mouse $CD8^+$ DC [102]. Recently, a subset of human mDC expressing BDCA3+ was found to internalize material from dead cells in vitro, and to cross-present exogenous antigens to CD8+ T cells upon treatment with poly(I:C) [103].

Activation of human T cells by Poly(I:C) is generally regarded as an indirect consequence of TLR3 DC stimulation. However, TLR3 can also be expressed by T cells, at least on gamma/delta T cells, and acts as co-stimulatory receptor to enhance proliferation and/or cytokine production of T-cell receptor-stimulated T lymphocytes [104].The clinical grade poly(I:C)-analogue (Ampligen) was reported to promote optimal human DC maturation and Th1-type T cell responses in vitro [105].

Moreover, Poly(I:C) was reported to induce $CD4^+$ human T cells synthesis of both IL-17A and IL-21 and was able to drive the differentiation of naive T helper cells into an IL-21-producing phenotype [106].TLR3 has also been described to directly increase IFN-gamma production by human Ag-specific CD8+ T cells [107]. Regarding human NK cells, in contrast to the initial description [108], their activation by dsRNA now appears to be secondary to IFN-gamma production by mDC in response to TLR3 stimulation [109, 110]. Thus, the combined activities of TLR3 on human mDC and T cells are likely to help developing Th1-polarized and strong cytotoxic T cells responses.

Indeed, syngeneic mouse tumor models have shown the importance of TLR3 expressed on non-cancer cells not only in tumor immunosurveillance but also for the control of tumor growth. Protection conferred by tumor vaccine including Poly(I:C) was mediated by primary and memory CD8+ T cells that has been robustly activated by antigen cross-presenting DC [111-115], and by IFN-I-activated NK cells [115]. Moreover, in a mouse model of established pulmonary metastasis, Poly(I:C) elicited a Th1-like, Th17-like, and cytotoxic immune environment following the activation of DCs and the production of IFN type [116]. Those animal models allowed also to show that combining Poly(I:C) with CD40 signaling dramatically increased the efficacy of mouse tumor vaccine [117, 118]. Such adjuvant combination was also able to convert mouse ovarian cancer-infiltrating dendritic cells from immunosuppressive to immunostimulatory cells [119]

TLR3 agonist might also restrain tumor-driven blood supply, as multiple human endothelial cell types express surface TLR3, and as dsRNA-induced TLR3 activation inhibits *in vitro* angiogenesis [120]. Moreover, siRNA was found to inhibit in a sequence-independent, and possibly TLR3-dependent manner, the dermal neovascularization in mice [121] and the proliferation and morphogenesis of endothelial cells in a mouse model of hepatocellular carcinoma in vivo [122].

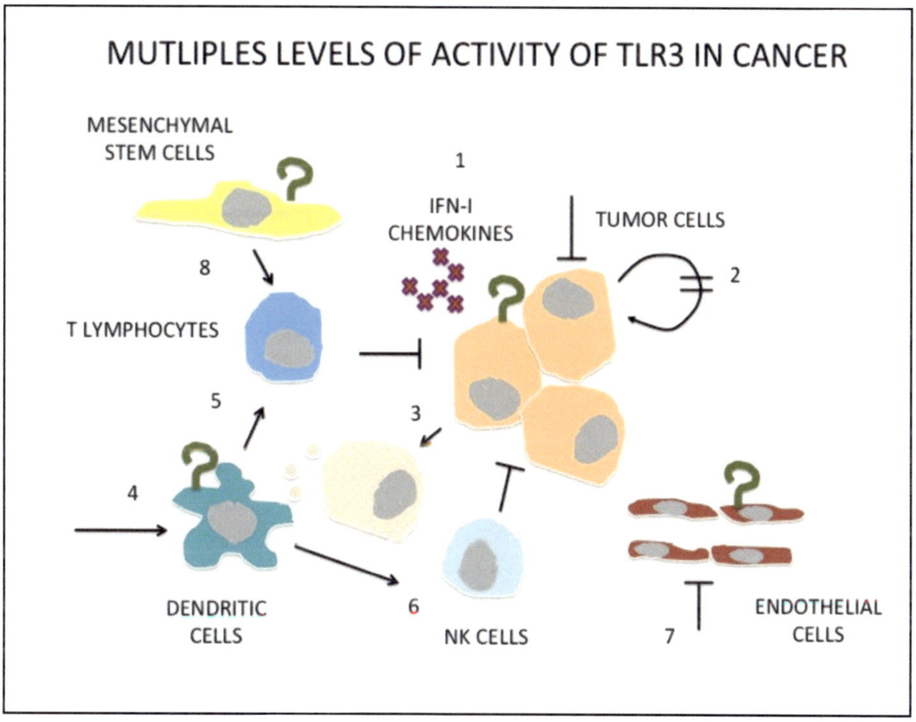

Figure 2. **(1)**TLR3 can stimulate cancer cells to secrete proinflammatory cytokine sand chemokines that attract and activate immune cells, respectively; **(2)**TLR3 can inhibit the proliferation of cancer cells; **(3)** TLR3 can trigger the apoptosis of cancer cells and the release of apoptotic bodies; **(4)**TLR3 can activate DC; **(5)** TLR3 can enhance the efficacy of DC to generate Th1 cells and cytotoxic T cells; **(6)** TLR3 can help NK cells to become cytotoxic; **(7)** TLR3 can inhibit tumor-driven neoangiogeneis; **(8)** TLR3 can switch MSC from immunosuppressive to immunosupportive phenotype.

Lastly, Toll-Like Receptor 3, which is strongly expressed by human mesenchymal stem cells (MSC), inhibits their Notch-dependent immunosuppressive effect on T cells [14]. In addition, in response to TLR3-triggering, MSC sustain and amplify the functions of neutrophils and may consequently contribute to local inflammation [123].

Many of the above-mentioned mechanisms summarized in figure 2 probably contribute to the remarkable activity of Poly(I:C) used as vaccine adjuvant in several mouse tumor models [113, 124].Indeed, compared with other TLR agonists, DC stimulated with poly(I:C) displayed the strongest activity in stimulating proinflammatory responses and the production of tumor-specific CD8(+) T cells in several mouse tumor models [125] Interestingly, the combination of TLR3 with TLR7 ligands increased the capacity of mouse DC to establish an in vivo anti-tumoral response [126].

5. Conclusions and prospectives

Since the first description of TLR in mouse, the members of this family of receptors have been linked to the activation of the innate immunity (Medzhitov et al., 1997). It was therefore natural to study the adjuvancy capabilities of TLR ligands for vaccines, including anti-tumor vaccines. However, the ongoing recognition of the multiple levels of action of TLR on immune and non-immune cells indicates that a better understanding of the result of these combined activities will be required to anticipate how TLR agonist might interfere with cancer progression.

Regarding TLR3 agonists, evidences coming not only from *in vitro* experiments and from preclinical mouse models, but also from clinical data strongly suggest that they could be useful in cancer. In particular, the discovery that TLR3 behaves as a death receptor selectively in cancer cells makes it similar to TRAIL receptors that are currently targeted in phase II clinical trials. However, answering a few key questions summarized in table1 will be required in order to determine whether and how TLR3 may become a successful target in cancer.

1. Which are the molecular mechanisms that underlie the sensitivity vs. the resistance of normal and cancer cells to TLR3-triggered apoptosis?
Answer to this question should help to identify a priori tumors that would benefit from TLR3 agonist treatment
2. What is the net effect of the pro-apoptotic activity on cancer cells and the immunostimulatory effect of TLR3 ligand on tumor progression?
This important question has not been addressed yet as, in contrast with human tumors, mouse tumor appears to be rather resistant to TLR3-triggerd apoptosis
3. Could TLR3 agonist synergize which (chemotherapeutic) drugs and allow increasing their efficacy while limiting their toxicity?
This question must also be addressed in a syngeneic tumor model that associates a tumor sensitive to TLR3-triggered apoptosis and a fully functional immune system

Table 1. Unsolved questions related to tlr3 and cancer

Author details

Yann Estornes, Toufic Renno and Serge Lebecque*
Cancer Research Center of Lyon, UMR5286 CNRS/INSERM/University Lyon 1 UCBL, Lyon, France

Olivier Micheau
U866 INSERM/University of Burgundi, Dijon, France

* Corresponding Author

6. References

[1] Zhang Z, Kim T, Bao M, Facchinetti V, Jung SY, Ghaffari AA, et al. DDX1, DDX21, and DHX36 Helicases Form a Complex with the Adaptor Molecule TRIF to Sense dsRNA in Dendritic Cells. Immunity 2011;34(6):866-78.

[2] Zhang Z, Yuan B, Lu N, Facchinetti V, Liu YJ. DHX9 pairs with IPS-1 to sense double-stranded RNA in myeloid dendritic cells. J Immunol 2011;187(9):4501-8.

[3] Alexopoulou L, Holt AC, Medzhitov R, Flavell RA. Recognition of double-stranded RNA and activation of NF-kappaB by Toll-like receptor 3. Nature 2001;413(6857):732-8.

[4] Vercammen E, Staal J, Beyaert R. Sensing of viral infection and activation of innate immunity by toll-like receptor 3. Clin Microbiol Rev 2008;21(1):13-25.

[5] Zhang SY, Jouanguy E, Ugolini S, Smahi A, Elain G, Romero P, et al. TLR3 deficiency in patients with herpes simplex encephalitis. Science 2007;317(5844):1522-7.

[6] Begon E, Michel L, Flageul B, Beaudoin I, Jean-Louis F, Bachelez H, et al. Expression, subcellular localization and cytokinic modulation of Toll-like receptors (TLRs) in normal human keratinocytes: TLR2 up-regulation in psoriatic skin. Eur J Dermatol 2007;17(6):497-506.

[7] Schreiner B, Voss J, Wischhusen J, Dombrowski Y, Steinle A, Lochmuller H, et al. Expression of toll-like receptors by human muscle cells in vitro and in vivo: TLR3 is highly expressed in inflammatory and HIV myopathies, mediates IL-8 release and up-regulation of NKG2D-ligands. Faseb J 2006;20(1):118-20.

[8] Wornle M, Schmid H, Banas B, Merkle M, Henger A, Roeder M, et al. Novel role of toll-like receptor 3 in hepatitis C-associated glomerulonephritis. Am J Pathol 2006;168(2):370-85.

[9] Ritter M, Mennerich D, Weith A, Seither P. Characterization of Toll-like receptors in primary lung epithelial cells: strong impact of the TLR3 ligand poly(I:C) on the regulation of Toll-like receptors, adaptor proteins and inflammatory response. J Inflamm (Lond) 2005;2:16.

[10] Cario E, Podolsky DK. Differential alteration in intestinal epithelial cell expression of toll-like receptor 3 (TLR3) and TLR4 in inflammatory bowel disease. Infect Immun 2000;68(12):7010-7.

[11] Salaun B, Coste I, Rissoan MC, Lebecque SJ, Renno T. TLR3 can directly trigger apoptosis in human cancer cells. J Immunol 2006;176(8):4894-901.

[12] Uehara A, Fujimoto Y, Fukase K, Takada H. Various human epithelial cells express functional Toll-like receptors, NOD1 and NOD2 to produce anti-microbial peptides, but not proinflammatory cytokines. Mol Immunol 2007;44(12):3100-11.

[13] Hultcrantz M, Huhn MH, Wolf M, Olsson A, Jacobson S, Williams BR, et al. Interferons induce an antiviral state in human pancreatic islet cells. Virology 2007;367(1):92-101.

[14] Liotta F, Angeli R, Cosmi L, Fili L, Manuelli C, Frosali F, et al. Toll-like receptors 3 and 4 are expressed by human bone marrow-derived mesenchymal stem cells and can inhibit their T-cell modulatory activity by impairing Notch signaling. Stem Cells 2008;26(1):279-89.

[15] Tissari J, Siren J, Meri S, Julkunen I, Matikainen S. IFN-alpha enhances TLR3-mediated antiviral cytokine expression in human endothelial and epithelial cells by up-regulating TLR3 expression. J Immunol 2005;174(7):4289-94.

[16] Lafon M, Megret F, Lafage M, Prehaud C. The innate immune facet of brain: human neurons express TLR-3 and sense viral dsRNA. J Mol Neurosci 2006;29(3):185-94.

[17] Limmon GV, Arredouani M, McCann KL, Corn Minor RA, Kobzik L, Imani F. Scavenger receptor class-A is a novel cell surface receptor for double-stranded RNA. Faseb J 2008;22(1):159-67.

[18] Jiang Z, Zamanian-Daryoush M, Nie H, Silva AM, Williams BR, Li X. Poly(I-C)-induced Toll-like receptor 3 (TLR3)-mediated activation of NFkappa B and MAP kinase is through an interleukin-1 receptor-associated kinase (IRAK)-independent pathway employing the signaling components TLR3-TRAF6-TAK1-TAB2-PKR. J Biol Chem 2003;278(19):16713-9.

[19] Silva AM, Whitmore M, Xu Z, Jiang Z, Li X, Williams BR. Protein kinase R (PKR) interacts with and activates mitogen-activated protein kinase kinase 6 (MKK6) in response to double-stranded RNA stimulation. J Biol Chem 2004;279(36):37670-6.

[20] Fitzgerald KA, McWhirter SM, Faia KL, Rowe DC, Latz E, Golenbock DT, et al. IKKepsilon and TBK1 are essential components of the IRF3 signaling pathway. Nat Immunol 2003;4(5):491-6.

[21] Häcker H, Redecke V, Blagoev B, Kratchmarova I, Hsu LC, Wang GG, et al. Specificity in Toll-like receptor signalling through distinct effector functions of TRAF3 and TRAF6. Nature 2006;439(7073):204-7.

[22] Sato M, Tanaka N, Hata N, Oda E, Taniguchi T. Involvement of the IRF family transcription factor IRF-3 in virus-induced activation of the IFN-beta gene. FEBS Lett 1998;425(1):112-6.

[23] Meylan E, Burns K, Hofmann K, Blancheteau V, Martinon F, Kelliher M, et al. RIP1 is an essential mediator of Toll-like receptor 3-induced NF-kappa B activation. Nat Immunol 2004;5(5):503-7.

[24] Cusson-Hermance N, Khurana S, Lee TH, Fitzgerald KA, Kelliher MA. Rip1 mediates the Trif-dependent toll-like receptor 3- and 4-induced NF-{kappa}B activation but does not contribute to interferon regulatory factor 3 activation. J Biol Chem 2005;280(44):36560-6.

[25] Salaun B, Zitvogel L, Asselin-Paturel C, Morel Y, Chemin K, Dubois C, et al. TLR3 as a biomarker for the therapeutic efficacy of double-stranded RNA in breast cancer. Cancer Res 2011;71(5):1607-14.

[26] Chuang HC, Huang CC, Chien CY, Chuang JH. Toll-like receptor 3-mediated tumor invasion in head and neck cancer. Oral Oncol 2012;48(3):226-32.

[27] Hasimu A, Ge L, Li QZ, Zhang RP, Guo X. Expressions of Toll-like receptors 3, 4, 7, and 9 in cervical lesions and their correlation with HPV16 infection in Uighur women. Chin J Cancer 2011;30(5):344-50.

[28] Zhou M, McFarland-Mancini MM, Funk HM, Husseinzadeh N, Mounajjed T, Drew AF. Toll-like receptor expression in normal ovary and ovarian tumors. Cancer Immunol Immunother 2009;58(9):1375-85.

[29] Rydberg C, Mansson A, Uddman R, Riesbeck K, Cardell LO. Toll-like receptor agonists induce inflammation and cell death in a model of head and neck squamous cell carcinomas. Immunology 2009;128(1 Suppl):e600-11.

[30] González-Reyes S, Fernández JM, González LO, Aguirre A, Suárez A, González JM, et al. Study of TLR3, TLR4, and TLR9 in prostate carcinomas and their association with biochemical recurrence. Cancer Immunol Immunother 2011;60(2):217-26.

[31] Salaun B, Lebecque S, Matikainen S, Rimoldi D, Romero P. Toll-like receptor 3 expressed by melanoma cells as a target for therapy? Clin Cancer Res 2007;13(15 Pt 1):4565-74.

[32] Goto Y, Arigami T, Kitago M, Nguyen SL, Narita N, Ferrone S, et al. Activation of Toll-like receptors 2, 3, and 4 on human melanoma cells induces inflammatory factors. Mol Cancer Ther 2008;7(11):3642-53.

[33] Sheyhidin I, Nabi G, Hasim A, Zhang RP, Ainiwaer J, Ma H, et al. Overexpression of TLR3, TLR4, TLR7 and TLR9 in esophageal squamous cell carcinoma. World J Gastroenterol 2011;17(32):3745-51.

[34] Matijevic T, Marjanovic M, Pavelic J. Functionally active toll-like receptor 3 on human primary and metastatic cancer cells. Scand J Immunol 2009;70(1):18-24.

[35] Chiron D, Jego G, Pellat-Deuceunynck C. Toll-like receptors: expression and involvement in multiple myeloma. Leuk Res 2010;34(12):1545-50.

[36] Galli R, Starace D, Busà R, Angelini DF, Paone A, De Cesaris P, et al. TLR stimulation of prostate tumor cells induces chemokine-mediated recruitment of specific immune cell types. J Immunol 2010;184(12):6658-69.

[37] Shojaei H, Oberg HH, Juricke M, Marischen L, Kunz M, Mundhenke C, et al. Toll-like Receptors 3 and 7 Agonists Enhance Tumor Cell Lysis by Human {gamma}{delta} T Cells. Cancer Res 2009.

[38] Zhang Y, Sun R, Liu B, Deng M, Zhang W, Li Y, et al. TLR3 activation inhibits nasopharyngeal carcinoma metastasis via downregulation of chemokine receptor CXCR4. Cancer Biol Ther 2009;8(19).

[39] Chiron D, Pellat-Deceunynck C, Amiot M, Bataille R, Jego G. TLR3 ligand induces NF-{kappa}B activation and various fates of multiple myeloma cells depending on IFN-{alpha} production. J Immunol 2009;182(7):4471-8.

[40] Pries R, Hogrefe L, Xie L, Frenzel H, Brocks C, Ditz C, et al. Induction of c-Myc-dependent cell proliferation through toll-like receptor 3 in head and neck cancer. Int J Mol Med 2008;21(2):209-15.

[41] McCall KD, Harii N, Lewis CJ, Malgor R, Kim WB, Saji M, et al. High basal levels of functional toll-like receptor 3 (TLR3) and noncanonical Wnt5a are expressed in papillary thyroid cancer and are coordinately decreased by phenylmethimazole together with cell proliferation and migration. Endocrinology 2007;148(9):4226-37.

[42] Yu M, Lam J, Rada B, Leto TL, Levine SJ. Double-stranded RNA induces shedding of the 34-kDa soluble TNFR1 from human airway epithelial cells via TLR3-TRIF-RIP1-dependent signaling: roles for dual oxidase 2- and caspase-dependent pathways. J Immunol 2011;186(2):1180-8.

[43] Whitson JM, Noonan EJ, Pookot D, Place RF, Dahiya R. Double stranded-RNA-mediated activation of P21 gene induced apoptosis and cell cycle arrest in renal cell carcinoma. Int J Cancer 2009;125(2):446-52.

[44] Weber A, Kirejczyk Z, Besch R, Potthoff S, Leverkus M, Hacker G. Proapoptotic signalling through Toll-like receptor-3 involves TRIF-dependent activation of caspase-8 and is under the control of inhibitor of apoptosis proteins in melanoma cells. Cell Death Differ 2009;17(6):942-51.

[45] Taura M, Fukuda R, Suico MA, Eguma A, Koga T, Shuto T, et al. TLR3 induction by anticancer drugs potentiates poly I:C-induced tumor cell apoptosis. Cancer Sci 2010;101(7):1610-7.

[46] Paone A, Starace D, Galli R, Padula F, De Cesaris P, Filippini A, et al. Toll-like receptor 3 triggers apoptosis of human prostate cancer cells through a PKC-alpha-dependent mechanism. Carcinogenesis 2008;29(7):1334-42.

[47] Morikawa T, Sugiyama A, Kume H, Ota S, Kashima T, Tomita K, et al. Identification of Toll-like receptor 3 as a potential therapeutic target in clear cell renal cell carcinoma. Clin Cancer Res 2007;13(19):5703-9.

[48] Jiang Q, Wei H, Tian Z. Poly I:C enhances cycloheximide-induced apoptosis of tumor cells through TLR3 pathway. BMC Cancer 2008;8:12.

[49] Friboulet L, Gourzones C, Tsao SW, Morel Y, Paturel C, Temam S, et al. Poly(I:C) induces intense expression of c-IAP2 and cooperates with an IAP inhibitor in induction of apoptosis in cancer cells. BMC Cancer 2010;10:327.

[50] Friboulet L, Pioche-Durieu C, Rodriguez S, Valent A, Souquere S, Ripoche H, et al. Recurrent overexpression of c-IAP2 in EBV-associated nasopharyngeal carcinomas: critical role in resistance to Toll-like receptor 3-mediated apoptosis. Neoplasia 2008;10(11):1183-94.

[51] Harashima N, Inao T, Imamura R, Okano S, Suda T, Harada M. Roles of the PI3K/Akt pathway and autophagy in TLR3 signaling-induced apoptosis and growth arrest of human prostate cancer cells. Cancer Immunol Immunother 2011; 61(5):667-76.

[52] Hasan UA, Caux C, Perrot I, Doffin AC, Menetrier-Caux C, Trinchieri G, et al. Cell proliferation and survival induced by Toll-like receptors is antagonized by type I IFNs. Proc Natl Acad Sci U S A 2007;104(19):8047-52.

[53] Kerr JF, Wyllie AH, Currie AR. Apoptosis: a basic biological phenomenon with wide-ranging implications in tissue kinetics. Br J Cancer 1972;26(4):239-57.

[54] Feoktistova M, Geserick P, Kellert B, Dimitrova DP, Langlais C, Hupe M, et al. cIAPs Block Ripoptosome Formation, a RIP1/Caspase-8 Containing Intracellular Cell Death Complex Differentially Regulated by cFLIP Isoforms. Mol Cell 2011;43(3):449-63.

[55] Estornes Y, Toscano F, Virard F, Jacquemin G, Pierrot A, Vanbervliet B, et al. dsRNA induces apoptosis through an atypical death complex associating TLR3 to caspase-8. Cell Death Differ 2012; 19(9):1482-94.

[56] Ruckdeschel K, Pfaffinger G, Haase R, Sing A, Weighardt H, Hacker G, et al. Signaling of apoptosis through TLRs critically involves toll/IL-1 receptor domain-containing adapter inducing IFN-beta, but not MyD88, in bacteria-infected murine macrophages. J Immunol 2004;173(5):3320-8.

[57] Kaiser WJ, Offermann MK. Apoptosis induced by the toll-like receptor adaptor TRIF is dependent on its receptor interacting protein homotypic interaction motif. J Immunol 2005;174(8):4942-52.

[58] Knox PG, Davies CC, Ioannou M, Eliopoulos AG. The death domain kinase RIP1 links the immunoregulatory CD40 receptor to apoptotic signaling in carcinomas. J Cell Biol 2011;192(3):391-9.

[59] Shikama Y, Yamada M, Miyashita T. Caspase-8 and caspase-10 activate NF-kappaB through RIP, NIK and IKKalpha kinases. Eur J Immunol 2003;33(7):1998-2006.

[60] Petersen SL, Wang L, Yalcin-Chin A, Li L, Peyton M, Minna J, et al. Autocrine TNFalpha signaling renders human cancer cells susceptible to Smac-mimetic-induced apoptosis. Cancer Cell 2007;12(5):445-56.

[61] Varfolomeev E, Blankenship JW, Wayson SM, Fedorova AV, Kayagaki N, Garg P, et al. IAP antagonists induce autoubiquitination of c-IAPs, NF-kappaB activation, and TNFalpha-dependent apoptosis. Cell 2007;131(4):669-81.

[62] Vince JE, Wong WW, Khan N, Feltham R, Chau D, Ahmed AU, et al. IAP antagonists target cIAP1 to induce TNFalpha-dependent apoptosis. Cell 2007;131(4):682-93.

[63] Bertrand MJ, Milutinovic S, Dickson KM, Ho WC, Boudreault A, Durkin J, et al. cIAP1 and cIAP2 facilitate cancer cell survival by functioning as E3 ligases that promote RIP1 ubiquitination. Mol Cell 2008;30(6):689-700.

[64] Varfolomeev E, Goncharov T, Fedorova AV, Dynek JN, Zobel K, Deshayes K, et al. c-IAP1 and c-IAP2 are critical mediators of tumor necrosis factor alpha (TNFalpha)-induced NF-kappaB activation. J Biol Chem 2008;283(36):24295-9.

[65] O'Donnell MA, Legarda Addison D, Skountzos P, Yeh WC, Ting AT. Ubiquitination of RIP1 regulates an NF-kappaB-independent cell-death switch in TNF signaling. Curr Biol 2007;17(5):418-24.

[66] Wang L, Du F, Wang X. TNF alpha induces two distinct caspase-8 activation pathways. Cell 2008;133(4):693-703.

[67] O'Donnell MA, Ting AT. RIP1 comes back to life as a cell death regulator in TNFR1 signaling. Febs J 2011;278(6):877-87.

[68] Ermolaeva MA, Michallet MC, Papadopoulou N, Utermohlen O, Kranidioti K, Kollias G, et al. Function of TRADD in tumor necrosis factor receptor 1 signaling and in TRIF-dependent inflammatory responses. Nat Immunol 2008;9(9):1037-46.

[69] Pobezinskaya YL, Kim YS, Choksi S, Morgan MJ, Li T, Liu C, et al. The function of TRADD in signaling through tumor necrosis factor receptor 1 and TRIF-dependent Toll-like receptors. Nat Immunol 2008;9(9):1047-54.

[70] Tenev T, Bianchi K, Darding M, Broemer M, Langlais C, Wallberg F, et al. The Ripoptosome, a Signaling Platform that Assembles in Response to Genotoxic Stress and Loss of IAPs. Mol Cell 2011;43(3):432-48.

[71] Irmler M, Thome M, Hahne M, Schneider P, Hofmann K, Steiner V, et al. Inhibition of death receptor signals by cellular FLIP. Nature 1997;388(6638):190-5.

[72] Sharp DA, Lawrence DA, Ashkenazi A. Selective knockdown of the long variant of cellular FLICE inhibitory protein augments death receptor-mediated caspase-8 activation and apoptosis. J Biol Chem 2005;280(19):19401-9.

[73] Micheau O, Lens S, Gaide O, Alevizopoulos K, Tschopp J. NF-kappaB signals induce the expression of c-FLIP. Mol Cell Biol 2001;21(16):5299-305.

[74] Boatright KM, Deis C, Denault JB, Sutherlin DP, Salvesen GS. Activation of caspases-8 and -10 by FLIP(L). Biochem J 2004;382:651-7.

[75] Umemura N, Zhu J, Mburu YK, Forero A, Hsieh PN, Muthuswamy R, et al. Defective NF-?B signaling in metastatic head and neck cancer cells leads to enhanced apoptosis by double-stranded RNA. Cancer Res 2012;72(1):45-55.

[76] Micheau O, Thome M, Schneider P, Holler N, Tschopp J, Nicholson DW, et al. The long form of FLIP is an activator of caspase-8 at the Fas death-inducing signaling complex. J Biol Chem 2002;277(47):45162-71.

[77] Pop C, Oberst A, Drag M, Van Raam BJ, Riedl SJ, Green DR, et al. FLIP(L) induces caspase 8 activity in the absence of interdomain caspase 8 cleavage and alters substrate specificity. Biochem J 2011;433(3):447-57.

[78] Oberst A, Dillon CP, Weinlich R, McCormick LL, Fitzgerald P, Pop C, et al. Catalytic activity of the caspase-8-FLIP(L) complex inhibits RIPK3-dependent necrosis. Nature 2011;471(7338):363-7.

[79] Varfolomeev EE, Schuchmann M, Luria V, Chiannilkulchai N, Beckmann JS, Mett IL, et al. Targeted disruption of the mouse Caspase 8 gene ablates cell death induction by the TNF receptors, Fas/Apo1, and DR3 and is lethal prenatally. Immunity 1998;9(2):267-76.

[80] Sakamaki K, Inoue T, Asano M, Sudo K, Kazama H, Sakagami J, et al. Ex vivo whole-embryo culture of caspase-8-deficient embryos normalize their aberrant phenotypes in the developing neural tube and heart. Cell Death Differ 2002;9(11):1196-206.

[81] Kaiser WJ, Upton JW, Long AB, Livingston-Rosanoff D, Daley-Bauer LP, Hakem R, et al. RIP3 mediates the embryonic lethality of caspase-8-deficient mice. Nature 2011;471(7338):368-72.

[82] Hitomi J, Christofferson DE, Ng A, Yao J, Degterev A, Xavier RJ, et al. Identification of a molecular signaling network that regulates a cellular necrotic cell death pathway. Cell 2008;135(7):1311-23.

[83] Cho YS, Challa S, Moquin D, Genga R, Ray TD, Guildford M, et al. Phosphorylation-driven assembly of the RIP1-RIP3 complex regulates programmed necrosis and virus-induced inflammation. Cell 2009;137(6):1112-23.

[84] O'Donnell MA, Perez-Jimenez E, Oberst A, Ng A, Massoumi R, Xavier R, et al. Caspase 8 inhibits programmed necrosis by processing CYLD. Nat Cell Biol 2011;13(12):1437-42.

[85] Degterev A, Hitomi J, Germscheid M, Ch'en IL, Korkina O, Teng X, et al. Identification of RIP1 kinase as a specific cellular target of necrostatins. Nat Chem Biol 2008;4(5):313-21.

[86] Green DR, Oberst A, Dillon CP, Weinlich R, Salvesen GS. RIPK-dependent necrosis and its regulation by caspases: a mystery in five acts. Mol Cell 2011;44(1):9-16.

[87] Vandenabeele P, Galluzzi L, Vanden Berghe T, Kroemer G. Molecular mechanisms of necroptosis: an ordered cellular explosion. Nat Rev Mol Cell Biol 2010;11(10):700-14.

[88] Vanlangenakker N, Vanden Berghe T, Vandenabeele P. Many stimuli pull the necrotic trigger, an overview. Cell Death Differ 2012;19(1):75-86.

[89] Nordlund JJ, Wolff SM, Levy HB. Inhibition of biologic activity of poly I: poly C by human plasma. Proc Soc Exp Biol Med 1970;133(2):439-44.

[90] Robinson RA, DeVita VT, Levy HB, Baron S, Hubbard SP, Levine AS. A phase I-II trial of multiple-dose polyriboinosic-polyribocytidylic acid in patieonts with leukemia or solid tumors. J Natl Cancer Inst 1976;57(3):599-602.

[91] Levy HB, Baer G, Baron S, Buckler CE, Gibbs CJ, Iadarola MJ, et al. A modified polyriboinosinic-polyribocytidylic acid complex that induces interferon in primates. J Infect Dis 1975;132(4):434-9.

[92] Strayer DR, Carter WA, Brodsky I, Cheney P, Peterson D, Salvato P, et al. A controlled clinical trial with a specifically configured RNA drug, poly(I).poly(C12U), in chronic fatigue syndrome. Clin Infect Dis 1994;18:S88-95.

[93] Gowen BB, Wong MH, Jung KH, Sanders AB, Mitchell WM, Alexopoulou L, et al. TLR3 is essential for the induction of protective immunity against Punta Toro Virus infection by the double-stranded RNA (dsRNA), poly(I:C12U), but not Poly(I:C): differential recognition of synthetic dsRNA molecules. J Immunol 2007;178(8):5200-8.

[94] Goutagny N, Estornes Y, Hasan U, Lebecque S, Caux C. Targeting pattern recognition receptors in cancer immunotherapy. Target Oncol 2012;7(1):29-54.

[95] Butowski N, Chang SM, Junck L, DeAngelis LM, Abrey L, Fink K, et al. A phase II clinical trial of poly-ICLC with radiation for adult patients with newly diagnosed supratentorial glioblastoma: a North American Brain Tumor Consortium (NABTC01-05). J Neurooncol 2009;91(2):175-82.

[96] Grossman SA, Ye X, Piantadosi S, Desideri S, Nabors LB, Rosenfeld M, et al. Survival of patients with newly diagnosed glioblastoma treated with radiation and temozolomide in research studies in the United States. Clin Cancer Res 2010;16(8):2443-9.

[97] Stupp R, Mason WP, van den Bent MJ, Weller M, Fisher B, Taphoorn MJ, et al. Radiotherapy plus concomitant and adjuvant temozolomide for glioblastoma. N Engl J Med 2005;352(10):987-96.

[98] Conforti R, Ma Y, Morel Y, Paturel C, Terme M, Viaud S, et al. Opposing effects of toll-like receptor (TLR3) signaling in tumors can be therapeutically uncoupled to optimize the anticancer efficacy of TLR3 ligands. Cancer Res 2010;70(2):490-500.

[99] Kadowaki N, Ho S, Antonenko S, Malefyt RW, Kastelein RA, Bazan F, et al. Subsets of human dendritic cell precursors express different toll-like receptors and respond to different microbial antigens. J Exp Med 2001;194(6):863-9

[100] Loré K, Betts MR, Brenchley JM, Kuruppu J, Khojasteh S, Perfetto S, et al. Toll-like receptor ligands modulate dendritic cells to augment cytomegalovirus- and HIV-1-specific T cell responses. J Immunol 2003;171(8):4320-8.

[101] Hovden AO, Karlsen M, Jonsson R, Appel S. The bacterial preparation OK432 induces IL-12p70 secretion in human dendritic cells in a TLR3 dependent manner. PLoS One 2012;Epub 2012 Feb 21.

[102] Schulz O, Diebold SS, Chen M, Naslund TI, Nolte MA, Alexopoulou L, et al. Toll-like receptor 3 promotes cross-priming to virus-infected cells. Nature 2005;433(7028):887-92.

[103] Poulin LF, Salio M, Griessinger E, Anjos-Afonso F, Craciun L, Chen JL, et al. Characterization of human DNGR-1+ BDCA3+ leukocytes as putative equivalents of mouse CD8alpha+ dendritic cells. J Exp Med 2010;207(6):1261-71.

[104] Wesch D, Beetz S, Oberg HH, Marget M, Krengel K, Kabelitz D. Direct costimulatory effect of TLR3 ligand poly(I:C) on human gamma delta T lymphocytes. J Immunol 2006;176(3):1348-54.

[105] Navabi H, Jasani B, Reece A, Clayton A, Tabi Z, Donninger C, et al. A clinical grade poly I:C-analogue (Ampligen) promotes optimal DC maturation and Th1-type T cell responses of healthy donors and cancer patients in vitro. Vaccine 2009;27(1):107-15.

[106] Holm CK, Petersen CC, Hvid M, Petersen L, Paludan SR, Deleuran B, et al. TLR3 ligand polyinosinic:polycytidylic acid induces IL-17A and IL-21 synthesis in human Th cells. J Immunol 2009;183(7):4422-31.

[107] Tabiasco J, Devevre E, Rufer N, Salaun B, Cerottini JC, Speiser D, et al. Human effector CD8+ T lymphocytes express TLR3 as a functional coreceptor. J Immunol 2006;177(12):8708-13.

[108] Schmidt KN, Leung B, Kwong M, Zarember KA, Satyal S, Navas TA, et al. APC-independent activation of NK cells by the Toll-like receptor 3 agonist double-stranded RNA. J Immunol 2004;172(1):138-43.

[109] Perrot I, Deauvieau F, Massacrier C, Hughes N, Garrone P, Durand I, et al. TLR3 and Rig-like receptor on myeloid dendritic cells and Rig-like receptor on human NK cells are both mandatory for production of IFN-gamma in response to double-stranded RNA. J Immunol 2010;185(4):2080-8.

[110] Eriksson M, Meadows SK, Basu S, Mselle TF, Wira CR, Sentman CL. TLRs mediate IFN-gamma production by human uterine NK cells in endometrium. J Immunol 2006;176(10):6219-24.

[111] Salem ML, Kadima AN, Cole DJ, Gillanders WE. Defining the antigen-specific T-cell response to vaccination and poly(I:C)/TLR3 signaling: evidence of enhanced primary

and memory CD8 T-cell responses and antitumor immunity. J Immunother 2005;28(3):220-8.

[112] Salaun B, Greutert M, Romero P. Toll-like receptor 3 is necessary for dsRNA adjuvant effects. Vaccine 2009;27(12):1841-7.

[113] Wick DA, Martin SD, Nelson BH, Webb JR. Profound CD8+ T cell immunity elicited by sequential daily immunization with exogenous antigen plus the TLR3 agonist poly(I:C). Vaccine 2011;29(5):984-93.

[114] Jelinek I, Leonard JN, Price GE, Brown KN, Meyer-Manlapat A, Goldsmith PK, et al. TLR3-specific double-stranded RNA oligonucleotide adjuvants induce dendritic cell cross-presentation, CTL responses, and antiviral protection. J Immunol 2011;186(4):2422-9.

[115] Park JS, Kim HS, Park HM, Kim CH, Kim TG. Efficient induction of anti-tumor immunity by a TAT-CEA fusion protein vaccine with poly(I:C) in a murine colorectal tumor model. Vaccine 2011;29(47):8642-8.

[116] Forte G, Rega A, Morello S, Luciano A, Arra C, Pinto A, et al. Polyinosinic Polycytidylic Acid Limits Tumor Outgrowth in a Mouse Model of Metastatic Lung Cancer. J Immunol 2012; 188(11):5357-64.

[117] Aranda F, Llopiz D, Díaz-Valdés N, Riezu-Boj JI, Bezunartea J, Ruiz M, et al. Adjuvant combination and antigen targeting as a strategy to induce polyfunctional and high-avidity T-cell responses against poorly immunogenic tumors. Cancer Res 2011;71(9):3214-24.

[118] Cho HI, Celis E. Optimized peptide vaccines eliciting extensive CD8 T-cell responses with therapeutic antitumor effects. Cancer Res 2009;69(23):9012-9.

[119] Scarlett UK, Cubillos-Ruiz JR, Nesbeth YC, Martinez DG, Engle X, Gewirtz AT, et al. In situ stimulation of CD40 and Toll-like receptor 3 transforms ovarian cancer-infiltrating dendritic cells from immunosuppressive to immunostimulatory cells. Cancer Res 2009;69(18):7329-37.

[120] Guo Z, Chen L, Zhu Y, Zhang Y, He S, Qin J, et al. Double-stranded RNA-induced TLR3 activation inhibits angiogenesis and triggers apoptosis of human hepatocellular carcinoma cells. Oncol Rep 2012;27(2):396-402.

[121] Kleinman ME, Yamada K, Takeda A, Chandrasekaran V, Nozaki M, Baffi JZ, et al. Sequence- and target-independent angiogenesis suppression by siRNA via TLR3. Nature 2008;452(7187):591-7.

[122] Bergé M, Bonnin P, Sulpice E, Vilar J, Allanic D, Silvestre JS, et al. Small interfering RNAs induce target-independent inhibition of tumor growth and vasculature remodeling in a mouse model of hepatocellular carcinoma. Am J Pathol 2010;177(6):3192-201.

[123] Cassatella MA, Mosna F, Micheletti A, Lisi V, Tamassia N, Cont C, et al. Toll-like receptor-3-activated human mesenchymal stromal cells significantly prolong the survival and function of neutrophils. Stem Cells 2011;29(6):1001-11.

[124] Zhu X, Nishimura F, Sasaki K, Fujita M, Dusak JE, Eguchi J, et al. Toll like receptor-3 ligand poly-ICLC promotes the efficacy of peripheral vaccinations with tumor antigen-derived peptide epitopes in murine CNS tumor models. J Transl Med 2007;5:10.

[125] Bogunovic D, Manches O, Godefroy E, Yewdall A, Gallois A, Salazar AM, et al. TLR4 engagement during TLR3-induced proinflammatory signaling in dendritic cells promotes IL-10-mediated suppression of antitumor immunity. Cancer Res 2011;71(16):5467-76.

[126] Warger T, Osterloh P, Rechtsteiner G, Fassbender M, Heib V, Schmid B, et al. Synergistic activation of dendritic cells by combined Toll-like receptor ligation induces superior CTL responses in vivo. Blood 2006;108(2):544-50.

Chapter 12

A Different Approach for Cellular Oncogene Identification Came from *Drosophila* Genetics

Laura Monica Magdalena and Lorand Savu

Additional information is available at the end of the chapter

http://dx.doi.org/10.5772/54150

1. Introduction

1.1. Cancer is a genetic disease

Cancer is a major health concern of our time, being responsible for more than 25% of deaths worldwide. The past two decades have produced strong evidence for the genetic basis of cancer. Cancer develops as a clonal disease occuring by the accumulation in multiple steps of genetic (or epigenetic) changes in oncogenes, tumor suppressor genes and "guardian" genes that support expansion of a new clone over the old one. Subsequently, it is the natural selection which helps expansion of a new clone carrying characteristics advantageous for proliferation [1, 2, 3].

Nevertheless, the events contributing to cancer are not restricted to the cancer cells. The most encountered example is the case of *NFkB* (nuclear factor kappa-light-chain-enhancer of activated B cells) which is a protein complex that controls the transcription of DNA, that may be up-regulated in hepatocytes through different changes in the expression of *TNF* (Tumor Necrosis Factor) from the neighboring stromal inflammatory cells, and thus can become a key contributor in many cancer cells [3].

Recently, it has been estimated that up to seven rate-limiting genetic / epigenetic events are needed for the development of a common human cancer [4]. These can appear in multiple different combinations depending on which particular tissue or cell-specific "anticancer" barriers are to be circumvented.

A lot of knowledge about cancer was obtained from studying rare familial "monogenic" cancer syndromes. Although the most of the cancer cases appear to be "sporadic", when cancer- causing gene mutations occurred only in adult somatic cells, these cases also proved to be important for understanding this intricate disease. Other important aspect refferes to the fact that many key molecular factors to cancer progression may not be deregulated at the gene level. Downstream signaling proteins may become up-regulated by alterations in upstream growth factor signaling, altered catabolism, genes inactivated by epigenetic factors, protein expression altered by enzyme activity, degradation, chaperones, etc [4].

The idea that genes determine the growth behavior of a cell is now widely accepted, with abnormal growth reflecting the action of abnormal genes. The transformation of a normal cell to a cancer cell starts with changes in growth regulatory genes, and in the course of tumor progression further escape from normal growth control is caused by additional alterations in genes that direct cell multiplication and cell survival. Therefore, either somatic or germline mutations are both considered the root cause of cancer. These heritable changes in cancer cells are subsequently the targets for current attempts to develop effective and specific therapies for this disease [2]. As a general rule, one can say that most things related to cancer are a matter of timing and are determined by many other factors like the cell of origin, the mutations accumulated and the environment, together referred to as the molecular "road map" leading to cancer.

At this time, more than 1% of all human genes are believed to be "cancer genes". Approximately 90% of them represent somatic mutations in cancer, 20% bear germ-line mutations that predispose to cancer and 10% show both somatic and germ-line mutations [1]. Therefore, it was assumed that there are far fewer "pathways" implicated in cancer than genes. The identification of disease-related genes has led to a number of available genetic tests that detect disease or an individual's risk of disease. Gene tests are available for different disorders and also in cancer testing, some good examples being for the *BRCA1* genes related to the breast cancer, or for MEN1 and RET genes which are linked with endocrine tumors. Once more disease linked-genes are discovered, more gene tests are expected to become available [1].

1.1.1. The origin of cancer

Cancer had been recognized throughout recorded history and was known to the ancient Egyptians, from around 1600 BC, but it was not studied until the seventeenth century, when the formal study of cancer (oncology) was first documented [1]. Nevertheless, only rather recently were registered spectacular progresses in describing the fundamental molecular basis of cancer, following the entry of molecular biology and especially of genetics.

Usually, cancer is behaving exactly as a clonal disease, beginning with a mutational episode in a single cell and then develops in multiple stages through the acquisition of further mutations which are inherited through division, by the progeny of that cell. As the same outcome can also arise by epigenetic factors that alter chromatin structure, without altering the coding DNA, mutations are not the only way in which a cancer cell acquires inactivation or activation of a key gene/ protein. Therefore, sometimes the term "epimutations" is used to encompass both major routes by which cancer cells acquire aberrant expression/activity of key genes and proteins.

The adult human has been estimated to contain in average as many as 10^{14} cells, most of which could theoretically become a cancer cell given the right sort of genetic (mutations) and epigenetic changes. Replicating cells may be most vulnerable to cancer-causing mutations. Even if some cell type, of which adult nerve cell are good examples, may avoid becoming cancer cell because they are essentially non-proliferating in the adult, most cells either regularly do or can at a pinch replicate [1]. It seems that most adult cells survive on average for 4-6 weeks and then have to be replaced. Also, over a thousand billion cells may die each day and are renewed either by replication of existing cells or from stem cells precursors. Given that every cell gets a significant amount of daily DNA damage and 10^{11} or more of them will replicate each day- that is a lot of potential cancer cells. Keeping this in mind a cancer might be expected to be a frequent incidence although so far this only happens in 1 in 3 people and usually even then only after 60 or 70 years of potentially mutation-causing events [1].

It was well documented that there is a geographical variation in cancer incidence and death, and this likely reflects socioeconomic factors. The different roles of genetic predisposition, gene-environment interaction and infectious agents shared importance in causing cancer. Recent research points to the considerable overlap between the behavior of cancer cells and that of cells during normal physiological wound healing and during embryogenesis. Similarities refers to replication, less differentiated state, invasion/migration, with the major differences reflecting the lack of control and the unscheduled nature of replication which characterizes cancer. One intrigued question addressed later was how the organism is able to distinguish between normal growth and tissue repair (normal cell cycle) on one hand and neoplastic growth (cancer cell cycles) on the other. Several theories [2, 3] sustain that for the initial expansion of a clone of cells more than one mutation is needed. Efforts in several science laboratories sustain that in certain cases the mutational route to cancer may be rather short (in molecular terms) with as few as two interlocking mutations required for initiation or progression of cancer- especially in animal models, unlike in man where at least one of these lesions involves particularly "dangerous" oncogenes such as c-*myc*. Therefore, it is believed that at least in some cases the genetic basis of a given cancer may be remarkably simple. Reference genome for man and other model organisms from the last decade has helped the explosion of new knowledge in human genetics.

1.2. The origin of oncogenes

An oncogene is a gene that contributes to converting a normal cell into a cancer cell when mutated or expressed at abnormally-high levels. Although the discovery of the origin of oncogenes came in parallel with the study of retroviruses, known in general as cancer inductors, not all retroviruses are tumor viruses [4, 5]. Even from early 1972 many researchers set out to explore the "oncogene hypothesis" proposed by Robert J. Huebner and George J. Todaro of the National Cancer Institute [6]. Looking for one mechanism to explain the induction of cancer by many different agents, Huebner and Todaro had suggested that there are the retroviral oncogenes as part of the genetic baggage of all cells, perhaps acquired through viral infection early in evolution. They supposed that the oncogenes would be innocuous as long as they remained quiescent. When stimulated into activity by a carcinogenic agent, however, they could convert cells to cancerous growth. It was reasoned that if the hypothesis was correct, the *src (sarcoma)* gene might be found in the DNA of normal cells. The copy of *src* could therefore be identified in the DNA from uninfected chickens and other birds. The next purpose was to find DNA related to *src* in mammals, including human beings, and in fishes. All vertebrates revealed to possess a gene related to *src*, and the oncogene hypothesis was consequently declared to be correct. But, on closer inspection, however, the gene that was discovered in vertebrates proved not to be a retrovirus gene at all. It was a cellular gene, which is now called *c-src*. The most convincing evidence for this conclusion came from the finding that the protein-encoding information of *c-src* is divided into several separate domains, called exons, by intervening regions known as introns. A split configuration of this kind is typical of animal-cell genes but not of the genes of retroviruses. Apart from their introns, the versions of *c-src* found in fishes, birds and mammals are all closely related to the viral gene *v-src* and to one another. It appears the vertebrate *src* gene has survived long periods of evolution without major change, implying that it is important to the well-being of the species in which it persists [6]. As a result, the genetic view of cancer-genes has for a long time its origins in virology. Retroviral oncogenes constitute the bridge between virus-induced tumors and tumors of all other etiologies: a cellular oncogene activated by viral transduction is a mere special example of the general phenomenon of genetic alterations that can convert important and useful growth regulators of the cell into driving forces of unbridled growth. Studies on tumor viruses had shown that viral genomes could carry individual genes that, when expressed in host cells, are both necessary and sufficient for the induction of oncogenic transformation. Such oncogenes became particularly interesting in retroviruses, because they turned out to be recent acquisitions from cellular genomes, pieces of host genetic information that were mutated, transduced and expressed as part of the viral life cycle.

It was thus supposed that the biologically active cellular oncogenes are mutant forms of normal proto-oncogenes that differ in the regulation of their expression or in the structure and function of their gene products. Nevertheless, biologically active cellular oncogenes were also identified by the ability of tumor DNAs to induce transformation in gene transfer assays. Such experiments have led to the identification of more than a dozen distinct human oncogenes that are activated either by point mutations or by DNA rearrangements in human neoplasm, or by DNA rearrangements that occur in the process of gene transfer. Both somatic mutations and DNA rearrangements of such oncogenes activated in human tumors suggest implication of cellular oncogene activation in the pathogenesis of human cancers. Accordingly, in the last decade, many researchers focused their attention to studies extremely helpful in elucidating these questionable aspects by implying model organisms.

1.2.1. Classification of cancer-genes

The genetic injure present in a parental tumorigenic cell, if not correctable, is maintained such that it is a heritable trait of all subsequent generations cells. Most, if not all cancer cells contain genetic damage that appears to be the responsible event leading to tumorigenesis. Two types of genetic damage are generally found in cancer cells:

A. Dominant genetic damage- and the involved genes have termed proto-oncogenes

A proto-oncogene is a gene whose altered protein product has the capacity to induce cellular transformation. The distinction between proto-oncogene and oncogene relates to the activity of the protein product of the gene. Therefore, an oncogene is believed to be a gene that has sustained some genetic damage and produces a protein capable of cellular transformation. The process of activation of proto-oncogenes to oncogenes can include retroviral transduction or retroviral or transposon integration, point mutations, insertion mutations, gene amplification, chromosomal translocation and/or protein-protein interactions. In general, proto-oncogenes have been classified based upon sequence homology to other known proteins or based on their normal function within cells [6]. As predicted, proto-oncogenes have been identified at all levels of the various signal transduction cascades that control cell growth, proliferation and differentiation. A common rule ascertains that proto-oncogenes which were originally identified as inhabitants in transforming retroviruses are designated as *c-* indicative of the cellular origin as opposed to *v-* to signify original identification in retroviruses. The list of proto-oncogenes identified to date is rather lengthy [3, 6].

B. Recessive genetic damage- and the involved genes are variously termed tumor suppressors/ growth suppressors/ recessive oncogenes or anti-oncogenes

There is an equally important category of cancer genes that contribute to tumorigenesis through a loss of function named tumor suppressor genes. In contrast to the growth stimulatory oncogenes, tumor suppressors normally function as attenuators and as inhibitors of growth. This category includes any gene that has the potential of becoming a constitutive growth stimulator and determinant of oncogenic cellular properties. The oncogenicity of these genes is therefore correlated with a gain of function.

The normal versions of both oncogenes and tumor suppressor genes serve in diverse regulatory systems of the cell. Most proto-oncogenes encode for components of signal transduction pathways that convert an extracellular stimulus into a programmed pattern of gene expression. A functional relatedness of tumor suppressors is less apparent; some domains of tumor suppressor gene action include cell surface properties, signal transduction, gene transcription, DNA repair, and checkpoints for cell division [6].

1.3. Identification of new target cancer related genes by insertional mutagenesis

Insertional mutagenesis is a good mechanism for identifying new cellular proto-oncogenes, especially when correlating with neoplasms induction by different viruses or transposons. The activation of a candidate oncogene by such an insertion not only provides a means of identifying such potential oncogenes, but also permits their isolation as molecular clones for subsequent investigation. After integrating its viral/ transposon DNA, the virus/ transposon itself represents a marker that could help to isolate surrounding molecular clones. These clones can furthermore provide the flanking genomic sequences, which can reveal the targeted proto-oncogene activated/ targeted by the insertion. A good example for this mechanism is provided by *wnt-1* (previously called *int-1*) which is usually activated upon integration of MMTV proviral DNA in mouse mammary carcinomas, first isolated in the laboratory by Harold Varmus in 1982 [7]. The MMTV virus LTR end usually acts as an enhancer to elevate *wnt-1* expression. The flanking DNA could have be cloned and then sequenced and it helped to elucidate the targeted *wnt-1* gene sequence. So it was revealed that the *wnt-1* genomic locus contains a transcriptional unit that was activated in tumors, either by upstream or downstream MMTV DNA insertion. The *wnt*-1 thus appeared to be a cellular oncogene because of its frequent activation by insertional viral spontaneous mutagenesis. But the designation of *wnt-1* as a real oncogene was later decided when it was shown that introduction of this gene into cultured mammary epithelial cells induced abnormal growth characteristic of neoplastic transformation [8]. Although it was initially identified by indirect criteria of structural alteration in tumors, this demonstration of the biological activity of *wnt*-1 provided important subsequent justification for this approach for oncogenes isolation. Provirus insertional mutagenesis was also implicated in activation of other cellular proto-oncogenes, encoding for different growth factors. For example, the gibbon ape leukemia cell line *MLA144* constitutively produces the *interleukin*-2 growth factor (T-cell growth factor), which appeared to be required for proliferation of these cells. Subsequent analysis of the interleukin-2 gene revealed that its constitutive expression is a consequence of the integration of gibbon ape leukemia virus DNA in the 3′ untranslated gene region [8].

Most recently studies revealed that one of the best examples of how a transposon insertion could facilitate for oncogene/ candidate-cancer gene identification is given by numerous studies from *Drosophila melanogaster*. Using genetic methods in *Drosophila* null alleles of the *P*-transposon tagged genes can be generated by remobilizing the transposons and screening for transposon's imprecise excisions. Different studies have also highlighted the power of *D. melanogaster P*-derivative transposons for examining cooperative interactions between tumor suppressors and oncogenes and for generating *in vivo* models of tumor development and metastasis [9]. Therefore, *Drosophila* is currently widely used as a model organism to explore the functions of different genes particularly those ones which are structural homologs of human oncogenes and tumor suppressor genes involved in a variety of tumors.

1.4. How similar are the fruit flies and humans

The fundamental aspects of the cellular biology, regulation the gene expression, neuronal connectivity, synaptogenesis, cellular signaling and cellular death are commonly accepted as being similar between humans and fruit flies. The structural homology between *Drosophila* and human genes has been revealed immediately after sequencing the *D.melanogaster* genome [10], and the human genome. Thereafter, the interest was focused on considerable studies using *Drosophila* as an experimental model for different human diseases. Numerous studies have been done to identify genes implicated in human pathologies that could be investigated in Drosophila. The most detailed study was done by

Reiter and collaborators [11] in 2001. Using the Online Mendelian Inheritance in Man (Homophila) database, Reiter and coworkers found that 714 of the 929 (77%) OMIM human disease gene entries have highly similar cognates in *Drosophila*, which were referring hereafter as "related genes". These data can be accessed through http://superfly.ucsd.edu/homophila, and the query can be made by key word, disease name, fly gene, and OMIM number (Table 1).

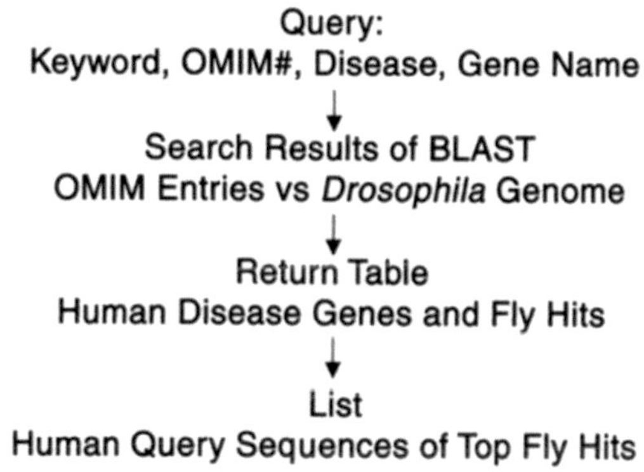

Table 1. How to query the Homophila database. The user enters the text query in the form of human disease name, OMIM number, fly gene name, or keyword search through the human disease entry box. A window with information on the disease name, and human and fly genes that match the key word query is opened. The user then can examine the details of an individual human-to-*Drosophila* BLAST comparison to get more information on the specific BLAST score, alignment, and other hits to this gene. In addition, transposons' (*P*-element) information is found at this level [after 11].

A list of disease phenotypes resulting from mutations in genes that are highly related to *Drosophila* genes has been categorized into various subclasses based on clinical phenotypes. A large number of human disease genes sharing *Drosophila* counterparts involved in different disorders such as: cancer, non-myelin associated neurological disorders, other developmental defects etc, has been therefore identified. Additional notable result of their study was that the great majority of *Drosophila* genes related to human disease genes (e.g. 395 genes out of 548) had not been analyzed by loss-of-function genetics by that time. Moreover, they found that many of these *Drosophila* related counterpart genes are marked by *P*-elements insertions in or near them (e.g., within 1 kb of the gene-coding region) and the *P*-element insertions were the only known alleles of those genes. Immediately after this study was published, using routine genetic methods in *Drosophila*, the possibility to create null alleles of these 56 *P* element tagged genes was starting in different laboratories by remobilizing the *P*-elements and screening for imprecise excisions that delete all or parts of the coding regions. Thus, loss-of-function analysis has become possible for identifying the function of these "related genes". Without the complete comparisons of the genomes in a database like *Homophila*, it would not be immediately obvious that genes e.g. responsible for human deafness could be functionally analyzed in an organism like *Drosophila* [11]. Surprisingly, the human genome is predicted to have only little over twice the number of genes found in flies and a comparison of both proteomes indicates 67% similarity at the amino acid level [10].

2. Why studying cancer in the fruit flies?

The expansion of human cancer is a multistep route, involving the cooperation of mutations in signaling, cell-cycle and cell-death pathways, as well as interactions between the tumor and the microenvironment. In this context, to *in vivo* explore the steps of tumorigenesis, simple animal models are needed. The genetically amenable, multicellular organism, the vinegar fly, *D.melanogaster*, can be used to elucidate the functions of different human structural homologues whose mutations were identified in different types of cancers [12]. This choice is not surprisingly taking into account the research history in *Drosophila* and the contributions of the *Drosophila* genetics for understanding the signaling pathways implicated in oncogenesis, such as: *Ras/MAPK, Notch, Wnt/wingless, hedgehog* and *BMP*.

D. melanogaster is an experimental model organism currently largely used for cancer research [13]. In 1916, decades before *Drosophila* would become one of the most popular models for studying many aspects of modern biology, the discovery of melanotic tumor-like granules in mutant larvae, by Bridges and Stark, first suggested that flies could develop tumors [14]. It took more than 50 years of genetic analysis to obtain convincing data which prove that insects can suffer from cancer [15]. Later, spontaneous mutations were identified causing the death of the animals at larval stages, because of overproliferation of certain internal tissues [16, 17]. Another study [18] showed that homozygous mutations in a series of genes from *Drosophila* can cause the appearance of tissue-specific tumors, which can affect either the embryonic or the larval development. Among these genes, the *lethal (2) giant larvae* (*l(2)gl*), has been the most studied. Homozygous mutations in *l(2)gl* produce malignant tumors in the brain and the imaginal discs. The *l(2)gl* gene was cloned, introduced back into the genome of l(2)gl-deficient animals and shown to restore the normal development [19], a process called "rescue-phenotype". A mosaic screen for over-proliferation mutants has been used successfully to identify several novel tumor suppressors in flies, including the large tumor suppressor (*lats;* also known as *wts*) gene. Somatic cells mutant for *lats* undergo extensive proliferation and form large tumor outgrowths with morphological characteristics similar to those of human tumors, confirming that *Drosophila* can grow tumors that are comparable with those found in humans. The human homolog of the *lats* gene (*LATS1*) could be used to suppress tumor growth and rescue developmental defects in *lats* mutant flies, including embryonic lethality [20]. Studies in *Drosophila* of such genes provided information that was directly relevant to tumorigenesis in humans.

In 2009, the second BioMed Conference from Barcelona entitled "Modelling Cancer in *Drosophila*" emphasizes again *Drosophila* as a model to elucidate human cancers. It was for the first time when a group of scientists came together to discuss the ways in which the fruit fly could provide novel contributions to the field of human cancers. For some of the presentations, discoveries in *Drosophila* were later validated in mammalian system or in humans [21]. So that, there is a large spectrum of candidate genes implicated in human pathologies that can be studied in *Drosophila*, and the lack of redundancy can simplify the analysis of biological process in the fly [22]. The functional orthology between *Drosophila* and human genes can be proved by rescue phenotype experiments (the equivalent of gene therapy) and it is working and gives surprising results.

2.1. Testing for preserved function between Drosophila genes and human counterparts

There are a number of ways to test the function of a foreign gene/ protein in transgenic *Drosophila*. Homologs of a fly gene for which mutants exist can be tested for the ability to rescue the fly mutant phenotype. If the fly counterpart has dominant effects or if one might expect dominant effects as a result of the function of the protein in vertebrates (such as for a dominant oncogene or disease gene), then another test is to determine whether the vertebrate homolog can induce similar dominant phenotypes in flies. There are examples of dominant oncogenic mutations leading to a form of the protein that also functions dominantly in the fly [23]. In some cases, expression of vertebrate/human genes in fruit flies has demonstrated that a conserved function of the vertebrate and fly genes is autoregulation; thus, the vertebrate protein (frequently a transcription factor) turns on expression of the endogenous fly counterpart. If one has mutants in the fly gene involved. Then, it is possible to test for functional conservation in the genetic background of a protein null mutant of the fly gene and, hence, address broader aspects of functional conservation.

Herein are presented some results of a study concerned on the clarification of the putative functional conservation between *DmManf* gene from *Drosophila* (previously called *ARP-like* for *arginine-rich protein-like*), and its counterpart- the human *Manf* gene (*Mesencephalic astrocyte-derived neuroptrophic factor*), which was found to be implicated in various human pathologies, including cancer.

2.2. Exploration of the DmManf in comparison with Manf putative oncogene from human

Mesencephalic astrocyte-derived neurotrophic factor, *DmManf* gene is referred in *FlyBase* by the symbol *CG7013* (*CG*, computed gene). It has the cytological map location 89B19, in the right arm of the 3rd chromosome. The molecular function is unknown. Previously, it was shown that a *P{EP}* transposon insertion at the position –157 upstream of the 5'UTR region of the *Manf* gene does not affect the *Manf* gene function [24].

The *DmManf* gene contains 1436 nucleotides and encodes for a protein of 173 amino acids. In the fruit-fly stock *EP(3)3171* the *DmManf* gene is associated with a *P* derivative transposon. In general, transposable elements insertion's are extremely powerful means of gene disruption. The transposon associated with *DmManf* gene was symbolized by *P{EP}EP3171* and was first inserted in the 5'UTR region of *DmManf* gene, and then, could be mobilized generating mutant alleles of the targeted gene.

The human *Manf* counterpart gene, previously named *ARP* (from Arginine-Rich Protein) is located in the chromosomal band 3p21.2, a region that is frequently deleted in a variety of solid tumors. It encodes for a protein highly conserved in evolution. First oncological information was given by Shridhar and coworkers [25, 12] who reported an ATG-to-AGG transversion in codon 50 of the *ARP* gene or deletion of codon 50 in different tumor types including 10 of 21 sporadic renal cell carcinomas. Later (1997), they observed the same mutations in 11 of 37 pancreatic tumors. Either of the changes abolishes a methionine residue and gives rise to an uninterrupted string of AGG trinucleotides in the *ARP* gene and arginines in its predicted protein product. The finding of 4 other nucleotide substitutions in codon 50 that replaced methionine with 4 different amino acids other than arginine suggested that loss of this methionine residue is critical to a carcinogenic role of this gene.

Their finding of an AGG-to-AAG (arg-to-lys) mutation in the adjacent codon 51 in 2 tumors emphasized further the importance of this region. Other evidence [25] suggested that only a single copy of the *ARP/Manf* gene is mutated in the cancer cells, indicating its possible causal role as an oncogene.

Mesencephalic astrocyte-derived neurotrophic factor sequences are referring to a family of small proteins of approximately 170 residues which contain four di-sulfide bridges that are highly conserved, from nematodes to humans (Table 2).

	Genes	Proteins
1	MANF, *H.sapiens* mesencephalic astrocyte-derived neurotrophic factor	NP_006001.3 182 aa
2	MANF, *P.troglodytes* mesencephalic astrocyte-derived neurotrophic factor	XP_001169644.1 246 aa
3	MANF, *C.lupus* mesencephalic astrocyte-derived neurotrophic factor	XP_850540.1 179 aa
4	MANF, *B.taurus* mesencephalic astrocyte-derived neurotrophic factor	NP_001094681.1 179 aa
5	Manf, *M.musculus* mesencephalic astrocyte-derived neurotrophic factor	NP_083379.2 179 aa
6	Manf, *R.norvegicus* mesencephalic astrocyte-derived neurotrophic factor	XP_236614.3 179 aa
7	Manf, *D.rerio* mesencephalic astrocyte-derived neurotrophic factor	NP_001070097.1 180 aa
9	Manf, *D.melanogaster* Mesencephalic astrocyte-derived neurotrophic factor	NP_477445.1 173 aa
10	AgaP_AGAP003016, *A.gambiae* AGAP003016-PA	XP_311862.3 180 aa
11	Y54G2A.23, *C.elegans* hypothetical protein	NP_500273.2 168 aa

Table 2. HomoloGene report showing the putative homologs of mesencephalic astrocyte-derived neurotrophic factor. The identification number of the protein, the size and their conserved domain architectures are are assigned (www.ncbi.nlm.nih.gov/homologene).

The amino acid sequences of this highly conserved protein in evolution shows 51% identity on average between *Drosophila Manf* gene and the human *Manf* (Fig. 1).

The higher homology revealed by the comparison of the whole aminoacid sequences of the *Drosophila* and human proteins (51% identity, 71% positives) as compared to the amino acids of the Saposin_like domains (41% identity, 58% positives) suggests that, in addition to the Saposin_like domain, there are other motifs which highlight the similarity or even identity between the compared aminoacid sequences. These motifs could be important for a particular function of the protein and suggest a similar function of the two proteins. This remark is in agreement with a similar situation that was encountered when *Drosophila lats* and human *LATS1* were compared [20]. Although the overall sequence similarity in the amino-terminal regions of these two proteins was lower (22% identity and 42% similarity) than in the kinase carboxy-terminal (74% sequence identity), stretches of highly conserved sequences have been identified in both proteins, and finally, they proved that the genes are even functionally conserved. Another similar study presents the case of *Mgstl* which encodes a protein similar to human *mGST*. Because the identity between both genes was 45% but their hydrophobic profiles were also very similar, the authors' expectation was that these genes share a functional similarity [26].

```
 Score =  174 bits (442),  Expect = 1e-59, Method: Compositional matrix adjust.
 Identities = 83/163 (51%), Positives = 116/163 (71%), Gaps = 1/163 (1%)

Query  10   LAVALALSVLPGSRALRPGDCEVCISYLGRFYQDLKDRDVTFSPATIENELIKFCREARG  69
            + +     ++    S AL+  DCEVC+   + RF    L D          IE     KFC+   +
Sbjct  8    VVIGFLATLAQTSLALKEEDCEVCVKTVRRFADSLDD-STKKDYKQIETAFKKFCKAQKN  66

Query  70   KENRLCYYIGATDDAATKIINEVSKPLAHHIPVEKICEKLKKKDSQICELKYDKQIDLST  129
            KE+R CYY+G  +++AT I+NE+SKPL+  +P EKICEKLKKKD+QIC+L+Y+KQIDL++
Sbjct  67   KEHRFCYYLGGLEESATGILNELSKPLSWSMPAEKICEKLKKKDAQICDLRYEKQIDLNS  126

Query  130  VDLKKLRVKELKKILDDWGETCKGCAEKSDYIRKINELMPKYA  172
            VDLKKL+V++LKKIL+DW E+C GC EK D+I++I EL PKY+
Sbjct  127  VDLKKLKVRDLKKILNDWDESCDGCLEKGDFIKRIEELKPKYS  169
```

Figure 1. Comparison between *D melanogaster Manf* and human *Manf* sequences. „Query"= protein from human and „Sbjct= protein from *Drosophila*. Amino acids from Saposin-like domain are surrounded by green; bordered in blue is EF-hand domain. For detailes, see text.

To study whether *DmManf* holds not only a structural, but also a true *in vivo* functional similarity with its human counterpart, we mobilized the *P{EP}EP3171*-element from the *EP(3)3171* line to obtain specific mutant alleles of the *DmManf* gene. Different mechanisms of repairing the double-strand break generated by the *P[EP]* excision induced a variety of new genetic variants, including loss-of-function *DmManf* alleles [27].

In this study we took advantage of our first reported loss-of-function mutant *DmManf* allele, namelythe *Manf*$^{\Delta 1151}$ (GenBank ID: DQ649527). The *Manf*$^{\Delta 1151}$ allele was isolated in *Ex.35* mutant line (Fig. 2). By DNA sequencing of the specific mutant amplicon we discovered that the *Ex.35* mutant line contains a deletion of 1278 bp that removes part of the intergenic region, the 5'UTR and almost the whole coding region of the *DmManf* gene, leaving behind the distal end of the last exon and the 3'UTR region (Fig.2 Ba) and is affecting only the *DmManf* gene.

The *Manf*$^{\Delta 1151}$ allele from *Ex.35* line proved to be homozygous lethal. To define the lethal phase during development, we took advantage of the *GFP* (*Green Fluorescent Protein*) marker present in the *Drosophila* balancer chromosome *TM3SerGFP*, which could help distinguishing,

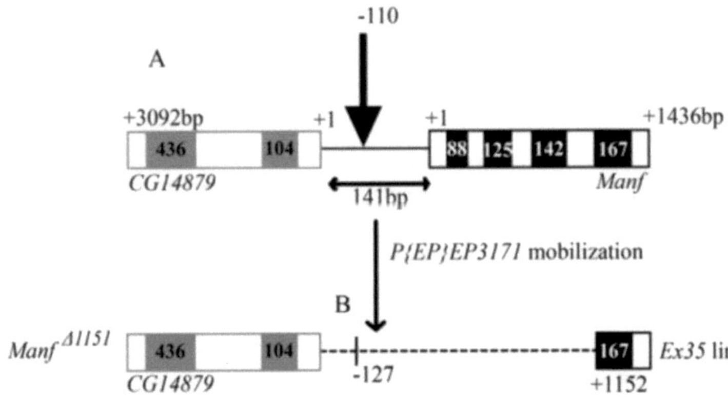

Figure 2. The structure and deletion breakpoints of *P{EP}EP3171* homozygous lethal allele found in *Ex.35* line. A: The genomic context including *Drosophila Manf* and *CG14879* genes separated by 141bp intergenic region and transcribed in opposite direction. Δ stands for *P{EP}EP3171* original insertion site. Exons are indicated by filled boxes, introns by empty boxes. Nucleotide numbers are assigned for the exons. B): The lethal *Manf*$^{\Delta1151}$ alele genomic deletion is indicated by the dashed line. The numbers of nucleotides are assigned for each exon [after 27].

under an UV source, the *GFP* heterozygous individuals and *non-GFP* homozygous individuals. Therefore, after letting *Drosophila* females from *Ex.35* line to lay eggs onto Petri dishes containing appropriate culture medium, we followed the development of the embryos and larvae comparing the numbers of the heterozygous and homozygous individuals. Starting with 594 embryos, we noticed that the number of the homozygotes was continuously decreasing during the subsequent developmental stages. As it revealed, the homozygous lethality was polyphasic, the homozygotes mostly died in the embryonic and 1st instar larval (L1) phases, although L2 stage escapers were also found. Among the counted 3rd stage larvae, two *non-GFP* excapers were found. One of them was transferred onto another culture plate and observed for several days. This mutant L3 larva contained some internal „holes", *i.e.* empty, transparent spaces similar to that "empty" spaces found in another *DmManf* specific mutant, from a similar study [23]. First these homozygous larvae atypically wander away from the food, and then move more slowly, and finally freeze immobilized but still responding to touch. It was unable to enter the pupal stage and died keeping the phenotype described before. Homozygous mutant adults for *Manf*$^{\Delta1151}$ allele were never found. These empty „holes" remained unchanged during the observation period, suggesting that the pupae died inside, probably after several unsuccessful encapsulation immune reactions by which lammellocytes should encapsulate melanise and kill the parasites, fungi or even abnormal cells- such as tumor cells (Fig. 3).

Most of the *Drosophila* overgrowing mutations are late larval or pupal lethal and affect the adult organ rudiments, imaginal discs, while leaving the other larval tissues necessary for larval survival mostly unaffected [28, 16]. The majority of such mutations display a prolonged larval period, also seen in the case of *Manf*$^{\Delta1151}$mutant, which can be explained by the presence of non-differentiating growing imaginal rudiments preventing ecdysone release [29].

While *DmManf* recently [23] was found to be required during the maturation of the embryonic nervous system for maintenance of neuronal connectivity, there were also indications (http://superfly.ucsd.edu/homophila/) of a possible role of *Manf /ARP* in human tumor formation [12, 25].

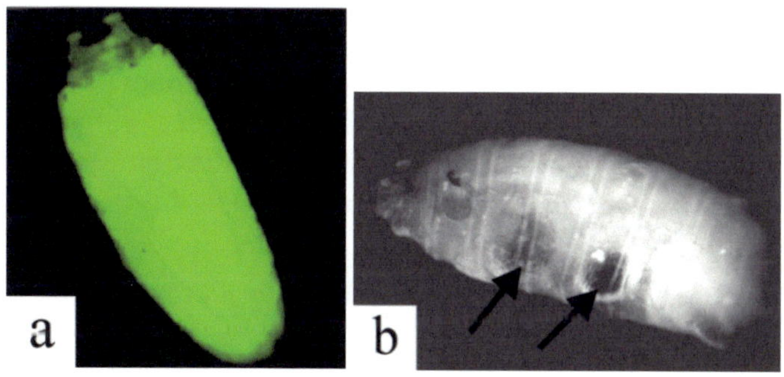

Figure 3. Heterozygote and homozygote pupae from *Ex.35* line. a) *Ex.35* heterozygous control pupae (genotype: *Manf*$^{\Delta 1151}$/TM3SerGFP); b) *Ex.35* homozygous pupae (genotype: *Manf*$^{\Delta 1151}$/ *Manf*$^{\Delta 1151}$); arrows show the internal holes in the dead pupa.

A wealth of data support the view that cancer is a multistage disease progressing via the accumulation of multiple genetic changes lesions that compromise the normal control of cell proliferation, survival, differentiation, migration and social interactions with neighboring cells [1]. It is also important to note that apparently phenotypically similar cancers may arise through different combinations of lesions: there are likely many different routes to cancer even in the same cell type. Many key cancer –relevant signaling pathways may be activated or inactivated by mutations at various points that could result in largely identical cell behavior.

From this point of view, interesting cancer-like phenotypes were observed for different mutants previously obtained after *P{EP}EP3171* transposon mobilization, from the *DmManf* gene vicinity [27]. The most aggressive cancer-like phenotypes which appeared in our mutants either killed the adult flies, e.g. in the case of *Ex.29* mutant (Fig. 4) or let the adults survive, although they expressed in all the body melanotic tissue/nodules, in both females and male, *e.g.* in the case of *Δ26.1* mutant (Fig. 6). Symbols and numbers in the mutant names designate different lines obtained from different *P{EP}EP3171* mobilization experiments [27].

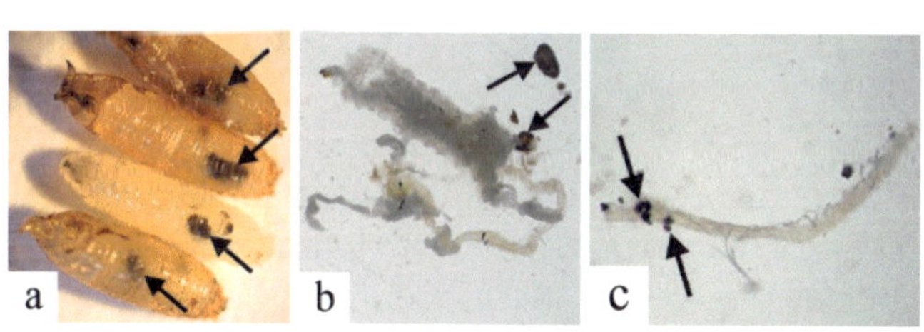

Figure 4. Larval and pupal phenotypes found in the *Ex.29* mutant. a. Larvae and pupae containing melanotic masses; b. dissected homozygous mutant larva in the *III*rd instar enclosing melanotic masses; c. The gut surrounded by melanotic masses. The arrows label melanotic masses. The *Ex.29/Ex.29* homozygote mutants never developed as adults.

The appearances of the melanotic masses in flies were extensively characterized. Although the *Toll* pathway seems to be responsible for the formation of melanotic masses in *Drosophila* [30], other genes could also be implicated upstream of downstream of this well characterized pathway. Spectacular results were obtained by investigating the ultra-structure of the interesting melanotic masses found in case of *Ex.29* mutant under the electron microscope. After dissecting normal and melanotic gut of the *Ex29/Ex29* homozygote mutant 3rd instar larvae, several sections were examined under the electron microscope (Fig. 5). We noticed that in the cells of control normal gut the nucleus revealed a typical structure with nuclear envelope, caryoplasm and nucleolus (Fig 5a). Caryoplasma, the fundamental substance of this nucleus appeared typical, as a protein gel with the embedded chromosomes and a nucleolus. Chromatin displayed a fibrillar structure, consisting mainly of DNA associated with histones and non-histone proteins. Chromatic substance of the nucleus become visible as a network, resulting from a strong despiralization, hydration, swelling, dragging and overlapping events of the chromosomes. In some parts, the chromatic substance disclosed more condensed probably corresponding to heterochromatic areas.

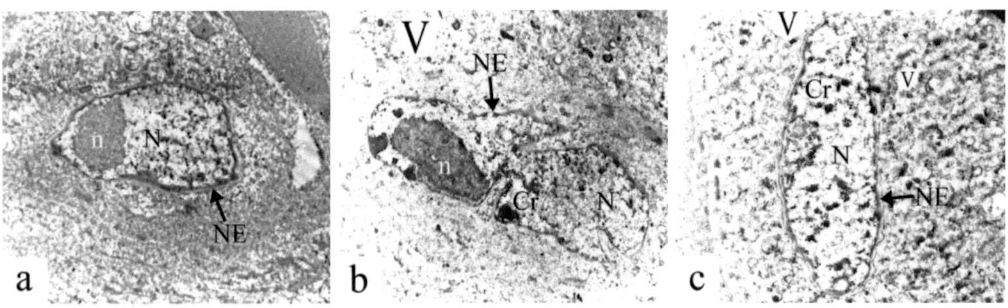

Figure 5. Electron microscopic images after micro-dissection of *Ex.29* homozygote 3rd instar larval gut; a. Nucleus and nucleolus of a normal gut cell. Magnification is 8640X; b. Dissection through melanotic "young tumor"- light black masses; the nucleus has a lobated edge, magnification 8640X; c. Dissection through melanotic "old tumor" -dark black masses, showing a nucleus without nucleolus. Magnifications 12400X. N- Nucleus; n- nucleolus; NE- nuclear envelope, V- vacuole; Cr- chromatin.

Nucleolus, another important cellular structure displayed an oval shape with irregular contour (Figs. 5a, 5b), without specific membrane, being surrounded by a network of chromatic filaments of nuclear origin which twisted into perinucleolar chromatin. As typical, is prearranged in a fibrillar-granular structure consisting of fibrils and ribo-nucleo-proteinic granules, like ribosomes.

In contrast, in the „old tumor" dark black masses, resembling senescent cells (Fig. 5c) appeared having ceased its function, many structural changes occurring probably due to the intensification of autolitic processes. As a result, the cytoplasmic content decreased significantly, most of the cellular volume being replaced by the vacuolar system. In this cell the nucleus still persists, although the nucleolus have disappeared. Only a few blocks of chromatin and an increased number of autolytic vacuoles can be detected. These changes lead to the idea that such a cell is doomed to apoptosis. Other notable melanotic-like nodule phenotype was observed in case of the *A26.3* mutant stock, which contains *DmManf*$^{A26.3}$ allele, carrying a residual part from the original *P* element insertion (GenBank ID: HQ623183). The stereomicroscopic examination of these mutants showed mild melanotic masses in the larvae (Fig. 6).

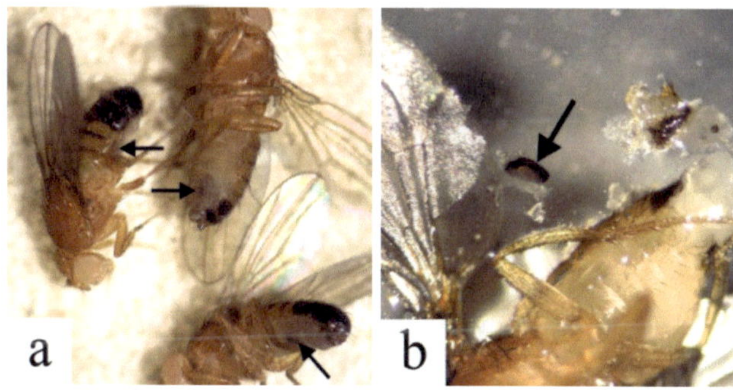

Figure 6. The *A26.3* mutant phenotype is shown. a. Melanotic nodules in the adult flies, both in males and females. b dissected adult female carrying black melanotic nodules/ pseudo-tumors.

Particular mutants expressing characteristic melanotic phenotype were also obtained in other insertional/ excisional *P* element mutagenesis experiments [31]. As it was shown previously, mutations in ~30 genes that regulate different pathways and developmental processes in *Drosophila* can cause a melanotic phenotype in larvae. The observed melanotic masses were generally linked to the hemocyte-mediated immune response. In general, the melanotic masses can be subdivided into melanotic nodules engaging the hemocyte-mediated encapsulation and into melanizations that are not encapsulated by hemocytes [31]. With rare exception, the encapsulation is carried out by lamellocytes. Encapsulated nodules are found in the hemocoel or in association with the lymph gland, while melanizations are located in the gut, salivary gland, and tracheae. These results can show that the phenotype of each mutant not only reflects its connection to a particular genetic pathway but also point to the tissue-specific role of the individual gene.

Half a century ago, melanotic tumors in *Drosophila* larvae and adults were viewed as the equivalent of cancer and as events of controlled histological differentiation that could be manipulated genetically. The participation of blood cells in the formation of some melanotic tumors was reported at about the same time [32, 33]. Black melanotic spots are found in a number of different mutants and have been called, interchangeably, melanotic tumors or pseudotumors. These "tumors" are usually not invasive and involve tumorous overgrowth only in some instances. Therefore it is generally accepted to use the term "melanotic masses" to describe the phenotype generally and "melanotic nodules" and "melanizations" to describe more specific phenotypes.

Experiments in our laboratory indicated that an artificial transposon, *P{EP}EP3171*, when mobilized [27] could induce variable mutant genotypes and phenotypes resulting in a polyallelic series of the *DmManf* and/ or other interactor genes, including melanotic masses and nodules. This is not particularly suprising, taking into account other genes, *e.g.* the deep orange (*dor*) gene, whose poly-alellic series affect different functions resulting in lethality, male sterility, sterility with maternal effect, or simple changes in the eye color [34]. We also found *Drosophila* mutants with paternal effect sterility, which could give away *DmManf* gene's pleiotropic functions. By investigating all these isolated alleles we can reach comprehensive understanding of the role of the *DmManf* gene.

2.3. Application of the rescue phenotype (gene therapy) technique in flies

Gene therapy consists of the insertion of genes into an individual's cells and tissues to treat a disease, and hereditary diseases, in which a defective mutant allele is replaced by a functional one. Although the technology is still in its infancy, the researchers have already successfully tested it in *Drosophila*, for homozygous lethal mutations of the *l(2)gl* [19] or the *lats* gene [35], which could be saved by the orthologous genes from human: *Hugl*-1, *scrib*, *dlg* [36] etc. Therefore, when expressing a foreign gene in the fly in a tissue that normally does not express any such gene, screening of interacting proteins will be useful for understanding the function of the gene in its normal cellular context. It is important to assess whether any phenotypic effects observed in the fly accurately reflect conserved functions of the vertebrate protein under scrutiny. For example, will vertebrate anti-apoptotic genes block *Drosophila* programmed cell death? Will the vertebrate homolog, like its fly counterpart, direct ectopic tissue formation in the fly? If the vertebrate cDNA induces a dominant effect, is that effect the result of elevated levels of a normal activity of the protein (a hypermorphic effect) or of a new activity of the protein that may have little to do with its normal function (a neomorphic effect). Neomorphic effects, for example, might be the result of subcellular mislocalization of the vertebrate protein in the fly. To what degree does the pathology of a human disease gene reflect biological effects known to occur in humans or vertebrate models, and can these effects be faithfully replicated in the fly model? These are, of course, specific issues that vary for any one gene of interest, and they are critical to consider.

2.3.1. DmManf is the true ortholog of the human Manf putative oncogene

To investigate whether human *Manf* is able to compensate for the loss of function of *DmManf* mutants, we carried out rescue experiments with *UAS-HsManf* transgenic flies. We applied the gene therapy (rescue phenotype) procedure to the *Ex.35* mutant which contains the loss-of-function allele *Manf*$^{\Delta 1151}$, and shows lethal phenotype. First, we verified if the *Manf*$^{\Delta 1151}$ mutant lethality was solely the result of the *DmManf* deletion, by inducing the ubiquitous ectopic expression of *UAS-DmManf* in the *DmManf*$^{\Delta 1151}$ homozygote mutant background using the Actin-GAL4 driver (Fig. 7). Then, the ubiquitous Actin-GAL4 *UAS-HsManf* expression was tested if it is also able to rescue the adult lethality of *DmManf*$^{\Delta 1151}$ homozygote mutants (Fig.7).

We proved that the lethality was only caused by deletion of *DmManf* demonstrating that *DmManf* is important at least for the normal development and essential for viability. The rescue percentage of adult flies was similarly obtained when using separately the *Drosophila* and the Human *Manf* transgenes, driven by the ActinGal4 driver. These results demonstrate that *DmManf* is the fruit fly functional ortholog of human *Manf*, and that fruit fly and human Manf share a yet unknown cognate receptor, essential for viability and normal development.

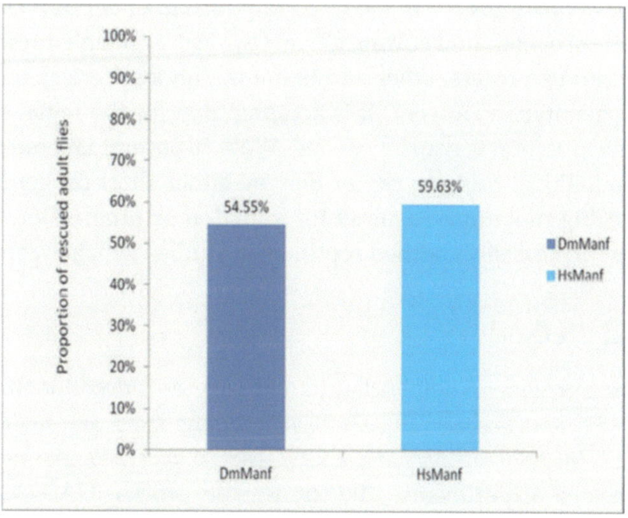

Figure 7. The lethality of $DmManf^{\Delta 115}$ adults is rescued by ectopic UAS-*DmManf* and UAS-*HsManf* expression with the ubiquitous Actin-GAL4 driver. The proportion of rescued adults relative to all adults is presented; 100% indicates the maximum expected value of complete rescue estimated by Mendelian inheritance.

Herein is described a pilot experiment that supports the evolutionary conservation of the *Manf* gene functions' in the fruit fly- *Drosophila melanogaster* and its important role in deciphering human pathologies. Our results complement previous results [23] when *DmManf* mutant (namely $DmManf^{\Delta 96}$) lethality rescue- phenotype experiment resulted in complete larval rescue up to the pupal stage [23]. These authors were using 69B-GAL4 driving the transgenic *DmManf* expression in epidermis and CNS, proving the importance of *DmManf* expression in both tissues in the fly. They also proved that *DmManf* is required for the maintenance of the DA neurites but not the neurites of serotonergic or the subpopulation of motoneurons. Surprisingly, despite the axonal degeneration in $DmManf^{\Delta 96}$ mutant larvae, the cell body of DA neurons persists. Moreover, some DA neurons but not their neurites persist even when their death was ectopically triggered by over expression of the proapoptotic proteins. Thus, programmed cell death in the *Drosophila* DA neurons seems to follow a "dying-back" pattern where the neurites degenerate first followed by the death of the cell body [23, 37]. Whether *DmManf* is a *bona fide* NTF promoting the survival of DA neurons remains, however, open as the mutant larvae died before it could be judged [23]. By TEM analysis, the elimination of *DmManf* causes cell death resembling caspase independent cell death, characterized by swelling of organelles, and the appearance of "empty" spaces [23, 38]. Similar observations were also found in the case of our mutant *Ex.35*, which contains the $DmManf^{\Delta 115}$ allele (see Fig. 3).

By the experiments involving *DmManf* gene from *Drosophila* presented here, some scientific data about the yet unknown role of this gene was obtained. We completed a first pilot phenotypic rescue of our *DmManf* deficient animals. It still remained unclear if the *DmManf* is a true oncogene or a tumor-suppressor gene. We assumed that a real cancerous phenotype could have not appeared in the *Ex.35* mutant, either because *DmManf* gene might not be a canonical oncogene, or because while *DmManf* although preserved a particular function in the cancerous process, other additional mutations were simultaneously needed for the cancerous phenotype to appear. It is accepted that for the initial expansion of a cell clone more than one mutation is usually needed. Work in several laboratories sustain that in certain cases the mutational route to cancer may be either short (in genetic terms) with as few as two interlocking mutations required for initiation or progression of cancer, or long, and these instances can be easily clarified routinely in studies which involve animal models.

3. Materials and methods

Drosophila strains: For genetic nomenclature, cytology and description of mutations and chromosomes see [39] and *Flybase* [40]. *Drosophila* strains used are: *w;EP(3)3171/TM3SbSer [24], w;TM3SerGFP/TM6TbSb, Ex.35/TM3, Ex.29/TM3, A26.3/TM3, Actin-GAL4/SM6Cy*. For the phenotypic rescue experiments, the transgenic stocks UAS-*DmManf* and UAS-*HumanManf* were received as gifts from Dr. T.I.Heino. Fly crosses were done on standard cornmeal-yeast-agar medium, at 25°C.

Phenotypic rescue experiments. The transgenic lines for UAS-*DmManf* and UAS-*HsManf* were recombined together with Actin-GAL4 driver, a GAL4 line of ubiquitous expression, on the *DmManf*$^{\Delta 115}$ mutant background. For each experiment 3 independent crosses were made and transferred twice to fresh vials; progeny from all vials of each cross was counted, and the proportion of rescued adults relative to all adults was calculated.

StereoMicroscopy and Image Analyses: Larval and pupal images were taken through an *Olympus SZX7* stereo-microscope equipped with an *Olympus* DP70 camera.

Electron Microscopy (EM) Analyses. The gut and melanotic tissues isolated from dissected *Ex.29* homozygous larvae were fixed in 4% glutar-aldehyde in 0.1M sodium cacodylate buffer, pH7.3, 4h at 40°C and post-fixed in 1.5 % osmium tetroxide in the same buffer. They were then dehydratated in a graded ethanol series (30%, 50%, 70%, 90%, 95% and 100%) and embedded in Epon 812. The samples were sectioned on an ultra microtome, stained in 4% aqueous uranyl acetate, post-stained with lead citrate and examined with a Philips 201 electron microscope.

4. Conclusions

Cancer can be measured as a complex multistep pathology that requires the accumulation of several mutations giving to cells an aberrant proliferative advantage, improved resistance to pro-apoptotic stimuli and loss of differentiation markers. Increasing evidences underline the importance of the tumor microenvironment in the growth of cancer cells. Since it has been shown to exert both pro- and anti-tumoral effects, the role of the immune system in fighting cancer progression has been contradictory. Due to the simplicity of genetic manipulations, *Drosophila* research could bring meaningful insights to our understanding of the mechanisms of communication between cancerous and normal cells, as well as between the tumor tissue and the immune system. Although it still remained unclear if the *Manf* gene from *Drosophila* is a true oncogene or a tumor-suppressor gene, we assumed that *DmManf* gene could play a particular function in the process and probably other additional mutations are simultaneously needed for the cancerous phenotype to become visible. Efforts to use *Drosophila* to explore issues specific to cancer will keep on growing. *Drosophila* is being used for what it does best: identifying novel oncogenes and tumor suppressors, and linking cancer-related genes together into complex signaling pathways [9]. The use of whole organisms *in vivo* is generally considered as being essential for understanding the tumorigenesis.

Author details

Laura Monica Magdalena*
Department of Genetics, University of Bucharest, Bucharest, Romania

Lorand Savu
Genetic Lab SRL, Bucharest, Romania

Acknowledgement

We owe our special thanks to Dr. J. Szidonya for kindly providing *EP(3)3171 and w;TM3SerGFP/TM6TbSb Drosophila* laboratory strains. We are grateful to Dr. T.I.Heino for providing UAS-*DmManf* and UAS-*HuManf* transgenic stocks. We are appreciative to C. Parvu for EM analysis, to A. Burcea for the help with the Figures and really indebted to Dr. I Kiss for kindly review this paper. This research was supported by UEFISCDI Romania, IDEAS grant no.1004/ 2009, ID code 1936/2009.

5. References

[1] Pelengaris S and Khan M (2006) The Molecular Biology of Cancer. Blackwell Publishing Ltd. 531p.

[2] Vogelstein B and Kinzler K W (2004) Cancer genes and the pathways they control. Nature Medicine 10 (8): 789-99.

[3] Pelengaris S, Khan M and Evan GI (2002) Suppression of MYC-induced apoptosis in beta cells exposes multiple oncogenic properties of Myc and triggers carcinogenic progression. Cell. 109 (3): 321-34.

* Corresponding Author

[4] Pitot H C (2002) Fundamentals of Oncology, Fourth edition, revised and expanded, Marcel Dekker Inc. 998p.

[5] Coffin J M, Hughes S H and Varmus H E (1997) Retroviruses. Cold Spring Harbor NY: Cold Spring Harbor Laboratory Press.

[6] Cooper G M (1995) Oncogenes, II-nd edition. Jones and Bartlett Publishers Inc. Boston. 384p.

[7] Nusse R (1991) Insertional mutagenesis in mouse mammary tumorigenesis. In: H. J. Kung and P. Vogt (Eds.), Retroviral insertion and oncogene activation. Curr. Top. Microbiol. Immunol. 171:43–65.

[8] Ymer S, Tucker W Q J, Sanderson C J, Hapel A J, Campbell, H D, and Young IG (1985) Constitutive synthesis of interleukin-3 by leukaemia cell line WEHI-3B is due to retroviral insertion near the gene. Nature 317: 255-258.

[9] Vidal M and Cagan R L (2006) Drosophila models for cancer research. Curr. Opin. Genet. Dev. 16(1): 10-16.

[10] Adams M D et. al. (2000). The Genome Sequence of Drosophila melanogaster, Science 24 March 2000: Vol. 287 no. 5461: 2185- 2195.

[11] Reiter LT et al. (2001) A Systematic Analysis of Human Disease-Associated Gene Sequences in Drosophila melanogaster. Cold Spring Harbor Laboratory Press. Genome Research 11: 1114-1125.

[12] Shridhar V et al. (1997) Mutations in the arginine-rich protein gene (ARP) in pancreatic cancer. Oncogene 14: 2213-2216.

[13] Fortini ME et al. (2000). A survey of human disease gene counterparts in the Drosophila genome. The Journal of Cell Biology. vol. 150. no.2. The Rockefeller University Press.

[14] Stark MB (1919) A Benign Tumor that is Hereditary in Drosophila. Proc Natl Acad Sci USA. 5(12): 573–580.

[15] Harshbarger J C and Taylor R L (1968) Neoplasms in insects. Annu. Rev. Entomol. 13: 159-190.

[16] Gateff E. (1978) Malignant neoplasms of genetic origin in Drosophila melanogaster. Science 200: 1448-1459.

[17] Mechler BM et al. (1985) Molecular cloning of lethal(2)giant larvae, a recessive oncogene of Drosophila melanogaster. E.M.B.O.J 4: 1551-1557.

[18] Merz R et al. (1990) Molecular Action of the l(2)gl Tumor Suppressor Gene of Drosophila melanogaster, Environmental Health Perspectives. Vol. 8:163-167.

[19] Mechler B. M. et al. (1991) Drosophila as a model system for molecular analysis of tumorigenesis, Environmental Health Perspectives. Vol. 93: 63-71.

[20] Tao W et al. (1999) Human homologue of the Drosophila melanogaster lats tumour suppressor modulates CDC2 activity. Nat. Genet. 21 (2): 177-81.

[21] Botas J (2007) Drosophila researchers focus on human disease. Nature Genetics. Vol. 39 No 5:589- 591.

[22] Sang TK and Jackson GR (2005) Drosophila Models of Neurodegenerative Disease, NeuroRx: The Journal of the American Society for Experimental NeuroTherapeutics Vol. 2: 438–446.

[23] Palgi M, Lindström R, Peränen J, Piepponen TP, Saarma M and Heino TI (2009) Evidence that DmMANF is an invertebrate neurotrophic factor supporting dopaminergic neurons. Proc. Natl. Acad.Sci. U.S.A. 106(7): 2429-2434.

[24] Georgescu LM, Ecovoiu Al, Graur M, Gavrila L (2005) P{EP}EP3171 allele of ARP-like gene from Drosophila melanogaster is not lethal, Romanian Biotechnological Letters 10 nr.1:1995-2000. (http://cachescan.bcub.ro/2010-03-27/576941.pdf).

[25] Shridhar V et al. (1996) A gene from human chromosomal band 3p21.1 encodes a highly conserved arginine-rich protein and is mutated in renal cell carcinomas. Oncogene 12: 1931-1939.

[26] Toba G, Ohsako T, Miyata N, Ohtsuka T, Seong KH and Aigaki T (1999) The gene search system: A method for efficient detection and rapid molecular identification of genes in Drosophila melanogaster. Genetics 1999. 151: 725-737.

[27] Magdalena LM, Savu L, Costache M, Kiss I (2011) Deletions and structural alterations of chromosome region 89B13 from Drosophila melanogaster, by induced transposition of PEP3171 element, Romanian Biotechnological Letters vol 16, nr.3: 6153-6161.

[28] Torok T, et al. (1993) P-lacW Insertional Mutagenesis on the Second Chromosome of Drosophila melanogaster: Isolation of Lethals With Different Overgrowth Phenotypes Genetics 135: 71-80.

[29] Poodry C A and Woods D F (1990) Control of the developmental timer for Drosophila pupariation. Roux's Arch. Dev. Biol. 199 219-227.

[30] Lemaitre B, Meister M, Govind S, Georgel P, Steward R et al. (1995) Functional analysis and regulation of nuclear import of dorsal during the immune response in Drosophila. EMBO J. 14: 536–545.

[31] Minakhina S and Steward R. (2006) Melanotic Mutants in Drosophila: Pathways and Phenotypes Genetics 174: 253–263.

[32] Oftedal P (1953) The histogenesis of a new tumor in Drosophila melanogaster, and a comparison with tumors of five other stocks. Z. Indukt. Abstamm. Vererbungsl. 85: 408–422.

[33] Rizki M T (1960) Melanotic tumor formation in Drosophila. J. Morphol. 106: 147–157.

[34] Wolfner MF and GoldbergML (1994) Harnessing the power of Drosophila genetics. Goldstein. Fyrberg: 33-80.

[35] Xu T et al. (1995) Identifying tumor suppressors in genetic mosaics: the Drosophila lats gene encodes a putative protein kinase. Development 121: 1053-1063.

[36] Grifoni D et al. (2004) The human protein Hugl-1 substitutes for Drosophila Lethal giant larvae tumour suppressor function in vivo Oncogene 23: 8688–8694.

[37] Raff M, Whitmore A, Finn J (2002) Axonal self-destruction and neurodegeneration. Science 296:868–871.

[38] Clarke PG (1990) Developmental cell death: morphological diversity and multiple mechanisms. Anat Embryol 195–213.

[39] Lindsley DL and Zimm GG (1992) The Genome of Drosophila melanogaster. Academic Press, San Diego.

[40] http://www.flybase.org, version FB2012_02, released March 2nd, 2012.

Section 5

Non Coding RNA and Micro RNA in Tumorigenesis

Chapter 13

Post-Transcriptional Regulation of Proto-Oncogene *c-fms* in Breast Cancer

Ho-Hyung Woo and Setsuko K. Chambers

Additional information is available at the end of the chapter

http://dx.doi.org/10.5772/53541

1. Introduction

1.1. *c-fms* and breast cancer

In the development and progression of breast cancers, both the *c-fms* proto-oncogene (which encodes the tyrosine kinase receptor for CSF-1) as well as CSF-1 (colony stimulating factor-1), play an important role. Evidence from transgenic models suggests that *c-fms* encodes for the sole receptor for CSF-1 (Dai *et al*, 2002). We and others have found that *c-fms* and/or CSF-1 are expressed by the tumor epithelium in several human epithelial cancers (Kacinski *et al*, 1988, 1990, 1991; Rettenmier *et al*, 1989; Filderman *et al*, 1992; Ide *et al*, 2002); elevated levels of *c-fms* and CSF-1 are associated with poor prognosis (Kacinski *et al*, 1988; Tang *et al*, 1990; Price *et al*, 1993; Chambers *et al*, 1997, 2009; Scholl *et al*, 1993; Kluger *et al*, 2004; Sapi 2004). In human breast cancer, 94% of *in situ* and invasive lesions express *c-fms* (Kacinski *et al*, 1991; Flick *et al*, 1997), while 36% express both CSF-1 and *c-fms* (Kacinski *et al*, 1991; Scholl *et al*, 1993). Among breast cancer patients, serum levels of CSF-1 are frequently elevated in those with metastases (Kacinski *et al*, 1991). In breast tumors, nuclear CSF-1 staining is associated with poor survival (Scholl *et al*, 1994), and *c-fms* expression confers an increased risk for local relapse (Maher *et al*, 1998). In a large breast cancer tissue array, *c-fms* (Kluger *et al*, 2004) is strongly associated with lymph node metastasis, and poor survival. This strong correlation with prognosis suggests an etiologic role for *c-fms*/CSF-1 in tumor invasion and metastasis.

Tumor-associated macrophages bearing CSF-1 promote progression of breast cancer (Pollard 2004). In mice bearing human breast cancer xenografts, targeting mouse (host) *c-fms* with siRNA, or CSF-1 with antisense, siRNA or antibody suppressed primary tumor growth by 40-50% (Aharinejad *et al*, 2004; Paulus *et al*, 2006), and improved their survival (Aharinejad *et al*, 2004). Hence, paracrine signaling by macrophages bearing CSF-1 also plays a critical role in breast cancer progression. Transgenic models suggest that the absence of CSF-1 results in delay of tumor invasion and metastasis, while targeting CSF-1 to mammary epithelium in these models enables macrophage infiltration and invasive breast cancer to develop and metastasize (Lin *et al,* 2001).

We have reported that glucocorticoids (GC) up-regulate *c-fms* expression both in breast cancer cells (Kacinski *et al,* 1991; Flick *et al,* 2002; Sapi *et al,* 1995), and in primary organ cultures of breast cancer specimens (Kacinski *et al,* 2001). In a study of 329 breast cancer patients, 52% of the breast cancer tissues had functional glucocorticoid receptor (GR) (Allegra *et al,* 1979). This allows for breast cancer responsiveness to circulating, endogenous GCs.

In the *in vivo* environment, with endogenous GCs, we observed extensive metastatic spread by breast cancer cells over-expressing *c-fms,* compared to controls (Toy *et al,* 2005). Parenchymal invasion was demonstrated only by the *c-fms* overexpressing cells. Interrupting the autocrine loop between *c-fms* and CSF-1 inhibits GC-stimulated invasiveness, motility, and adhesiveness *in vitro* of breast cancer cells (Toy *et al,* 2010). This mechanism of increasing *c-fms* by GC becomes aberrantly up-regulated in invasive, metastatic breast cancer.

1.2. Regulation of *c-fms* expression

Regulation of *c-fms* expression is a complex process. Both transcriptional and post-transcriptional regulations are involved to maintain a proper level of *c-fms* expression. This chapter summarizes the research over the last 20 years concerning post-transcriptional regulation of *c-fms* and its expression in breast cancer.

1.3. Stability of *c-fms* transcripts in breast cancer cells

c-fms expression is high in metastatic breast cancer cells, but not detectable in the normal breast cells and non-invasive precursors of breast neoplasms (Kacinski *et al,* 1988, 1990). Unusually long half-life of *c-fms* mRNA partially contributes high expression in metastatic breast cancer cells (Chambers *et al,* 1994, Woo et al, 2011). GCs increase the *c-fms* mRNA half-life from 9.6 h to 18.9 h in BT20 breast cancer cells (Woo et al, 2011). In highly invasive MDA-MB-231 breast cancer cells, *c-fms* mRNA half-life increases up to 27 h in response to GC treatment (Figure 1).

1.4. Post-transcriptional regulation of *c-fms* expression by 3′UTR

mRNA 3′UTR contains *cis*-acting regulatory sequences which are involved in regulation of mRNA stability and polyadenylation (Mignone *et al,* 2003; Bashirullah *et al,* 2001), mRNA degradation (Bevilacqua *et al,* 2003), translation, and subcellular localization of mRNAs (Loya *et al,* 2008; Jansen, 2001). Mutations in 3′UTR could result in diseases and are proposed as 'a molecular hotspot for pathology (Chen *et al,* 2006; Conne *et al,* 2000). Post-transcriptional regulation exerted by 3′UTR is considered an important counterpart to transcriptional regulation for maintaining the proper level of gene products in the cell.

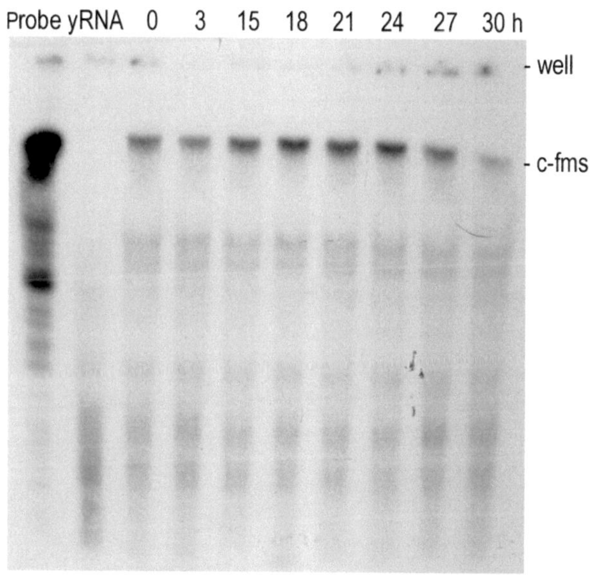

Probe – free probe, yRNA – yeast RNA as negative control, Total RNA was isolated after dexamethasone treatment at the indicated time.

Figure 1. RNase protection analysis of *c-fms* mRNA in MDA-MB-231 cells treated by 400 nM dexamethasone.

Human *c-fms* mRNA 3'UTR encodes 774 nt and contains unique regions including a non-AU-rich-69 nt sequence (3499-3567) which we have described and characterized (Woo *et al*, 2009, 2011), and also several putative target sequences for miRNA binding (Figure 2). The 69 nt sequence contains 3 islets of pyrimidine-rich sequences (CUUU). Mutations in these pyrimidine-rich sequences in 69 nt disrupted vigilin and HuR binding (Woo *et al*, 2009, 2011).

In metazoans, the 69 nt sequence within the 3'-UTR of *c-fms* mRNA is partially conserved between human, mouse, and rat (Figure 2). This region does not contain conventional AU-rich elements (ARE) (Woo *et al*, 2009). Overall, the 69 nt sequence is slightly pyrimidine-rich (>57-61%) and we proposed that primary sequence as well as loop structure may be important for protein binding (Woo *et al*, 2011; Kanamori *et al*, 1998). Indeed, this 69 nt region is predicted to form a stable loop structure (Figure 3).

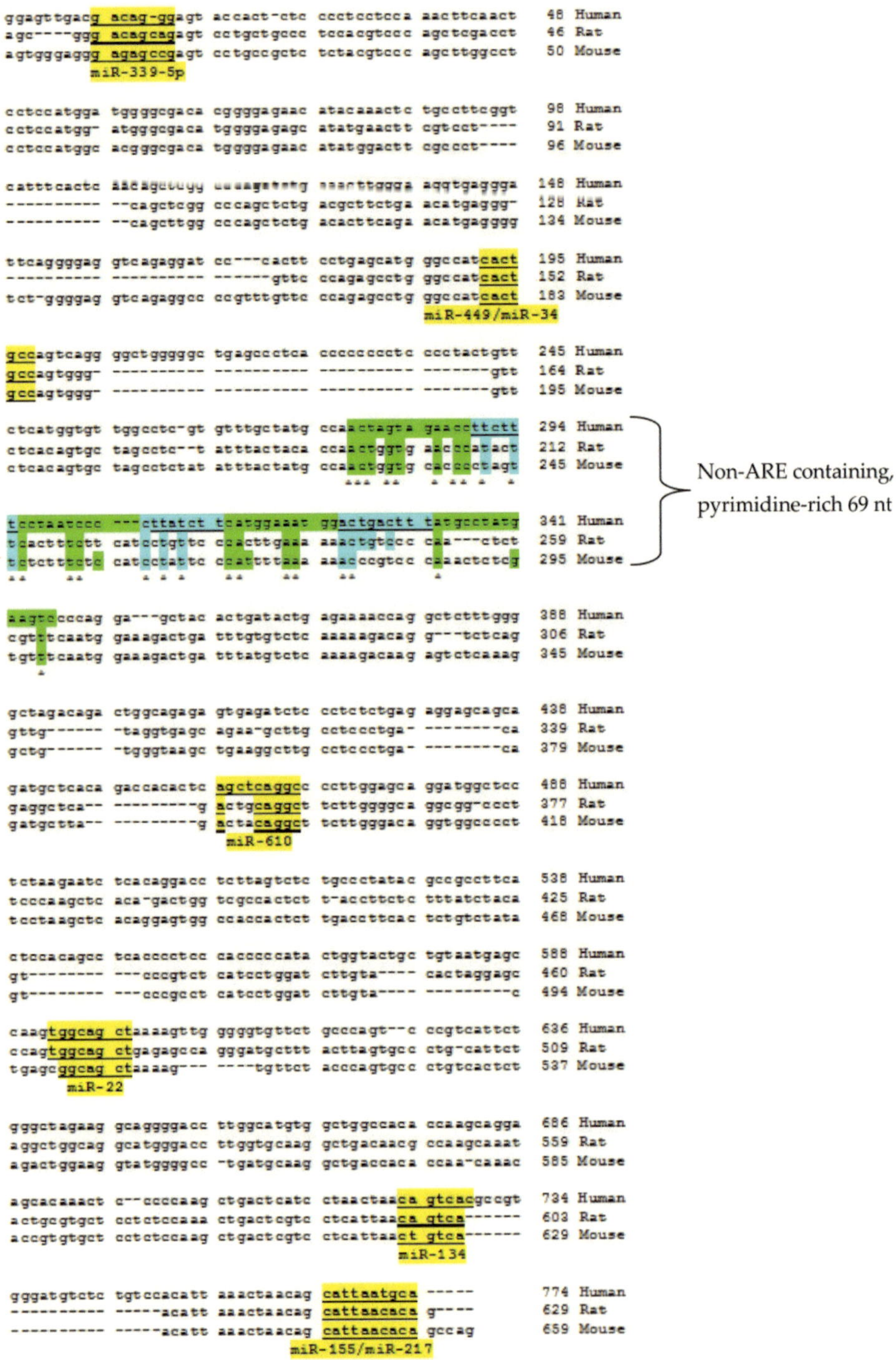

The 69 nt sequence (3499-3567) is partially conserved in human, rat, and mouse.

Figure 2. Alignment of *c-fms* mRNA 3'UTRs of human, rat, and mouse. Six regions are predicted as targets by eight miRNAs.

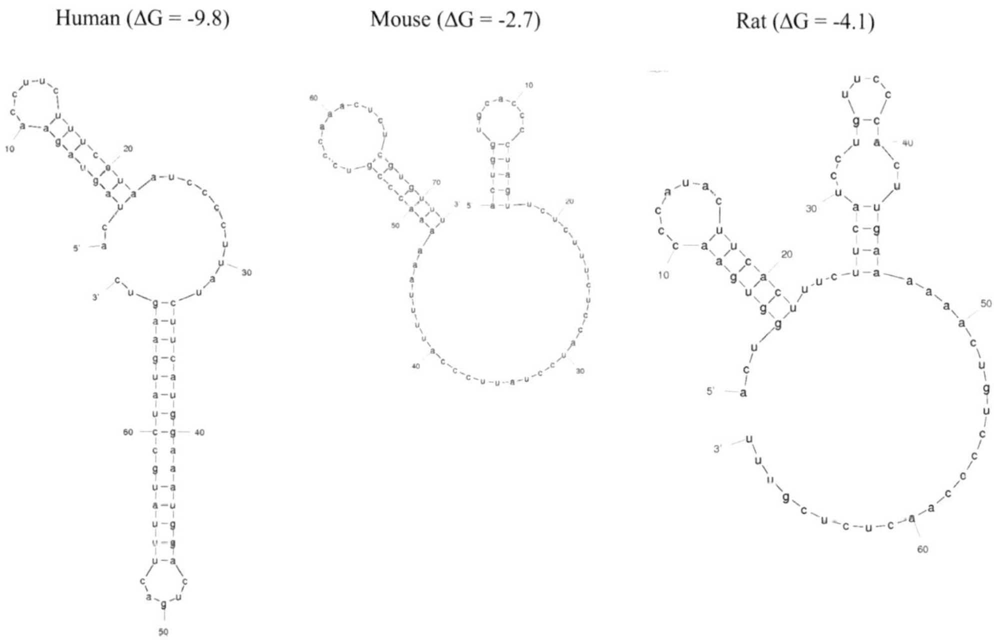

Figure 3. RNA loops of 69 nt are predicted by mfold (http://mfold.rna.albany.edu/?q=mfold).

1.5. microRNAs for *c-fms* mRNA regulation

MicroRNAs (miRNAs) are 21-23 nucleotide single-stranded RNAs, that in general down-regulate translation and enhance mRNA degradation (Huntzinger and Izaurralde, 2011; Braun *et al*, 2011). As a consequence, miRNAs are involved in the regulation of several biological functions (differentiation, hematopoiesis, tumorigenesis, apoptosis, development, proliferation, and growth) (Kim, 2005). They are predicted to regulate more than 60% of human mRNA (Friedman *et al*, 2009). It has been found that mRNAs with long 3′UTRs are more susceptible to miRNA regulation than those with short 3′UTRs as the latter lack the number of binding sites necessary for multiple miRNA binding and regulation (Stark *et al*, 2005).

Bioinformatics analysis predicted eight miRNAs (miR-339-5p, miR-449, miR-34, miR-610, miR-22, miR-134, miR-155, and miR-217) targeting six regions in *c-fms* mRNA 3′UTR (Figure 2). These six target regions are also highly conserved in human, mouse and rat. Among those, two miRNAs (miR-610 and miR-155) were selected by us for further analysis. *C-fms* mRNA level is higher in BT20 epithelial breast cancer cells than in Hey epithelial ovarian cancer cells (Figure 4). In contrast, miR-610 and miR-155 RNA levels show opposite expression patterns with their RNA levels lower in BT20 than in Hey cells. Using a luciferase RNA-fused *c-fms* mRNA 3′UTR reporter system, introduction of miR-610 inhibitors in BT20 cells increased luciferase RNA level by 5.5-fold and luciferase activity by 1.3-fold. The down-regulation of mir-610 has more effects on luciferase RNA levels than translational repression. Some reports describe miRNA effects to be mainly on translational repression, while others describe an effect primarily on mRNA decay. Guo *et al* (2010) reported that the predominant effect of mammalian miRNAs is on mRNA decay which results reduced translation. In contrast, in zebrafish, miR-430 reduced translation initiation prior to inducing mRNA decay (Bazzini *et al*, 2012). Djuranovic *et al* (2012) reported miRNA-mediated translational repression is followed by mRNA deadenylation. Recently, the concept of mRNA destabilization by miRNAs gained support by genome-wide observation studies (Huntzinger and Izaurralde, 2011).

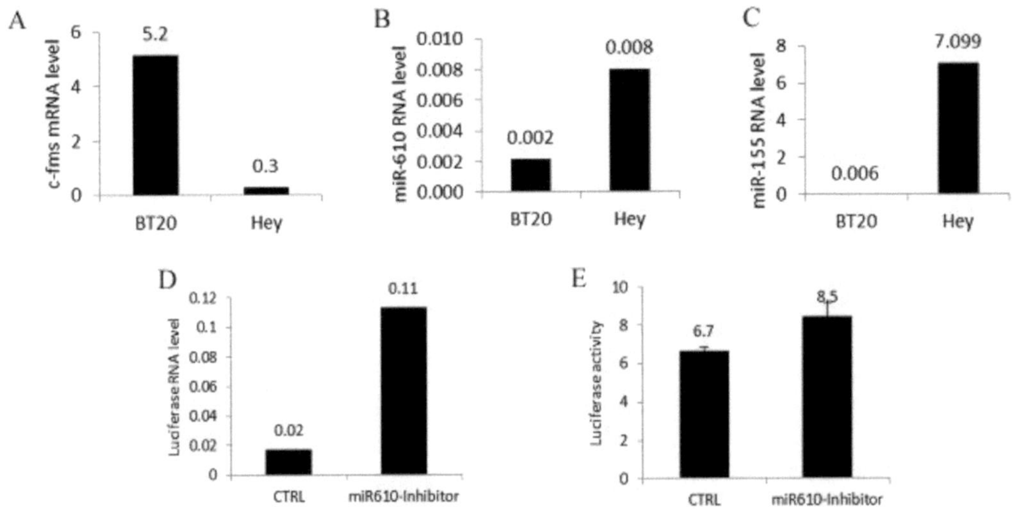

Figure 4. (A) *c-fms* mRNA level is higher in BT20 than in Hey cells. (B) miR-610 RNA level is higher in Hey than in BT20 cells. (C) miR-155 RNA level is higher in Hey than BT20 cells. (D) Using a luciferase RNA-fused *c-fms* mRNA 3'UTR reporter system, introduction of miR-610 inhibitor increased luciferase RNA level by 5.5-fold and (E) luciferase activity by 1.3-fold in BT20 cells.

1.6. RNA-binding proteins for *c-fms* mRNA metabolism and translation

The first evidence supporting post-transcriptional regulation of *c-fms* mRNA by RNA-binding proteins was reported in human monocytes (HL-60 cells) (Weber *et al*, 1989). In their study, TPA (12-*O*-tetradecanoylphorbol-13-acetate)-induced monocytic differentiation did not change *c-fms* transcription, but increased *c-fms* mRNA level. In addition, treatment of protein synthesis inhibitor cycloheximide decreased half-life of *c-fms* mRNA in TPA-induced HL-60 cells. From this observation, they proposed that a labile protein(s) is involved in stabilization of *c-fms* mRNA.

Chambers *et al*. (1993) reported the existence of mRNA regulatory proteins involved in *c-fms* mRNA destabilization in dexamethasone (Dex) or cyclosporin A (CsA) treated HL-60 cells. Dex or CsA blocked TPA-induced monocytic differentiation as well as TPA-induced adherence and further differentiated morphology. In TPA-induced HL-60 cells, *c-fms* mRNA half life was decreased after the addition of Dex or CsA. The effects of cycloheximide of *c-fms* mRNA decay in this setting suggested the existence of labile destabilizing protein(s).

Furthermore, in breast carcinoma cells (BT20 and SKBR3), Dex-treatment at later time points increased *c-fms* mRNA level without affecting *c-fms* transcription. Addition of protein synthesis inhibitors prevented Dex-induced increase of *c-fms* mRNA level suggesting the presence of Dex-inducible stabilizing protein(s) in breast carcinoma cells (Chambers *et al*, 1994).

RNA-binding proteins: About 1,500 RNA-binding proteins (RBPs) have been identified, which bind to mRNA and modulate mRNA stability and translation. mRNA primary sequences as well as loop structures are known to facilitate regulatory protein binding for post-transcriptional regulation.

HuR – HuR, one of the most extensively studied RBPs, encoded by ELAVL1 (embryonic lethal, abnormal vision, *Drosophila*-like 1) binds *cis*-acting AU-rich elements (AREs) (Barreau *et al*, 2005) and also non-ARE-containing sequences including pyrimidine-rich sequences (Woo *et al*, 2009) in target mRNAs. HuR stabilizes and increases half-life of target mRNAs and therefore enhances their translation (Srikantan and Gorospe, 2011). Our study indicates that HuR binds *c-fms* mRNA 3'UTR and enhances mRNA stability and translation (Woo *et al*, 2009).

In human breast-cancer tissues, HuR is expressed mostly in nucleus (>90%), but expression in cytoplasm is also found. High nuclear expression of HuR is a poor prognostic factor both in breast and ovarian cancer (Woo *et al*, 2009; Yi *et al*, 2009).

Vigilin – Vigilin, a high-density lipoprotein-binding protein, contains 15 K-homology (KH) domains (Goolsby and Shapiro, 2003). The KH domain protein family interacts with ARE-containing mRNAs and enhances mRNA degradation and consequently down-regulates

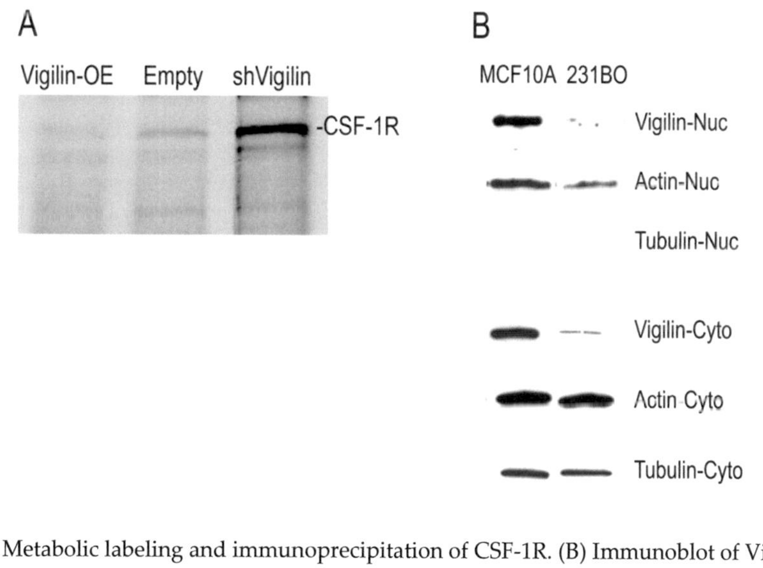

Figure 5. (A) Metabolic labeling and immunoprecipitation of CSF-1R. (B) Immunoblot of Vigilin in both nuclear (Nuc) and cytoplasmic (Cyto) fractions of MCF10A and MDA-MB-231BO cells. Absence of tubulin in nuclear fraction and presence of tubulin in cytoplasmic fraction indicate no cross-contamination in both fractions.

translation (Gherzi *et al*, 2004). In contrast, vigilin interacts largely with unstructured pyrimidine-rich sequences in mRNA 3'UTR (Kanamori *et al*, 1998; Woo *et al*, 2011). We found that vigilin decreases *c-fms* mRNA half-life and down-regulates translation. Ectopic expression of vigilin in breast cancer cells showed that the effects of down-regulation is more pronounced on *c-fms* protein level than on the mRNA level (Woo *et al*, 2011). Metabolic labeling and immunoprecipitation of *c-fms* protein showed that vigilin overexpression down-regulated *c-fms* protein level in BT20 cells (Figure 5A). In contrast, suppression of vigilin by shRNA up-regulated *c-fms* protein level.

Furthermore, immunoblot analysis showed that vigilin expression was lower in metastatic breast cancer MDA-MB-231BO cells than in non-tumorigenic epithelial breast MCF10A cells (Figure 5B). This indicates that a possible suppressive role of vigilin in invasive characters of breast cancer cells.

Both *in vitro* and *in vivo* studies indicate that vigilin and HuR competitively bind to the pyrimidine-rich 69 nt sequence of *c-fms* mRNA 3'UTR (Figure 4, Woo *et al*, 2009, 2011). *In vitro* competition assay showed that affinity of vigilin to the 69 nt sequence is at least 3-fold higher than that of HuR (Figure 6).

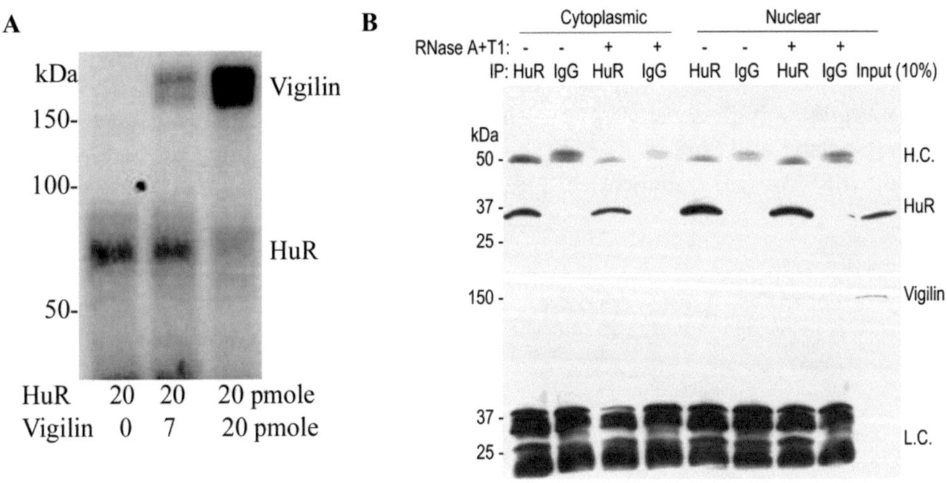

Figure 6. (A) Competition assay between vigilin and HuR by UV crosslink. (B) Co-immunoprecipitation assay. Vigilin and HuR do not present in the same mRNP complexes. IP assays were carried out using cellular lysates from MDA-MB-231 cells in either RNase-free or RNase-treated conditions using anti-human HuR mAb, or IgG. The presence of HuR in the IP materials was monitored by immunoblot. H.C. – heavy chain of IgG. L.C. – Light chain of IgG.

1.7. Effects of HuR and vigilin on invasiveness of breast cancer cells

Increased *c-fms*/CSF-1 levels correlate with the invasive breast cancer phenotype, and with prognosis (Toy, 2005; Toy *et al*, 2010; Sapi, 2004; Kluger *et al*, 2004; Scholl *et al*, 1994, 1993; Maher *et al*, 1998). We studied the ability of BT20 breast cancer cells to invade through a human derived simple matrix *in vitro*. The invasion of BT20 cells was significantly inhibited by the over-expression of vigilin, resulting in a 48% decrease compared to control (Figure 7). In contrast, over-expression of HuR increased invasiveness by 34%. Our findings suggest that vigilin can negatively impact, through suppression of *c-fms* expression, breast cancer cell invasiveness. In contrast, HuR enhances breast cancer cell invasiveness.

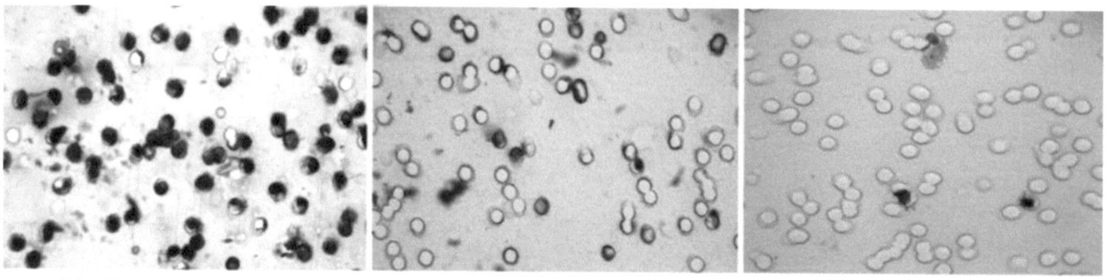

Figure 7. Vigilin and HuR regulate *in vitro* invasiveness of BT20 breast cancer cells. This findings correlate with relative *c-fms* expression.

1.8. Post-translational modification: dimerization and tyrosine-phosphorylation of CSF-1R activation of PIP3/Akt signal transduction pathway

Activation of CSF-1R, product of the *c-fms* gene, requires ligand-induced non-covalent dimerization and phosphorylation of tyrosine residues in CSF-1R (Xiong *et al*, 2011; Li and Stanley, 1991). Here, we focus on one of the major signaling transduction pathways which result from CSF-1R activation. Phosphorylated CSF-1R interacts with PI3K (Phosphatidylinositol 3-kinases) (Shurtleff *et al*, 1990). In turn, PI3K converts PIP2 (Phosphatidylinositol-3,4-bisphosphate) to PIP3 (Phosphatidylinositol-3,4,5 tisphosphate). PIP3 interacts with Akt (protein kinase B, PBK), and activates downstream components in the PIP3/Akt signaling pathway. As a result, several physiological consequences are regulated including cell proliferation, apoptosis, and growth. An activated PIP3/Akt pathway is a common event in human cancer. (Arcaro and Guerreiro, 2007).

In breast cancer cells, multiple components are known to activate phosphorylation of CSF-1R. Endogenous cytokine CSF-1, functioning as an autocrine signal, can bind to the extracellular domain of CSF-1R and activate the cytoplasmic kinase domain leading to autophosphorylation of tyrosine-residues in CSF-1R. There is evidence to suggest that endogenous CSF-1 can also bind CSF-1R without interaction on the membrane surface. Exogenous CSF-1, from other sources such as macrophages, osteoclasts, or fibroblasts, can function in a paracrine manner to activate CSF-1R on the membrane surface. Consequently, phosphorylation of tyrosine residues in CSF-1R activates cell proliferation and invasive potential (Yu *et al*, 2012; Sapi *et al*, 1996). Our study indicates glucocorticoids (dexamethasone) and starvation also activate CSF-1R auto-phosphorylation (Figure 8).

CSF-1R is localized both in the cytoplasm, plasma membrane, and nuclear envelope (Zwaenepoel *et al*, 2012). CSF-1R in the nuclear envelope becomes phosphorylated in response to CSF-1. Phosphorylated CSF-1R in the nuclear envelope triggers the phosphorylation of Akt and p27 inside the nucleus.

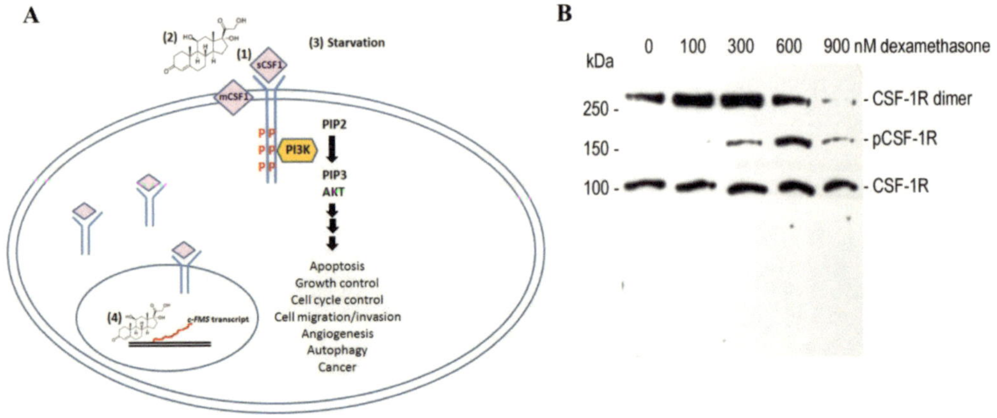

Figure 8. (A) Signal transduction through pCSF-1R/PI3K regulates cell growth and angiogenesis. Both autocrine and paracrine signals (sCSF-1, glucocorticoids, and starvation) trigger dimerization and autophosphorylation of CSF-1R, which interacts with PI3K. The PI3K generates PIP3, which binds to Akt. Activation of PIP3/Akt activates downstream components and regulates growth, apoptosis and cell cycle. (B) Dexamethasone induces autophosphorylation of CSF-1R in starved MDA-MB-231 cells.

2. Discussion

Post-transcriptional and translational regulation of *c-fms* expression by vigilin and HuR in breast cancer cells: mRNA translation and decay are complex multi-staged processes. Mature mRNAs either enter translation or degradation pathways depending on the developmental stages of the cell. We have reported vigilin and HuR, both nuclear-cytoplasmic shuttling RNA-binding proteins, to be involved in post-transcriptional as well as translational regulation of *c-fms* mRNA (Woo *et al*, 2009, 2011). Vigilin binds the pyrimidine-rich 69 nt sequence in the *c-fms* mRNA 3′UTR, to which HuR also binds. Both *in vitro* and *in cell* studies indicate that they compete for the same 69 nt sequence in the *c-fms* mRNA 3′UTR and that dynamic changes in the ratio of vigilin to HuR can influence their ability to associate with the *c-fms* mRNA and post-transcriptionally regulate cellular *c-fms* levels. While vigilin down-regulates *c-fms* translation as well as mRNA stability, HuR, in contrast, has opposite effect on *c-fms* levels; i.e., HuR up-regulates *c-fms* mRNA stability resulting increased *c-fms* protein levels. In our previous study, the polysome profile indicates vigilin is associated with free mRNPs and low MW monosomes. In contrast, HuR was detected with high MW polysomes (Woo *et al*, 2011). Vigilin also represses translation of reporter RNA (luciferase RNA fused with *c-fms* mRNA 3′UTR sequence) in the rabbit reticulocyte lysate cell-free translation system (Woo *et al*, 2011).

Translation can be divided in three phases; initiation, elongation, and termination. Translation initiation is a complicated process for which a large number of eukaryotic initiation factors (eIFs) have been identified (Sonnenberg and Hinnebusch, 2009). Translation initiation starts with the assembly of a 48S quaternary initiation complex comprised of the 40S ribosomal subunit, eIFs, $tRNA_{Met}$, and m^7G cap of the mRNA. In general, this 48S initiation complex scans and base pairs with the AUG initiation codon in

5'UTR of mRNA. This results in formation of the 80S ribosome and is continued in the elongation step of peptide synthesis.

In a 'closed-loop' mRNP model for cap-dependent translational regulation, PABPs bind both to the poly A+ tail at the 3'UTR and eIF4G of the translation initiation complex at the 5'-cap (Huntzinger and Izaurralde, 2011). This mRNA circularization attracts ribosomes to form a translation initiation complex. Subsequently, after translation termination, joining of the 5'- and 3'-ends of the mRNA facilitates the transfer of ribosomal subunits from the 3' to the 5'-end.

Our results have demonstrated presence of vigilin in free mRNP fractions in human BT20 breast cancer cells. While vigilin association with free mRNPs may prevent 'closed-loop' formation and consequently inhibit *c-fms* protein translation, it was also found to associate with tRNAs and elongation factors (Kruse *et al*, 2003; Vollbrandt *et al*, 2004). Binding of vigilin with these components may deplete the available tRNAs and elongation factors for translation elongation. We propose a model that the impaired translation resulting from vigilin binding may expose both 5'- and 3'-ends of the mRNA through reduced circularization and increase its rate of degradation (Figure 9). In contrast, we propose that HuR binding to *c-fms* mRNA 3'UTR may enhance 'closed-loop' formation which increases the *c-fms* mRNA stability and also translation initiation efficiency. Immunoblot analysis indicates that vigilin is, in general, less expressed in breast cancer cells than in non-tumorigenic breast cells (Woo *et al*, 2011). This indicates that down-regulation of vigilin may be partly responsible for increased *c-fms* level in breast cancer cells. In summary, RNA binding proteins, such as vigilin and HuR are critical regulators for determining the fate of proto-oncogene *c-fms* mRNA, either to be translated or decayed.

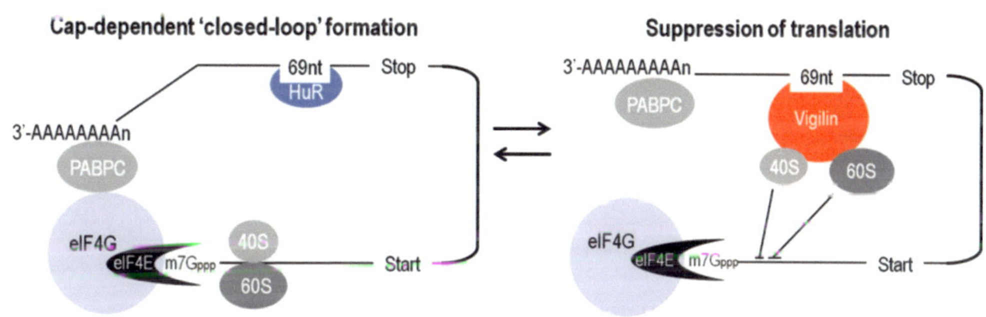

Figure 9. Competition between HuR and vigilin for binding 69 nt of *c-fms* mRNA 3'UTR regulates translational machinery formation. Binding of HuR to 69 nt may induce 'closed-loop' formation. In contrast, binding of vigilin to 69 nt could prevent 'closed-loop' formation.

Future research in post-transcriptional and translational regulation of *c-fms* in breast cancer: Translational inhibition and mRNA degradation are coordinated processes in which translation initiation is inhibited and translation factors (eIFs) are exchanged with repression/degradation complex (hDcp1/2, Hedls) (Fenger *et al*, 2005), resulting in mRNA degradation by exonucleases (Xrn1 and exosomes) (Balagopal and Parker, 2009). In general, 3'-deadenylation leads to 5'-decapping followed by exonucleolytic digestion at either ends of mammalian poly-A⁺-mRNAs (Franks and Lykke-Anderson, 2008; Zheng *et al,* 2008). In human cells, deadenylation is initiated by deadenylase complex (Pan2/3, Caf1, and Ccr4) (Zheng *et al,* 2008). Deadenylated oligo(A) mRNPs are further processed by decapping complex (including Xrn1 for 5′-to-3′ decay) or exosomes (for 3′-to-5′ decay). In yeast, decapping activators (Dhh1, Pat1, Lsm1-7, Edc1-3, Scd6) were identified which enhance decapping (Nissan *et al,* 2010). Mutated or excess nontranslating mRNAs are stored and degraded in processing bodies (P-bodies, GW-bodies, or Dcp-bodies) and/or stress granules (SGs). During inhibition of translation initiation, elevated numbers of P-bodies and SGs are observed (Shyu *et al,* 2008). Nontranslating mRNPs accumulate both in P-bodies and SGs. Decapping complex (hDcp1/2, Hedls) and mRNA decay fragments are found in P-bodies suggesting presence of 5′-to-3′ exonuclease activities (Xrn1). Deadenylation complex (Pan2/3, Caf1, Ccr4) is also present in mouse P-bodies. On the other hand, translation initiation components (eIFs) and RNA-binding proteins (Ataxin-2, Pab1, TIA-R, TIA-1) are found in SGs (Buchan and Parker, 2009). Another very important aspect of mRNA stability is mRNA binding proteins. They can stimulate decapping and degradation processes. Over-expression of cold-inducible RNA-binding protein (CIRP), which represses translation, induces SGs (De Leeuw *et al,* 2007). In contrast, HuR was shown to release translational repression by helping human mRNA associated with P-bodies to re-enter polysomes (Bhattacharyya *et al,* 2006). In mammalian cells, P-bodies and SGs often dock together during translation inhibition. Since vigilin was shown to repress *c-fms* translation, it is crucial to understand mechanisms of transitions of *c-fms* mRNPs between P-bodies, SGs and

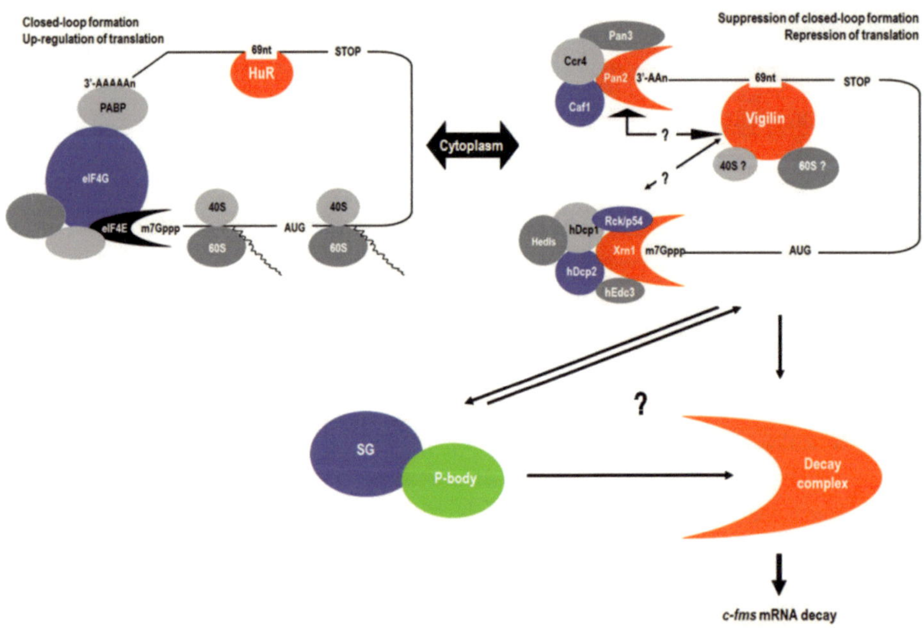

Figure 10. Proposed model for post-transcriptional regulation of *c-fms* by HuR and vigilin. HuR enhances closed-loop formation and increases *c-fms* mRNA stability and translation. In contrast, vigilin prevent closed-loop formation and attracts mRNA degradation complex and down-regulates translation. SG – stress granule

polysomes. A model for these mechanisms is proposed in Figure 10. Elucidating the molecular mechanisms of these exchanges from one state to another is critical to the understanding of regulation of *c-fms* protein levels in breast cancer.

3. Conclusion

In the design of clinical therapeutics, suppression of pathogenic gene expression requires high specificity to prevent off-target toxicity. In order to achieve this, detailed regulatory mechanisms of target gene expression should be elucidated. Understanding the regulatory mechanisms and specific proteins through which vigilin effects translational down-regulation of proto-oncogene *c-fms* in breast cancer can result in more accurate control of its expression.

Based on information available from the last 20 years of research and our recent data, it is now possible to elucidate vigilin's role in translational down-regulation of *c-fms* mRNA in breast cancer. Information obtained from this research will support a model on the manner in which interaction between a specific mRNA (*c-fms*) and proteins (vigilin and HuR) regulates *c-fms* at a translational level. These findings will bring us one step closer to development of a targeted therapy based on these mechanisms.

4. Methods

4.1. Cell culture

A human breast carcinoma cell line BT20 was maintained in MEM (Sigma) supplemented with 0.1 mM non-essential amino acids, 2 mM L glutamine, 1 mM sodium pyruvate, 1.5 g/L sodium bicarbonate, and 10% fetal bovine serum (Invitrogen) in 5% CO_2 at 37°C. A human breast carcinoma cell line MDA-MB-231 was cultured in DMEM (Sigma) supplemented with 10% fetal bovine serum. For studies using glucocorticoids, cells were grown in starvation medium with 100 nM Dex (Sigma-Aldrich) for 72 h and collected for immunoblot analysis. A human ovarian cancer cell line Hey was grown in DMEM/F12 (Sigma) supplemented with 10% fetal bovine serum.

4.2. Total RNA isolation for semi-quantitative real-time RT-PCR analysis

Cells were grown in 6-well plate for 2-3 days before harvesting. Total RNA was extracted with 500 ul Trizol (Invitrogen) per well. After Trizol extraction, 150 ul of supernatant was carefully removed to avoid genomic DNA contamination. Supernatant was re-extracted by equal volume of chloroform and 100 ul of supernatant was carefully removed and ethanol precipitated for cDNA synthesis.

4.3. Semi-quantitative real-time RT-PCR analysis for *c-fms* mRNAs

Total RNA was oligo-dT_{18} primed by M-MuLV reverse transcriptase (New England Biolab). For PCR analysis, reverse transcriptase reaction was diluted by 10-fold and 2 ul was used for

20 ul PCR reaction. GAPDH mRNA was amplified in PCR reaction as internal loading control.

c-fms PCR primers (forward primer = 5′-GGAGTTGACGACAGGGAGTACCAC-3′, reverse primer = 5′- ACGAGGCCAACACCATGAGAACAG-3′).

GAPDH PCR primers (forward primer = 5′ CGGGAAACTGTGGCGTGATGGC-3′, reverse primer = 5′-AGGAGACCACCTGGTGCTCAGTG-3′).

c-fms mRNA expression level was calculated with the ΔΔCT method (Schmittgen and Livak, 2008).

4.4. Stem-loop real-time RT-PCR analysis for miR-610 and miR-155 quantification

miRNA expression was determined by the stem-loop qRT-PCR analysis to increase the specificity of miRNA amplification (Chen *et al,* 2005). cDNAs for miR-610, miR-155, and tRNAGlu specific were synthesized using sequence specific stem-loop forming primers. After 10-fold dilution of reverse transcriptase reaction, 2 ul was used for 20 ul real-time PCR. tRNAGlu was used as internal loading control.

miR-610 reverse transcription primer = 5′-gtcgtatccagtgcagggtccgaggtattcgcact ggatacgactcccag-3′)

miR-610 PCR primers (forward primer = 5′- GGCGCTGAGCTAAATGTGTGC-3′, reverse primer = 5′- GTGCAGGGTCCGAGGT-3′)

miR-155 reverse transcription primer = 5′- gtcgtatccagtgcagggtccgaggtattcgcact ggatacgacacccct-3′

miR-155 PCR primers (forward primer = 5′- GGCGCTTAATGCTAATCGTGATAG-3′, reverse primer = 5′- GTGCAGGGTCCGAGGT-3′)

tRNAGlu reverse transcription primer = 5′- GTCGTATCCAGTGCAGGGTCCGAGGTATTCGCACT GGATACGAC GGTGAAAG-3′

tRNAGlu PCR primers (forward primer = 5′- CTGGTTAGTACTTGGACGGGAGAC -3′, reverse primer = 5′- gtgcagggtccgaggt -3′)

4.5. Analysis of *c-fms* mRNA Half Life

The *c-fms* mRNA half-life was determined by RNase protection assay (RPA) (Bordonaro *et al,* 1994). Radioactive-labeled antisense RNA probes of *c-fms* mRNA was generated by *in vitro* transcription. *c-fms* cDNA (237nt, 1789-2025) with 67nt random sequence and 23nt T7 promoter at 3′-end was generated by PCR and used as a templete for *in vitro* transcription. Probes with specific activity of $1x10^5$ cpm were hybridized with 10 μg of total RNA in hybridization buffer (80% deionized formamide, 40 mM PIPES pH6.4, 400 mM NaCl, and 1 mM EDTA) at 42°C overnight. Next morning, unbound RNA was digested by RNase A and

T1 at 37°C for 1 h. After proteinase K treatment at 37°C for 30 min, samples were extracted by phenol-chloroform and precipitated in ethanol. Samples were analyzed on a 5% acrylamide/8M urea gel and exposed on X-ray film.

4.6. Metabolic labeling and immunoprecipitation of *c-fms* proteins

The BT20 cultures at 75-80% confluence were washed with PBS and incubated in labeling medium (Met,Cys-free RPMI1640 (Sigma R-7513), 5% dialyzed FCS, 500ug/ml Glutamine) for 40 min to deplete endogenous methionine and cysteine in cell. For metabolic labeling, 5 ml labeling medium and 50 ul (500 uCi) of 35S-Methionine/35S-Cysteine per T75 flask was added and incubated for 30-40 min. After brief chase in chase medium (labeling medium with 500μg/ml Cysteine-HCl and 100μg/ml Methionine), cells were harvested and lysed in IP buffer (1% Triton x-100, 0.05% NP-40 in TBS, protease inhibitors). For immunoprecipitation of c-fms proteins, 5 ug of *c-fms* monoclonal antibody and 50 μl of Protein A/G-agarose (50% slurrry) (Santa Cruz) were added to cell lysates and incubated overnight at 4°C. Next morning, agarose beads was washed extensively with IP buffer and protein was eluted by SDS sample buffer. Labeled protein was analyzed in 10% SDS-PAGE.

4.7. Gain-of-function and loss-of-function assay

Plasmids encoding a control shRNA or shRNA directed against vigilin were purchased from Origene. The shRNAs correspond to coding region nucleotides 614–642 (5'-AAGCTCG GAAGGACATTGTTGCTAGACTG-3') and 829–863 (5'-CATGAAGTCTTACTCATCTCTG CCGAGCAGGACAA-3'), respectively, of human vigilin (GenBank BC001179). An shRNA containing a non-specific 29nt GFP sequence (TR30003, Origene) was used as a transfection control (Empty). For RNAi, 5 ×106 cells were transfected with 10 μg shRNA plasmid using Fugene HD (Roche) according to the manufacturer's instructions. Transfected cells were maintained in culture medium for 3-4 days to permit knockdown before assays.

For vigilin overexpression, pTetCMV-Fo(AS)-vigilin (Cunningham et al, 2000) was transfected using Fugene HD (Roche). The BT20 cells at 75-80% confluence in 6-well plates were transfected with 5 μg of plasmids. The overexpression effects were monitored for 3-4 days by qRT-PCR and western blot analyses.

4.8. UV crosslinking and label transfer with *c-fms* mRNA 3′UTR

UV cross-linking of HuR and vigilin was performed as described previously (Urlaub *et al*, 2000) with modifications. RNAs of *c*-fms 3′UTR labeled with 32P UTP were incubated with recombinant HuR or recombinant vigilin proteins. The 15 μl reaction mixture contained 5 mM HEPESpH7.6, 1.25 mM MgCl2, 3.8% glycerol, 0.02 mM DTT, 1 mM EDTA, 25 mM KCl, 50 ng yeast tRNA, 50 ng heparin, 1 mM ATP, and ^{32}P-labeled RNA probe (50,000 cpm). After incubation at 30°C for 20 min, reaction mixture in a 96-well polystyrene plate on ice was illuminated at 254 nm, 125 mJoule for 120 seconds using a GS Gene Linker UV Chamber (Bio-Rad). After crosslink, excess RNA was digested by RNase A for 30 min at 37°C. Crosslinked protein was fractionated in 10% SDS-PAGE.

4.9. Invasion assay

The Membrane Invasion Culture System (MICS chamber) was used to quantitate, the degree of invasion of MDA-MB-231 transiently transfected vigilin or HuR overexpressing clones. Breast cancer cells were cultured in the presence of 100 nM Dex and remained under starved conditions for transfection duration prior to the invasion assays. Parent or transfected cells, $1x10^5$ per well in a 6-well plate, were seeded onto 10-µm pore filters coated with a human defined matrix containing 50 µg/ml human laminin, 50 µg/ml human collagen IV, and 2 mg/ml gelatin in 10 mM acetic acid.

Author details

Ho-Hyung Woo and Setsuko K. Chambers
Arizona Cancer Center, University of Arizona, Tucson, AZ, USA

Acknowledgement

This work was supported by Department of Defense grant DAMD 17-02-1-0633 (to S.K.C), by Arizona Biomedical Research Commission grant 07-061 (to S.K.C.), and the Rodel Foundation (to S.K.C.).

5. References

Aharinejad, S., Paulus, P., Sioud, M., Hofmann, M., Zins, K., Schafer, R., Stanley, E.R., Abraham, D. (2004). Colony-stimulating factor-1 blockade by antisense oligonucleotides and small interfering RNAs suppresses growth of human mammary tumor xenografts in mice. *Cancer Res.* 64: 5378-5384.

Allegra, J.C., Lippman, M.E., Thompson, E.B., Simon, R., Barlock, A., Green, L., Huff , K.K., Do, H.M. & Aitken, S.C. (1979). Distribution, frequency, and quantitative analysis of estrogen, progesterone, androgen, and glucocorticoids receptors in human breast cancer. *Cancer Res.* 39: 1447-1454.

Arcaro, A. & Guerreiro, A.S. (2007). The Phosphoinositide 3-kinase pathway in human cancer: genetic alterations and therapeutic implications. *Current Genomics* 8: 271-306.

Balagopal, V. & Parker R. (2009). Polysomes, P bodies and stress granules: states and fates of eukaryotic mRNAs. *Curr. Op. Cell Biol.* 21: 403-408.

Barreau, C., Paillard, L. & Osborne, B. (2005). AU-rich elements and associated factors: are there unifying principles? *Nucleic Acids Res.* 33: 7138-7150.

Bashirullah, A, Cooperstock, R.L. & Lipshitz, H.D. (2001). Spatial and temporal control of RNA stability. *PNAS* 98: 7025–7028.

Bazzini, A., Lee, M.T. & Giraldez A.J. (2012). Ribosome profiling shows that miR-430 reduces translation before causing mRNA decay in Zebrafish. *Science* 336: 233-237.

Bevilacqua, A., Cerian, M.C. Capaccioli, S. & Nicolin, A. (2003). Post-transcriptional regulation of gene expression by degradation of messenger RNAs. *J. Cell. Physiol.* 195: 356-372.

Bhattacharyya, S.N., Habermacher, R., Martine, U., Closs, E.I. & Filipowicz, W. (2006). Relief of microRNA-mediated translational repression in human cells subjected to stress. *Cell* 125: 1111-1124.

Bordonaro, M., F. Saccomanno, C.F., L. Nordstrom, J.L. (1994) An improved T1/A ribonuclease protection assay, BioTechniques 16, 428-430.

Buchan, J.R. & Parker R. (2009) Eukaryotic stress granules: the ins and outs of translation. *Mol. Cell* 36: 932-941.

Chambers, S.K. (2009). Role of CSF-1 in progression of epithelial ovarian cancer. *Future Oncol.* 5: 1429-1440.

Chambers, S.K., Kacinski, B.M., Ivins, C.M. & Carcangiu, M.L. (1997). Overexpression of epithelial CSF-1 and CSF-1 receptor: a poor prognostic factor in epithelial ovarian cancer; contrasted to a protective effect of stromal CSF-1. *Clin. Cancer Res.* 3: 999-1007.

Chambers, S.K., Gilmore-Hebert, M., Wang, Y., Rodov, S., Benz, E.J. Jr, & Kacinski, B.M. (1993). Posttranscriptional regulation of colony-stimulating factor-1 (CSF-1) and CSF-1 receptor gene expression during inhibition of phorbol-ester-induced monocytic differentiation by dexamethasone and cyclosporin A: potential involvement of a destabilizing protein. *Exp Hematol.* 21: 1328-1334.

Chambers, S.K., Wang, Y., Gilmore-Hebert, M., & Kacinski, M. (1994). Post-transcriptional regulation of *c-fms* proto-oncogene expression by dexamethasone and of CSF-1 in human breast carcinomas in vitro. *Steroids* 59: 514-522.

Chen, C., Ridzon, D.A., Broomer, AJ, *et al.* (2005). Real-time quantification of microRNAs by stem-loop RT-PCR. *Nucleic Acids Res* 33: e179.

Chen J-M, Fe´rec. & Cooper D.N. (2006). A systematic analysis of disease-associated variants in the 3′ regulatory regions of human protein-coding genes II: the importance of mRNA secondary structure in assessing the functionality of 3′ UTR variants. *Hum Genet* 120: 301–333.

Conne, B., Stutz, A. & Vassalli J.-D. (2000). The 3′ untranslated region of messenger RNA: A molecular 'hotspot' for pathology? *Nature Med* 6: 637-641.

Cunningham, K. S., Dodson, R.E., Nagel, M.A., Shapiro, D.J. & Schoenberg D.R. (2000). Vigilin binding selectively inhibits cleavage of the vitellogenin mRNA 3′-untranslated region by the mRNA endonucleases polysomal ribonuclease 1. *PNAS* 97: 12498-12502.

Dai, X-M., Ryan, G.R., Hapel, A.J., Dominguez, M.G., Russell, R.G., Kapp, S., Sylvestre, V. & Stanley, E.R. (2002). Targeted disruption of the mouse colony-stimulating factor 1 receptor gene results in osteopetrosis, mononuclear phagocyte deficiency, increased primitive progenitor cell frequencies, and reproductive defects. *Blood* 99: 111-120.

De Leeuw, F., Zhang, T., Wauquier, C., Huez, G., Kruys, V. & Gueydan, C. (2007). The cold-inducible RNA-binding protein migrates from the nucleus to cytoplasmic stress granules by a methylation-dependent mechanism and acts as a translational repressor. *Exp. Cell Res.* 313: 4130-4144.

Djuranovic, S., Nahvi, A., & Green R. (2012). miRNA-mediated gene silencing by translational repression followed by mRNA deadenylation and decay. *Science* 336: 237-240.

Fenger, M., Fillman, C., Norrild, B. & Lykke-Anderson, J. (2005). Multiple processing body factors and the ARE binding protein TTP activate mRNA decapping. *Mol. Cell* 20: 905-915.

Filderman, A.E., Bruckner, A., Kacinski, B.M., Deng, N. & Remold, H.G. (1992). Macrophage colony-stimulating factor (CSF-1) enhances invasiveness in CSF-1 receptor-positive carcinoma cell lines. *Cancer Res.* 52: 3661-3666.

Flick, M.B., Sapi, E., Perrotta, P.L., Maher, M.G., Halaban, R., Carter, D. & Kacinski, B.M. (1997). Recognition of activated CSF-1 receptor in breast carcinomas by a tyrosine 723 phosphospecific antibody. *Oncogene* 14: 2553-2561.

Flick, M.B., Sapi, E. & Kacinski, B.M. (2002). Hormonal regulation of the c-fms proto-oncogene in breast cancer cells is mediated by a composite glucocorticoid response element. *J Cell Biochem.* 85: 10-23.

Franks, T.M. & Lykke-Anderson J. (2008). The control of mRNA decapping and P-body formation. *Mol. Cell* 32: 605-615.

Friedman, R.C., Farh, K.K., Burge, C.B. & Bartel, D.P. (2009). Most mammalian mRNAs are conserved targets of microRNAs. *Genome Res.* 19: 92-105.

Gherzi, R., K. Y. Lee, P. Briata, D. Wegmüller, C. Moroni, M. Karin. & Chen C.Y. (2004). A KH domain RNA binding protein, KSRP, promotes ARE-directed mRNA turnover by recruiting the degradation machinery. *Mol. Cell* 14: 571-583.

Goolsby, K.M., Shapiro, D.J. (2003). RNAi-mediated depletion of the 15 KH domain protein, vigilin, induces death of dividing and non-dividing human cells but does not initially inhibit protein synthesis. *Nucleic Acids Res.* 31: 5644–5653.

Guo, H, Ingolia NT, Weissman JS, Bartel D.P. (2010). Mammalian microRNAs predominantly act to decrease target mRNA levels. *Nature* 466: 835-840.

Huntzinger, E, Izaurralde E. (2011). Gene silencing by microRNAs: contributions of translational repression and mRNA decay. *Nature Reviews: Genetics* 12: 99-110.

Ide, H., Seligson, D.B., Memarzadeh, S., Xin, L., Horvath, S., Dubey, P., Flick, M.B., Kacinski, B.M., Palotie, A., Witte, O.N. (2002). Expression of colony-stimulating factor 1 receptor during prostate development and prostate cancer progression. *PNAS.* 99: 14404-14409.

Jansen, R.-P. (2001). mRNA localization: message on the move. *Nature Reviews* 2: 247-256.

Kacinski, B.M., Flick, M.B. & Sapi, E. (2001). RU-486 can abolish glucocorticoid-induced increases in CSF-1 receptor expression in primary human breast carcinoma specimens. *J Soc Gynecol Investig.* 8: 114-116.

Kacinski, B.M., Carter, D., Mittal, K., Kohorn, E.I., Bloodgood, R.S., Donahue, J., Donofrio, L., Edwards, R., Schwartz, P.E., Chambers, J.T. & Chambers, S.K. (1988). High level expression of fms proto-oncogene mRNA is observed in clinically aggressive human endometrial adenocarcinomas. *Int. J. Radiat. Oncol. Biol. Phys.* 15: 823-829.

Kacinski, B.M., Carter, D., Mittal, K., Yee, L.D., Scata, K.A., Donofrio, L., Chambers, S.K., Wang, K., Yang-Feng, T., Rohrschneider, L.R. & Rothwell, V.M. (1990). Ovarian adenocarcinomas express *fms*-complementary transcripts and *fms* antigen, often with coexpression of CSF-1. *Am. J. Pathol.* 137: 135-147.

Kacinski, B.M., Scata, K.A., Carter, D., Yee, L.D., Sapi, E., King, B.L., Chambers, S.K., Jones, M.A., Pirro, M.H., Stanley, E.R. & Rohrschneider, L.R. (1991). FMS (CSF-1 receptor) and CSF-1 transcripts and protein are expressed by human breast carcinomas in vivo and in vitro. *Oncogene* 6: 941-952.

Kanamori, H., Dodson, R.E. & Shapiro, D.J. (1998). *In vitro* genetic analysis of the RNA binding site of vigilin, a multi-KH-domain protein. *Mol. Cell. Biol.* 18, 3991–4003

Kim, V.N. (2005). MicroRNA biogenesis: coordinated cropping and dicing. *Nat Rev Mol Cell Biol*. 6: 376-385.

Kluger, H. M., Dolled-Filhart, M.D., Rodov, S., Kacinski, B.M., Camp, R.L. & Rimm, D.L. (2004). Macrophage colony-stimulating factor-1 receptor expression is associated with poor outcome in breast cancer by large cohort tissue microarray analysis. *Clin. Cancer Res*. 10: 173-177.

Kruse, C., Willkomm, D., Gebken, J., Schuh, A., Stossberg, H., Vollbrandt, T., & Müller, P.K. (2003). The multi-KH protein vigilin associates with free and membrane-bound ribosomes. *Cell Mol. Life Sci.* 60: 2219-2227.

Li, W. & Stanley, E.R. (1991). Role of dimerization and modification of the CSF-1 receptor in its activation and internalization during the CSF-1 response. *The EMBO J.* 10: 277-288.

Lin, E.Y., Nguyen, A.V., Russell, R.G., Pollard, J.W. (2001). Colony-stimulating factor 1 promotes progression of mammary tumors to malignancy. *J Exp Med*. 193: 727-739.

Loya, A., Pnueli, L., Yosefzon, Y., Wexler, Y., Ziv-Ukelson, M. & Arava, Y. (2008). The 39-UTR mediates the cellular localization of an mRNA encoding a short plasma membrane protein. *RNA* 14:1352–1365.

Maher, M.G., Sapi, E., Turner, B., Gumbs, A., Perrotta, P.L., Carter, D., Kacinski, B.M. & Haffty B.G. (1998) Prognostic significance of colony-stimulating factor receptor expression in Ipsilateral breast cancer recurrence. *Clin. Cancer Res*. 4: 1851-1856.

Mignone, F., Gissi, C., Liuni, S. & Pesole, G. (2003). Untranslated regions of mRNAs. *Genome Biology* 3: 0004.1–0004.10.

Moncini, S., Bevilacqua, A., Venturin, M., Fallini, C., Ratti, A., Nicolin, A. & Riva, P. (2007). The 3' untranslated region of human cyclin-dependent kinase 5 regulatory subunit 1 contains regulatory elements affecting transcript stability. *BMC Molecular Biology* 8: 111.

Nissan, T., Rajyaguru, P., She, M., Song, H. & Parker, R. (2010). Decapping activators in *Saccharomyces cerevisiae* act by multiple mechanisms. *Mol. Cell* 39: 773-783.

Paulus, P., Stanley, E.R., Schafer, R., Abraham, D., Aharinejad, S. (2006). Colony-Stimulating Factor-1 Antibody Reverses Chemoresistance in Human MCF-7 Breast Cancer Xenografts. *Cancer Res.* 66: 4349-4356.

Pollard, J.W., Stanley, E.R., Paul, M.W. (1996). Pleiotropic roles for CSF-1 in development defined by the mouse mutation osteopetrotic. *Adv. Dev. Biochem*. 4: 153-193.

Pollard, J.W. (2004). Tumour-educated macrophages promote tumour progression and metastasis. *Nat. Rev. Cancer* 4: 71-78.

Price, F.V., Chambers, S.K., Chambers, J.T., Carcangiu, M.L., Schwartz, P.E., Kohorn, E.I., Stanley, E.R., Kacinski, B.M. (1993). CSF-1 concentration in primary ascites of ovarian cancer is a significant predictor of survival. *Am J Obstet Gynecol.* 168: 520-527.

Rettenmier, C.W., Sacca, R., Furman, W.L., Roussel, M.F., Holt, J.T., Nienhuis, A.W., Stanley, E.R. & Sherr, C.J. (1989). Expression of the human c-fms proto-oncogene product (colony-stimulating factor-1 receptor) on peripheral blood mononuclear cells and choriocarcinoma cell lines. *J Clin Invest*. 77: 1740-1746.

Roberts, W.M., Shapiro, L.H., Ashmun, R.A. & Look, A.T. (1992). Transcription of the human colony-stimulating factor-1 receptor gene is regulated by separate tissue-specific promoters. *Blood* 79: 586-593.

Sapi, E., Flick, M.B., Rodov, S., Gilmore-Hebert, M., Kelley, M., Rockwell, S. & Kacinski, B.M. (1996). Independent regulation of invasion and anchorage-independent growth by different autophosphorylation sites of the macrophage colony-stimulating factor 1 receptor. *Cancer Res*. 56: 5704-5712.

Sapi, E., Flick, M.B., Gilmore-Hebert M., Rodov, S. & Kacinski, B.M. (1995). Transcriptional regulation of the *c-fms* (CSF-1R) proto-oncogene in human breast carcinoma cells by glucocorticoids. *Oncogene* 10: 529-42.

Sapi, E. (2004). The role of CSF-1 in normal physiology of mammary gland and breast cancer: an update. *Exp Biol Med* 229(1): 1-11.

Schmittgen, T.D. & Livak, K.J. (2008). Analyzing real-time PCR data by the comparative CT method. *Nature Protocol* 3: 1101-1108.

Scholl, S.M., Mosseri, V., Tang, R., Beuvon, F., Palud, C., Lidereau, R. & Pouillart, P. (1993). Expression of colony-stimulating factor-1 and its receptor (the protein product of c-fms) in invasive breast tumor cells. Induction of urokinase production via this pathway? *Ann N Y Acad Sci.* 698: 131-135.

Scholl, S.M., Pallud, C., Beuvon, F., Hacene, K., Stanley, E.R., Rohrschneider, L., Tang, R., Pouillart, P. & Lidereau, R. (1994). Anti-colony stimulating factor-1 antibody staining in primary breast adenocarcinomas correlates with marked inflammatory cell infiltrates and prognosis. *J Natl Cancer Inst.* 86: 120-126.

Shurtleff, S.A., Downing, JR., Rock, C.O., Hawkins, S.A., Roussel, M.F. & Sherr, C.J. (1990). Structural features of the colony-stimulating factor receptor that affect its association with phosphatidylinositol 3-kinase. *The EMBO J.* 9: 2415 – 2421.

Shyu, A.B., Wilkinson, M.F. & van Hoof, A. (2008). Messenger RNA regulation: to translate or to degrade. *EMBO J.* 27: 471-481.

Sonenberg N. & Hinnebusch A.G. (2009). Regulation of translation initiation in eukaryotes: mechanisms and biological targets. *Cell* 136: 731-745.

Srikantan, S. & Gorospe, M. (2011) Unclipsing HuR nuclear function. *Mol. Cell*. 43: 319-321.

Stark, A., Brennecke, J., Bushati, N., Russell, R.B. & Cohen, S.M. (2005). Animal MicroRNAs confer robustness to gene expression and have a significant impact on 3'UTR evolution. *Cell* 123: 1133-1146.

Tang, R., Kacinski, B., Validire, P., Beuvon, F., Sastre, X., Benoit, P., de la Rochefordiere, A., Mosseri, V., Pouillart, P., Scholl, S. (1990). Oncogene amplification correlates with dense lymphocyte infiltration in human breast cancers: a role for hematopoietic growth factor release by tumor cells? *J. Cell Biochem.* 44: 189-198.

Toy, E.P., Bonafe, N., Savlu, A., Zeiss, C., Zheng, W., Flick, M., Chambers, S.K. (2005). Correlation of tumor phenotype with c-fms proto-oncogene expression in an in vivo intraperitoneal model for experimental human breast cancer metastasis. *Clin. Exp. Metastasis.* 22: 1-9.

Toy, E.P., Lamb, L., Azodi, M., Roy, W.J, Woo, H.H. & Chambers, S.K. (2010). Inhibition of the *c-fms* proto-oncogene autocrine loop and tumor phenotype in glucocorticoid stimulated human breast carcinoma cells. *Breast Cancer Res. Treat* 129: 411-419.

Urlaub, H., Hartmuth, K., Kostka, S., Grelle, G.M. & Luhrmann, R. (2000). A general approach for identification of RNA-protein cross-linking sites within native human spliceosomal small nuclear ribonucleoproteins (snRNPs). Analysis of RNA-protein contacts in native U1 and U4/U6.U5 snRNPs. *J Biol Chem.* 275: 41458-41468.

Vollbrandt, T., Willkomm, D., Stossberg, H., Kruse, C. (2004). Vigilin is co-localized with 80S ribosomes and binds to the ribosomal complex through its C-terminal domain. *Int. J. Biochem. Cell Biol.* 36: 1306-1318.

Weber, B., Horiguchi, J., Luebbers, R., Sherman, M., & Kufe, D. (1989). Posttranscriptional stabilization of *c-fms* mRNA by a labile protein during human monocytic differentiation. *Mol. Cell Biol.* 9: 769-775.

Woo, H.H., Zhou, Y., Yi, X., David, C.L., Zheng, W., Gilmore-Hebert, M., Klugger, H.M., Ulukus, E.C., Baker, T., Stoffer, J.B. & Chambers, S.K. (2009). Regulation of non-AU-rich element containing *c-fms* proto-oncogene expression by HuR in breast cancer. *Oncogene* 28: 1176-1186.

Woo, H.H., Yi, X., Lamb, T., Menzl, I., Baker, T, Shapiro, D.J. & Chambers, S.K. (2011). Posttranscriptional suppression of proto-oncogene *c-fms* expression by vigilin in breast cancer. *Mol. Cell. Biol.* 31: 215-225.

Xiong, Y., Song, D., Cai, Y., Yu, W., Yeung, Y.-G. & Stanley, E.R. (2011). A CSF-1 Receptor Phosphotyrosine 559 Signaling Pathway regulates Receptor ubiquitination and tyrosine phosphorylation. *JBC.* 286: 952–960.

Yu, W., Chen, J, Xiong, Y., Pixley, F.J., Yeung, Y.-G. & Stanley, E.R. (2012).Macrophage proliferation is regulated through CSF-1 receptor tyrosines 544, 559 and 807. *JBC.* M112.355610.

Yi, X., Zhou, Y., Zheng, W. & Chambers, S. (2009). HuR expression in the nucleus correlates with high histological grade and poor disease-free survival in ovarian cancer. *Australian and New Zealand J Obstetrics and Gynaecology* 49: 93-98.

Zwaenepoel, O., Tzenaki, N., Vergetaki, A., Makrigiannakis, A., Vanhaesebroeck, B. & Papakonstanti, E.A. (2012). Functional CSF-1 receptors are located at the nuclear envelope and activated via the p110δ isoform of PI 3-kinase. *The FASEB J.* 26: 691-706.

Zheng, D., Ezzeddine, N., Chen, C.Y., Zhu, W., He, X. & Shyu, A.B. (2008). Deadenylation is prerequisite for P-body formation and mRNA decay in mammalian cells. *JCB.* 182: 89-101.

Chapter 14

Non-Coding RNAs and Cancer

Gianpiero Di Leva and Michela Garofalo

Additional information is available at the end of the chapter

http://dx.doi.org/10.5772/54997

1. Introduction

The question of which regions of the human genome constitute its functional elements—those expressed as genes or serving as regulatory elements—has long been a central topic in biology. In the 1970s and 1980s, early cloning-based methods revealed the presence of more than 7000 genes in human genome [1], and large-scale analyses of expressed sequence tags (ESTs) in the 1990s suggested that the estimated number of human genes range from 35,000 to 100,000 [2]. The completion of the human genome project narrowed the focus considerably by highlighting the surprisingly small number of protein-coding genes, which is now conventionally cited as less than 25,000 [3]. While the number of protein-coding genes (20,000–25,000) has maintained broad consensus, recent studies of the human transcriptome have revealed an astounding number of non-coding RNAs (ncRNAs) [4-6]. In fact, the increased sensitivity of genome tiling arrays provides an even more detailed view, revealing that the extent of non-coding sequence transcription is at least four times greater than coding sequence, and that the abundance of non-coding transcripts had been previously overlooked. The RNA world hypothesis proposes that early life was based on RNAs, which subsequently devolved the storage of information to more stable DNA, and catalytic functions to more versatile proteins. Consequently, despite crucial roles in the ancient processes of translation and splicing, RNA is assumed to have been largely relegated to an intermediate between gene and protein, encapsulated in the central dogma 'DNA makes RNA makes protein' [7]. However, the finding that most of the genome in complex organisms is transcribed and the discovery of new classes of regulatory non-coding RNAs (ncRNAs) challenges this assumption and suggests that RNAs have continued to evolve and expand alongside proteins and DNA.

ncRNAs are considered as RNA transcripts that do not encode for a protein. In the past decade, a great diversity of ncRNAs has been observed. Depending on the type of ncRNA, transcription can occur by any of the three RNA polymerases (RNA Pol I, RNA Pol II, or RNA Pol III). General conventions divide ncRNAs into two main categories: small ncRNAs less than 200 bp and long ncRNAs greater than 200 bps [8]. Within these two categories, there are also many individual classes of ncRNAs (**Table1**), although the degree of biological and experimental support for each class ranges substantially and should be evaluated individually. The relevance of ncRNAs in gene regulation has been rapidly unveiling during the last decade. However, the functional elements in the primary sequence of noncoding genes that determine their role as RNA molecules remain unknown. Protein-coding genes have a defined language with a set of grammatical rules: three nucleotides forms a codon that translates into a specific amino acid [9]. Aberrations in codons of a protein-coding gene can be interpreted in terms of the amino acids they encode. We can recognize a mutation in a codon and determine its contribution to a given disease. In contrast to the genetic code for protein synthesis, 'the ncRNA alphabet' – a specific set of RNA sequences or structural motifs important for ncRNA function – remains to be largely elucidated. However, it has become increasingly apparent that the ncRNAs are of crucial functional importance for normal development, physiology and disease [10]. The functional relevance of the ncRNAs is particularly evident for a class of small non-coding RNAs called microRNAs (miRNAs) [11-12]. In human diseases, particularly cancer, it has been shown that epigenetic and genetic defects in miRNAs and their processing machinery are a common hallmark of disease [13-16]. However, miRNAs are just the tip of the iceberg, and other ncRNAs such as small nucleolar RNAs (snoRNAs), PIWI-interacting RNAs (piRNAs), large intergenic non-coding RNAs (lincRNAs) and, overall, the heterogeneous group of long non-coding RNAs (lncRNAs), might also contribute to the development of many different human disorders. Here we discuss the most recent genetic studies on ncRNAs and their related proteins in the context of cancer and we will analyze the new regulatory elements of the noncoding language to interpret their contribution to the pathogenesis of cancer.

2. MicroRNAs

In 1993, Victor Ambros and colleagues discovered a gene, *lin-4,* that affected development in *Caenorhabditis elegans* and found that its product was a small nonprotein-coding RNA [31]. The number of known small RNAs in different organisms such as *Caenorhabditis elegans, Drosophila melanogaster,* plants, and mammals—including humans—has since expanded substantially, mainly as a result of the cloning and sequencing of size-fractionated RNAs. MiRNAs are single stranded RNAs (ssRNAs) of 19–25 nucleotides in length that are generated from endogenous hairpin transcripts [32]. They play an important role in the negative regulation of gene expression by base-pairing to partially complementary sites on the target messenger RNAs (mRNAs), usually in the 3' untranslated region (UTR). Binding of a miRNA to the target mRNA typically leads to translational repression and exonucleolytic mRNA decay, although highly complementary targets can be cleaved endonucleolytically. A genomic analysis of miRNAs has revealed that more than 50% of mammalian miRNAs are located within the intronic regions of annotated protein-coding or non-protein-coding genes [33]. These miRNAs could therefore use their host gene transcripts as carriers, although it remains possible that some are actually transcribed separately from internal promoters. Other miRNAs, located in intergenic regions, apparently have their own transcriptional regulatory elements and thus constitute

Category	Name	Supporting data	Function	Role in cancer	Refs.
Housekeeping RNAs	Ribosomal RNAs (rRNA)	high	ribosome structure	no	17-18
	Transfer RNAs (tRNA)	high	protein translation	no	17-18
	Small nuclear RNAs (snRNA)	high	splicing	no	17-18
	Small nucleolar RNAs (snoRNA)	high	post-translational modification	yes	17-18
Short non coding RNAs (above 200nt in size)	MicroRNAs	high	translational repression	yes	20,21
	Tiny transcription initiation RNAs	high	may regulate gene expression	not known	18
	Repeat associated small interfering RNAs	high	gene regulation, transposon control and viral defence	not known	18
	Promoter-associated short RNAs	high	may regulate gene expression at chromatin level	not known	18, 22,24
	Termini-associated short RNAs	high	may regulate gene expression at chromatin level	not known	18, 22,24
	Antisense termini associated short	high	may regulate gene expression at chromatin level	not known	17, 22,24
	Piwi-interacting RNAs	high	regulate transposon activity and chromatin state	yes	23
	Transcription start site antisense RNAs	moderate	may regulate transcription	not known	17
	Retrotraspon-derived RNAs	high	may regulate transcription	not known	24
	3'UTR-derived RNAs	moderate	may regulate transcription	not known	17
	Splice-site RNAs	poor	not known	not known	18
Long non coding RNAs (over 200nt in size)	Long or large intergenic ncRNAs	high	epigenetic regulation, protein complex subcellular compartments or localization	yes	25,26
	Transcribed ultraconserved regions	high	not known	yes	27
	Pseudogenes	high	competitive endogenous RNAs	yes	25, 28
	Enhancer RNAs	high	not known	yes	29
	Long intronic ncRNAs	moderate	not known	not known	17,18
	Repeat associated ncRNAs	high	not known	not known	23
	Antisense RNAs	high	gene expression	not known	28
	Promoter associated long RNAs	moderate	may regulate gene expression at chromatin level	not known	22, 30
	Long stress-induced non-coding transcripts	moderate	epigenetic regulation, protein complex subcellular compartments or localization	yes	17, 18

Table 1. Non coding RNA in human genome.

independent transcription units. Animal miRNAs are processed from longer primary transcripts (pri-miRNAs) that can contain multiple miRNAs [34,35]. Few pri-miRNA transcripts have been studied in detail, but in general miRNAs are regulated and transcribed similar to protein encoding genes by (Pol) II with the exception of the rapidly evolving RNA polymerase (Pol) III transcribed miRNA cluster [36]. MiRNA processing occurs in three essential steps (**Figure 1**). First, the nuclear endoribonuclease protein Drosha recognizes the miRNA hairpins in the primary transcript and cleaves each hairpin ~11 nt from its base [37-38]. It has been proposed that Drosha may recognize the pri-miRNA through the stem-loop structure and then cleave the stem at a fixed distance from the loop to liberate the pre-miRNA. How is the Drosha enzyme able to discriminate the pri-miRNA stem-loop structure from the other stem-loop cellular RNAs? Both cell culture experiments and in vitro Drosha cleavage assays have shown that proteins associated with Drosha confer specificity to this process. In fact, Drosha has been found to be part of a large, ~650-kDa protein complex known as the Microprocessor [39], where Drosha interacts with its cofactor DGCR8 (the DiGeorge syndrome critical region gene 8 protein) in the human and interacts with Pasha in *Drosophila melanogaster* [40]. The next step in miRNA biogenesis is recognition of the ~60 nt pre-miRNA by exportin-5 and export into the cytoplasm in a ran-guanine-GTP-dependent manner [41-43]. The Exp5/Ran-GTP complex has a high affinity for pre-miRNAs,

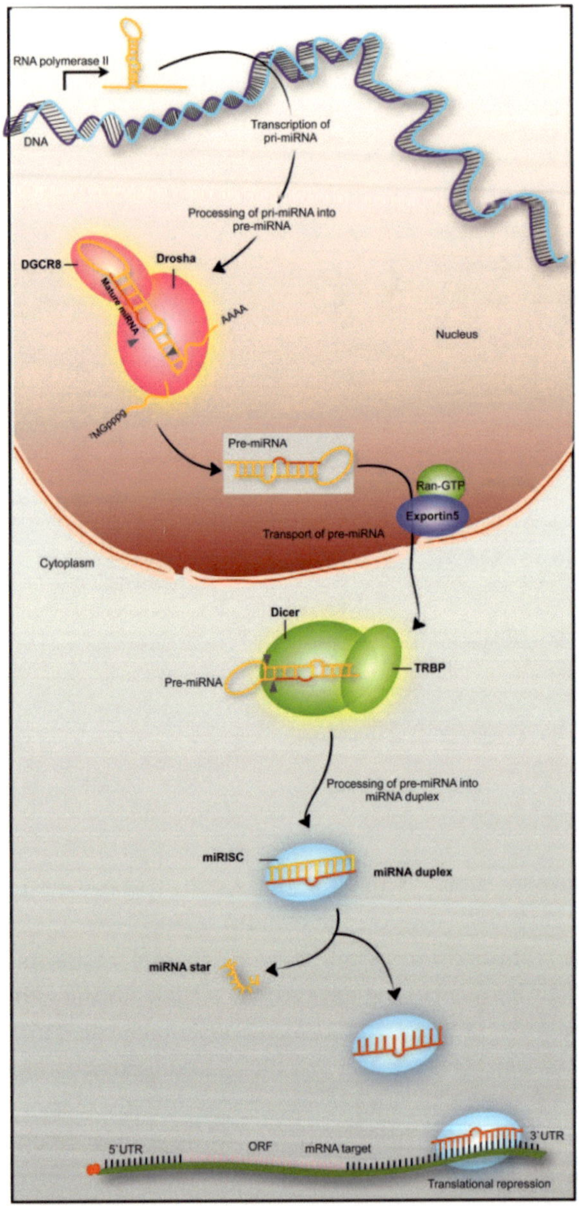

Figure 1. miRNA biogenesis and function. The primary miRNA (pri-miRNA) is transcribed by RNA pol II from its genomic location and cleaved by the microprocessor complex, which comprises Drosha and DGCR8. The resulting pre-miRNA is actively transported to the cytoplasm by exportin 5 (Expt.5), where the pre-miRNA undergoes further processing into the mature miRNA by Dicer and its co-factors, protein activator of interferon-induced protein kinase (PACT) and TAR RNA binding protein (TRBP). Normally, one strand of this duplex is degraded (miRNA star), whereas the other strand accumulates as a mature miRNA. From the miRNA-miRNA duplex, only the miRNA enters preferentially in the protein effector complex, formed by the RNA-induced silencing complex (RISC) and miRgonaute and binds with partial complementarity to the 3′ untranslated region (UTR) of target messenger RNAs (mRNAs) to mediate translational repression.

protecting them from the moment they are generated in the nucleus until they are ready for the next cleavage step in the cytoplasm, where GTP is hydrolyzed to guanosine diphosphate (GDP); at that point, the Exp5/Ran-GDP complex releases its cargo. Third, the endoribonuclease protein Dicer cleaves the pre-miRNA into ~22 nt duplexes and, with the help of cofactors such as TAR RNA binding protein (TRBP) and protein activator of the interferon-induced protein kinase (PACT), preferentially incorporates one of the duplex strands Into the RNA induced-silencing complex (RISC) [44-50]. The final product is a miRNA-miRNA duplex that needs to be unwound to act as a single-stranded guide in the RISC to recognize its target mRNAs. It was originally proposed that an ATP-dependent helicase (known as unwindase) separates the two small RNA strands, after which the resulting single-stranded guide is loaded into Ago proteins. However, it was later shown that *Drosophila* Ago2 [51], as well as human Ago2 [52], directly receive double-stranded small RNA from the RISC-loading complex. Ago2 then cleaves the passenger strand, thereby liberating the single-stranded guide to form mature Ago2-RISC. In mammals, miRNAs guide the RISC to complementary target sites in mRNAs, where endonucleolytically active Ago proteins cleave the RNA [53] (**Figure 1**). Finally, RISC can cleave [54-55] degrade [56-57] or suppress translation [58-59] of target mRNAs depending on the complementarity between miRNA and mRNA. Imperfect base pairing between small RNAs and their target mRNAs leads to repression of translation and/or deadenylation (removal of the polyA tail of the target), followed by destabilization of the target [60], whereas perfect base pairing usually leads to mRNA degradation.

3. MicroRNAs and cancer

Cancer is a multistep process in which normal cells experience genetic changes that progress them through a series of pre-malignant states (initiation) into invasive cancer (progression) that can spread throughout the body (metastasis). The dysregulation of genes involved in cell proliferation, differentiation and/or apoptosis is associated with cancer initiation and progression. Genes linked with cancer development are characterized as oncogenes and tumor suppressors. Recently, the definition of oncogenes and tumor suppressors has been expanded from the classical protein coding genes to include miRNAs [61-62]. MiRNAs have been found to regulate more than 60% of mRNAs and have roles in fundamental processes, such as development [63], differentiation [64], cell proliferation [65], apoptosis [66], and stress responses [67]. Over the past few years, many miRNAs have been implicated in various human cancers. The first evidence that miRNAs are involved in cancer comes from the finding that miR-15 and miR-16 are downregulated or deleted in most patients with chronic lymphocytic leukemia [68]. This discovery has projected miRNAs to the center stage of molecular oncology and, in the past few years, a myriad of genome-wide miRNA expression profiling analyses have shown a general dysregulation of miRNA expression in all tumors (**Table 2**) [69]. Surprisingly, the use of miRNA profiles is newly becoming highly preferred to the traditional mRNA signature for a variety of reasons. First, the remarkable stability of miRNAs, due to their short length, has allowed scientists to perform analyses also in samples considered to be technically challenging, such as formalin fixed specimens. High sensitive and refined miRNA detection technique provide high reliability in the use of miRNAs as a diagnostic tools. Finally, miRNA fingerprints have demonstrated the ability to identify the tissue of origin for cancer that have already spread in multiple metastatic sites, thereby reducing patient's psychological burden and overall procedure costs. To date, over 1000 miRNAs have been reported in humans (miRbase: 1527 at November 2011), and both loss and gain of miRNA functions contribute to cancer development through a range of different mechanisms that we will discuss in the following sections.

Cancer	*Authors*	*Samples*	*Main findings*	*miRNA signature*
	Iorio et al. 2005	10 normal 76 tumors	First miRNA signature of breast cancer. 15 miRNAs predict the nature of the sample analyzed with 100% accuracy.	**miR-21**, **-155** were up-regulated while **miR-10b**, **-125b**, **-145** were down-regulated.
	Mattie et al. 2006	20 tumors	Unique sets of miRNAs are associated with ErbB2 and ER/PR status.	ErbB2 status (**let-7f**, **let-7g**, **miR-107**, **-10b**, **-126**, **-154**, **-195**) ER/PR status (**miR-142-5p**, **-200a**, **-205**, **-25**).
	Blenkiron et al. 2007	93 tumors	Striking differences in miRNA expression between breast tumor molecular subtypes (luminal A, luminal B, basal-like, HER2+ and normal breast-like).	-
Breast Cancer	Sempere et al. 2007	> 100 pairs tumor-normal	In situ hybridization method to reveal the spatial distribution of miRNA expression in archived formalin-fixed breast tumors	20 miRNAs differentiate matched normal/tumor. **miR-21** up-regulated in all tumor specimens, **miR-145** and **miR-451** were the only miRs high expressed in normal specimens and low expressed in tumor specimens. **let-7a**, **miR-21**,**-141**, **-214** preferentially expressed in luminal cells, **miR-145** and **-205** in myoepithelial cells.
	Foekens et al. 2008	299 tumors	Identification of miRNAs associated with metastatic capability.	**miR-7**, **-128a**, **-210**, **-516–3p** associated with tumor aggressiveness in ER-positive patients with lymph node-negative disease. **miR-210** associated with early relapse in ER-negative patients with lymph node-negative disease and with poor outcome.
	Volinia et al 2012	80 IDC 8 DCIS 6 normal	Identification of miRNA dysregulation during the transition from ductal carcinoma in situ to invasive ductal carcinoma	**Let-7d**, **miR-210**, and **-221** down-regulated in DCIS and up-regulated in IDC. **miR-210**, **-21**, **-106b***, **-197**, and **let-7i** associated with prognosis. Only miR-210involved in the invasive transition.
	Yanaihara et al. 2006	104 pairs tumor-normal	miRNA expression profiles are diagnostic and prognostic markers of lung cancer.	43 miRNAs discriminate between normal ad tumors. **let-7a-2**, **mir-155**, **-17-3p**, **-145**, **-21** were associated with adenocarcinoma patients survival.
	Raponi et al. 2009	10 normal 61 squamous	miRNAs may have greater clinical utility in predicting the prognosis of patients with squamous cell lung carcinomas than mRNA-based signatures.	15 miRNAs that were differentially expressed including **miR-17/92** cluster, **miR-155**, **let-7**. **miR-146b** has the strongest prediction accuracy for stratifying prognostic groups.
	Landi et al. 2010	290 tumors 165AC-125SQ	miRNA expression profiles can distinguish adenocarcinoma (AC) from squamous carcinoma (SQ) and predict survival.	**let-7g** and **miR-26** were the most down-regulated in SQ versus AC. **miR-25**, **-34c-5p**, **-34a**, **-191** and **let-7e** strongly predicted SQ survival for the 107 male smokers with early-stage SQ tumors. **miR-21** is overexpresssed in AC and may be a marker of tumor progression in adenocarcinoma.
Lung Cancer	Tan et al. 2011	34 pairs tumors-normal	miRNA expression profiles of squamous carcinoma vs normal tissues.	**miR-210**, **-182**, **-486-5p**, **-30a**, **-140-3p** discriminate between cancerous and normal lung tissues. **miR-31** was associated with poor survival in squamous cell carcinoma.
	Lu et al. 2012	527 tumors	Identification of miRNA signatures that predict prognosis of stage I NSCLC.	Two miRNA signatures that are highly predictive of recurrence/ relapse free survival were identified. The first contained 34 miRNAs derived from 357 stage I NSCLC patients independent of cancer subtype, whereas the second containing 27 miRNAs was adenocarcinoma specific.
	Guan et al. 2012	14 different dataset	A meta-analysis reviews 14 microRNA expression profiling studies that compared the microRNAs expression profiles in lung cancer tissues with those in normal lung tissues.	184 miRNAs discriminate lung cancer tissues from normal tissues; 61 miRNAs were reported in at least two studies. Up-regulated miRNA: **miR-210** was reported in 9 studies and **miR-21** in 7 studies.Down-regulated miRNA: **miR-126** was reported in 10 studies and **miR-30a** in 8 studies.
	Pallante et al. 2006	10 normals 30 tumors	Identification of the miRNA expression profile of papillary carcinomas.	A significant increase in **miR-221**, **-222** and **-181b** was detected in papillary carcinomas in comparison with normal thyroid tissue.
	Visone et. al 2007	10 normals 76 tumors	Identification of the miRNA expression profile of anaplastic carcinomas from normal thyroid tissues.	A significant decrease in **miR-30d**, **-125b**, **-26a**, **-30a-5p** was detected in anaplastic carcinomas compared to normal thyroid tissue.
Thyroid Cancer	Nikiforova et al. 2008	60 normals 60 tumors	Identification of miRNA signature for the different thyroid tumors subtypes: Oncocytic, conventional follicular, papillary and medullary carcinomas.	**miR-187**, **-221**, **-222**, **-146b**, **-155**, **-224**, **-197** were the most differentially overexpressed in thyroid tumors vs. hyperplastic nodules and combination of them classified the different subtypes.
	Yip et al. 2011	32 tumors	Identification of a specific signature in aggressive (17) compared with nonaggressive papillary carcinomas (15).	Upregulation of **miR-146b**, **-221**, **-222**, **-155**, **-31** and downregulation of **miR-1**, **-34b**, **-130b**, **-138** downregulation. **miR-146** overexpression was associated with aggressive behavior in BRAF-positive tumors.
	Kitano et al 2011	47 tumors	miRNAs expression signature for samples representing difficult to diagnose histologic subtypes of thyroid neoplasm (21 benign, 26 malignant).	Out of 34 differentially expressed miRNA, **miR-126** and **miR-7** had high diagnostic accuracy and could be helpful in the classification of benign and malignant thyroid tumors.

a

Cancer	*Authors*	*Samples*	*Main findings*	*miRNA signature*
Colon Cancer	Schetter et al. 2008	84 pairs tumor-normal	miRNA expression profiles and clinical correlation for colon cancer.	37 miRNAs differentially expressed in tumors: high **miR-21** was in adenomas and tumors with more advanced TNM staging. High **miR-21** expression was also associated with poor survival and therapeutic outcome.
	Schepeler et al. 2008	10 normals 49 tumors	miRNA expression profiles of colon cancer with different microsatellite status and prognosis.	**miR-145** showing the lowest expression in cancer relative to normal tissue. **miR-142-3p**, **-212**, **-151**, **-144** were associated with tumor microsatellite status. High expression of **miR-320** or **-498** associated with good prognosis.
	Arndt et al. 2009	8 cell lines 4 normals 45 tumors	miRNA expression profiles for colon cancer.	37 miRNAs discriminate between colorectal cancer and normal tissues. 22 miRNAs were differentially expressed between normal and early stage cancer including increases in **miR-21** and **-224** and decreases in **miR-133a** and **-145**. A differential expression in **miR-31**, **-7**, **-99b**, **-378***, **-133a**, **-125a** discriminates between early and late stage.
Prostate Cancer	Ambs et al. 2008	16 normals 60 tumors	First miRNA expression profiles for prostate cancer.	Up-regulated miRs: **miR 32**, **-182**, **-31**, **-26a**, **-200c**, **-196a**, **-106b/25** cluster; down-regulated miRNAs included **miR-520h**, **-494**, **-490**, **-1/133a** cluster.
	Tong et al. 2009	40 pairs normal-tumor	miRNA expression profiles of paired microdissected malignant and non-involved areas from stage T2a/b, early relapse and non-relapse cancer patients.	**miR-23b**, **-100**, **-145**, **-221**, **-222** were significantly downregulated in malignant tissues. Patients with post-surgery elevation of prostate-specific antigen (chemical relapse) displayed a distinct profile of 16 miRNAs, as compared with those with non-relapse disease.
	Schaefer et al. 2010	76 pairs normal-tumor	miRNA expression profiles for prostate cancer and clinical correlation.	**miR-16**, **-31**, **-125b**, **-145**, **-149**, **-181b**, **-184**, **-205**, **-221**, **-222** were downregulated and **miR-96**, **-182**, **-182**, **-183**, **-375** were upregulated. Expression of 5 miRNAs correlated with Gleason score or pathological tumor stage.
Liver Cancer	Murakami et al. 2006	25 pairs normal-tumor	miRNA expression profiles in hepatocellular carcinoma and non-tumorous tissues.	**miR-18**, precursor **miR-18**, **-224**, **-199a***, **-195**, **-199a**, **-200a**, **-125a** differentially expressed between cancer and normal tissues; **miR-92**, **-20**, **-18** and precursor **miR-18** were significantly higher in poorly differentiated tumors. In contrast, **miR-99a** exhibited a positive correlation between expression levels and degree of tumor differentiation.
	Budhu et al. 2008	241 pairs normal-tumor	miRNA expression profiles in liver cancer predict metastasis.	A unique 20-miRNA metastasis signature was identified that could predict primary neoplastic tissues with venous metastases from metastasis-free solitary tumors. **mir-219-1**, **-207**, and **-338** were most highly up-regulated, whereas **mir-34a**, **-30c-1**, **-148a** were most highly down-regulated in metastasis cases.
	Wang et al. 2008	4 normals 46 tumors	miRNA expression profiles in hepatocellular carcinoma and non-tumorous tissues.	**miR-224** overexpression identified in all tumors and **miR-200c**, **-200**, **-21**, **-224**, **-10b**, **-222** specific deregulation in benign or malignant tumors. **miR-96** was overexpressed in HBV tumors, and **miR-126*** was down-regulated in alcohol-related hepatocellular carcinoma. Down-regulations of **miR-107** and **miR-375** were specifically associated with HNF1alpha and beta catenin gene mutations, respectively.
	Ji et al. 2009	241 pairs normal-tumor	miRNA expression profiles in hepatocellular carcinoma and non-tumorous tissues and significant correlation to survival.	Reduced **miR-26** in tumors and the expression of **miR-26a** and **miR-26b** in nontumor liver tissue was higher in women than in men. Low **miR-26** is associated to a short overall survival but a better response to interferon therapy.
	Toffanin et al. 2011	89 tumors	miRNA expression profiles in hepatocellular carcinoma and non-tumorous tissues: identification of tumor subtypes and new oncomiRs.	3 main clusters of hepatocellular carcinoma: beta catenin gene mutated tumors (36%), interferon-response–related genes (33%), and tumors with abnormal activation of IGF and mTOR-(PI)3K pathways (31%). A subset of tumors in last subclass (9%) overexpressed a family of miRNAs from chr19q13.42: **miR-517a** and **miR-520c** (from ch19q13.42) increased proliferation, migration, and invasion of HCC cells in vitro.

b

Cancer	Authors	Samples	Main findings	miRNA signature
Ovarian Cancer	Iorio et al. 2007	5 cell lines 15 normals 69 tumors	miRNA expression profiles of ovarian cancer vs normal and tumor subtype-specific miRNA signature.	29 miRNAs differentially expressed between normal and tumor with a classification rate of 89%. 4 up-modulated: miR-200a, -200b, -200c, -141; 25 down-modulated: miR-199a, -140, -145, -125b-1 among the most significant.
	Yang et al. 2008	10 normal cells 10 tumors	miRNA expression profiles of ovarian cancer vs normal ephitelial cells.	Up-regulation of miR-214, -199a*, -200a and down-regulation of miR-100; alterations of the first three miRNAs is associated with late-stage and high-grade ovarian tumors. miR-214 induces cell survival and cisplatin resistance by targeting the PTEN/Akt pathway.
	Wu et al. 2009	10 pairs normal-tumor	miRNA expression profiles of endometrioid ovarian cancer vs normal tissues.	17 up regulated (miR-205, -449, -429) and 6 down-regulated (miR-204, -99b, -193b) miRNAs in endometrioid adenocarcinoma samples.
	Marchini et al. 2011	144 tumors	miRNA expression profiles of stage I ephitelial ovarian cancer assess the existence of a miRNA signature associated with overall and progression-free survival.	34 miRNAs were associated with survival. Between them miR-200c, -199a-3p, -199a-5p were highly associated with overall and progression-free survival.
	Devor et al. 2011	4 normal 23 tumors	miRNA signature in ovarian cancer vs normal and in serous (9) and endometrioid (14) subtypes	7 miRNAs was down-regulated and 13 miRNAs up-regulated in both adenocarcinomas. miR-133b the most repressed miRNA in both adenocarcinomas; miR-205 the most expressed miRNA. miR-135b, -200a, -200b, -200c, -141, -429 significantly overexpressed in both types of endometrial cancers.
Gastric Cancer	Luo et al. 2009	2 cell lines 3 normals 24 tumors	miRNA expression profiles of gastric cancer vs normal.	19 miRNAs down-regulated and 7 miRNAs up-regulated. miR-433 and miR-9 were remarkably down-regulated in the carcinoma samples.
	Ueda et al. 2010	160 pairs normal-tumor	miRNA expression profiles of gastric cancer vs normal and miRNA signature in histological subtypes	22 miRNAs upregulated and 13 downregulated in gastric cancer. Diffuse-type and intestinal-type subtypes were discriminated by miRNA expression. miR-125b, -199a, -100 were the most important microRNAs involved progression signature. Low let-7g and miR-433 and high expression of miR-214 were associated with unfavourable outcome in overall survival independent of clinical covariates, including depth of invasion, lymph-node metastasis, and stage.
	Brenner et al. 2011	45 tumors	miRNA expression profiles of primary tumor of patients with recurrent and non-recurrent gastric cancer.	miR-451, -199a-3p, -195 differentially expressed in gastric tumors from patients with good prognosis vs bad prognosis. High expression of each miR was associated with poorer prognosis for both recurrence and survival. miR-451 showed a positive predictive value for non-recurrence of 100%.
	Kim et al. 2011	34 normals 90 tumors	miRNA signature distinguishes gastric cancer from normal stomach epithelium from healthy volunteers, and a chemo-reresistance miRNA signature that is correlated with time to progression after cisplatin/fluorouracil therapy	30 miRNAs inversely correlated with time to progression of disease after chemotherapy whereas 28 miRNAs positively correlated. Among the upregulated miRNAs associated with chemosensitivity: let-7g, miR-342, -16, -181, -1, -34 known to regulate apoptosis.
Esophageal Cancer	Guo et al. 2008	31 pairs normal-tumor	miRNA expression profiles of esophageal cancer vs normal tissues.	46 miRNAs differently expressed between the cancerous and adjacent normal tissues. A minimal set of 7 distinguishes malignant from normal esophageal tissues: miR-25, -424, -151 showed up-regulation and miR-100, -99a, -29c, -140* showed down-regulation. High miR-103/107 correlated with poor survival.
	Yang et al. 2009	32 pairs normal-tumor	miRNA expression profiles of esophageal cancer progression from Barret's low to high grade dysplasia to adenocarcinoma.	111 miRNAs differentiated the adenocarcinoma tissues with 100% accuracy. 11 miRNAs may be important in the progression from low-grade to high-grade dysplasia. let-7b/a/c/f, miR-345, -494, -193a were modulated in the progression from high-grade dysplasia to adenocarcinoma, and all of them were down-regulated in esophageal adenocarcinoma.
	Mathe et al. 2009	170 tumors	Identification of miRNAs involved in major histologic types of esophageal carcinoma and significant associations with prognosis.	In adenocarcinoma patients: high expression of miR-21, -223, -192, -194 and low miR-203 levels. In squamous carcinoma: high expression of miR-21 and low miR-375 levels. High miR-21 in normal tissue of squoamous carcinoma and low levels of miR-375 in cancerous tissue of adenocarcinoma patients with Barrett's were strongly associated with worse prognosis.
	Fassan et al. 2011	14 normals 23 dysplasias	miRNA expression profiles in Barrett's subtypes (7 low grade dysplasia, 5 high grade dysplasia, 11 Barrett's adenocarcinomas)	Up-regulation of miR-215, -560, -615-3p, -192, -326, -147 and down-regulation of miR-100, -23a, -605, -99a, -205, let-7c, -203.
	Feber et al. 2011	45 tumors	miRNA expression profiles provide prognostic utility in staging esophagus cancer patients and elucidate steps in the metastatic pathway and allow for development of targeted therapy.	Up-regulation of miR-143, -199a_3p, -199a_5p, -100, -99a predicted a worse survival. miR-99b, -199a_3p and _5p also associated with the presence of lymph node metastasis.

c

Table 2. miRNA profiling in cancer.

4. Oncogenic microRNAs

Although studies linking miRNA dysfunctions to human diseases are in their infancy, a great deal of data already exists, establishing an important role for miRNAs in the pathogenesis of cancer. Many miRNAs have been shown to function as oncogenes in the majority of cancers profiled to date (**Table 3**). *MiR-21* displays a strong evolutionary conservation across a wide range of vertebrate species in mammalian, avian and fish clades [70]. It has been demonstrated that a primary transcript containing *miR-21* (i.e., *pri-miR-21*) is independently transcribed from a conserved promoter that is located within the intron of the overlapping protein-coding gene *TMEM49* [71]. Several studies suggest that this miRNA is oncogenic [72-74] and that it may act as an antiapoptotic factor. For example, Chan et al. have found that miR-21 is commonly and markedly up-regulated in human glioblastoma and that inhibiting miR-21 expression leads to caspase activation and associated apoptotic cell death [72]. Moreover, Zhu and collaborators provided the first evidence that *miR-21* regulates invasion and metastasis, at least in part, by targeting metastasis-related tumor suppressor genes such as TPM1, programmed cell death 4 (PDCD4) and maspin [73]. Furthermore, examination of human breast tumor specimens revealed an inverse correlation of *miR-21* with PDCD4 and maspin [74]. The final proof of miR-21 oncogenic activity came from the Slack laboratory where the first conditional knock-in of miR-21 overexpressing mice was generated. The mice developed a severe pre-B-cell lymphoma but when miR-21 was reduced to endogenous levels, the mouse tumors completely disappeared, defining the concept of "oncomiR addition" [75].

Another important oncogenic miRNA is represented by *miR-155*. Several groups have shown that *miR-155* is highly expressed in pediatric Burkitt's lymphoma [76], Hodgkin's disease [77], primary mediastinal non-Hodgkin's lymphoma [77], chronic lymphocytic leukemia (CLL) [78], acute myelogenous leukemia (AML) [79], lung cancer [80], pancreatic cancer [81], and breast cancer [80]. Dr. Croce laboratory reported that *miR-155* transgenic mice develop acute lymphoblastic leukemia/high-grade lymphoma and that most of these leukemias start at approximately nine months, irrespective of the mouse strain, preceded by a polyclonal pre-B-cell proliferation [82].

Another example of "oncomiR" is represented by *miR-221&222* cluster that is highly upregulated in a variety of solid tumors, including thyroid cancer [83], hepatocarcinoma [84], estrogen receptor negative breast tumor [85], and melanoma [86]. Elevated *miR-221&222* expression has been causally linked to proliferation [85-87], apoptosis [88-89], and migration [89] of several cancer cell lines. We recently reported that the hepatocyte growth factor receptor (MET) oncogene, through c-Jun transcriptional activation, upregulates *miR-221&222* expression, which, in turn, by targeting *PTEN* and *TIMP3*, confers resistance to tumor necrosis factor–related apoptosis-inducing ligand (TRAIL) and enhances tumorigenicity of lung and liver cancer cells [89]. The results suggest that therapeutic intervention involving the use of miRNAs should not only sensitize tumor cells to drug-inducing apoptosis but also inhibit their survival, proliferation, and invasion [89].

The miR-106b-25 polycistron is composed of the highly conserved miR-106b, miR-93, and miR-25 that accumulate in different types of cancer, including gastric, prostate, and pancreatic neuroendocrine tumors, as well as neuroblastoma and multiple myeloma. Petrocca and collaborators [90] demonstrated that E2F1 regulates miR-106b, miR-93, and miR-25, inducing their accumulation in gastric tumors. Conversely, miR-106b and miR-93 control E2F1 expression, establishing a negative feedback loop that may be important in preventing E2F1 self-activation and apoptosis. On the other hand, miR-106b, miR-93, and

miRNA	*Target*	*Tumor*
	PTEN	cholangiocarcinoma
	TPM1	breast cancer
	PDCD4	breast cancer
	SPRY1	
miR-21	RECK, TIMP3	glioblastoma
	p63, JMY, TOPORS, TP53BP2, DAXX, HNRPK, TGFβRII	glioblastoma
	MARKS	prostate cancer
	ANP32A, SMARCA4	prostate cancer
	SOCS1	breast cancer
	CEBPB, PU.1 ,CUTL1, PICALM	AML
	BACH1, ZIC3	
	ETS1, MEIS1	human cord blood CD34+
	C-MAF	lymphocytes
	HGAL	diffuse large B-cell lymphoma
miR-155	JMJD1A	nasopharyngeal carcinoma
	WEE1	breast cancer
	TP53INP1	pancreatic cancer
	SMAD1, SMAD5, HIVEP2, CEBPB, RUNX2, MYO10	
	FOXO3A	breast cancer
	hMSH2, hMSH6, hMLH1	colon cancer
	SMAD5	diffuse large B-cell lymphoma
	p27(KIP1)	glioblastoma, prostate and thyroid carcinoma
	p57 (KIP2)	normal fibroblast
	PTEN, TIMP3	non small cell lung cancer and hepatocellular carcinoma
	FOXO3A	breast cancer
	KIT	Endotelial cells
miR-221/222	ESR1	breast cancer
	PUMA	glioblastoma
	TRSP1	breast cancer
	PTPμ	glioblastoma
	DICER	breast cancer
	APAF1	non small cell lung cancer
	BIM, p21	gastric cancer
miR-106a~363 *miR-106b~25*	E2F1	prostate cancer
	PTEN	prostate cancer
	TSP-1, CTGF	colon
	E2F2, E2F3	prostate/Burkitt lymphoma/testis carcinoma/
	BIM PTEN	c-Myc induced lymphoma
	HIF1α	lung cancer
	PTPRO	cervix tumor cell line
	p63	myeloid cells
miR-17-92	BIM, PTEN, PRKAA1, PPP2R5e,	T-cell acute lymphoblastic leukaemia
	JAK1	endothelial cells
	HBP1	breast cancer
	p21(WAF1)	Ras induced senescent-fibroblasts
	TGFβII, SMAD4	glioblastoma
	MnSOD, GPX2, TRXR2	prostate
	HOXB1, HOXB3	pancreatic cancer
	HOXD10	breast cancer
miR-10a/10b	KLF4	esophageal cancer
	TIAM1	breast cancer
	NF1	Ewing's sarcoma

Table 3. *-oncomiRs*

miR-25 overexpression causes a decreased response of gastric cancer cells to TGFβ by downregulating p21 and Bim, the two most downstream effectors of TGFβ-dependent cell cycle arrest and apoptosis, respectively.

Another example of a miRNA locus with oncogenic properties is represented by the *miR-17-92* cluster, which consists of six miRNAs: miR-17-5p, -18, -19a, -19b, -20a, and -92-1. The miR-17-92 cluster is located in a region frequently amplified in several types of lymphoma and solid tumors [91-92]. It has been shown that mice deficient for miR-17-92 die shortly after birth with lung hypoplasia and a ventricular septal defect. This cluster is also essential for B cell development; its absence, in fact, leads to increased levels of the proapoptotic protein Bim and inhibits B cell development at the pro-B-to-pre-B transition [93]. All together these studies indicate that many miRNAs have oncogenic activity. Importantly, their knockdown through the use of antisense oligonucleotides, inhibits the development of cancer-associated phenotypes, laying the groundwork for the creation of miRNA-based therapies [94-96].

5. Tumor suppressor microRNAs

The first evidence that miRNAs are involved in cancer comes from the finding that miR-15 and miR-16 are downregulated or deleted in most patients with chronic lymphocytic leukemia (CLL) (**Table 4**) [68]. They are transcribed as a cluster (*miR-15a–miR-16-1*) that resides in the 13q14 chromosomal region. Deletions or point mutations in region 13q14 occur at high frequency in CLL, lymphoma, and several solid tumors [97]. Their expression is inversely correlated to *BCL2* expression in CLL [98]. The tumor suppressor function of *miR-15a/16-1* has also been addressed in vivo. In immunocompromised nude mice, ectopic expression of *miR-15a/16-1* was found to cause dramatic suppression of tumorigenicity of MEG-01 leukemic cells that exhibited a loss of endogenous expression of *miR-15a/16-1*. Furthermore, Klein et al. [99] generated transgenic mice with a deletion of the *miR-15a–miR-16-1* cluster, causing development of indolent B-cell-autonomous, clonal lymphoproliferative disorders, recapitulating the spectrum of CLL-associated phenotypes observed in humans. Recently, Bonci et al. reported that the *miR-15a–miR-16-1* cluster targets not only *BCL2* but also *CCND1* (encoding cyclin D1) and *WNT3A* mRNA, which promote several prostate tumorigenic features, including survival, proliferation, and invasion [100]. Together, these data suggest that *miR 15a/16-1* genes are natural antisense interactors of *BCL2* and probably other oncogenes and that they can be used to suppress tumor growth in therapeutic application for a variety of tumors [100].

In mammalians, the miR-34 family comprises three processed miRNAs that are encoded by two different genes: miR-34a is encoded by its own transcript, whereas miR-34b and miR-34c share a common primary transcript. The miR-34 family has been shown to form part of the p53 tumor-suppressor network: their expression is directly induced by p53 in response to DNA damage or oncogenic stress [101-102]. He et al. identified different miR-34 targets such as cyclin E2 (CCNE2), CDK4, and MET. Silencing these selected miR-34 targets through the use of small interfering RNAs (siRNAs) led to a substantial cell cycle arrest in G1.

Moreover, ectopic miR-34 delivery caused a decrease in levels of phosphorylated retinoblastoma gene product (Rb), consistent with lowered activity of both CDK4 and CCNE2 complexes [102]. BCL2 and MYCN were also identified as miR-34a targets and likely mediators of the tumor suppressor phenotypic effect in neuroblastoma [103]. It has been also reported that p53 activation suppressed the EMT-inducing transcription factor SNAIL via induction of the miR-34a/b/c genes. In fact, suppression of miR-34a/b/c by anti-miRs caused up-regulation of SNAIL and cells displayed EMT markers, enhanced migration and invasion [104].

MicroRNA-122 (miR-122) is a liver-specific microRNA and is frequently downregulated in liver cancer [105]. Xu et al. reported that restoration of miR-122 in hepatocellular carcinoma cells could render cells sensitive to chemotherapeutic agents adriamycin or vincristine through downregulating antiapoptotic gene Bcl-w and cell cycle related gene cyclin B1 [106]. Another group found that over-expression of miR-122 inhibits hepatocellular carcinoma cell growth and promotes the cell apoptosis by affecting Wnt/β-catenin signalling pathway [107]. Coulouarn et al. showed that miR-122 is specifically repressed in a subset of primary hepatocellular tumors that are characterized by poor prognosis [108]. They further reported that loss of miR-122 resulted in an increase of cell migration and invasion and that restoration of miR-122 reverses this phenotype [108]. The final understanding of the tumor suppressor role for mir-122 role in liver cancer came from a recent study where miR-122 knockout mice were studied. When miR-122 KO mice aged, hepatic inflammation ensued, preceding the progressive onset of fibrosis and, eventually, tumors resembling human liver cancer. These pathologic manifestations were associated with hyperactivity of oncogenic pathways and hepatic infiltration of inflammatory cells that produce pro-tumorigenic cytokines, including IL-6 and TNF [109].

miRNA	***Target***	***Tumor***
	BCL2	CLL
	COX-2	colon cancer
	CHEK1	follicolar lymphoma
	CEBPβ, CDC25a, CCNE1	fibroblast
	VEGF, VEGFR2, FGFR1	fibroblast
miR-15/16	FGF2, FGFR1	cancer associated fibroblast
	CCNE1	
	FGFR1, PI3KCa, MDM4, VEGFa	multiple myeloma
	WIP1	
	BMI-1	ovarian cancer
	CCND1, CCND2, CCNE1	lung cancer
	SIRT1	colon cancer
	BCL2, NOTCH, HMGA2	
	MYC	fibroblast
miR-34	AXL	lung cancer
	MET	ovarian cancer
	NANOG, SOX2, MYCN	embryonic fibroblast
	SNAIL	colon cancer

Table 4. Tumor suppressor *miRS*

6. MetastamiRs

Metastasis is the result of cancer cells detaching from a primary tumor, consequently adapting to distant tissues and organs, and forming a secondary tumor [110] and this ability of cancer cells to metastasize is a hallmark of malignant tumors [111-112]. To successfully metastasize, a tumor cell must complete a complex set of processes, including invasion, survival and arrest in the circulatory system, and colonization of foreign organs. Despite great advancements in knowledge of metastasis biology, the molecular mechanisms are still not completely understood. Several miRNAs have been shown to initiate invasion and metastasis by targeting multiple proteins that are major players in these cellular events, thus they have been denominated as metastamiRs (**Table 5**). It seems that these metastasis-associated miRNAs do not influence primary tumor either in development or initiation steps of tumorigenesis, but they regulate key steps in the metastatic program and processes, such as epithelial-mesenchymal transition (EMT), apoptosis, and angiogenesis. Ma et. al reported that miR-10b is highly expressed in metastatic breast cancer cells and positively regulates cell migration and invasion. Overexpression of miR-10b in otherwise non-metastatic breast tumors initiates robust invasion and metastasis [113]. The team led by Joan Massague found that miR-335, miR-126, and miR-206 are metastasis-suppressors in breast cancer [114]. MiR-126 and miR-206 restoration reduced overall tumor growth and proliferation, whereas miR-335 inhibits metastatic cell invasion through targeting of the progenitor cell transcription factor *SOX4* and extracellular matrix component tenascin C [114]. Others miRNAs with prominent roles in breast cancer metastasis have been reported. It has been reported that miR-31 inhibited multiple steps of metastasis including invasion, anoikis, and colonization leading to almost complete reduction of lung metastasis [115]. Clinically, miR-31 levels were lower in breast cancer patients with metastasis. In addition, miR-9, which is up-regulated in breast cancer cells, directly targets CDH1, the E-cadherin-encoding messenger RNA, leading to increased cell motility and invasiveness [116].

Another important aspect of the metastatic dissemination is represented by the epithelial-to-mesenchymal transition (EMT) that allow neoplastic cells to abandon their primary site and survive in the new tissue. During EMT, an epithelial neoplastic cell looses cell adhesion by repressing E-cadherin expression and thereby the cell increases its motility. Numerous studies have shown that different microRNAs are modulated during EMT and one of the best-studied example is represented by the miR-200 family. These miRs are commonly lost in aggressive tumors such as lung, prostate, and pancreatic cancer. It has been shown that miR-200 family members directly target ZEB1 and ZEB2, transcription repressors of E-cadherin [117]. In fact, in the highly aggressive mouse lung cancer model where KRAS is constitutively activated and p53 function is perturbed, miR-200 ectopic expression prevented metastasis by repressing ZEB1 and ZEB2 and preventing E-cadherin down-regulation [117]. However, overexpression of the miR-200 family is associated with an increased risk of metastasis in breast cancer and this overexpression promotes metastatic colonization in mouse models, phenotypes that cannot be explained by E-cadherin expression alone [118]. By using proteomic profiling of the targets of mesenchymal-to-ephitelial (MET)-inducing miR-200, the authors discovered that miR-200 globally targets secreted proteins in breast cancer cells. Between the 38 modulated target genes, Sec23a, which is involved in transporting protein cargo from the endoplasmic reticulum to the Golgi, shows a superior association with human metastatic breast cancer as compared to the currently recognized miR-200 targets ZEB1 and the EMT marker E-cadherin. EMT is first acquired in the onset of transmigration and then reversed in the new metastatic site. Korpal et al. have shown that the miR-200 status predicts predisposition of the cancer to successful metastasis [119].

miRNA	*Target*	*Tumor*
miR-10a/10b	HOXB1, HOXB3	pancreatic cancer
	HOXD10	breast cancer
	KLF4	esophageal cancer
	TIAM1	breast cancer
	NF1	Ewing's sarcoma
miR-9	PRDM1/BLIMP-1	lymphomas
	CDH1	breast cancer
	CAMTA	glioblastoma
miR-31	ITGA5, RDX, RHOA FZD3, M-RIP, MMP16	breast cancer
	SATB2	cancer associated fibroblast
miR-200 family	ZEB1, ZEB2	breast cancer
	ERRFI-1	bladder cancer
	ZEB1, CTNNB1	nasopharyngeal carcinoma
	BMI-1	pancreatic cancer
	PLCγ1	breast cancer
	FAP1	
	SUZ12	breast cancer
	FLT1/VEGFR1	lung cancer
	JAG1, MALM2, MALM3	
	FN1, LEPR, NTRK2, ARHGAP19	breast and endometrial cancer
	p38α	ovarian cancer

Table 5. *metastamiRS*

7. Other non-coding RNAs: Biology and implications in cancer

7.1. snoRNAs: From post-transcriptional modification to cancer

Small nucleolar RNAs (snoRNAs) have, for many years, been considered one of the best-characterized classes of non-coding RNAs (ncRNAs) [120-123] but despite the common assumption that snoRNAs only have cellular housekeeping functions, in the past few years, independent reports have converged in implicating snoRNAs in the control of cell fate and oncogenesis [124-130]. SnoRNAs are small RNAs of 60-300nt in lenght that specifically accumulate in the nucleolar compartment of the cell where are in charge of the 2′-O-ribose methylation and pseudouridylation of specific ribosomal RNA nucleotides, essential modification for the efficient and accurate production of the ribosome [120-122]. The snoRNAs carry out their function in the form of small nucleolar ribonucleoproteins (snoRNPs), each of which consists of a box C/D or box H/ACA guide RNA, and four associated C/D or H/ACA snoRNP proteins (**Figure 2**). In both cases, snoRNAs hybridize specifically to the complementary sequence in the rRNAs, and the associated protein complexes then carry out the appropriate modification on the nucleotide that is identified by the snoRNAs. Biogenesis of vertebrate snoRNPs is remarkable and highly variable: in fact snoRNA gene organization ranges from independently transcribed genes, endowed with their own promoter elements, to intronic coding units lacking an independent promoter. In both yeast and animals, processing of intron-encoded snoRNAs is largely splicing-dependent; in contrast, the production of plant snoRNAs from introns seems to rely on a splicing-independent process [131]. Moreover, in both contexts (intergenic or intronic), genes can be either single or part of clusters. In the latter case, the generation of individual snoRNAs involves the enzymatic processing of polycistronic precursor RNAs. Such a processing, at least in yeast, appears to involve the same combination of endo- and exoribonucleases required for the maturation of monocistronic pre-snoRNAs [132-134]. The first indication that snoRNAs might have important roles in human disease was provided by the genetic studies on Prader–Willi syndrome (PWS), an inherited human disorder characterized by a complex phenotype, including mental retardation, decreased muscle tone and failure to thrive at birth, short stature, hypogonadism, sleep apnea, behavioral problems and hyperphagia (an insatiable appetite) that can lead to severe obesity [135]. The disease is caused by the genomic loss of the imprinted chromosomic 15q11-q13 locus which is normally only active on the paternal allele. The only characterized and conserved genes within this 121-kb-long genomic interval are the numerous HBII-85 snoRNA gene copies, thus suggesting that loss of expression of these repeated small C/D RNA genes might play a role in conferring some (or even all) phenotypes of the human disease and PWS-like phenotypes in mice (neonatal lethality, growth retardation and hypotonia). In fact, it has been shown that a site-specific deletion of the entire murine MBII-85 gene cluster led to post-natal growth retardation with low postnatal lethality (<15%) only seen in some genetic backgrounds, but no obesity [136]. Although all the imprinted C/D RNAs that have been tested accumulate within the nucleolus, none of them appear to act as RNA guides to modify rRNAs or spliceosomal U-snRNAs; they are called 'orphan C/D RNAs'. So far, the MBII-52 gene clusters have attracted much attention, given that the neuronal-specific MBII-52 small RNA is predicted to interfere (A-to-I RNA editing and/or alternative RNA splicing) with the post-transcriptional regulation of the pre mRNA that encodes the 5-HT_{2C} (5-hydroxytryptamine 2C) receptor, playing a key role in regulating serotonergic signal transduction [137-138]. These observations raised the possibility that snoRNAs could have functions completely independent from their traditional activities and carry out other regulatory roles. The first insights into the potential roles of snoRNAs in cancer began with a study that identified C/D box snoRNA U50 and its host gene U50HG at the breakpoint in the t(3;6) (q21;q15) translocation in a diffuse large B cell lymphoma [139]. Moreover, snoRNAU50 gene has been found to undergo to a frequent copy number loss and a transcriptional downregulation in breast and prostate cancer samples [139,140]. In addition, a 2-bp deletion in U50 sequence also occurred both somatically and in germline, leading to increased incidence of homozygosity for the deletion in cancer cells [140].

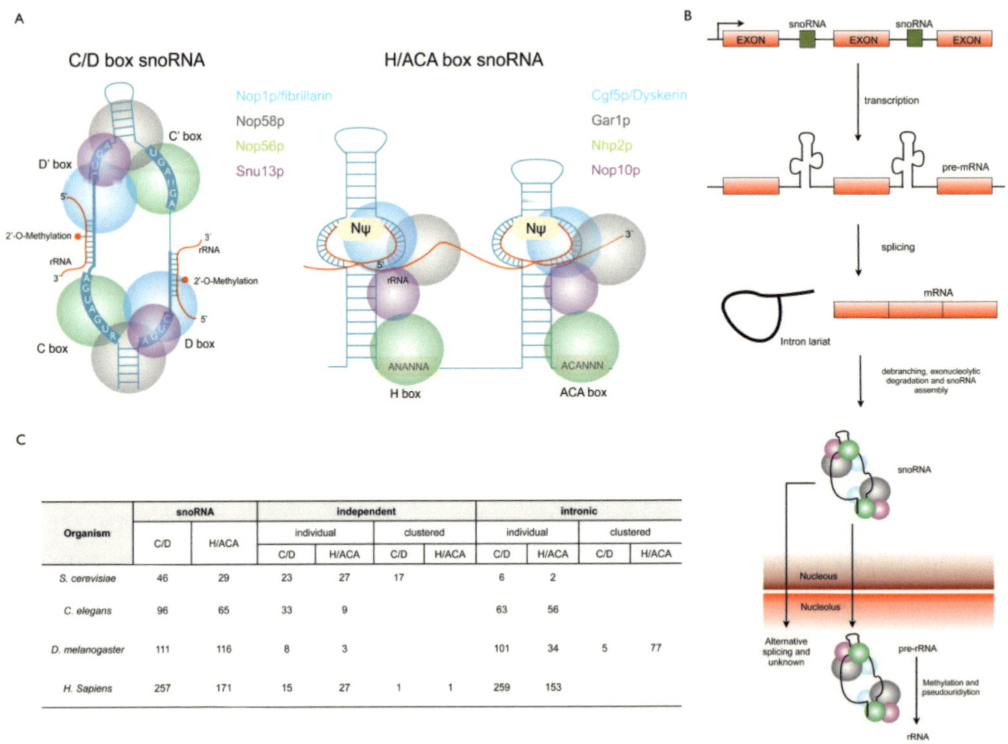

Organism	snoRNA		independent				intronic			
			individual		clustered		individual		clustered	
	C/D	H/ACA	C/D	H/ACA	C/D	H/ACA	C/D	H/ACA	C/D	H/ACA
S. cerevisiae	46	29	23	27	17		6	2		
C. elegans	96	65	33	9			63	56		
D. melanogaster	111	116	8	3			101	34	5	77
H. Sapiens	257	171	15	27	1	1	259	153		

Figure 2. snoRNAs. A. Boxed sequences C and D (named from conserved, nuclease-resistant sequences that were originally identified in snoRNA U3) are hallmarks of the C/D box snoRNAs; boxed sequences H (Hinge region) and ACA are hallmarks of the H/ACA box snoRNAs. These conserved boxed sequences are important for the associations with protein components that are required to form the functional small nucleolar ribonucleoprotein (snoRNP) complexes and for accumulation in the nucleolus. C/D box snoRNAs associate with several proteins, including fibrillarin, which is the methyl transferase that is involved in the 2′-O-methylation of particular ribonucleotides, and H/ACA box snoRNAs associate with proteins such as the pseudouridine synthase dyskerin. Antisense sequences within the C/D box and H/ACA box snoRNAs guide the snoRNP complex to the appropriate nucleotide within the target RNA (most often ribosomal RNA). In a minority of cases both C/D-associated and C′D′-associated antisense sequences within the same C/D box snoRNA can act as guides for 2′-O-methylation of the target RNA. The eukaryotic H/ACA box snoRNAs contain two hairpin domains with complementary regions flanking the uridine to be converted in the target rRNA, at a position 14–16 nucleotides upstream of the conserved H and/or ACA box. Most mammalian snoRNAs are encoded within the introns of genes producing 5′ terminal oligopyrimidine (5′TOP) RNAs. **B.** Organization of snoRNA genes in representative eukaryotic genomes **C.** Small nucleolar RNAs (snoRNAs) in vertebrate are predominantly located in introns. Following splicing, debranching and trimming, mature snoRNAs are either exported, in which case they function in ribosomal RNA (rRNA) processing, or remain in the nucleus, where they are involved in alternative splicing and additional yet unknown functions.

SnoRNA42 (SNORA42) is located on chromosome 1q22 which is a commonly frequent amplified genomic region in lung cancer and overexpression of SNORA42 is frequently and remarkably found in NSCLC cells [141]. In addition, SNORA42 exhibited close correlations between its increases of copy number and expression level, suggesting that SNORA42 overexpression could be activated through its amplification. Importantly, engineered repression of SNORA42 caused marked repression of lung cancer growth in vitro and in vivo and it is associated with increased apoptosis by a p53-dependent pathway. Although not exhibiting apoptosis, p53 null and mutant p53 cancer cells with reduced levels of SNORA42 also show inhibited proliferation and growth, suggesting that SNORA42 knockdown can inhibit cell proliferation in p53-dependent or -independent manner. These independent studies on U50 and SNORA42 provide evidence for the functional importance of snoRNAs in cancer, and they show that snoRNAs can promote, as well as suppress, tumour development. In 2002, Wu and coworkers demonstrated that the expression of snoRNAs 5S was differentially displayed in different tissues and noticeably was highly expressed in normal brain, but its expression drastically decreased in meningioma [142]. Recently, genome-wide approaches identified six snoRNAs (SNORD33, SNORD66, SNORD73B, SNORD76, SNORD78, and SNORA42) that were statistically differently expressed between the non small cell lung cancer tumor and paired noncancerous samples [143]. Specifically, all these snoRNAs displayed a strong up-regulation in lung tumor specimens and the majority of them is located in commonly frequent genomic amplified regions in lung cancer: SNORD33 is located in chromosome 19q13.3 that contain potential oncogenes in lung cancer, while SNORD66 and SNORD76 are situated in chromosomal regions 3q27.1 and 1q25.1, respectively 3q27.1 and 1q25.1 are two of the most frequently amplified chromosomal segments in solid tumors, particularly NSCLC [143].

As well as the initial evidence that snoRNAs are involved in cancer development, there are some preliminary data showing that the genes that host snoRNAs might also contribute to the aetiology of this disease. A research screening for potential tumor-suppressor genes identified that Growth arrest-specific transcript 5 (gas5) gene as almost undetectable in actively growing cells but highly expressed in cells undergoing serum starvation or density arrest [144-145]. Gas5 is a multi-snoRNA host gene which encodes 9 (in mouse) or 10 (in human) snoRNAs and like all known snoRNA host genes exhibit characteristics which belong to the class of genes encoding 5′ terminal oligopyrimidine (5′TOP) mRNAs [146]. The first and stronger evidence that GAS5 is related to cancer is the identification that GAS5 transcript levels are significantly reduced in breast cancer samples relative to adjacent unaffected normal breast epithelial tissues and some, but not all, GAS5 transcripts sensitize mammalian cells to apoptosis inducers [147]. Other studies have also showed that GAS5 reduced expression is associated with poor prognosis in both breast cancer and head and neck squamous cell carcinoma [148]. Of note, GAS5 has been also identified as a novel partner of the BCL6 in a patient with diffuse large B-cell lymphoma, harboring the t(1;3)(q25;q27) [149]. Another example of a mature spliced transcript that harbors C/D-box snoRNAs and can function independently of the snoRNAs is represented by the transcript Zfas1 [150]. This gene intronically hosts three C/D box snoRNAs (Snord12, Snord12b, and Snord12c) and has been identified as one of the most differentially expressed gene during mouse mammary development. siRNA-mediated downregulation of Zfas1 mRNA in a mouse mammary cell line increased proliferation and differentiation without substantially affecting the levels of the snoRNA hosted within its intron. The human homologue, ZFAS1 (also known as ZNFX1-AS1), which is predicted to share secondary structural features with mouse Zfas1, is expressed at high levels in the mammary gland and is downregulated in breast cancer. Taken together, these findings indicates that snoRNA host genes might have important functions in regulating cellular homeostasis and, potentially, cancer biology but more studies are needed to understand their involvement in molecular basis of disease and classify them as sources of potential biomarkers and therapeutic targets.

Another important aspect of the association between snoRNAs and tumorigenesis is represented by the involvement of their associated proteins in cancer. A point mutations in the DKC1 gene is the cause of a rare X-linked recessive disease, the dyskeratosis congenita (DC) [151-152]. Individuals with DC display features of premature aging, as well as nail dystrophy, mucosal leukoplakia, interstitial fibrosis of the lung, and increased susceptibility to cancer. DKC1 codes for dyskerin, a putative pseudouridine synthase, which carries out two separate functions, both fundamental for proliferating cells. One function is the pseudo-uridylation of ribosomal RNA (rRNA) molecules as a part of the H/ACA ribonucleoprotein complex, and the other is the stabilization of the telomerase RNA component necessary for telomerase activity. Dkc1 mutant mice recapitulate the major features of DC, including an increased susceptibility to tumor formation. Early generation (G1 and G2) of Dkc1 mutant mice showed a full spectrum of DC and presented alterations in rRNA modification, whereas defects in telomere length were not evident until G4 mice, suggesting that deregulated ribosome function is important for the initiation of DC and that impairment in telomerase activity in Dkc1 mutant mice may modify and/or exacerbate the disease in later generations. To this regard, DKC1 was identified as one of only seventy genes that, collectively, constitute a gene expression profile that strongly correlates with the development of aneuploidy and is associated with poor clinical prognosis in a variety of human cancers. Therefore, one hypothesis is that an alteration of physiologic dyskerin function, irrespective of the mechanism, may perturb mitosis and contribute to tumorigenesis but this idea will require more detailed investigation. Another possibility is related to the strong effect of dyskerin loss on H/ACA accumulation. Recent finding in fact have shown that some H/ACA box and C/D box can be processed to produce small RNAs, at least some of which can function like miRNAs [153]. Such processing may be of crucial importance, as miRNAs have important roles in the development of many cancers as previously discussed. To date, Xiao and colleagues have recently reported that an H/ACA box snoRNA- derived miRNA, miR-605, has a key role in stress-induced stabilization of the p53 tumour suppressor protein [154]. p53 transcriptionally activates its negative regulator, MDM2, in addition to miR-605. miR-605 counteracts MDM2 through post-transcriptional repression; under conditions of stress, this snoRNA-derived miRNA offsets the MDM2 negative-feedback loop, generating a positive-feedback loop to enable the rapid accumulation of p53. However, whether this regulation of p53 by miR-605 is relevant to cancer biology has not yet been addressed. Like dyskerin, NHP2 and NOP10 proteins, both components of the H/ACA snoRNPs, are also significantly up-regulated in sporadic cancers and high levels may be associated with poor clinical prognosis. Moreover, germline NHP2 and NOP10 mutations give rise to autosomal recessive forms of dyskeratosis congenita, and cancer susceptibility is also a feature of these genetic forms of the disease. Since the functions of several snoRNAs have not yet been identified (orphan snoRNAs), it is possible that disruption of snoRNP biogenesis by any mechanism may affect an array of important cellular processes, and could potentiate cancer development and/or progression.

7.2. piRNAs: Guardians of the genome

Piwi-interacting RNAs (piRNAs) are germline-specific small silencing RNAs of 24–30 nt in length, that suppress transposable elements (TE) activity and maintain genome integrity during germline development, a role highly conserved across animal species [155-156]. TEs are genomic parasites that threaten the genomic integrity of the host genome: they are able to move to new sites by insertion or transposition and thereby disrupt genes and alter the genome [157]. In animals, endogenous siRNAs also silence TEs, but the piRNA pathway is at the forefront of defense against transposons in germ cells [158]. piRNAs specifically associate with PIWI proteins, which are germline-specific members of the AGO protein family, AGO3, Aubergine (Aub) and Piwi, and form a piRNA-induced silencing complex (piRISC) which will guide the TE silencing [159-162]. Any mutations in each of the three members of the PIWI family lead to transposon derepression in the germline, indicating that they act non-redundantly during TE silencing. Initial screening of piRNA sequences revealed that there are hundreds of thousands, if not millions, of individual piRNA sequences [163-165]. Furthermore, they are characterized by the absence of specific sequence motifs or secondary structures such as miRNA precursors. Despite their large diversity, most piRNAs can be mapped to a relatively small number of genomic regions called piRNA clusters. Each cluster extends from several to more than 200 kilobases, it contains multiple sequences that generate piRNAs and some piRNAs map to both genomic strands, suggesting bidirectional transcription [163-165] Indeed, analysis of piRNA clusters in different *Drosophila* species has shown that, although the clusters locations are conserved, their sequence content has evolved very quickly suggesting adjustments in the piRNAs patrimony in order to suppress new active transposons invading the species. Therefore, piRNA clusters may be considered as repositories of information, enabling production of many mature piRNAs that target diverse TEs. Two main pathways, highly conserved in many animal species, have been discovered to be responsible for the biogenesis of the piRNAs: the primary pathways and the Ping-Pong amplification (**Figure 3**) [166-168]. First, the primary piRNA biogenesis pathway provides an initial pool of piRNAs that target multiple TEs. Next, the Ping-Pong cycle further shapes the piRNA population by amplifying sequences that target active transposons. It is currently unclear how primary piRNAs are produced from piRNA clusters but it is likely that piRNA precursors are single-stranded and therefore do not require Dicer for their processing. Interestingly, piRNAs that associate with each member of the PIWI protein family have a distinct size, suggesting that PIWI proteins can act as 'rulers' that define the size of mature piRNAs. Several additional proteins (e.s. Zucchini, Armitage and Yb) have also been identified that are involved in primary piRNA biogenesis and mutations in and/or depletion of any of these three proteins eliminates primary piRNAs associated with PIWI proteins. In some cell types, such as somatic follicle cells of the *D. melanogaster* ovary, primary piRNA biogenesis is the only mechanism that generates piRNAs. However, in germline cells of the *D. melanogaster* ovary and in the pre-meiotic spermatogonia in mice, there is another mechanism called the Ping-Pong cycle that amplifies specific sequences generated by the primary biogenesis pathway

[163,169]. Mainly the Ping-Pong pathway engages AGO3 and Aubergine, both of which are accumulated in perinuclear structures located at the cytoplasmic face of the nuclear envelope in animal germline cells, named "nuage". The pathway depends on the endoribonuclease or Slicer activity of AGO3 and Aubergine, which act catalytically one after the other, leading to a cleavage of the target RNAs between their tenth and eleventh nucleotides relative to the 'guide' small RNAs. This process results in the generation of repeated rounds of piRNA production having exactly the same sequence of the original primary piRNA. The ping-pong pathway amplifies piRNAs in *D. melanogaster* testes, especially those originating from TEs. Non-TE-derived piRNAs seem to be barely amplified by the amplification loop. This two steps of piRNA biogenesis can be compared with the function of the adaptive immune system in protecting against pathogens. The primary piRNA biogenesis pathway resembles the initial generation of the hypervariable antibody repertoire, whereas the amplification loop is analogous to antigen-directed clonal expansion of antibody-producing lymphocytes during the acute immune response. An emerging number of studies highlight the role of piRNAs or PIWI proteins in the regulation of tumorigenesis. First examples of the piRNA involvement in cancer is represented by the up-regulation of HIWI, one of the four human Piwi homologues, in about 60 % of seminomas [170]. In fact, HIWI maps to a locus known as a germ cell tumor susceptibility locus (12aq24.33). HIWI overexpression has also been found in somatic cells such as soft-tissue sarcomas or ductal pancreas adenocarcinoma, and strongly correlates with bad prognosis and high incidence of tumor-related death, providing an example for a potential tumorigenic role of a piRNA-related protein in somatic cells [171,172]. In some cancers, PIWIL2 overexpression has been suggested to induced resistance in cells to cisplatin, which might arise because of increased chromatin condensation that prevents the normal process of DNA repair [173]. Furthermore, new high-throughput sequencing data revealed the presence of piRNAs in somotic cells, such as HeLa cells. These somatic piRNAs appear located in the nucleolus and in the cytoplasmic area surrounding the nuclear envolope and in contrast with the large population of known piRNAs in male germ cells, this population of piRNAs is dramatically smaller [174]. Another recent study demonstrated that the level of piR-651 is significantly higher in several cancer histotype including lung, mesothelium, breast, liver, and cervical cancer compared to non-cancerous adjacent tissues and inhibition of piR-651 induced block of gastric cancer cells at the G2/M phase [175,176]. Another example is represented by the downregulation of piR-823 in gastric cancer tissues; its enforced expression inhibited gastric cancer cell growth in vitro and in vivo, suggesting a tumor suppressive properties for piR-823 [177]. Interestingly, piRNAs not are only involved in direct regulation by degradation of TE but they have also been linked to DNA methylation of the retrotraspon regions, extending piRNA functions beyond post-transcriptional silencing. In fact, CpG DNA methylation, which is required for efficient transcriptional silencing of LINE and LTR retrotransposons in the genome, is decreased in the male germ line of mice with defective PIWI proteins. Specifically, mice with defective PIWI proteins fail to establish de novo methylation of TE sequences during spermatogenesis, leading to the hypothesis that the piRISC can also guide the *de novo* methylation machinery to TE loci. In this scenerio, piRNAs may present a perfect guide for discriminating TE sequences from normal protein-coding genes and marking them for DNA methylation; however, the biochemical details of how these two mechanisms of piRNA

action might be linked have not yet been revealed [178,179]. All together, these data revealed that PIWI-associated RNAs and PIWI pathway has a more profound function outside germline cells than was originally thought but many more studies are needed to clarify their specific role in tumorigenesis.

A

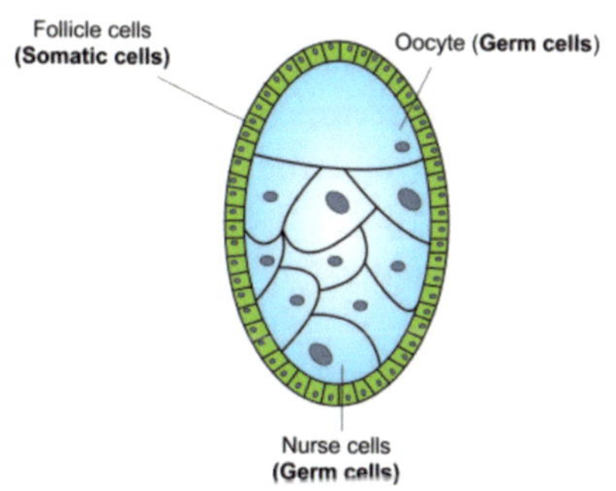

B

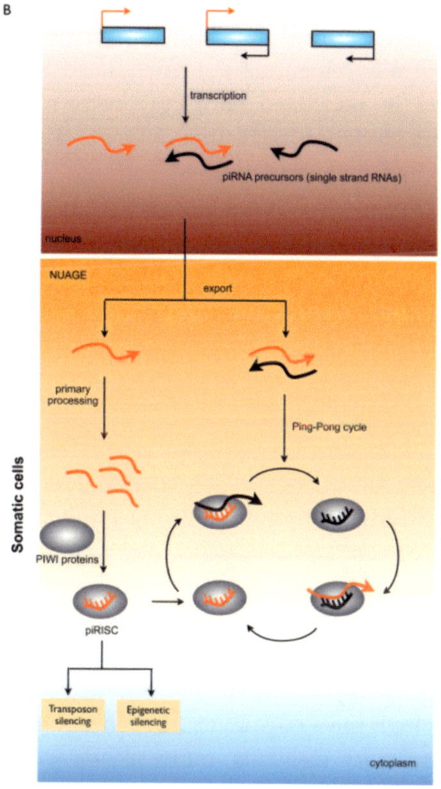

C

Organism	number of clusters	total number of piRNAs		
			plus strand	minus strand
H. Sapiens	89	15241	6057	9174
M. musculus	111	43213	18707	23506
R. norvegicus	179	48478	22529	25949
D. melanogaster	569	202370	98748	103622

Figure 3. piRNAs. A, schematic representation of the Drosophila egg chamber. **B,**piRNAs (which are 24–32 nt in length) are processed from single-stranded RNA precursors that are transcribed largely from mono- or bidirectional intergenic repetitive elements known as piRNA clusters. Unlike miRNAs and siRNAs, piRNAs do not require Dicer for their processing. First, primary piRNAs are produced through the primary processing pathway and are amplified through the ping-pong pathway, which requires Slicer activity of PIWI proteins. Subsequently, additional piRNAs are produced through a PIWI-protein-catalysed amplification loop (called the 'ping-pong cycle') via sense and antisense intermediates. Primary piRNA processing and loading onto mouse PIWI proteins might occur in the cytoplasm. The PIWI ribonucleoprotein (piRISC) complex functions in transposon repression through target degradation and epigenetic silencing. **C,** total number of piRNA clusters in different animal species according to the piRNA Database (http://pirnabank.ibab.ac.in/).

8. The emergence of long non-coding RNAs

Over the last decade, advances in genome-wide analyses of the eukaryotic transcriptome have revealed that most of the human genome is transcribed, generating a large repertoire of (>200 nt) long non-coding RNAs (lncRNA or lincRNA, for long intergenic ncRNA) that map to intronic and intergenic regions [181,181]. Given their unexpected abundance, lncRNAs were initially thought to be spurious transcriptional noise resulting from low RNA polymerase fidelity [182]. However, the restricted expression of many long ncRNAs to particular developmental contexts, the often exhibiting precise subcellular localization and the binding of transcription factors to non-coding loci, suggested that a significant portion of ncRNAs fulfills functional roles beyond transcriptional remodelling [183-187]. lncRNA typically refers to a polyadenylated long ncRNA that is transcribed by RNA polymerase II and is associated with epigenetic signatures common to protein-coding genes, such as trimethylation of histone 3 lysine 4 (H3K4me3) at the transcriptional start site (TSS) and trimethylation of histone 3 lysine 36 (H3K36me3) throughout the gene body [188-189]. lncRNAs also commonly exhibit splicing of multiple exons into a mature transcript, and their transcription occurs from an independent gene promoter and is not coupled to the transcription of a nearby or associated parental gene. RNA-Seq studies now suggest that several thousand uncharacterized lncRNAs are present in any given cell type [188-189], and that the human genome may harbor nearly as many lncRNAs as protein-coding genes (perhaps ~15,000 lncRNAs), although only a fraction is expressed in a given cell type. One main characteristic of the lncRNAs is their very low sequence conservation that had fueled the idea that they are not functional. This assertion needs to be carefully considered and takes in consideration several points. First, a recent study identified the presence of 1,600 lncRNAs that show a strong evolutionary conservation and function ranging from from embryonic stem cell pluripotency to cell proliferation [189]. In contrast to the protein coding genes, long ncRNAs can exhibit shorter stretches of sequence that are conserved to maintain functional domains and structures. Indeed, many long ncRNAs with a known function, such as *Xist*, only exhibit high conservation over short sections of their length [190]. Third, rather than being indicative of non-functionality, low sequence conservation can also be explained by high rates of primary sequence evolution if long ncRNAs have, like promoters and other regulatory elements, more plastic structure–function constraints than proteins [190]. The diverse selection pressures acting on long ncRNAs probably reflect the wide range of their functions which can be regrouped in three major subclasses: chromatin remodeling, transcriptional modulation and nuclear architecture/subnuclear localization.

long ncRNAs can mediate epigenetic changes by recruiting chromatin remodelling complexes to specific genomic loci resolving the paradox of how a small repertoire of chromatin remodelling complexes are able To specify the large array of chromatin modifications without any apparent specificity for the genomic loci [191,192]. A recent study found that 20% of 3300 human long non coding RNAs are bound by Polycomb Repressive Complex 2 (PRC2) [193]. Although the specific molecular mechanisms are not defined, there are several examples that can illustrate the silencing potential of lncRNAs (**Figure 4**). The first most known example is represented by the X-chromosome inactivation which is carried out by a number of lncRNAs including Xist and RepA, which bind PRC2 complex, and the antogonist of Xist, Tsix [194]. In pre-X-inactivation cells, Tsix competes with RepA for the binding of PRC2 complex; when the X-inactivation starts Tsix is downregulated and PRC2 becomes available to RepA which can actively induced the transcription of Xist. The up-regulated Xist in turn preferentially binds to PRC2 and spreads across the chromosome X inducing PCR2-mediated trimethylated histone H3 lysine27. Another important example is represented by the hundreds of long ncRNAs which are sequentially expressed along the temporal and spatial developmental axes of the human homeobox (Hox) loci, where they define chromatin domains of differential histone methylation and RNA polymerase accessibility [195]. One of these ncRNAs, Hox transcript antisense RNA (HOTAIR), originates from the HOXC locus and silences transcription across 40 kb of the HOXD locus in trans by inducing a repressive chromatin state, which is proposed to occur by recruitment of the Polycomb chromatin remodelling complex PRC2 by HOTAIR (**Figure 4**). Recently, it has been proposed that HOTAIR has the ability to bind other histone-modifying enzymes such as the demethylase LSD1 [196]. In fact, knockdown of HOTAIR induces a rapid loss of LSD1 or PRC2 at hundreds of gene loci with the corresponding increase in expression. This model fits other chromatin modifying complexes, such as Mll, PcG, and G9a methyltransferase, which can be similarly directed by their associated ncRNAs [196]. As modulator of epigenetic landmark, it has been shown that HOTAIR has a profound effect on tumorigenesis. In fact, HOTAIR is upregulated in breast carcinoma and colon cancer and its correlates with metastasis and poor prognosis [197] Enforced expression of HOTAIR consistently changed the pattern of occupancy of Polycomb proteins from the typical epithelial mammary cells pattern to that of embryonic fibroblasts [198]. Another important effect of lncRNAs on chromatin modification that can highlight their impact on cancer is the relationship between the lncRNA ANRIL and the INK4b/ARF/INK4a locus, encoding for three tumor-suppressor genes highly deleted or silenced in a large cohort of tumors [199]. ANRIL, which is transcribed antisense to the protein coding genes of the locus, controls the epigenetic status of the locus by interacting with subunits of PRC1 and PRC2. High expression of ANRIL is found in some cancer tissues and is associated to a high levels of PCR-mediated trimethylated histone H3 lysine27. Inhibition of ANRIL releases PRC1 and PRC2 complexes from the locus, decreases the histone methylation status with the following increase of the protein coding gene transcription. Many other tumor suppressor genes that are frequently silenced by epigenetic mechanisms in cancer also have antisense partners, which can affect gene expression with different other mechanism. First, antisense ncRNAs can mask key cis-elements in mRNA by the formation of RNA duplexes, as in the case of the Zeb2 antisense RNA, which complements the 5′ splice site of an intron of Zeb2 mRNA [200]. Expression of the ncRNA prevents the splicing of the intron that contains an internal ribosome entry site required for efficient translation and expression of the ZEB2 protein with a further efficient translation (**Figure 4**). In this context, it has been evaluated that the prevalence of lncRNAs are antisense to introns, hypothesizing their role in the regulation of splicing or capable of generating mRNA duplexes that fuel the RISC machinery to silence gene expression. One major emergent theme is the involvement of the lncRNAs in the assembly or activity of transcription factors functioning as a scaffold for the docking of many proteins, mimicking functional DNA elements or modulation of PolII itself. The first example is represented by the suppression of CCND1 mediated by the lncRNAs through the recruitment and integration of the RNA binding protein TLS into a transcriptional programme. DNA damage signals induce the expression of long ncRNAs associated with the cyclin D1 gene promoter, where they act cooperatively to recruit the RNA binding

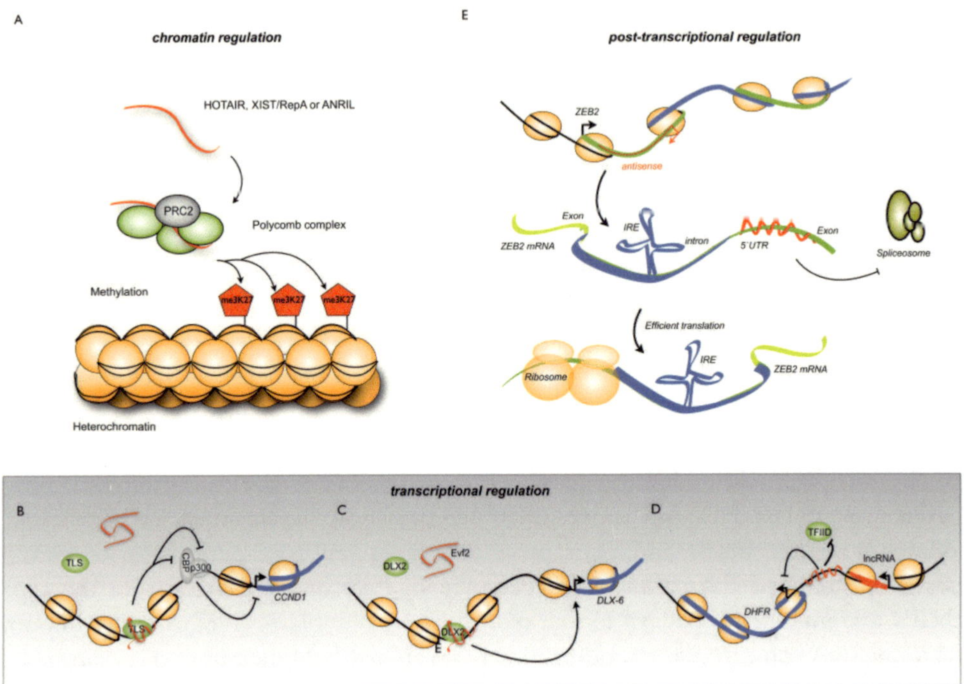

Figure 4. lncRNAs. Schematic representation of the control operated on protein coding gene by the lncRNAs at the level of chromatin remodelling, transcriptional control and post-transcriptional processing. **A**, lncRNAs (Xist, HOTAIR, ANRIL, etc) can recruit chromatin modifying complexes to specific genomic loci to localize their catalytic activity. In this case, the lncRNA recruits the Polycomb complex by inducing trimethylation of the lysine 27 residues (me3K27) of histone H3 to produce heterochromatin formation and repress gene expression. **B, C, D,** lncRNAs can regulate the transcriptional process through a range of mechanisms. First, lncRNAs tethered to the promoter of the cyclin D1 gene recruit the RNA binding protein TLS to modulate the histone acetyltransferase activity of CREB binding protein (CBP) and p300 to repress gene transcription. Second, an ultraconserved enhancer is transcribed as a long ncRNA, Evf2, which subsequently acts as a co-activator to the transcription factor DLX2, to regulate the Dlx6 gene transcription. Third, a lncRNA transcribed from the DHFR minor promoter form a triplex at the major promoter to reduce the access of the general transcription factor TFIID, and thereby suppress DHFR gene expression. **E**, a lncRNA is antisense to Zeb2 mRNA and mask the 5′ splice site resulting in intron retention. This retention results in an efficient Zeb2 translation related to the presence of an internal ribosome entry site (IRE) in the retained intron.

protein TLS. The modified and promoter-docked TLS inhibits the histone acetyltransferase activities of CReB binding protein and p300 inducing the silencing of cyclin D1 expression (Figure 4) [201]. A different co-activator activity mediated by lncRNAs is also evident in the regulation of Dlx genes, important modulators of neuronal development and patterning [202]. Dlx5-6 expression is regulated by two ultraconserved enhancers one of which is transcribed in a lncRNA, named Evf-2. Evf2 forms a stable complex with the homodomein protein DLX-2 which in turn acts as a transcriptional enhancer of Dxl5-6 gene (Figure 4). In some cases, lncRNAs can also affect RNA polymerase activity by influencing the initiation complex in the choice of the promoter. For example, in humans, a ncRNA transcribed from an upstream region of the dihydrofolate reductase (DHFR) locus forms a triplex in the major promoter of DHFR to prevent the binding of the transcriptional co-factor TFIID (Figure 4). This could be a widespread mechanism for controlling promoter usage as thousands of triplex structures exist in eukaryotic chromosomes. Recently, lncRNAs have also shown their tumorigenic potential by modulating the transcriptional program of p53 [203]. An 3kb lncRNAs, linc-RNA-p21, transcriptionally activated by p53, has been shown to collaborate with p53 in order to control the gene expression in response to DNA damage. Specifically, silencing of lincRNA-p21 derepresses the expression of hundred of genes which are also derepressed following p53 knockdown. It has also been discovered that lincRNA-p21 interacts with hnRNPK and this binding is essential for the modulation of p53 activity.

The final category of lncRNAs is represented by those molecules capable to generate the formation of compartmentalized nuclear organelles, subnuclear membraneless nuclear bodies whose funtion is relative unknown. One of them is represented by cell-cycle regulated nuclear foci, named paraspeckles. In addition to protein components, two lncRNAs, NEAT1 and Men epsilon, have been detected as essential part of the paraspeckles. While depletion of NEAT or Men epsilon disrupts the paraspeckles, their overexpression strongly increases their number. There is a number of different lncRNAs that localize to different nuclear regions [204]. Metastasis-associated lung adenocarcinoma transcript 1 (MALAT1) localizes to the splicing speckles, Xist and Kcnq1ot1 both, localize to the perinucleolar region during the S phase of the cell cycle, a class of repeat-associated lncRNAs (es SatIII) are associated to nuclear stress bodies which are produced on specifc pericentromeric heterochromatic domains containing SatIII gene itself.

9. Conclusions

Alterations in microRNAs and other short or long non-coding RNA (ncRNA) are involved in the initiation, progression, and metastasis of human cancer. Over the last decade, a growing number of non-coding transcripts have been found to have roles in gene regulation and RNA processing. The most well known small non-coding RNAs are the microRNAs, but the network of long and short non-coding transcripts is complex and is likely to contain as yet unidentified classes of molecules that form transcriptional regulatory networks. The field of small and long non coding RNAs is rapidly advancing toward in vivo delivery for therapeutic purposes. Advanced molecular therapies aimed at downmodulating or upmodulating the level of a given miRNA in model organisms have been successfully established. RNA-based gene therapy can be used to treat cancer by using RNA or DNA molecules as therapy against the mRNA of genes involved in cancer pathogenesis or by directly targeting the ncRNAs that participate in pathogenesis. The use of miRNAs is still being evaluated preclinically; no clinical or toxicologic studies have been published but the future is promising. Kota and collegues reported that systemic administration of this miRNA in a mouse model of HCC using adeno-associated virus (AAV) results in inhibition of cancer cell proliferation, induction of tumor-specific apoptosis, and dramatic protection from disease progression without toxicity (116). Recently, Pineau et al. (117) identified DNA damage-inducible transcript 4 (DDIT4), a modulator of the mTor pathway, as a bona fide target of miR-221. They introduced into liver cancer cells, by lipofection, LNA-modified oligonucleotides specifically designed for miR-221 (antimiR-221) and miR-222 (antimiR-222) knockdown. Treatment by antagomiRs, but not scrambled oligonucleotide, reduced cell growth in liver cancer cell lines that overexpressed miR-221 and miR-222 by 35% and 22%, respectively. Thus the use of synthetic inhibitors of miR-221 may prove to be a promising approach to liver cancer treatment (117). Despite recent progress in silencing of miRNAs in rodents, the development of effective and safe approaches for sequence-specific antagonism of miRNAs in vivo remains a significant scientific and therapeutic challenge. Recently, Elmen and collaborators (118) showed for the first time, that the simple systemic delivery of an unconjugated, PBS-formulated LNA-antimiR effectively antagonizes the liver-expressed miR-122 in nonhuman primates. Administration by intravenous injections of LNA-antimiR into African green monkeys resulted in the formation of stable heteroduplexes between the LNA-antimiR and miR-122, accompanied by depletion of mature miR-122 and dose-dependent lowering of plasma cholesterol. These findings demonstrate the utility of systemically administered LNA-antimiRs in exploring miRNA functions in primates and show the impressive potential of this strategy to overcome a major hurdle for clinical miRNA therapy. In conclusion, the discovery of small RNAs and their functions has revitalized the prospect of controlling expression of specific genes in vivo, with the ultimate hope of building a new class of gene-specific medical therapies. Just how significant are the ncRNAs? They appear to be doing something important and highly sophisticated; there are so many of them, their sequences are so highly conserved, their expression is tissue specific, and they have recognition sites on more than 30% of the entire transcriptome. It seems that ncRNAs were overlooked in the past simply because researchers were specifically looking for RNAs that code proteins. The above discussed data highlight that the complexity of genomic control operated by the ncRNAs is somewhat greater than previously imagined, and that they could represent a total new order of genomic control. In this scenario, understanding the precise roles of ncRNAs is a key challenge. The targeting of other ncRNAs, in addition to miRNAs, is still in its infancy, but new important developments are expected in this area. Therefore, small RNAs could become powerful therapeutic tools in the near future.

Author details

Gianpiero Di Leva and Michela Garofalo*

The Ohio State University, Department of Molecular Immunology, Virology and Medical Genetics. Columbus, OH, USA

10. References

[1] Matsubara K, Okubo K. (1993). Identification of new genes by systematic analysis of cDNAs and database construction. Curr Opin Biotechnol. 4:672-677.

[2] Liang F, Holt I, Pertea G, Karamycheva S, Salzberg SL, Quackenbush J. (2000). Gene index analysis of the human genome estimates approximately 120,000 genes. Nat Genet. 25:239-240.

* Corresponding Author

[3] Lander ES, Linton LM, Birren B, Nusbaum C, Zody MC, Baldwin J, Devon K, Dewar K, Doyle M, FitzHugh W, Funke R, Gage D, Harris K, Heaford A, Howland J, Kann L, Lehoczky J, LeVine R, McEwan P, McKernan K, Meldrim J, Mesirov JP, Miranda C, Morris W, Naylor J, Raymond C, Rosetti M, Santos R, Sheridan A, Sougnez C, Stange-Thomann N, Stojanovic N, Subramanian A, Wyman D, Rogers J, Sulston J, Ainscough R, Beck S, Bentley D, Burton J, Clee C, Carter N, Coulson A, Deadman R, Deloukas P, Dunham A, Dunham I, Durbin R, French L, Grafham D, Gregory S, Hubbard T, Humphray S, Hunt A, Jones M, Lloyd C, McMurray A, Matthews L, Mercer S, Milne S, Mullikin JC, Mungall A, Plumb R, Ross M, Shownkeen R, Sims S, Waterston RH, Wilson RK, Hillier LW, McPherson JD, Marra MA, Mardis ER, Fulton LA, Chinwalla AT, Pepin KH, Gish WR, Chissoe SL, Wendl MC, Delehaunty KD, Miner TL, Delehaunty A, Kramer JB, Cook LL, Fulton RS, Johnson DL, Minx PJ, Clifton SW, Hawkins T, Branscomb E, Predki P, Richardson P, Wenning S, Slezak T, Doggett N, Cheng JF, Olsen A, Lucas S, Elkin C, Uberbacher E, Frazier M, Gibbs RA, Muzny DM, Scherer SE, Bouck JB, Sodergren EJ, Worley KC, Rives CM, Gorrell JH, Metzker ML, Naylor SL, Kucherlapati RS, Nelson DL, Weinstock GM, Sakaki Y, Fujiyama A, Hattori M, Yada T, Toyoda A, Itoh T, Kawagoe C, Watanabe H, Totoki Y, Taylor T, Weissenbach J, Heilig R, Saurin W, Artiguenave F, Brottier P, Bruls T, Pelletier E, Robert C, Wincker P, Smith DR, Doucette-Stamm L, Rubenfield M, Weinstock K, Lee HM, Dubois J, Rosenthal A, Platzer M, Nyakatura G, Taudien S, Rump A, Yang H, Yu J, Wang J, Huang G, Gu J, Hood L, Rowen L, Madan A, Qin S, Davis RW, Federspiel NA, Abola AP, Proctor MJ, Myers RM, Schmutz J, Dickson M, Grimwood J, Cox DR, Olson MV, Kaul R, Raymond C, Shimizu N, Kawasaki K, Minoshima S, Evans GA, Athanasiou M, Schultz R, Roe BA, Chen F, Pan H, Ramser J, Lehrach H, Reinhardt R, McCombie WR, de la Bastide M, Dedhia N, Blöcker H, Hornischer K, Nordsiek G, Agarwala R, Aravind L, Bailey JA, Bateman A, Batzoglou S, Birney E, Bork P, Brown DG, Burge CB, Cerutti L, Chen HC, Church D, Clamp M, Copley RR, Doerks T, Eddy SR, Eichler EE, Furey TS, Galagan J, Gilbert JG, Harmon C, Hayashizaki Y, Haussler D, Hermjakob H, Hokamp K, Jang W, Johnson LS, Jones TA, Kasif S, Kaspryzk A, Kennedy S, Kent WJ, Kitts P, Koonin EV, Korf I, Kulp D, Lancet D, Lowe TM, McLysaght A, Mikkelsen T, Moran JV, Mulder N, Pollara VJ, Ponting CP, Schuler G, Schultz J, Slater G, Smit AF, Stupka E, Szustakowski J, Thierry-Mieg D, Thierry-Mieg J, Wagner L, Wallis J, Wheeler R, Williams A, Wolf YI, Wolfe KH, Yang SP, Yeh RF, Collins F, Guyer MS, Peterson J, Felsenfeld A, Wetterstrand KA, Patrinos A, Morgan MJ, de Jong P, Catanese JJ, Osoegawa K, Shizuya H, Choi S, Chen YJ. (2001). International Human Genome Sequencing Consortium. Initial sequencing and analysis of the human genome. Nature. 409:860-921.

[4] Guttman M, Amit I, Garber M, French C, Lin MF, Feldser D, Huarte M, Zuk O, Carey BW, Cassady JP, Cabili MN, Jaenisch R, Mikkelsen TS, Jacks T, Hacohen N, Bernstein BE, Kellis M, Regev A, Rinn JL, Lander ES. (2009). Chromatin signature reveals over a thousand highly conserved large non-coding RNAs in mammals. Nature. 458:223–227

[5] Guttman M, Garber M, Levin JZ, Donaghey J, Robinson J, Adiconis X, Fan L, Koziol MJ, Gnirke A, Nusbaum C, Rinn JL, Lander ES, Regev A. (2010). Ab initio reconstruction of

cell type-specific transcriptomes in mouse reveals the conserved multi-exonic structure of lincRNAs. Nat. Biotechnol. 28:503–510.

[6] Marques AC, Ponting CP. (2009). Catalogues of mammalian long noncoding RNAs: modest conservation and incompleteness. Genome Biol.10:R124.

[7] Cech TR. (2009). Crawling out of the RNA world. Cell. 136:599-602.

[8] Kapranov P, Cheng J, Dike S, Nix DA, Duttagupta R, Willingham AT, Stadler PF, Hertel J, Hackermüller J, Hofacker IL, Bell I, Cheung E, Drenkow J, Dumais E, Patel S, Helt G, Ganesh M, Ghosh S, Piccolboni A, Sementchenko V, Tammana H, Gingeras TR. (2007). RNA maps reveal new RNA classes and a possible function for pervasive transcription. Science. 316:1484–1488.

[9] Crick FH, Barnett L, Brenner S, Watts-Tobin RJ. (1961). General nature of the genetic code for proteins. Nature. 192:1227–1232.

[10] Mercer TR, Dinger ME, Mattick JS. (2009) Long non-coding RNAs insight into functions. Nature Rev. Genet. 10:155–159.

[11] He L, Hannon GJ. (2004). MicroRNAs: small RNAs with a big role in gene regulation. Nature Rev. Genet. 5:522–531.

[12] Mendell JT. (2005). MicroRNAs: critical regulators of development, cellular physiology and malignancy. Cell Cycle 4:1179–1184.

[13] Esquela-Kerscher A, Slack FJ. (2006). OncomiRs — microRNAs with a role in cancer. Nature Rev. Cancer 6:259–269.

[14] Hammond SM. (2007). MicroRNAs as tumor suppressors. Nature Genet. 39:582–583.

[15] Croce CM. (2009). Causes and consequences of microRNA dysregulation in cancer. Nature Rev. Genet. 10:704–714.

[16] Nicoloso M S, Spizzo R, Shimizu M, Rossi S, Calin GA. (2009). MicroRNAs — the micro steering wheel of tumour metastases. Nature Rev. Cancer. 9:293–302.

[17] Carninci P, Kasukawa T, Katayama S, Gough J, Frith MC, Maeda N, Oyama R, Ravasi T, Lenhard B, Wells C, Kodzius R, Shimokawa K, Bajic VB, Brenner SE, Batalov S, Forrest AR, Zavolan M, Davis MJ, Wilming LG, Aidinis V, Allen JE, Ambesi-Impiombato A, Apweiler R, Aturaliya RN, Bailey TL, Bansal M, Baxter L, Beisel KW, Bersano T, Bono H, Chalk AM, Chiu KP, Choudhary V, Christoffels A, Clutterbuck DR, Crowe ML, Dalla E, Dalrymple BP, de Bono B, Della Gatta G, di Bernardo D, Down T, Engstrom P, Fagiolini M, Faulkner G, Fletcher CF, Fukushima T, Furuno M, Futaki S, Gariboldi M, Georgii-Hemming P, Gingeras TR, Gojobori T, Green RE, Gustincich S, Harbers M, Hayashi Y, Hensch TK, Hirokawa N, Hill D, Huminiecki L, Iacono M, Ikeo K, Iwama A, Ishikawa T, Jakt M, Kanapin A, Katoh M, Kawasawa Y, Kelso J, Kitamura H, Kitano H, Kollias G, Krishnan SP, Kruger A, Kummerfeld SK, Kurochkin IV, Lareau LF, Lazarevic D, Lipovich L, Liu J, Liuni S, McWilliam S, Madan Babu M, Madera M, Marchionni L, Matsuda H, Matsuzawa S, Miki H, Mignone F, Miyake S, Morris K, Mottagui-Tabar S, Mulder N, Nakano N, Nakauchi H, Ng P, Nilsson R, Nishiguchi S, Nishikawa S, Nori F, Ohara O, Okazaki Y, Orlando V, Pang KC, Pavan WJ, Pavesi G, Pesole G, Petrovsky N, Piazza S, Reed J, Reid JF, Ring BZ, Ringwald M, Rost B, Ruan Y, Salzberg SL, Sandelin A, Schneider C, Schönbach C, Sekiguchi K, Semple CA, Seno S, Sessa L, Sheng Y, Shibata Y, Shimada H, Shimada K, Silva D, Sinclair B, Sperling S, Stupka E, Sugiura K, Sultana R, Takenaka Y, Taki K, Tammoja K, Tan SL, Tang S, Taylor MS, Tegner J,

Teichmann SA, Ueda HR, van Nimwegen E, Verardo R, Wei CL, Yagi K, Yamanishi H, Zabarovsky E, Zhu S, Zimmer A, Hide W, Bult C, Grimmond SM, Teasdale RD, Liu ET, Brusic V, Quackenbush J, Wahlestedt C, Mattick JS, Hume DA, Kai C, Sasaki D, Tomaru Y, Fukuda S, Kanamori-Katayama M, Suzuki M, Aoki J, Arakawa T, Iida J, Imamura K, Itoh M, Kato T, Kawaji H, Kawagashira N, Kawashima T, Kojima M, Kondo S, Konno H, Nakano K, Ninomiya N, Nishio T, Okada M, Plessy C, Shibata K, Shiraki T, Suzuki S, Tagami M, Waki K, Watahiki A, Okamura-Oho Y, Suzuki H, Kawai J, Hayashizaki Y; FANTOM Consortium; RIKEN Genome Exploration Research Group and Genome Science Group (Genome Network Project Core Group).(2005). The transcriptional landscape of the mammalian genome. Science. 309:1559–1563.

[18] Gibb EA, Brown CJ, Lam WL. (2011). The functional role of long non-coding RNA in human carcinomas. Mol Cancer 10:38.

[19] Taft RJ, Pang KC, MErcer TR, Dinger M, Mattick JS. (2010) Non-coding RNAs: regulators of disease. J Pathol.220:126-39.

[20] Di Leva G, Croce CM. (2010). Roles of small RNAs in tumor formation. Trends Mol Med.16:257-67.

[21] Garofalo M, Croce CM. (2011). microRNAs: Master regulators as potential therapeutics in cancer. Annu Rev Pharmacol Toxicol. 51:25-43.

[22] ENCODE Project Consortium, Birney E, Stamatoyannopoulos JA, Dutta A, Guigó R, Gingeras TR, Margulies EH, Weng Z, Snyder M, Dermitzakis ET, Thurman RE, Kuehn MS, Taylor CM, Neph S, Koch CM, Asthana S, Malhotra A, Adzhubei I, Greenbaum JA, Andrews RM, Flicek P, Boyle PJ, Cao H, Carter NP, Clelland GK, Davis S, Day N, Dhami P, Dillon SC, Dorschner MO, Fiegler H, Giresi PG, Goldy J, Hawrylycz M, Haydock A, Humbert R, James KD, Johnson BE, Johnson EM, Frum TT, Rosenzweig ER, Karnani N, Lee K, Lefebvre GC, Navas PA, Neri F, Parker SC, Sabo PJ, Sandstrom R, Shafer A, Vetrie D, Weaver M, Wilcox S, Yu M, Collins FS, Dekker J, Lieb JD, Tullius TD, Crawford GE, Sunyaev S, Noble WS, Dunham I, Denoeud F, Reymond A, Kapranov P, Rozowsky J, Zheng D, Castelo R, Frankish A, Harrow J, Ghosh S, Sandelin A, Hofacker IL, Baertsch R, Keefe D, Dike S, Cheng J, Hirsch HA, Sekinger EA, Lagarde J, Abril JF, Shahab A, Flamm C, Fried C, Hackermüller J, Hertel J, Lindemeyer M, Missal K, Tanzer A, Washietl S, Korbel J, Emanuelsson O, Pedersen JS, Holroyd N, Taylor R, Swarbreck D, Matthews N, Dickson MC, Thomas DJ, Weirauch MT, Gilbert J, Drenkow J, Bell I, Zhao X, Srinivasan KG, Sung WK, Ooi HS, Chiu KP, Foissac S, Alioto T, Brent M, Pachter L, Tress ML, Valencia A, Choo SW, Choo CY, Ucla C, Manzano C, Wyss C, Cheung E, Clark TG, Brown JB, Ganesh M, Patel S, Tammana H, Chrast J, Henrichsen CN, Kai C, Kawai J, Nagalakshmi U, Wu J, Lian Z, Lian J, Newburger P, Zhang X, Bickel P, Mattick JS, Carninci P, Hayashizaki Y, Weissman S, Hubbard T, Myers RM, Rogers J, Stadler PF, Lowe TM, Wei CL, Ruan Y, Struhl K, Gerstein M, Antonarakis SE, Fu Y, Green ED, Karaöz U, Siepel A, Taylor J, Liefer LA, Wetterstrand KA, Good PJ, Feingold EA, Guyer MS, Cooper GM, Asimenos G, Dewey CN, Hou M, Nikolaev S, Montoya-Burgos JI, Löytynoja A, Whelan S, Pardi F, Massingham T, Huang H, Zhang NR, Holmes I, Mullikin JC, Ureta-Vidal A, Paten B, Seringhaus M, Church D, Rosenbloom K, Kent WJ, Stone EA; NISC Comparative Sequencing Program; Baylor College of Medicine Human Genome Sequencing Center; Washington University

Genome Sequencing Center; Broad Institute; Children's Hospital Oakland Research Institute, Batzoglou S, Goldman N, Hardison RC, Haussler D, Miller W, Sidow A, Trinklein ND, Zhang ZD, Barrera L, Stuart R, King DC, Ameur A, Enroth S, Bieda MC, Kim J, Bhinge AA, Jiang N, Liu J, Yao F, Vega VB, Lee CW, Ng P, Shahab A, Yang A, Moqtaderi Z, Zhu Z, Xu X, Squazzo S, Oberley MJ, Inman D, Singer MA, Richmond TA, Munn KJ, Rada-Iglesias A, Wallerman O, Komorowski J, Fowler JC, Couttet P, Bruce AW, Dovey OM, Ellis PD, Langford CF, Nix DA, Euskirchen G, Hartman S, Urban AE, Kraus P, Van Calcar S, Heintzman N, Kim TH, Wang K, Qu C, Hon G, Luna R, Glass CK, Rosenfeld MG, Aldred SF, Cooper SJ, Halees A, Lin JM, Shulha HP, Zhang X, Xu M, Haidar JN, Yu Y, Ruan Y, Iyer VR, Green RD, Wadelius C, Farnham PJ, Ren B, Harte RA, Hinrichs AS, Trumbower H, Clawson H, Hillman-Jackson J, Zweig AS, Smith K, Thakkapallayil A, Barber G, Kuhn RM, Karolchik D, Armengol L, Bird CP, de Bakker PI, Kern AD, Lopez-Bigas N, Martin JD, Stranger BE, Woodroffe A, Davydov E, Dimas A, Eyras E, Hallgrímsdóttir IB, Huppert J, Zody MC, Abecasis GR, Estivill X, Bouffard GG, Guan X, Hansen NF, Idol JR, Maduro VV, Maskeri B, McDowell JC, Park M, Thomas PJ, Young AC, Blakesley RW, Muzny DM, Sodergren E, Wheeler DA, Worley KC, Jiang H, Weinstock GM, Gibbs RA, Graves T, Fulton R, Mardis ER, Wilson RK, Clamp M, Cuff J, Gnerre S, Jaffe DB, Chang JL, Lindblad-Toh K, Lander ES, Koriabine M, Nefedov M, Osoegawa K, Yoshinaga Y, Zhu B, de Jong PJ. Identification and analysis of functional elements in 1% of the human genome by the ENCODE pilot project.(2007). Nature.447:799-816.

[23] Siomi MC, Sato K, Pezic D, Aravin AA. (2011). PIWI-interacting small RNAs: the vanguard of genome defence. Nat Rev Mol Cell Biol.12:246-58.

[24] Faulkner GJ, Kimura Y, Daub CO, Wani S, Plessy C, Irvine KM, Schroder K, Cloonan N, Steptoe AL, Lassmann T, Waki K, Hornig N, Arakawa T, Takahashi H, Kawai J, Forrest AR, Suzuki H, Hayashizaki Y, Hume DA, Orlando V, Grimmond SM, Carninci P. (2009). The regulated retrotransposon transcriptome of mammalian cells. Nat Genet. 41:563-71.

[25] Huarte M, Rinn JL. (2010). Large non-coding RNAs: missing links in cancer? Hum Mol Genet. 19:R152-61.

[26] Pauli A, Rinn JL, Schier AF. (2011). Non-coding RNAs as regulators of embryogenesis. Nat Rev Genet.12:136–49.

[27] Calin GA, Liu CG, Ferracin M, Hyslop T, Spizzo R, Sevignani C, Fabbri M, Cimmino A, Lee EJ, Wojcik SE, Shimizu M, Tili E, Rossi S, Taccioli C, Pichiorri F, Liu X, Zupo S, Herlea V, Gramantieri L, Lanza G, Alder H, Rassenti L, Volinia S, Schmittgen TD, Kipps TJ, Negrini M, Croce CM. (2007). Ultraconserved regions encoding ncRNAs are altered in human leukemias and carcinomas. Cancer Cell. 12:215-29.

[28] Poliseno L, Salmena L, Zhang J, Carver B, Haveman WJ, Pandolfi PP. (2010). A coding-independent function of gene and pseudogene mRNAs regulates tumour biology. Nature. 465:1033-8.

[29] He Y, Vogelstein B, Velculescu VE, Papadopoulos N, Kinzler KW. (2008). The antisense transcriptomes of human cells. Science. 322:1855-7.

[30] Kim TK, Hemberg M, Gray JM, Costa AM, Bear DM, Wu J, Harmin DA, Laptewicz M, Barbara-Haley K, Kuersten S, Markenscoff-Papadimitriou E, Kuhl D, Bito H, Worley PF,

Kreiman G, Greenberg ME. (2010). Widespread transcription at neuronal activity-regulated enhancers. Nature. 465:182-7.

[31] Lee RC, Feinbaum RL, Ambros V. (1993). The C. elegans heterochronic gene lin-4 encodes small RNAs with antisense complementarity to lin-14. Cell. 75:843–54.

[32] Kim VN. 2005. MicroRNA biogenesis: coordinated cropping and dicing. Nat. Rev. Mol. Cell Biol. 6:376–85.

[33] Rodriguez A, Griffiths-Jones S, Ashurst JL, Bradley A. (2004). Identification of mammalian microRNA host genes and transcription units. Genome Res. 14:1902–10.

[34] Lagos-Quintana M, Rauhut R, Yalcin A, Meyer J, Lendeckel W, Tuschl T. (2002). Identification of tissue-specific microRNAs from mouse. Curr Biol. 12: 735–739.

[35] Altuvia Y, Landgraf P, Lithwick G, Elefant N, Pfeffer S, Aravin A, Brownstein MJ, Tuschl T, Margalit H.(2005). Clustering and conservation patterns of human microRNAs. Nucleic Acids Res 33: 2697–2706.

[36] Borchert GM, Lanier W, Davidson BL. (2006). RNA polymerase III transcribes human microRNAs. Nat Struct Mol Biol. 13: 1097–1101.

[37] Han J, Lee Y, Yeom KH, Nam JW, Heo I, Rhee JK, Sohn SY, Cho Y, Zhang BT, Kim VN. (2006). Molecular basis for the recognition of primary microRNAs by the Drosha-DGCR8 complex. Cell 125: 887–901.

[38] Saetrom P, Snove O, Nedland M, Grunfeld TB, Lin Y, Bass MB, Cannon JR. (2006). Conserved microRNA characteristics in mammals. Oligonucleotides. 16:115-44.

[39] Gregory RI, Yan KP, Amuthan G, Chendrimada T, Doratotaj B, Cooch N, Shiekhattar R. (2004). The Microprocessor complex mediates the genesis of microRNAs. Nature 432:235–40.

[40] Han J, Lee Y, Yeom KH, Kim YK, Jin H, Kim VN. (2004). The Drosha-DGCR8 complex in primary microRNA processing. Genes Dev. 18:3016–27.

[41] Yi R, Qin Y, Macara IG, Cullen BR. (2003). Exportin-5 mediates the nuclear export of pre-microRNAs and short hairpin RNAs. Genes Dev. 17:3011–3016.

[42] Lund E, Guttinger S, Calado A, Dahlberg JE, Kutay U. (2004). Nuclear export of microRNA precursors. Science. 303:95–98.

[43] Bohnsack MT, Czaplinski K, Gorlich D. (2004). Exportin 5 is a RanGTP-dependent dsRNA-binding protein that mediates nuclear export of pre-miRNAs. RNA. 10:185–191.

[44] Maniataki E, Mourelatos Z. (2005). A human, ATP-independent, RISC assembly machine fueled by pre-miRNA. Genes Dev. 19:2979–2990.

[45] Lee Y, Hur I, Park SY, Kim YK, Suh MR, Kim VN. (2006). The role of PACT in the RNA silencing pathway. EMBO J. 25:522–532.

[46] Haase AD, Jaskiewicz L, Zhang H, Laine S, Sack R, Gatignol A, Filipowicz W. (2005). TRBP, a regulator of cellular PKR and HIV-1 virus expression, interacts with Dicer and functions in RNA silencing. EMBO Rep 6: 961–967.

[47] Gregory RI, Chendrimada TP, Cooch N, Shiekhattar R. (2005). Human RISC couples microRNA biogenesis and posttranscriptional gene silencing. Cell. 123:631–640.

[48] Forstemann K, Tomari Y, Du T, Vagin VV, Denli AM, Bratu DP, Klattenhoff C, Theurkauf WE, Zamore PD. (2005). Normal microRNA maturation and germ-line stem cell maintenance requires Loquacious, a double-stranded RNA-binding domain protein. PLoS Biol. 3:e236.

[49] Chendrimada TP, Gregory RI, Kumaraswamy E, Norman J, Cooch N, Nishikura K,Nishikura K, Shiekhattar R. (2005). TRBP recruits the Dicer complex to Ago2 for microRNA processing and gene silencing. Nature. 436: 740–744.

[50] Castanotto D, Sakurai K, Lingeman R, Li H, Shively L, Aagaard L, Soifer H, Gatignol A, Riggs A, Rossi JJ. (2007). Combinatorial delivery of small interfering RNAs reduces RNAi efficacy by selective incorporation into RISC. Nucleic Acids Res. 35:5154-64.

[51] Rand TA, Petersen S, Du F, Wang X. (2005). Argonaute2 cleaves the anti-guide strand of siRNA during RISC activation. Cell. 123:621–29.

[52] Leuschner PJ, Ameres SL, Kueng S, Martinez J. (2006). Cleavage of the siRNA passenger strand during RISC assembly in human cells. EMBO Rep. 7:314–20.

[53] Martinez J, Patkaniowska A, UrlaubH, Luhrmann R, Tuschl T. (2002). Single-stranded antisense siRNAs guide target RNA cleavage in RNAi. Cell. 110:563–74.

[54] Zamore PD, Tuschl T, Sharp PA, Bartel DP. (2000). RNAi: double-stranded RNA directs the ATP-dependent cleavage of mRNA at 21 to 23 nucleotide intervals. Cell. 101: 25–33.

[55] Yekta S, Shih IH, Bartel DP. (2004). MicroRNA-directed cleavage of HOXB8 mRNA. Science. 304: 594–596.

[56] Wu L, Fan J, Belasco JG. (2006). MicroRNAs direct rapid deadenylation of mRNA. Proc Natl Acad Sci USA. 103: 4034–4039.

[57] Bagga S, Bracht J, Hunter S, Massirer K, Holtz J, Eachus R, Pasquinelli AE. (2005). Regulation by let-7 and lin-4 miRNAs results in target mRNA degradation. Cell. 122: 553–563.

[58] Reinhart BJ, Slack FJ, Basson M, Pasquinelli AE, Bettinger JC, Rougvie AE, Horvitz HR, Ruvkun G. (2000). The 21-nucleotide let-7 RNA regulates developmental timing in Caenorhabditis elegans. Nature 403: 901–906.

[59] Olsen PH, Ambros V. (1999). The lin-4 regulatory RNA controls developmental timing in Caenorhabditis elegans by blocking LIN-14 protein synthesis after the initiation of translation. Dev Biol. 216: 671–680.

[60] Pillai RS, Bhattacharyya SN, Filipowicz W. (2007). Repression of protein synthesis by miRNAs: how many mechanisms? Trends Cell Biol. 17:118–26.

[61] Garzon R, Fabbri M, Cimmino A, Calin GA, Croce CM. (2006). MicroRNA expression and function in cancer. Trends Mol. Med. 12:580-587.

[62] Wu W, Sun M, Zou GM, Chen J. (2007). MicroRNA and cancer: Current status and prospective. Int. J. Cancer.120: 953-960.

[63] Boettger T, Braun T. (2012). A New Level of Complexity: The Role of MicroRNAs in Cardiovascular Development. Circ Res.110:1000-1013.

[64] Han R, Kan Q, Sun Y, Wang S, Zhang G, Peng T, Jia Y. (2012). MiR-9 promotes the neural differentiation of mouse bone marrow mesenchymal stem cells via targeting zinc finger protein 521. Neurosci Lett. Ahead of print.

[65] D'Urso PI, D'Urso OF, Storelli C, Mallardo M, Gianfreda CD, Montinaro A, Cimmino A, Pietro C, Marsigliante S. (2012). miR-155 is up-regulated in primary and secondary glioblastoma and promotes tumour growth by inhibiting GABA receptors. Int J Oncol. doi: 10.3892/ijo.2012.1420.

[66] Garofalo M, Romano G, Di Leva G, Nuovo G, Jeon YJ, Ngankeu A, Sun J, Lovat F, Alder H, Condorelli G, Engelman JA, Ono M, Rho JK, Cascione L, Volinia S, Nephew KP,

Croce CM. (2011). EGFR and MET receptor tyrosine kinase-altered microRNA expression induces tumorigenesis and gefitinib resistance in lung cancers. Nat Med.18:74-82.

[67] Frank D, Gantenberg J, Boomgaarden I, Kuhn C, Will R, Jarr KU, Eden M, Kramer K, Luedde M, Mairbäurl H, Katus HA, Frey N. (2012). MicroRNA-20a inhibits stress-induced cardiomyocyte apoptosis involving its novel target Egln3/PHD3. J Mol Cell Cardiol. 52:711-717.

[68] Calin GA, DumitruCD, ShimizuM,BichiR, Zupo S, Noch E, Aldler H, Rattan S, Keating M, Rai K, Rassenti L, Kipps T, Negrini M, Bullrich F, Croce CM. (2002). Frequent deletions and down-regulation of micro-RNA genes miR15 and miR16 at 13q14 in chronic lymphocytic leukemia. Proc. Natl. Acad. Sci. USA. 99:15524–29

[69] Calin GA, Croce CM. (2006). MicroRNA signatures in human cancers. Nat Rev Cancer. 6:857–866.

[70] Cai X, Hagedorn CH, Cullen BR. (2004). Human microRNAs are processed from capped, polyadenylated transcripts that can also function as mRNAs. RNA. 10:1957–1966.

[71] Cai X, Hagedorn CH, Cullen BR. (2004). Human microRNAs are processed from capped, polyadenylated transcripts that can also function as mRNAs. RNA. 10:1957–1966.

[72] Chan JA, Krichevsky AM, Kosik KS. 2005. MicroRNA-21 is an antiapoptotic factor in human glioblastoma cells. Cancer Res. 65:6029–6033.

[73] Zhu S, Wu H, Wu F, Nie D, Sheng S, Mo YY. (2008). MicroRNA-21 targets tumor suppressor genes in invasion and metastasis. Cell Res. 18:350–359.

[74] Zhu Q, Wang Z, Hu Y, Li J, Li X, Zhou L, Huang Y. (2012). miR-21 promotes migration and invasion by the miR-21-PDCD4-AP-1 feedback loop in human hepatocellular carcinoma. Oncol Rep.27:1660-1668.

[75] Medina PP, Nolde M, Slack FJ. (2010). OncomiR addiction in an in vivo model of microRNA-21-induced pre-B-cell lymphoma. Nature. 467:86-90.

[76] Metzler M, Wilda M, Busch K, Viehmann S, Borkhardt A. (2004). High expression of precursor microRNA-155/BIC RNA in children with Burkitt lymphoma. Genes Chromosom. Cancer. 39:167–169.

[77] Kluiver J, Poppema S, de Jong D, Blokzijl T, Harms G, Jacobs S, Kroesen BJ, van den Berg A. (2005). BIC and miR-155 are highly expressed in Hodgkin, primary mediastinal and diffuse large B cell lymphomas. J. Pathol. 207:243–249.

[78] Calin GA, Ferracin M, Cimmino A, Di Leva G, Shimizu M, Wojcik SE, Iorio MV, Visone R, Sever NI, Fabbri M, Iuliano R, Palumbo T, Pichiorri F, Roldo C, Garzon R, Sevignani C, Rassenti L, Alder H, Volinia S, Liu CG, Kipps TJ, Negrini M, Croce CM.(2005). A microRNA signature associated with prognosis and progression in chronic lymphocytic leukemia. N. Engl. J. Med. 353:1793–1801.

[79] Garzon R, Volinia S, Liu CG, Fernandez-Cymering C, Palumbo T, Pichiorri F, Fabbri M, Coombes K, Alder H, Nakamura T, Flomenberg N, Marcucci G, Calin GA, Kornblau SM, Kantarjian H, Bloomfield CD, Andreeff M, Croce CM. (2008). MicroRNA signatures associated with cytogenetics and prognosis in acute myeloid leukemia. Blood. 111:3183–3189.

[80] Volinia S, Calin GA, Liu CG, Ambs S, Cimmino A, Petrocca F, Visone R, Iorio M, Roldo C, Ferracin M, Prueitt RL, Yanaihara N, Lanza G, Scarpa A, Vecchione A, Negrini M, Harris CC, Croce CM. (2006). A microRNA expression signature of human solid tumors defines cancer gene targets. Proc. Natl. Acad. Sci. USA. 103:2257–2261.

[81] Greither T, Grochola LF, Udelnow A, Lautenschlager C, W¨url P, Taubert H. (2010). Elevated expression of microRNAs 155, 203, 210 and 222 in pancreatic tumors is associated with poorer survival. Int. J. Cancer. 126:73–80.

[82] Costinean S, Zanesi N, Pekarsky Y, Tili E, Volinia S, Heerema N, Croce CM. (2006). Pre-B cell proliferation and lymphoblastic leukemia/high-grade lymphoma in E(mu)-miR155 transgenic mice. Proc Natl Acad Sci U S A. 103:7024-7029.

[83] Pallante P, Visone R, Ferracin M, Ferraro A, Berlingieri MT, Troncone G, Chiappetta G, Liu CG, Santoro M, Negrini M, Croce CM, Fusco A. (2006). MicroRNA deregulation in human thyroid papillary carcinomas. Endocr. Relat. Cancer. 13:497–508.

[84] Fornari F, Gramantieri L, Ferracin M, Veronese A, Sabbioni S, Calin GA, Grazi GL, Giovannini C, Croce CM, Bolondi L, Negrini M. (2008). MiR-221 control CDKN1C/p57 and CDKN1B/p27 expression in human hepatocellular carcinoma. Oncogene. 27:5651–5661.

[85] Di Leva G, Gasparini P, Piovan C, Ngankeu A, Garofalo M, Taccioli C, Iorio MV, Li M, Volinia S, Alder H, Nakamura T, Nuovo G, Liu Y, Nephew KP, Croce CM. (2010). MicroRNA cluster 221–222 and estrogen receptor αinteractions in breast cancer. J. Natl. Cancer Inst. 102:706–721.

[86] Felicetti F, Errico MC, Bottero L, Segnalini P, Stoppacciaro A, Biffoni M, Felli N, Mattia G, Petrini M, Colombo MP, Peschle C, Carè A. (2008). The promyelocytic leukemia zinc finger–microRNA-221/-222 pathway controls melanoma progression through multiple oncogenic mechanisms. Cancer Res. 68:2745–2754.

[87] le Sage C, Nagel R, Egan DA, Schrier M, Mesman E, Mangiola A, Anile C, Maira G, Mercatelli N, Ciafrè SA, Farace MG, Agami R. (2007). Regulation of the p27Kip1 tumor suppressor by miR-221 and miR-222 promotes cancer cell proliferation. EMBO J. 26:3699–3708.

[88] Garofalo M, Quintavalle C, Di Leva G, Zanca C, Romano G, Taccioli C, Liu CG, Croce CM, Condorelli G. (2008). MicroRNA signatures of TRAIL resistance in human non-small cell lung cancer. Oncogene. 27:3845–3855.

[89] Garofalo M, Di Leva G, Romano G, Nuovo G, Suh SS, Ngankeu A, Taccioli C, Pichiorri F, Alder H, Secchiero P, Gasparini P, Gonelli A, Costinean S, Acunzo M, Condorelli G, Croce CM. (2009). miR-221&222 regulate TRAIL resistance and enhance tumorigenicity through PTEN and TIMP3 downregulation. Cancer Cell. 16:498–509.

[90] Petrocca F, Visone R, Onelli MR, Shah MH, Nicoloso MS, de Martino I, Iliopoulos D, Pilozzi E, Liu CG, Negrini M, Cavazzini L, Volinia S, Alder H, Ruco LP, Baldassarre G, Croce CM, Vecchione A. (2008). E2F1-regulated microRNAs impair TGFβ-dependent cell-cycle arrest and apoptosis in gastric cancer. Cancer Cell. 13:272–286.

[91] Ota A, Tagawa H, Karnan S, Tsuzuki S, Karpas A, Kira S, Yoshida Y, Seto M. (2004). Identification and characterization of a novel gene, C13orf25, as a target for 13q31-q32 amplification in malignant lymphoma. Cancer Res. 64:3087–3095.

[92] Hayashita Y, Osada H, Tatematsu Y, Yamada H, Yanagisawa K, Tomida S, Yatabe Y, Kawahara K, Sekido Y, Takahashi T. (2005). A polycistronic microRNA cluster, miR-17-92, is overexpressed in human lung cancers and enhances cell proliferation. Cancer Res. 65:9628–9632.

[93] Ventura A, Young AG, Winslow MM, Lintault L, Meissner A, Erkeland SJ, Newman J, Bronson RT, Crowley D, Stone JR, Jaenisch R, Sharp PA, Jacks T. (2008). Targeted deletion reveals essential and overlapping functions of the miR-17 through 92 family of miRNA clusters. Cell.132:875-886.

[94] Park JK, Lee EJ, Esau C, Schmittgen TD. (2009). Antisense inhibition of microRNA-21 or -221 arrests cell cycle, induces apoptosis, and sensitizes the effects of gemcitabine in pancreatic adenocarcinoma. Pancreas. 38:e190–199.

[95] Inomata M, Tagawa H, Guo YM, Kameoka Y, Takahashi N, Sawada K. (2009). MicroRNA-17-92 downregulates expression of distinct targets in different B-cell lymphoma subtypes. Blood. 113:396–402.

[96] Wang PY, Li YJ, Zhang S, Li ZL, Yue Z, Xie N, Xie SY. (2010). Regulating A549 cells growth by ASO inhibiting miRNA expression. Mol. Cell. Biochem. 339:163–171.

[97] Bandi N, Zbinden S, Gugger M, Arnold M, Kocher V, Hasan L, Kappeler A, Brunner T, Vassella E. (2009). miR-15a and miR-16 are implicated in cell cycle regulation in a Rb-dependent manner and are frequently deleted or down-regulated in non–small cell lung cancer. Cancer Res. 69:5553–5559.

[98] Cimmino A, Calin GA, Fabbri M, Iorio MV, Ferracin M, Shimizu M, Wojcik SE, Aqeilan RI, Zupo S, Dono M, Rassenti L, Alder H, Volinia S, Liu CG, Kipps TJ, Negrini M, Croce CM. (2005). miR-15 and miR-16 induce apoptosis by targeting BCL2. Proc. Natl. Acad. Sci. USA.102:13944–13949.

[99] Klein U, Lia M, Crespo M, Siegel R, Shen Q, Mo T, Ambesi-Impiombato A, Califano A, Migliazza A, Bhagat G, Dalla-Favera R. (2010). The DLEU2/miR-15a/16-1 cluster controls B cell proliferation and its deletion leads to chronic lymphocytic leukemia. Cancer Cell 17:28–40.

[100] Bonci D, Coppola V, Musumeci M, Addario A, Giuffrida R, Memeo L, D'Urso L, Pagliuca A, Biffoni M, Labbaye C, Bartucci M, Muto G, Peschle C, De Maria R. (2008). The miR-15a–miR-16-1 cluster controls prostate cancer by targeting multiple oncogenic activities. Nat. Med. 14:1271–1277.

[101] He X, He L, Hannon GJ. (2007). The guardian's little helper: microRNAs in the p53 tumor suppressor network. Cancer Res.67:11099-11101.

[102] He L, He X, Lim LP, de Stanchina E, Xuan Z, Liang Y, Xue W, Zender L, Magnus J, Ridzon D, Jackson AL, Linsley PS, Chen C, Lowe SW, Cleary MA, Hannon GJ. (2007). A microRNA component of the p53 tumour suppressor network. Nature. 447:1130-1134.

[103] Cole KA, Attiyeh EF, Mosse YP, Laquaglia MJ, Diskin SJ, Brodeur GM, Maris JM. (2008). A functional screen identifies miR-34a as a candidate neuroblastoma tumor suppressor gene. Mol. Cancer Res. 6:735–742.

[104] Siemens H, Jackstadt R, Hünten S, Kaller M, Menssen A, Götz U, Hermeking H. (2011). miR-34 and SNAIL form a double-negative feedback loop to regulate epithelial-mesenchymal transitions. Cell Cycle.10:4256-4271.

[105] Tsai WC, Hsu PW, Lai TC, Chau GY, Lin CW, Chen CM, Lin CD, Liao YL, Wang JL, Chau YP, Hsu MT, Hsiao M, Huang HD, Tsou AP. (2009). MicroRNA-122, a tumor suppressor microRNA that regulates intrahepatic metastasis of hepatocellular carcinoma. Hepatology. 49:1571-1582.

[106] Xu Y, Xia F, Ma L, Shan J, Shen J, Yang Z, Liu J, Cui Y, Bian X, Bie P, Qian C. (2011). MicroRNA-122 sensitizes HCC cancer cells to adriamycin and vincristine through modulating expression of MDR and inducing cell cycle arrest. Cancer Lett. 310:160-169.

[107] Xu J, Zhu X, Wu L, Yang R, Yang Z, Wang Q, Wu F. (2012). MicroRNA-122 suppresses cell proliferation and induces cell apoptosis in hepatocellular carcinoma by directly targeting Wnt/β-catenin pathway. Liver Int. 32:752-760.

[108] Coulouarn C, Factor VM, Andersen JB, Durkin ME, Thorgeirsson SS. (2009). Loss of miR-122 expression in liver cancer correlates with suppression of the hepatic phenotype and gain of metastatic properties. Oncogene. 28:3526-3536.

[109] Hsu SH, Wang B, Kota J, Yu J, Costinean S, Kutay H, Yu L, Bai S, La Perle K, Chivukula RR, Mao H, Wei M, Clark KR, Mendell JR, Caligiuri MA, Jacob ST, Mendell JT, Ghoshal K. (2012). Essential metabolic, anti-inflammatory, and anti-tumorigenic functions of miR-122 in liver. J Clin Invest.122:2871-2883.

[110] Nguyen DX, Bos PD, Massague J. (2009). Metastasis: From dissemination to organ-specific colonization. Nat. Rev. Cancer.9:274–284.

[111] Hanahan D, Weinberg RA. (2000). The hallmarks of cancer. Cell.100:57–70.

[112] Steeg PS. (2006). Tumor metastasis: Mechanistic insights and clinical challenges. Nat. Med.12:895–904.

[113] Ma L, Reinhardt F, Pan E, Soutschek J, Bhat B, Marcusson EG, Teruya-Feldstein J, Bell GW, Weinberg RA. (2010). Therapeutic silencing of miR-10b inhibits metastasis in a mouse mammary tumor model. Nat. Biotechnol.28:341–347

[114] Tavazoie SF, Alarcon C, Oskarsson T, Padua D, Wang Q, Bos PD, Gerald WL, Massagué J. (2008). Endogenous human microRNAs that suppress breast cancer metastasis. Nature. 451:147–52.

[115] Valastyan S, Reinhardt F, Benaich N, Calogrias D, Szász AM, Wang ZC, Brock JE, Richardson AL, Weinberg RA. (2009). A pleiotropically acting microRNA, miR-31, inhibits breast cancer metastasis. Cell. 137:1032–1046.

[116] Ma L, Young J, Prabhala H, Pan E, Mestdagh P, Muth D, Teruya-Feldstein J, Reinhardt F, Onder TT, Valastyan S, Westermann F, Speleman F, Vandesompele J, Weinberg RA. (2010). MiR-9, a MYC/MYCN-activated microRNA, regulates E-cadherin and cancer metastasis. Nat. Cell Biol.12: 247–256.

[117] Gregory, P.A., et al., The miR-200 family and miR-205 regulate epithelial to mesenchymal transition by targeting ZEB1 and SIP1. Nat Cell Biol, 2008. 10(5): p. 593-601.

[118] Gibbons, D.L., et al., Contextual extracellular cues promote tumor cell EMT and metastasis by regulating miR-200 family expression. Genes Dev, 2009. 23(18): p. 2140-51.

[119] Korpal, M., et al., Direct targeting of Sec23a by miR-200s influences cancer cell secretome and promotes metastatic colonization. Nat Med, 2011. 17(9): p. 1101-8.

[120] Kiss-Laszlo, Z., Henry, Y., Bachellerie, J., Caizergues- Ferrer, M. & Kiss, T. (1996). Site-specific ribose methylation of preribosomal RNA: a novel function for small nucleolar RNAs. Cell. 85:1077–1088.

[121] Tollervey, D. & Kiss, T. (1997). Function and synthesis of small nucleolar RNAs. Curr. Opin. Cell Biol. 9:337–342.

[122] Weinstein L. B., Steitz J. A. (1999). Guided tours: from precursor snoRNA to functional snoRNP. Curr. Opin. Cell Biol. 11: 378–384.

[123] Williams GT, Hughes JP, Stoneman V, Anderson CL, McCarthy NJ, Mourtada-Maarabouni M, Pickard M, Hedge VL, Trayner I, Farzaneh F. (2006). Isolation of genes controlling apoptosis through their effects on cell survival. Gene Ther. Mol. Biol.10B:255–261.

[124] Mourtada-Maarabouni M, Hedge VL, Kirkham L, Farzaneh F, Williams GT. (2008). Growth arrest in human T-cells is controlled by the non-coding RNA growth-arrest-specific transcript 5 (GAS5). J. Cell Sci. 121:939–946.

[125] Mourtada-Maarabouni M, Pickard MR, Hedge VL, Farzaneh F, Williams GT. (2009) GAS5, a non-protein-coding RNA, controls apoptosis and is downregulated in breast cancer. Oncogene. 28:195–208.

[126] Dong XY, Guo P, Boyd J, Sun X, Li Q, Zhou W, Dong JT. (2009). Implication of snoRNA U50 in human breast cancer. J. Genet. Genomics 36:447–454.

[127] Dong XY, Rodriguez C, Guo P, Sun X, Talbot JT, Zhou W, Petros J, Li Q, Vessella RL, Kibel AS, Stevens VL, Calle EE, Dong JT. (2008). SnoRNA U50 is a candidate tumor-suppressor gene at 6q14.3 with a mutation associated with clinically significant prostate cancer. Hum. Mol. Genet. 17:1031–1042.

[128] Gee HE, Buffa FM, Camps C, Ramachandran A, Leek R, Taylor M, Patil M, Sheldon H, Betts G, Homer J, West C, Ragoussis J, Harris AL. (2011). The small-nucleolar RNAs commonly used for microRNA normalisation correlate with tumour pathology and prognosis. Br. J. Cancer. 104:1168–1177.

[129] Liao J, Yu L, Mei Y, Guarnera M, Shen J, Li R, Liu Z, Jiang F. (2010). Small nucleolar RNA signatures as biomarkers for non-small-cell lung cancer. Mol. Cancer. 9:198.

[130] Martens-Uzunova ES, Jalava SE, Dits NF, van Leenders GJ, Møller S, Trapman J, Bangma CH, Litman T, Visakorpi T, Jenster G. (2011). Diagnostic and prognostic signatures from the small non-coding RNA transcriptome in prostate cancer. Oncogene. 31:978-991.

[131] Brown JW, Marshall DF, Echeverria M. (2008). Intronic noncoding RNAs and splicing. Trends Plant Sci.13:335–342.

[132] Chanfreau G, Legrain P, Jacquier A. (1998). Yeast RNase III as a key processing enzyme in small nucleolar RNAs metabolism. J. Mol. Biol. 284:975–988.

[133] Pettalski E, Dandekar T, Henry Y, Tollervey D. (1998). Processing of the precursors to small nucleolar RNAs and rRNAs requires common components. Mol. Cell. Biol.18:1181–1189.

[134] Qu LH, Henras A, Lu YL, Zhou H, Zhou WX, Zhu YQ, Zhao J, Henry Y, Caizergues-Ferrer M, Bachellerie JP. (1999). Seven novel methylation guide small nucleolar RNAs are processed from a common polycistronic transcript by Rat1p and RNase III in yeast Mol. Cell. Biol.19:1144–1158.

[135] Nicholls RD, Knepper JL. (2001). Genome organization, function, and imprinting in Prader—Willi and Angelman syndromes Annu. Rev. Genomics Hum. Genet. 2:153–175.

[136] Skryabin BV, Gubar LV, Seeger B, Pfeiffer J, Handel S, Robeck T, Karpova E, Rozhdestvensky TS, Brosius J. (2007). Deletion of the MBII-85 snoRNA gene cluster in mice results in postnatal growth retardation. PLoS Genet. 3:e235.

[137] Gurevich I, Englander MT, Adlerberg M, Siegal NB, Schmauss C. (2002). Modulation of serotonin 2C receptor editing by sustained changes in serotonergic neurotransmission J. Neurosci.22:10529–1053.

[138] Burns CM, Chu H, Rueter SM, Hutchinson LK, Canton H, Sanders-Bush E, Emeson RB. (1997). Regulation of serotonin-2C receptor G-protein coupling by RNA editing Nature. 387:303–308.

[139] Tanaka R, Satoh H, Moriyama M, Satoh K, Morishita Y, Yoshida S, Watanabe T, Nakamura Y, Mori S. (2000). Intronic U50 small-nucleolar-RNA (snoRNA) host gene of no protein-coding potential is mapped at the chromosome breakpoint t(3;6) (q27;q15) of human B-cell lymphoma. Genes Cells. 5:277–287.

[140] Dong XY, Rodriguez C, Guo P, Sun X, Talbot JT, Zhou W, Petros W, Li Q, Vessella RL, Kibel AS, Stevens VL, Calle EE, Dong DJ. (2008). SnoRNA U50 is a candidate tumor-suppressor gene at 6q14.3 with a mutation associated with clinically significant prostate cancer Hum. Mol. Genet.17:1031-1042.

[141] Mei YP, Liao JP, Shen JP, Yu L, Liu BL, Liu L, Li RY, Ji L, Dorsey SG, Jiang ZR, Katz RL, Wang JY, Jiang F. (2011). Small nucleolar RNA 42 acts as an oncogene in lung tumorigenesis. Oncogene.(doi:10.1038/onc.2011.449).

[142] Chang LS, Lin S Y, Lieu AS, Wu TL. (2002). Differential expression of human 5S snoRNA genes. Biochem. Biophys. Res. Commun. 299:196–200.

[143] Liao J, Yu L, Mei Y, Guarnera M, Shen J. (2010). Small nucleolar RNA signatures as biomarkers for non-small-cell lung cancer. Mol. Cancer. 9:198.

[144] Li R, Wang H, Bekele BN, Yin Z, Caraway NP, Katz RL, Stass SA, Jiang F.(2006). Identification of putative oncogenes in lung adenocarcinoma by a comprehensive functional genomic approach. Oncogene.18:2628–2635.

[145] Schneider C, King RM, Philipson L. Genes specifically expressed at growth arrest of mammalian cells. Cell. 1988;54:787–793.

[146] Amaldi F, Pierandrei-Amaldi P. (1997). TOP genes: a translationaly controlled class of genes including those coding for ribosomal proteins. In: Jeanteur P, editor. Progress in molecular and subcellular biology. Vol. 18. Springer-Verlag; Berlin, Germany: pp. 1–17.

[147] Mourtada-Maarabouni M, Pickard MR, Hedge VL, Farzaneh F, Williams GT. (2009). GAS5, a non-protein-coding RNA, controls apoptosis and is downregulated in breast cancerGAS5 regulates apoptosis. Oncogene. 28:195-208.

[148] Gee HE, Buffa FM, Camps C, Ramachandran A, Leek R, Taylor M, Patil M, Sheldon H, Betts G, Homer J, West C, Ragoussis J, Harris AL. (2011). The small-nucleolar RNAs commonly used for microRNA normalisation correlate with tumour pathology and prognosis. Br. J. Cancer. 104, 1168–1177.

[149] Nakamura Y, Takahashi N, Kakegawa E, Yoshida K, Ito Y, Kayano H, Niitsu N, Jinnai I, Bessho M. (2008). The GAS5 (growth arrest-specific transcript 5) gene fuses to BCL6 as

a result of t(1;3)(q25;q27) in a patient with B-cell lymphoma. Cancer Genetics and Cytogenetics.182:144-149.

[150] Askarian-Amiri ME, Crawford J, French JD, Smart CE, Smith MA, Clark MB, Ru K, Mercer TR, Thompson ER, Lakhani SR, Vargas AC, Campbell IG, Brown MA, Dinger ME, Mattick JS. (2011). SNORD-host RNA Zfas1 is a regulator of mammary development and a potential marker for breast cancer RNA. 17:878-891.

[151] Gupta V, Kumar A. (2010). Dyskeratosis congenita. Adv Exp Med Biol.685:215-219.

[152] Ruggero D, Grisendi S, Piazza F, Rego E, Mari F, Rao PH, Cordon-Cardo C, Pandolfi PP. (2003). Dyskeratosis congenita and cancer in mice deficient in ribosomal RNA modification. Science. 299:259-62.

[153] Ono M, Scott MS, Yamada K, Avolio F, Barton GJ, Lamond AI. (2011). Identification of human miRNA precursors that resemble box C/D snoRNAs. Nucleic Acids Res.39:3879-3891.

[154] Xiao J, Lin H, Luo X, Luo X, Wang Z. (2011). miR-605 joins p53 network to form a p53:miR-605:Mdm2 positive feedback loop in response to stress. EMBO J.30:5021.

[155] Siomi MC, Sato K, Pezic D, Aravin AA. (2011). PIWI-interacting small RNAs: the vanguard of genome defence. Nat Rev Mol Cell Biol.12:246-258.

[156] Ishizu H, Nagao A, Siomi H. (2011). Gatekeepers for Piwi-piRNA complexes to enter the nucleus. Curr Opin Genet Dev. 21:484-490.

[157] Kazazian HH Jr. (2004). Mobile elements: drivers of genome evolution. Science 303:1626–1632.

[158] Saito K, Siomi MC. (2010). Small RNA-mediated quiescence of transposable elements in animals. Dev. Cell. 19:687–697.

[159] Vagin VV, Klenov MS, Kalmykova AI, Stolyarenko AD, Kotelnikov RN, Gvozdev VA. (2004). The RNA interference proteins and vasa locus are involved in the silencing of retrotransposons in the female germline of Drosophila melanogaster. RNA Biol. 1:54–58.17.

[160] Kalmykova AI, Klenov MS, Gvozdev VA. (2005). Argonaute protein PIWI controls mobilization of retrotransposons in the Drosophila male germline. Nucleic Acids Res. 33:2052–2059.

[161] Savitsky M, Kwon D, Georgiev P, Kalmykova A, Gvozdev V. (2006). Telomere elongation is under the control of the RNAi-based mechanism in the Drosophila germline. Genes Dev. 20:345–354.

[162] Li C, Vagin VV, Lee S, Xu J, Ma S, Xi H, Seitz H, Horwich MD, Syrzycka M, Honda BM, Kittler EL, Zapp ML, Klattenhoff C, Schulz N, Theurkauf WE, Weng Z, Zamore PD. (2009). Collapse of germline piRNAs in the absence of Argonaute3 reveals somatic piRNAs in flies. Cell. 137:509–521.

[163] Aravin A, Gaidatzis D, Pfeffer S, Lagos-Quintana M, Landgraf P, Iovino N, Morris P, Brownstein MJ, Kuramochi-Miyagawa S, Nakano T, Chien M, Russo JJ, Ju J, Sheridan R, Sander C, Zavolan M, Tuschl T. (2006). A novel class of small RNAs bind to MILI protein in mouse testes. Nature. 442:203–207.

[164] Girard A, Sachidanandam R, Hannon GJ, Carmell MA. (2006) A germline-specific class of small RNAs binds mammalian Piwi proteins. Nature. 442:199–202.

[165] Brennecke J, Aravin AA, Stark A, Dus M, Kellis M, Sachidanandam R, Hannon GJ. (2007). Discrete small RNA-generating loci as master regulators of transposon activity in Drosophila. Cell. 128:1089–1103.

[166] Lau NC, Seto AG, Kim J, Kuramochi-Miyagawa S, Nakano T, Bartel DP, Kingston RE. (2006). Characterization of the piRNA complex from rat testes. Science 313, 363–367

[167] Houwing S, Berezikov E, Ketting RF. (2008). Zili is required for germ cell differentiation and meiosis in zebrafish. EMBO J. 27:2702–2711.

[168] Robine N, Lau NC, Balla S, Jin Z, Okamura K, Kuramochi-Miyagawa S, Blower MD, Lai EC. (2009) A broadly conserved pathway generates 3'UTR-directed primary piRNAs. Curr. Biol. 19:2066–2076.

[169] Aravin AA, Sachidanandam R, Bourc'his D, Schaefer C, Pezic D, Toth KF, Bestor T, Hannon GJ. (2008). A piRNA pathway primed by individual transposons is linked to de novo DNA methylation in mice. Mol. Cell. 31:785–799.

[170] Qiao D, Zeeman AM, Deng W, Looijenga LH, Lin H. (2002). Molecular characterization of hiwi, a human member of the piwi gene family whose overexpression is correlated to seminomas. Oncogene.21:3988-3999.

[171] Taubert H, Würl P, Greither T, Kappler M, Bache M, Bartel F, Kehlen A, Lautenschläger C, Harris LC, Kaushal D, Füssel S, Meye A, Böhnke A, Schmidt H, Holzhausen HJ, Hauptmann S. (2007). Stem cell-associated genes are extremely poor prognostic factors for soft-tissue sarcoma patients. Oncogene. 26:7170-7174.

[172] Taubert H, Greither T, Kaushal D, Würl P, Bache M, Bartel F, Kehlen A, Lautenschläger C, Harris L, Kraemer K, Meye A, Kappler M, Schmidt H, Holzhausen HJ, Hauptmann S. (2007) Expression of the stem cell self-renewal gene Hiwi and risk of tumour-related death in patients with soft-tissue sarcoma. Oncogene.26:1098-1100.

[173] Wang QE, Han C, Milum K, Wani AA. (2011). Stem cell protein Piwil2 modulates chromatin modifications upon cisplatin treatment. Mutat Res.708:59-68.

[174] Lu Y, Li C, Zhang K, Sun H, Tao D, Liu Y, Zhang S, Ma Y. (2010). Identification of piRNAs in Hela cells by massive parallel sequencing. BMB Rep.43:635-41.

[175] Cui L, Lou Y, Zhang X, Zhou H, Deng H, Song H, Yu X, Xiao B, Wang W, Guo J. (2011). Detection of circulating tumor cells in peripheral blood from patients with gastric cancer using piRNAs as markers. Clin Biochem. 44:1050-1057.

[176] Cheng J, Guo JM, Xiao BX, Miao Y, Jiang Z, Zhou H, Li QN. (2011). piRNA, the new non-coding RNA, is aberrantly expressed in human cancer cells. Clin Chim Acta. 412:1621-1625.

[177] Cheng J, Deng H, Xiao B, Zhou H, Zhou F, Shen Z, Guo J. (2012). piR-823, a novel non-coding small RNA, demonstrates in vitro and in vivo tumor suppressive activity in human gastric cancer cells. Cancer Lett. 315:12-17

[178] Reuter M, Chuma S, Tanaka T, Franz T, Stark A, Pillai RS. (2009). Loss of the Mili-interacting Tudor domain-containing protein-1 activates transposons and alters the Mili-associated small RNA profile. Nature Struct. Mol. Biol. 16:639–646.

[179] Shoji M, Tanaka T, Hosokawa M, Reuter M, Stark A, Kato Y, Kondoh G, Okawa K, Chujo T, Suzuki T, Hata K, Martin SL, Noce T, Kuramochi-Miyagawa S, Nakano T, Sasaki H, Pillai RS, Nakatsuji N, Chuma S. (2009) The TDRD9-MIWI2 complex is

essential for piRNA-mediated retrotransposon silencing in the mouse male germline. Dev. Cell 17:775–787.

[180] Struhl, K. (2007). Transcriptional noise and the fidelity of initiation by RNA polymerase II. Nature Struct. Mol. Biol. 14:103–105.

[181] Amaral PP, Mattick JS. (2008). Noncoding RNA in development. Mamm. Genome. 19:454–492.

[182] Dinger ME, Amaral PP, Mercer TR, Pang KC, Bruce SJ, Gardiner BB, Askarian-Amiri ME, Ru K, Soldà G, Simons C, Sunkin SM, Crowe ML, Grimmond SM, Perkins AC, Mattick JS. (2008). Long noncoding RNAs in mouse embryonic stem cell pluripotency and differentiation. Genome Res. 18:1433–1445.

[183] Mercer TR, Dinger ME, Sunkin SM, Mehler MF, Mattick JS. (2008). Specific expression of long noncoding RNAs in the adult mouse brain. Proc. Natl Acad. Sci. USA. 105:716–721.

[184] Cawley S, Bekiranov S, Ng HH, Kapranov P, Sekinger EA, Kampa D, Piccolboni A, Sementchenko V, Cheng J, Williams AJ, Wheeler R, Wong B, Drenkow J, Yamanaka M, Patel S, Brubaker S, Tammana H, Helt G, Struhl K, Gingeras TR. (2004). Unbiased mapping of transcription factor binding sites along human chromosomes 21 and 22 points to widespread regulation of noncoding RNAs. Cell.116:499–509.

[185] Ponjavic J, Ponting CP, Lunter G. (2007). Functionality or transcriptional noise? Evidence for selection within long noncoding RNAs. Genome Res. 17:556–565.

[186] Faulkner GJ, Kimura Y, Daub CO, Wani S, Plessy C, Irvine KM, Schroder K, Cloonan N, Steptoe AL, Lassmann T, Waki K, Hornig N, Arakawa T, Takahashi H, Kawai J, Forrest AR, Suzuki H, Hayashizaki Y, Hume DA, Orlando V, Grimmond SM, Carninci P. (2009). The regulated retrotransposon transcriptome of mammalian cells. Nat Genet. 41:563–71.

[187] Guttman M, Amit I, Garber M, French C, Lin MF, Feldser D, Huarte M, Zuk O, Carey BW, Cassady JP, Cabili MN, Jaenisch R, Mikkelsen TS, Jacks T, Hacohen N, Bernstein BE, Kellis M, Regev A, Rinn JL, Lander ES. (2009). Chromatin signature reveals over a thousand highly conserved large non-coding RNAs in mammals. Nature.458:223–227.

[188] Pang KC, Frith MC, Mattick JS. (2006). Rapid evolution of noncoding RNAs: lack of conservation does not mean lack of function. Trends Genet. 22.1–5.

[189] Cheng LL, Carmichael GG. (2010). Decoding the function of nuclear long non-coding RNAs. Curr Opinion in Cell Biology. 22:357-364.

[190] Kugel JF, Goodrich JA. (2012). Non-coding RNAs: key regulators of mammalian transcription. Trends in Biochemical Sciences. 37:144-151.

[191] Khalil AM, Guttman M, Huarte M. Garber M Ray A. Rivea Morales D. Thomas K, Presser A. (2009). Many human large intergenic noncoding RNAs associated with chromatin-modifying complexes and affect gene expression. Proc Natl Acad Sci USA. 106:11667-11672.

[192] Zhao J, Sun BK, Erwin JA, Song JJ, Lee JT. (2008). Polycomb proteins targeted by a short repeat RNA to the mouse X chromosome. Science 322:750-756.

[193] Rinn JL, Kertesz M, Wang JK, Squazzo SL, Xu X, Brugmann SA, Goodnough LH, Helms JA, Farnham PJ, Segal E, Chang HY.(2007) Functional demarcation of active and silent chromatin domains in human HOX loci by noncoding RNAs. Cell 129, 1311–1323.

[194] Tsai MC, Manor O, Wan Y, Mosammaparast N, Wang JK, Lan F, Shi Y, Segal E, Chang HY. (2010). Long noncoding RNA as modular scaffold of histone modification complexes. Sciences. 329:689-693.

[195] Morris KV, Santoso S, Turner AM, Pastori C, Hawkins PG. (2008). Bidirectional transcription directs both transcriptional gene activation and suppression in human cells. PLoS Genet. 4:e1000258.

[196] Nagano T, Mitchell JA, Sanz LA, Pauler FM, Ferguson-Smith AC, Feil R, Fraser P. (2008).The Air noncoding RNA epigenetically silences transcription by targeting G9a to chromatin. Science. 322:1717–1720.

[197] Gupta RA, Shah N, Wang KC, Kim J, Horlings HM, Wong DJ, Tsai MC, Hung T, Argani P, Rinn JL, Wang Y, Brzoska P, Kong B, Li R, West RB, van de Vijver MJ, Sukumar S, Chang HY. (2010). Long non-coding RNA HOTAIR reprograms chromatin state to promote cancer metastasis. Nature. 464:1071-1076.

[198] Kogo R, Shimamura T, Mimori K, Kawahara K, Imoto S, Sudo T, Tanaka F, Shibata K, Suzuki A, Komune S, Miyano S, Mori M. (2011). Long non-coding RNA HOTAIR regulates Polycomb-dependent chromatin modification and is associated with poor prognosis in colorectal cancers. Cancer Res.71: 6320-6326.

[199] Yap KL, Li S, Muñoz-Cabello AM, Raguz S, Zeng L, Mujtaba S, Gil J, Walsh MJ, Zhou MM. (2010). Molecular interplay of the non coding RNA ANRIL and methylated histone H3 lysine 27 by polycomb CBX7 in transcriptional silencing of INK4a. Mol Cell. 38:662-674.

[200] Beltran M, Puig I, Peña C, García JM, Alvarez AB, Peña R, Bonilla F, de Herreros AG. (2008). A natural antisense transcript regulates Zeb2/Sip1 gene expression during Snail1-induced epithelial–mesenchymal transition. Genes Dev. 22:756–769.

[201] Wang X, Arai S, Song X, Reichart D, Du K, Pascual G, Tempst P, Rosenfeld MG, Glass CK, Kurokawa R. (2008). Induced ncRNAs allosterically modify RNA-binding proteins in cis to inhibit transcription. Nature. 454:126–130.

[202] Feng J, Bi C, Clark BS, Mady R, Shah P, Kohtz JD. (2006). The Evf-2 noncoding RNA is transcribed from the Dlx-5/6 ultraconserved region and functions as a Dlx-2 transcriptional coactivator. Genes Dev. 20:1470–1484.

[203] Huarte M, Guttman M, Feldser D, Garber M, Koziol MJ, Kenzelmann-Broz D, Khalil AM, Zuk O, Amit I, Rabani M, Attardi LD, Regev A, Lander ES, Jacks T, Rinn JL. (2010). A large intergenic noncoding RNA induced by p53 mediates global gene repression in the p53 response. Cell. 142:409-419.

[204] Bond CS, Fox AH. (2009). Paraspeckles: nuclear bodies built on long noncoding RNA. J Cell Biol. 186:637-644.

Chapter 15

MiRNA and Proline Metabolism in Cancer

Wei Liu and James M. Phang

Additional information is available at the end of the chapter

http://dx.doi.org/10.5772/55139

1. Introduction

Tumor metabolism and bioenergetics are important areas for cancer research and present promising targets for anticancer therapy. Growing tumors alter their metabolic profiles to meet the bioenergetic and biosynthetic demands of increased cell growth and proliferation. These alterations include the well-known aerobic glycolysis, the Warburg effect, which has been considered as the central tenet of cancer cell metabolism for more than 80 years [1]. Interest in cancer cell metabolism has been refueled by recent advances in the study of signaling pathways involving known oncogene and tumor suppressor genes, which reveal their close interaction with metabolic pathways [2-4]. For example, recent studies document an important role of glutamine catabolism in tumor stimulated by the oncogenic transcriptional factor c-MYC (herein termed MYC) which has been previously shown to stimulate glycolysis [5, 6]. Although glucose and glutamine serve as the main metabolic substrate for tumor cells, proline as a microenvironmental stress substrate has attracted lots of attention due to its unique metabolic system, its availability in tumor microenvironments and its responses to various stresses.

1.1. Special features of proline metabolism

Proline is the only proteinogenic secondary amino acid, and it has special functions in biology [7-11]. Proline metabolism is distinct from that of primary amino acids. The inclusion of an alpha-nitrogen within its pyrrolidine ring precludes its being the substrate for the usual amino acid-metabolizing enzymes, such as, the decarboxylases, aminotransferases, and racemases. Instead, proline metabolism has its own family of enzymes with their tissue and subcellular localization and their own regulatory mechanisms. As shown in the schematic of proline metabolic pathway (Figure 1), these enzymes include proline dehydrogenase/oxidase (PRODH/POX) and pyrroline-5-carboxylate reductase (PYCR) catalyzing the interconversion of proline and Δ^1-pyrroline-5-carboxylate (P5C), P5C dehydrogenase (P5CDH) and P5C synthase (P5CS) mediating the interconversion of P5C and glutamate, and ornithine aminotransferase (OAT) catalyzing the interconversion of P5C and ornithine. Glutamate can be converted to α-ketoglutarate (α-KG) entering the tricarboxylic acid (TCA) cycle, which is also the main pathway of glutamine catabolism. Ornithine can be converted to arginine entering the urea cycle. Thus proline metabolism is closely related with glutamine metabolism, TCA cycle, and urea cycle, the main metabolic pathways in human body.

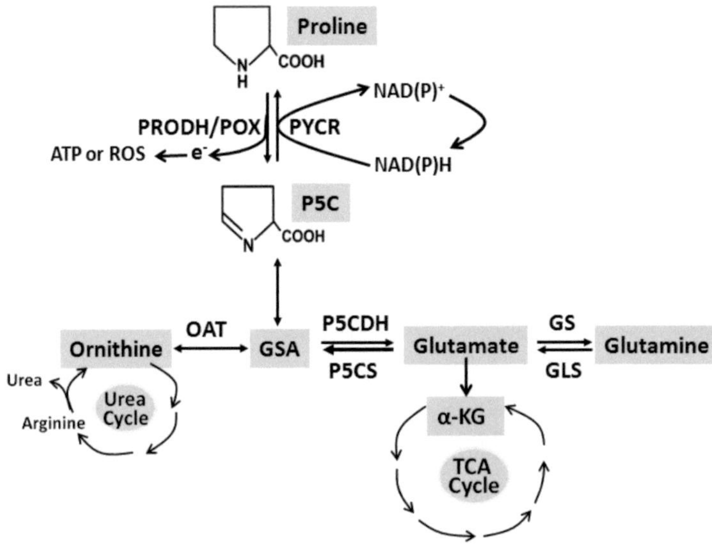

Figure 1. Proline metabolic pathway. Proline metabolism is closely related with glutamine metabolism, TCA cycle, urea cycle and pentose phosphate pathway (PPP). Abbreviations: P5C, Δ1 -pyrroline-5-carboxylate; GSA, glutamic-gamma-semialdehyde; PRODH/POX, proline dehydrogenase/oxidase; PYCR, P5C reductase; P5CDH, P5C dehydrogenase; GS, glutamine synthase; GLS, glutaminase; P5CS, P5C Synthase; OAT, ornithine aminotransferase. The interconversion between P5C and GSA is spontaneous.

Importantly, the interconversion between proline and P5C, catalyzed by PRODH/POX and PYCR, respectively, forms the "proline cycle" in the cytosol and mitochondria as shown in Figure 2, which acts as a redox shuttle transferring reducing and oxidizing potential. In the mitochondria, during the degradation of proline to P5C, PRODH/POX, the flavin adenine dinucleotide-containing enzyme tightly bound to mitochondrial inner membranes, donates electrons through its intervening flavine adenine dinucleotide into the electron transport chain (ETC) to generate ATP or ROS [7, 12, 13]. This characteristic of PRODH/POX serves as the basis of its function in human cancers, which will be discussed in detail in the following sections. P5C produced from the oxidation of proline, emerges from mitochondria and is converted back to proline in the cytosol using NADPH or NADH as cofactor, which interlock with the pentose phosphate pathway (Figure 1) or other metabolic pathways.

Proline metabolism has been shown to play an important role in various human physiologic and pathologic situations. For example, in the early 1970s, P5C, the immediate product of proline catabolism was found to be also the immediate biosynthetic precursor [7]. And in the 1980s, the conversion of P5C to proline was recognized to regulate redox homeostasis as mentioned above [8, 14, 15]. A variety of evidence has shown the inborn errors of the proline metabolic pathway in several human genetic diseases and their potential roles [11, 16], such as familial hyperprolinemias [11, 17], mutations of PRODH/POX in neuropsychiatric diseases [18, 19], mutations of PYCR1 in cutis laxa [20], mutations of P5CS in hyperammonemia [21, 22], and so on. During the last decade, our understanding of the roles of proline metabolism as represented by the regulation and functions of PRODH/POX in tumorigenesis and tumor progression has made significant advances, which will be main focus in this chapter.

1.2. Proline availability in tumor microenvironment

Proline is one of the most abundant amino acids in the cellular microenvironment. Together with hydroxyproline, proline constitutes more than 25% of residues in collagen, the predominant protein (80%) in the extracellular matrix (ECM) of the human body. Although proline can be obtained from the dietary proteins, an important source of proline is from the degradation of collagen in the ECM by sequential enzymatic catalysis of matrix metalloproteinases (MMPs) and prolidase [9, 23]. The upregulation of MMPs in tumors has been considered a critical step for tumor progression and invasion [24-26]. A number of reports have shown that proline concentration is increased in various tumors, which may result from the upregulated MMPs degrading collagen. Previous work from our lab showed that glucose depletion activated MMP-2 and MMP-9 in cancer cells, which accompanied an increase in intracellular proline levels [27].

Autophagy-induced degradation of the intracellular protein, which has been shown to regulate cancer development and progression as a survival strategy of cancer cells [28, 29], may also provide an important source of free proline. Furthermore, proline can be biosynthesized from either glutamate or ornithine as shown in Figure 1 and Figure 2. Our latest finding showed that a large part of products from glutamine catabolism stimulated by MYC is proline [30], suggesting proline biosynthesis might serve as an additional source of proline availability in cancer. Taken together, the ample sources of proline in tumor microenvironment ensure its availability as an important stress substrate for metabolism in human cancers.

2. PRODH/POX as a mitochondrial tumor suppressor

2.1. PRODH/POX induces apoptosis through ROS generation

PRODH, the gene encoding PRODH/POX was discovered to be a p53-induced gene in a screening study in 1997 [31]. Importantly, the p53-initiated apoptosis was later found to depend on the induction of PRODH/POX [32]. To further study the function of PRODH/POX, we developed a DLD1-POX colorectal cancer cell line (designated as DLD1-POX tet-off cell line), which was stably transfected with the *PRODH* gene under the control of a tetracycline-controllable promoter [33]. When doxycycline (DOX) was removed from the culture medium and the expression of PRODH/POX was induced, apoptotic cell death was initiated.

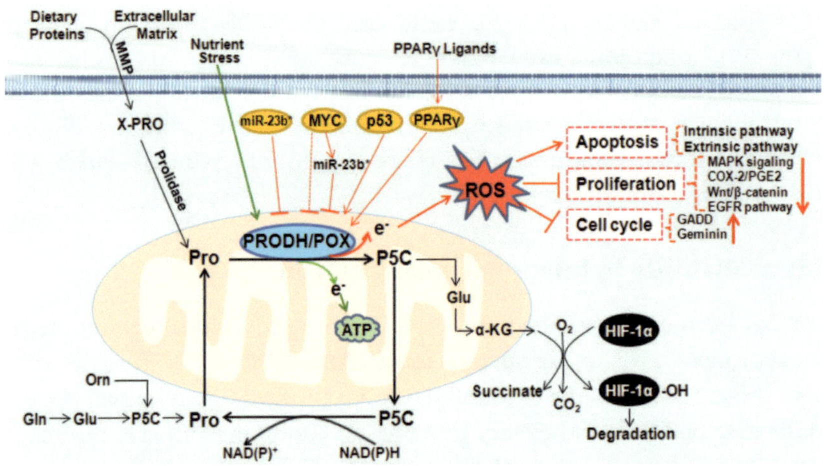

Figure 2. Proline metabolism in cancer. 1. Proline cycle: Interconversion of proline and P5C forms the proline cycle in the cytosol and mitochondria. Proline cycle acts as a redox shuttle transferring reducing potential generated by the pentose phosphate pathway or other metabolic pathway into mitochondria for the production of either ROS or ATP responding to different stresses. 2. Proline availability in human tumor microenvironment: dietary proteins, glutamate and ornithine catabolism, and degradation of extracellular matrix by matrix metalloproteinases (MMPs) are all important sources of proline, especially the last one. 3. The central enzyme of proline metabolism, PRODH/POX, localized in the mitochondrial inner membrane, function as a mitochondrial tumor suppressor. PRODH/POX is induced by p53, PPARγ and its ligands, and suppressed by miR-23b* and oncogenic protein MYC. PRODH/POX overexpression could initiate apoptosis, inhibit proliferation and induce G2 cell cycle arrest through ROS generation, and suppress HIF-1 signaling through increasing α-KG production. Abbreviations: X-PRO, x-prolyl dipeptide; Pro, proline; Orn, ornithine; Gln, glutamine; Glu, glutamate.

ROS, which include superoxide radical ($O_2^{-}\cdot$), hydroxyl radicals (OH·) and the non-radical hydrogen peroxide (H_2O_2), play an important role in the induction of apoptosis [34]. PRODH/POX could donate electron to the ETC to generate ROS. In cells overexpressing PRODH/POX, the addition of proline increased ROS generation in a concentration-dependent manner, and the proline-dependent ROS increased with PRODH/POX expression [35]. N-acetyl cysteine (NAC), a widely used antioxidant agent, dramatically reduced PRODH/POX-induced apoptosis, indicating PRODH/POX induces apoptosis through ROS generation [13]. By introducing the recombinant adenoviruses containing different antioxidant enzymes, such as manganese superoxide dismutase (MnSOD), Cu/Zn superoxide dismutase (CuZnSOD) or catalase (CAT) into the DLD1-POX tet-off cells, we found that only the expression of MnSOD, which localizes in the mitochondria, inhibited PRODH/POX-induced apoptosis, suggesting that it is superoxide as the form of ROS initially mediating PRODH/POX-induced apoptosis [13].

Further investigation on the molecular signaling involved in PRODH/POX-induced apoptosis showed that PRODH/POX activated both intrinsic and extrinsic apoptotic pathways [35, 36]. The DLD-1-POX cells overproducing PRODH/POX exhibited the mitochondria (intrinsic pathway) and death receptor (extrinsic pathway)-mediated apoptotic responses in a proline-dependent manner [35]. Intrinsic pathway induced by PRODH/POX includes the release of cytochrome c, activation of caspase-9, chromatin condensation, DNA fragmentation, and cell shrinkage. Extrinsic pathway induced by PRODH/POX involves the stimulation of the expression of tumor necrosis factor-related apoptosis inducing ligand (TRAIL), and death receptor 5 (DR5) and then cleavage of caspase-8 [36]. Both pathways culminate in the activation of caspase-3 and cleavage of substrates. NFATc1, a member of the nuclear factor of activated T cells (NFAT) family of transcription factors is partially responsible for the TRAIL activity stimulated by PRODH/POX [36]. All of these effects mediated by PRODH/POX could be partially reversed by MnSOD, further confirming the role of ROS/superoxides in PRODH/POX-induced apoptosis [36].

Parallel studies showed that peroxisome proliferator activated receptor gamma (PPARγ) is another critical regulator of PRODH/POX, besides p53. PPARγ belongs to the nuclear hormone receptor superfamily and functions as a ligand-dependent transcription factor [37]. It is widely expressed in many malignant tissues, and its ligands can induce terminal differentiation, apoptosis, and cell growth inhibition in a variety of cancer cells [38-40]. Using a *PRODH*-promoter luciferase construct [41], we found that PPARγ was the most potent effector activating the *PRODH* promoter. PRODH/POX contributes greatly to apoptosis induced by the pharmacologic ligands of PPARγ through ROS signaling in human colorectal cancer cells and non-small cell lung carcinoma cells [41, 42].

More recently, we found that PRODH/POX was upregulated to contribute to ATP production under nutrient stress, such as glucose deprivation [27]. Under hypoxic conditions [43] or high levels of oxidized low-density lipoproteins (oxLDLs) [44], ROS produced by PRODH/POX contributes to autophagy as a survival signal. These effects seem paradoxical with PRODH/POX-induced apoptosis, but they can be well understood considering the temporal and spatial development of the evolving tumor, like the "two faces" of tumor suppressor p53 [45]. A detailed description of this point can be found in our recent review [9].

2.2. PRODH/POX inhibits tumor cell growth through ROS generation

In addition to initiating apoptosis, PRODH/POX also inhibits tumor cell growth and proliferation. In DLD1-POX tet-off cells, soft agar colony formation assays showed that the cells readily formed clones when PRODH/POX expression was inhibited by DOX, whereas the cloning ability of the cells was totally blocked when POX was overexpressed [46].

Several signaling pathways associated with tumor growth are downregulated by PRODH/POX. First, PRODH/POX suppresses the phosphorylation of three major subtypes of the mitogen-activated protein kinase (MAPK) pathways, including MEK/ERK, JNK, p38 [36]. In fact, MAPK pathways play an important role in a variety of cellular responses, including proliferation, differentiation, development, transformation, and apoptosis. The inhibition of MEK/ERK pathway is involved in PRODH/POX-induced apoptosis. Secondly,

PRODH/POX markedly reduces the expression of cyclooxygenase-2 (COX-2), and thus suppresses the production of prostaglandin E_2 (PGE_2) [47]. The addition of PGE_2 partially reverses the apoptosis and inhibits tumor growth induced by PRODH/POX. Cyclooxygenase is an enzyme that catalyzes the key step of the conversion of free arachidonic acid to prostaglandins. It has been widely accepted that elevated COX2/PGE_2 signaling plays a critical role in the initiation and development of various solid tumors, especially colorectal cancer [48-50]. Thirdly, PRODH/POX inhibits the phosphorylation of epidermal growth factor receptor (EGFR). Activating mutants and overexpression of EGFR signaling contributes to carcinogenesis of various tumors by inducing cell proliferation and counteracting apoptosis [51]. Fourthly, Wnt/β-catenin signaling is decreased by PRODH/POX [47]. Constitutive activation of this signaling pathway is found in many human cancers, which regulates proliferation, differentiation and cell fate [52]. Phosphorylation of β-catenin by GSK-3β leads to its ubiquitination and proteasomal degradation. PRODH/POX decreases phosphorylation of GSK-3β and thereby increases phosphorylation of β-catenin, resulting in the reduced activity of Wnt/ β-catenin signaling. All of aforementioned changes induced by PRODH/POX are partially reversed by MnSOD, further indicating the critical role of ROS/superoxides in PRODH/POX-mediated effects.

Furthermore, PRODH/POX induces G2 cell cycle arrest through affecting the regulators of cell cycle, such as geminin, cyclin-dependent kinase (CDC), and growth arrest and DNA damage inducible proteins (GADDs) [46]. Geminin is a nuclear protein that inhibits DNA replication, and has been used as a marker for G2 phase [53]. Its expression is up-regulated by PRODH/POX. CDC2 normally drives cells into mitosis and is the ultimate target of pathways that mediate rapid G2 arrest in response to DNA damage [54]. Although total CDC2 did not change with PRODH/POX expression, the phosphorylated CDC2 at tyrosine 15 increased, whereas phosphorylation at threonine 161 decreased when PRODH/POX was overexpressed, indicating that CDC2 is in an inactive status. CDC25C, the phosphatase that removes the inhibitory phosphates from CDC2 and activates cyclinB-CDC2, is downregulated by PRODH/POX. Additionally, the most important regulators of G2 cell cycle arrest, GADDs [55] also play a role in PRODH/POX-induced G2 cell cycle arrest, including GADD34, GADD45a, GADDh, GADDg [46].

2.3. PRODH/POX inhibits HIF signaling mainly through increasing α-KG production

The above described PRODH/POX-mediated induction of apoptosis together with the suppression of cell growth suggests that PRODH/POX could function as a tumor suppressor. PRODH/POX protein is located in the mitochondrial inner membrane, and has an anaplerotic role through glutamate and α-KG for the TCA cycle (Fig.1). The identification of several mitochondrial tumor suppressors has demonstrated that one of the critical ways they exert their antitumor effects is through hypoxia inducible factor-1 (HIF-1) signaling, which mediates the transcriptional response to hypoxia as a transcriptional factor and plays an important role in angiogenesis and tumor growth [56, 57]. Similarly, PRODH/POX also downregulates HIF-1 signaling including its downstream gene VEGF in both normoxic and hypoxic conditions [46]. This is another mechanism, along with those described above, by which PRODH/POX exerts its tumor-suppressing role. However, unlike the effects of PRODH/POX on other signaling pathways, its effect on HIF-1 signaling could not be reversed by MnSOD, suggesting ROS is not the mediator for HIF inhibition.

The stability and transcriptional activity of HIF-1α are regulated through oxygen-sensitive modifications. Briefly, the posttranslational hydroxylation of specific prolyl and asparaginal residues in its α-subunits of HIF-1, catalyzed by prolyl hydroxylases (PHD), results in the degradation of HIF-1 through ubiquitinal and proteasomal degradation systems [58]. As an important substrate of PHD, the members of the 2-oxoglutarate (α-KG) dioxygenase family could increase the hydroxylation and degradation of HIF-1α [58]. HPLC analysis showed that α-KG was increased by overexpression of PRODH/POX [46]. When PRODH/POX expression is high, P5C, glutamate and α-KG are sequentially produced from proline, forming an important link between proline and the TCA cycle. The widely used cell-permeating α-KG analogue, dimethyloxalylglycine, was shown to block the inhibition of HIF-1 signaling by PRODH/POX, suggesting the pivotal role of α-KG in the down-regulation of HIF by PRODH/POX.

In addition, several TCA cycle intermediates and glycolytic metabolites, such as succinate and fumarate, have been revealed to inhibit PHD activity and stabilize HIF-1 signaling [58-61]. PRODH/POX expression could decrease succinate, fumarate and lactate as measured by gas chromatography-mass spectrometry (GC-MS) [46], which may also contribute to the impaired HIF-1 signaling.

2.4. PRODH/POX suppresses tumor formation *in vivo* and is downregulated in human tumors

The inhibitory effects of PRODH/POX on tumor cell growth are corroborated in a human colon cancer mouse xenograft model [46]. DLD-1 POX Tet-off cells were injected into immunodeficient mice. The expression of PRODH/POX was controlled by giving mice doxycycline in their drinking water. When PRODH/POX was suppressed by doxycycline, tumors readily formed in all the mice within a few days. By contrast, when PRODH/POX was overexpressed by removal of doxycycline in their drinking water, tumor development was greatly reduced and none of the mice developed tumors

Further investigation on a variety of cancer tissues along with normal tissue counterparts including kidney, bladder, stomach, colon and rectum, liver, pancreas, breast, prostate, ovary, brain, lung, skin, etc., showed that 61% of all tumors had decreased expression of PRODH/POX compared to normal tissues, especially the tumor from kidney and digestive tract [46, 47, 62], suggesting tumor could eliminate the tumor suppressor roles of PRODH/POX. Suppression of PRODH/POX was more significant in kidney and digestive tract. More interestingly, PRODH/POX protein levels showed more striking decrease than mRNA levels in renal cancers, implicating that PRODH/POX might be regulated at the post-transcriptional level.

Sequencing the *PRODH* gene showed no somatic mutation or functionally significant single nucleotide polymorphisms (SNP) in tumor tissues. Hypermethylation analysis also didn't show any differences of PRODH genomic DNA between tumor and normal tissues. Therefore, PRODH does not satisfy the canonical requisite for tumor suppressor genes which often show genetic or epigenetic mutations in human cancers. With the discovery of microRNAs (miRNAs), a new mechanism to regulate protein expression has been revealed. Considering the inconsistency between PRODH/POX mRNA and protein expression and the importance of miRNAs in cancer, the regulation of miRNAs on PRODH/POX represented a very promising hypothesis.

3. MiRNA in cancer

3.1. Biogenesis and function of miRNAs

3.1.1. Discovery of miRNAs

MiRNAs are a class of post-transcriptional regulators. They are conserved, endogenously expressed, non-coding small RNAs of 18-25 nucleotides in length. MiRNAs were first discovered in 1993 by Lee RC *et al.* [63] and Wightman R *et al.* [64] in the nematode *Caenorhabditis elegans (C. elegans)* as a regulator of developmental timing regarding the gene lin-14. They found that the lin-14 could be regulated by the small RNA products from lin-4, a gene that does not code for any protein but instead produces a pair of small RNAs. These lin-4 RNAs had antisense complementarity to multiple sites in the 3′ UTR of the lin-14 mRNA. However, it did not attract substantial attention until seven years later when let-7 was discovered to repress the expression of several mRNAs including lin-14 during transition in developmental stages in *C. elegans* [65]. Since then over 4000 miRNAs have been identified in eukaryotes including mammals, fungi and plants. More than 700 miRNAs have been found in humans.

3.1.2. Processing and biogenesis of miRNAs

In mammals, miRNA genes are usually transcribed as long primary transcripts (pri-miRNAs) by RNA polymerase II from DNA [66]. The pri-miRNAs then are cropped into the hairpin-shaped miRNA precursors (pre-miRNAs) by the RNase III enzyme Drosha [67, 68]. A single pri-miRNA may contain one to six pre-miRNAs which are composed of about 70 nucleotides. They are exported from the nucleus to the cytoplasm by exportin-5 (XPO5), a member of the Ran-dependent nuclear transport receptor family [69-71]. In cytoplasm, the pre-miRNA hairpin is subsequently cleaved by the endonuclease Dicer [72] into an imperfect miRNA:miRNA* duplex. Usually, only one strand of the duplex is incorporated into the RNA induced silencing complex (RISC) where the miRNA and its mRNA target interact. The thermodynamic stability, strength of base-pairing and the position of the stem-loop determine which strand becomes mature miRNA to incorporate into the RISC [73-75]. The other strand is normally degraded and is denoted with an asterisk (*) due to its lower levels in the steady state. However, recent evidence indicates that both strands of duplex are viable and become functional miRNA that target different mRNA populations [62, 76-78].

RISC is a multiprotein complex that incorporates mature miRNA to recognize complementary target mRNA. Once binding to target mRNA, miRNAs inhibit their target genes with the help of RISC. The key component of the RISC complex is the Argonaute (Ago) proteins, which are consistently found in RISC complexes from a variety of organisms [79]. Ago proteins directly interact with the miRNA [80, 81]. They are needed for miRNA-induced silencing and contain two conserved RNA binding domains: a PAZ domain, that can bind the single stranded 3′ end of the mature miRNA, and a PIWI domain, that structurally resembles ribonuclease-H (RNaseH) and functions in slicer activity through interacting with the 5′ end of the guide strand [82]. Most eukaryotes contain multiple Ago family members, with different Ago often specialized for distinct functions [83]. The human genome encodes four Ago proteins and Ago2 is the only Ago capable of endonuclease cleavage of target transcripts directly [84, 85].

Additional components of RISC involved in miRNA processing include the Vasa intronic gene (VIG) protein, the fragile X mental retardation protein (FMRP), human immunodeficiency virus transactivating response RNA binding protein (TARBP), protein activator of the interferon induced protein kinase (PACT), the SMN complex, Gemin3 and DICER1, and so on [86-92]. However their generality or precise function in miRNA silencing remains to be determined.

3.1.3. Stability of miRNAs

Turnover of mature miRNA is needed for rapid changes in miRNA expression profiles. Besides inducing the cleavage of the target mRNAs, Ago proteins have been recently reported to regulate the stability of miRNAs [93-98]. Mature miRNAs are stabilized after incorporation into Ago proteins, and release from this complex leaves miRNAs vulnerable to decay by exonucleases [94, 95]. Ectopic overexpression of Ago proteins prevents degradation of miRNAs, and loss of Ago2 significantly reduces miRNA stability and differentially regulates miRNAs production [93, 96].

In addition to taking refuge in protein complexes, mature miRNAs can undergo protective modifications [97]. For example, as indicated by work in the model organism *Arabidopsis thaliana*, mature plant miRNAs appear to be stabilized by the addition of methyl groups at the 3' end which prevents uridylation of miRNAs [99]. The addition of adenines to 3′ end of miRNAs detected in many different plant and animal miRNAs also has a stabilizing effect on miRNAs [100-104].

3.1.4. Function of miRNAs

MiRNAs inhibit the expression of their target genes through three different mechanisms [105, 106]. The first one is direct endonucleolytic cleavage of mRNAs supported by the slicer activity of specific Ago proteins present within RISC. As mentioned above, Ago2 is the only one of the four mammalian Ago proteins capable of directing cleavage [84, 85]. This mechanism is generally favored by a complete match of the so called seed-sequence of the miRNA (nucleotides 2-7 of 5′ end of miRNAs) and target mRNA [107], although some mismatches can be tolerated and still allow cleavage to occur [108, 109]. The complementarity of the seed region defines the targets of the miRNA because the seed region binds to the mRNA as governed by binding of complementary nucleotides. The second mechanism is by inhibiting protein translation but without degradation of the mRNA [110-112]. It seems to be the most prevalent in mammals [113]. In this mechanism, the seed region of the miRNA does not need to be fully complementary; yet, efficient translation repression by miRNAs often requires multiple miRNA-binding sites, as suggested by the observations that the identified mRNA targets of miRNAs contained multiple sites for miRNA binding, either the same miRNA or a combination of several different miRNAs [114, 115]. However, many predicted mRNA targets of miRNAs contain only a single miRNA-binding site in their 3′UTR [107], indicating that such single sites may lead to fine "tuning" of mRNA function [116]. Distinct from the slicer activity of the specific Ago in the first manner, translation repression by miRNAs is common to all members of the Ago protein family. The third mechanism is called mRNA decay independent of slicer [117, 118]. In this manner, miRNAs either promote mRNAs decapping and 5′ to 3′ degradation, or target mRNAs by an unknown decay pathway. In the former way, the protecting poly-A-tail and ''cap'' of the mRNAs are removed, resulting in their rapid destruction by RNA splicing enzymes.

MiRNAs are now known to target thousands of genes. Bioinformatics analyses estimated that up to 30% of known human genes are under miRNAs' control [107], whereas later reports increased this number to 74~92% [119]. A key issue in miRNAs function is the specificity of their interactions with their target mRNAs and how each interaction leads to discrete downstream consequences. Some miRNAs regulate specific individual targets, while others can function as master regulators of a process. Key miRNAs regulate the expression levels of hundreds of genes simultaneously, and many types of miRNAs regulate their targets cooperatively. Because of their potent and wide action on gene expression, miRNAs become critical regulators of cellular functions. They are involved in modulating a variety of biological processes, including cellular proliferation, differentiation, metabolic signaling, apoptosis and development. The aberrant expression or alteration of miRNAs has been linked to a range of human diseases, especially cancers.

3.2. Dysregulation of miRNA in cancer

In 2002, Calin *et al.* first demonstrated that miR-15 and miIR-16 are frequently deleted or down-regulated in chronic lymphocytic leukemia [120]. Subsequently, aberrant miRNA expression, and amplification or deletion of miRNAs are observed in various human tumors [121, 122]. MiRNAs are differentially expressed in cancer cells, in which they form distinct and unique miRNA expression patterns [123]. These properties make miRNAs become potential biomarkers for cancer diagnosis, in particular for the early detection of cancer [124]. The control of gene expression by miRNAs is seen in virtually all cancer cells. Their target genes are usually important proteins such as oncogenic factors (i.e., MYC, RAS), tumor suppressors (i.e., p53), or proteins regulating the cell cycle (i.e., the cyclin family). Even small changes in these crucial proteins can have profound effects on tumorigenesis or tumor development. Conversely, miRNAs are often critical downstream effectors of classic oncogene/tumor suppressor networks, such as MYC and p53 described below.

miRNAs can act as oncogenes or tumor suppressor genes in tumorigenesis depending on the targets they regulate. Oncogenic miRNAs repress known tumor suppressors, whereas tumor-suppressor miRNAs often negatively regulate protein-coding oncogenes (this has been reviewed in detail by others [125-127]). Oncogenic miRNAs are overexpressed in various human cancers. For example, the miR-17-92 cluster miRNAs which are transcribed as a polycistronic unit, are highly expressed in B-cell lymphoma and various solid cancer, such as breast, colon, lung, pancreas, prostate and stomach [128-130]. They function as oncogenes to promote proliferation, inhibit apoptosis, induce tumor angiogenesis, and augment the oncogenic effects of MYC [131-134]. Their effects on cell cycle and proliferation are at least in part through its regulation of E2F transcription factors [130, 135], and anti-apoptotic effects are through their inhibition of BIM, PTEN and p21 [135]. MiR-221 and miR-222 are frequently overexpressed in lung, liver and ERα- breast cancers. Their overexpression has been demonstrated to enhance tumorigenicity through suppressing the expression of different tumor suppressors, such as CDKN1B/C, BIM, PTEN, TIMP3 and FOXO3 [136, 137]. Overexpression of miR-504 promotes tumorgenicity of colon cancer *in vivo*, which directly targets tumor suppressor p53 and functions in apoptosis and cell cycle [138].

On the other hand, miRNAs that act as tumor suppressors are often found to be deleted or mutated in various human cancers. For example, Let-7 family miRNAs are frequently down-regulated in various cancers, including lung and colorectal cancers [139]. They can directly suppress the expression of oncogenes, including RAS and MYC, and therefore show tumor suppressive functions [139, 140]. MiR-15a and miR-16-1 are often deleted or down-regulated in B-cell chronic lymphocytic leukemia (B-CLL). They negatively regulate anti-apoptotic protein BCL2. Therefore, decreased expression of miR-15a and miR-16-1 up-regulates BCL2 levels and reduces apoptosis, contributing to malignant transformation [141].

Based on the critical role of miRNAs in tumorigenesis, recent research efforts are directed towards translating these basic discoveries into clinical applications in diagnosis, prognosis and therapy through identifying and targeting dysregulated miRNAs. Both silencing the oncogenic miRNAs and restoring the expression of silenced tumor-suppressor miRNAs have yielded positive results in mouse models of cancer and thus becomes promising therapeutic strategy for cancer [142, 143]. The silencing of oncogenic miRNAs can be achieved by using antisense oligonucleotides (antagomirs or anti-miRs), sponges or locked nucleic acid (LNA) constructs [144]. By contrast, the restoration of tumor-suppressor miRNA expression can be achieved by the use of synthetic miRNA mimics, adenovirus vectors, and pharmacological agents [144]. Although the drug delivery, proper drug composition and off-target effects are still the current challenges in the clinical application of miRNAs, the future is bright for miRNA-based therapy.

3.3. MiRNAs regulated by transcriptional factors, genetic and epigenetic changes

3.3.1. MiRNAs regulated by oncogenic transcriptional factor MYC

MiRNAs can be dysregulated by multiple transcription factors in cancer. Oncogenic transcriptional factor MYC regulates a variety of gene expression affecting a series of cellular processes in cancer including cell growth and proliferation, metabolism, cell-cycle, differentiation, apoptosis, angiogenesis and metastasis [145-147]. Recently, it was found that MYC is also an important regulator of miRNAs. Consistent with their ability to potently influence cancer phenotypes, the regulation of miRNAs by MYC affects virtually all aspects of the MYC oncogenic program.

MYC directly activates the transcription of miR-17-92 polycistronic cluster though binding to an E-box within the first intron of the gene encoding the miR-17-92 primary transcript [148, 149]. Given its oncogenic role, the inhibition of key targets of miR-17-92 contributes to MYC-induced tumorigenesis. MiR-9 could also be activated directly by MYC, which regulates E-cadherin and cancer metastasis [150]. In contrast, MYC activity also results in repression of numerous miRNAs [151]. This repression involves the downregulation of miRNAs with antiproliferative, antitumorigenic and pro-apoptotic activity, such as let-7, miR-15a/16-1, miR-26a miR-29 or miR-34 family members [143, 151-153]. MiR-23a/b is an additional important example to be directly suppressed by MYC, which targets glutaminase to enhance glutamine catabolism [5]. MYC-driven reprogramming of miRNA expression patterns was shown to be a contributing factor in hepatoblastoma (HB), a rare embryonal neoplasm derived from liver progenitor cells [154]. Like an embryonic stem cell expression profile, undifferentiated aggressive HBs overexpress the miR-371-3 cluster with concomitant down-regulation of the miR-100/let-7a-2/miR-125b-1 cluster, which exerts antagonistic effects on cell proliferation and tumorigenicity. Chromatin immunoprecipitation (ChIP) and MYC inhibition assays in hepatoma cells demonstrated that both miR clusters are regulated by MYC in an opposite manner.

Although further investigation is necessary, the current studies have indicated that MYC uses both transcriptional and post-transcriptional mechanisms to modulate miRNA expression [151, 155]. Primary transcript mapping and ChIP revealed that MYC associates directly with evolutionarily conserved promoter regions upstream of several miRNAs [151], such as the direct activation of miR-17-92 cluster and direct suppression of miR-23a/b described above. MYC is also able to modulate the maturation of specific miRNAs without affecting transcription of the pri-miRNAs. For example, MYC activity results in repression of mature let-7 miRNAs while the expression of let-7 primary transcripts is unchanged [151, 156]. This phenomenon could be due to Lin28A and Lin28B being the direct target of MYC, which interacts with let-7 pre-miRNA stem-loops and may regulate let-7 at multiple levels including Drosha and Dicer processing [156, 157]. Additionally, interaction of Lin28A and Lin28B recruits the 3′ terminal uridylyl transferase 4 (TUT4) to pre-let-7, resulting in uridylation and subsequent decay of the pre-miRNA [158, 159].

3.3.2. MiRNAs regulated by tumor suppressor p53

The tumor suppressor p53 is another transcription factor that regulate the expression of a group of miRNAs mediating a variety of anti-proliferative processes [160]. The miR-34 family, which consists of miR-34a, miR-34b and miR-34c, was initially reported to be induced directly by p53 [161] and mediate some of the p53 effects. ChIP and luciferase assays showed that p53 binds to p53 response elements (REs) in miR-34 promoters and activates their transcription [162]. MiR-34 family members directly repress the expression of several targets involved in the regulation of cell cycle and in the promotion of cell proliferation and survival. These targets include cyclin E2, cyclin-dependent kinases 4 and 6 (CDK4 and CDK6), BCL2 and hepatocyte growth factor receptor c-Met [161]. Later on, p53 was reported to directly regulate the transcriptional expression of several additional miRNAs, including miR-145, miR-107, miR-192 and miR215, miR-149* [160, 163]. MiR-145 negatively regulates oncogene *MYC*, which accounts partially for the miR-145-mediated inhibition of tumor cell growth both *in vitro* and *in vivo* [164]. MiR-107 contributes to the role of p53 in the regulation of hypoxia signaling and anti-angiogenesis through repressing the expression of HIF-1β, which interacts with HIF-1α subunits to form a HIF-1 complex, a key player in tumor formation. MiR-192 and miR-215 induce cell cycle arrest and reduce tumor cell growth through targeting a number of regulators of DNA synthesis and cell cycle checkpoints, such as CDC7, MDA2L1 and CUL5 [165]. MiRNA-149* targets glycogen synthase kinase-3α, resulting in increased expression of Mcl-1 and resistance to apoptosis in melanoma cells [163].

Moreover, p53 also enhances the post-transcriptional maturation of miRNAs. In response to doxorubicin, P53 interacts with the Drosha processing complex through the association with DEAD box RNA helicases p68 (also known as DDX5) and p72 (also known as DDX17), and facilitates the Drosha-mediated processing of pri-miRNAs to pre-miRNAs. These miRNAs include miR-16-1, miR-143 and miR-145 with growth-suppressive functions. Transcriptionally inactive p53 mutants interfere with a functional assembly between Drosha complex and p68, leading to attenuation of miRNA processing activity [166].

3.3.3. *MiRNAs regulated by other transcription factors*

Estrogen receptor alpha (ERα), a member of the nuclear receptor superfamily of transcription factors, was found to negatively regulate expression of miR-221 and miR-222 by promoter binding and recruiting the corepressors NCoR and SMRT [137]. Overexpression of miR-221 and miR-222 conversely suppresses the expression of ERα, conferring estrogen-independent growth. They also suppress the expression of different tumor suppressors, such as CDKN1B, CDKN1C, BIM, PTEN, TIMP3, DNA damage-inducible transcript 4, and FOXO3, to promote high proliferation [137]. Transcription factor c-Jun could also activate miR-221 and miR-222 [136].

Microarray-based expression profiles reveal that a specific spectrum of miRNAs is induced in response to low oxygen, at least some via a HIF-dependent mechanism, such as miR-210, miR-26a-2, miR-24 and miR-181c [167]. Of these, miR-210 as a direct transcriptional target of HIF-1α has emerged as a critical element of the cellular hypoxia response in a broad variety of cell types ranging from cancer cell lines to human umbilical vein endothelial cells [168-170]. MiR-210 has diverse functions, including modulating angiogenesis [171], stem cell survival [172], and hypoxia-induced cell cycle arrest [173]. MiR-143 and miR-145 could be repressed by RAS-responsive element-binding protein 1 (RREB1), a zinc finger transcription factor which binds to RAS-responsive elements (RREs) of their promoters. Thus these two miRNAs are embedded in KRAS oncogenic network [174].

In general, miRNAs can be dysregulated by transcription factors and, therefore, genetic or epigenetic alterations that result in the dysregulation of transcription factors can cause miRNA dysregulation. Importantly, miRNAs can also be directly regulated by genetic or epigenetic alterations.

3.3.4. MiRNAs regulated by genetic and epigenetic changes

MiRNAs are frequently located in fragile regions of the chromosomes, such as common chromosomal-breakpoints that are associated with the development of cancer [175, 176]. These fragile regions are often missing, amplified or mutated in cancer cells, resulting in the genetic alterations of miRNAs. The genetic alterations can affect the production of the primary miRNA transcript, their processing to mature miRNAs and/or interactions with mRNA targets. The dysregulation of miR-15 and miR-16 in most B cell chronic lymphocytic leukemias, one of the first observations between miRNAs and cancer development, is the result from chromosome 13q14 deletion [120]. Interestingly, somatic translocations in miRNA target sites can also occur, representing a drastic means of altering miRNA function [177, 178].

In addition to the structural genetic alterations, dysregulation of miRNAs in cancer can occur through epigenetic changes, such as methylation of the CpG islands of their promoters, the modification of histone [179-181]. As the example, miR-127 is silenced by promoter methylation, which leads to the overexpression of BCL6, an oncogene involved in the development of diffuse large B cell lymphoma [179]. The expression of miR-127 could be restored by using hypomethylating agents such as azacytidine. MiRNA-200 family could serve as another example. The miR-200 family can be shifted to hypermethylated or unmethylated 5'-CpG island status corresponding to the epithelial-mesenchymal transition (EMT) and mesenchymal-epithelial transition (MET) phenotypes, respectively, which contributes to the evolving and adapting phenotypes of human tumors [181].

4. miR-23b* targets PRODH/POX

Although numerous targets of miRNAs have been identified, miRNA regulators of critical cancer proteins and pathways remain largely unknown. As described above, PRODH/POX is frequently reduced in a variety of human cancers, including renal cancer, and PRODH/POX protein but not mRNA level is markedly down-regulated in renal cancers [46, 62]. The fact that miRNAs are critical post-transcriptional regulators, and miRNAs function as oncogenes to inhibit the expression of tumor suppressors raises attractive possibility that some specific miRNAs may regulate PRODH/POX and proline catabolism. Target-prediction algorithms have been used to identify the protein targets of miRNAs or miRNAs regulators of known protein, followed by experimental validation to eliminate false positives [141]. The bioinformatic analysis according to target-prediction algorithms predicted that 91 potential miRNAs could target PRODH/POX mRNA 3'UTR [62]. In miRNA microarrays, 10 miRNAs showed an increased expression in renal cancer cells relative to normal cells. However, only miR-23b* was shown to significantly inhibit

PRODH/POX protein expression, but not mRNA level. This is consistent with many previous reports, that is, in mammals, miRNAs more often inhibit protein translation of the target mRNA, other than inducing its degradation [113]. Subsequently, miR-23b* directly binding to PRODH/POX mRNA 3′UTR was experimentally confirmed through luciferase assays by co-transfecting the mimic miR-23b* and the luciferase reporter containing 3′UTR of PRODH/POX mRNA. Functional analysis showed that this miRNA impaired PRODH/POX functions, including PRODH/POX-mediated ROS generation, apoptosis, and PRODH/POX-inhibited HIF-1 signaling [62]. In contrast, the inhibitory antagomir of miR-23b* increased the expression of PRODH/POX protein in renal cancer cells. As a result, ROS production, the percentage of cells undergoing apoptosis increased, and HIF-1 signaling decreased.

The clinical relevance of these *in vitro* findings was substantiated by the data obtained in human renal carcinoma tissues *in vivo* [62]. There were statistical significant differences in both miR-23b* and PRODH/POX protein expression between carcinoma tissues and corresponding normal tissues, but not PRODH/POX mRNA levels. A negative correlation between miR-23b* and PRODH/POX protein was found.

In summary, PRODH/POX is subject to the negative regulation of miR-23b*, which is a novel mechanism for cells to regulate PRODH/POX protein level and functions. The increased miR-23b* might contribute to renal oncogenesis and progression by downregulating tumor suppressor PRODH/POX. This provides a possible strategic opening to inhibit tumor growth by decreasing the levels of miR-23b* or by blocking its function.

5. Regulation of miR-23b* in cancer

5.1. MiR-23b* regulation by oncogenic protein MYC

Recently, the oncogenic transcription factor MYC has been reported to transcriptionally suppress miR-23b to stimulate mitochondrial glutaminase expression and glutamine metabolism in lymphoma cells [5]. MiR-23b and miR-23b* are sibling miRNAs processed from the same transcript. Thus, this finding attracted our attention and compelled us to seek the potential effect of MYC on miR-23b* and related PRODH/POX expression and proline metabolism. As described above, MYC is a critical regulator of miRNAs expression at both transcriptional and post-transcriptional levels. Furthermore, proline and glutamine metabolism are closely related: not only their interconversions, but also both can be anaplerotic in the TCA cycle as an important energy source, as mentioned above. These facts strengthened our hypothesis that MYC may regulate the expression of miR-23b*, thereby PRODH/POX, and link proline and glutamine metabolism.

Using human Burkitt lymphoma model P493 cells that bear a tetracycline-repressible *MYC* construct, we found that MYC upregulated the expression of miR-23b* [30]. In PC3 prostate cancer cells which overexpress MYC, the same result was obtained, i.e., MYC knockdown by siRNA resulted in the decrease of miR-23b* expression. These results are distinct from the previous report which showed MYC directly bound to the transcriptional unit encompassing miR-23b, and regulated its expression at the transcriptional level [5]. Re-examination of the expression of miR-23b*, miR-23b, and their primary transcript (pri-miR23b) showed that pri-miR23b increased about 50% with MYC suppression by tetracycline and then decreased on MYC re-induction in P493 cells [30]. Similarly, in PC3 prostate cancer cells, with MYC knockdown by siRNA, miR-23b* decreased 68%, while miR-23b and Pri-miR-23b increased 51% and 70%, respectively [30]. Thus, the level of miR-23b* is higher than miR-23b in cells without MYC knockdown. These results support previous work that MYC suppresses miR-23b expression at the transcriptional level. Considering the fact that MYC enhances the expression of miR-23b*, the sibling of miR-23b, we hypothesized that differential effects of MYC on the sibling miRNAs may be due to their differential stabilization and/or degradation mediated by MYC. As a consequence, even if MYC suppressed the expression of miR-23b primary transcript, its effects on miR-23b* stabilization and/or degradation could account for net higher levels of miR-23b* as observed in this report.

The mechanisms responsible for stabilized miRNA expression have been largely elusive. As mentioned above, Ago proteins, the key players in miRNA processing and function, recently have been shown to regulate miRNA stability [93-96]. Ago2 differentially regulates miRNAs expression [93, 96]. Not surprisingly, MYC significantly upregulated the expression of Ago2 [30]. Knockdown of Ago2 in P493 MYC-overexpressed cells, the expression of miR-23b* and miR-23b were differentially decreased (76% vs. 42%, respectively), but not Pri-23b. Although the differential effects on miR-23b* and miR-23b resulted from Ago2 regulation by MYC do not completely account for the observed differential effects of MYC, they do support our hypothesis that MYC may regulate miRNA levels by differential effects on the stabilization of miRNAs, which can serve as a model for the effects on sibling miRNAs.

Since a large number of RISC components are involved in the miRNA processing [86]. It is likely that MYC with its multitude of target genes may affect many proteins like Ago2 and differentially affect miR-23b* and miR-23b expression. In fact, several reports have described the regulation of MYC on other RISCs or accessory RISCs, such as the upregulation of XPO5 and DEAD box protein 5 (DDX5) [86, 182, 183], and the aforementioned Lin28A and Lin28B regulation by MYC which affects the expression of mature let-7 miRNAs at multiple levels including their processing and modification [151, 156-159], but further studies are needed to elucidate how they affect the final expression of mature miRNAs and their interaction.

5.2. miR-23b* regulation by other factors

As mentioned above, PRODH/POX is encoded by a p53-induced gene [31]. Maxwell SA *et al.* reported that reduced expression of PRODH/POX mRNA in renal cancer was due to a p53 mutation [184]. On the other hand, p53 is a critical regulator of miRNAs. Thus, the possibility exists that wild-type p53 may regulate the expression of PRODH/POX by both direct and indirect (miR-23b*-dependent) mechanism. Interestingly, the experiment showed that ectopic expression of p53 in p53-mutant renal cancer cell line TK10 increased the expression of miR-23b* [62]. This suggests that the upregulation of miR-23b* by p53 may counteract the direct induction of p53 on PRODH/POX gene expression in clear cell renal cell carcinoma. This interaction might also account for discrepancies between PRODH/POX mRNA and protein expression.

In addition, current evidence suggests that miR-23b* could be regulated by factors other than p53 and MYC. For example, as discussed above, several reports have shown the link between upregulation of miR-23b and hypoxia [167, 185, 186]. As miR-23b and miR-23b* share the same precursor, miR-23b* could also be regulated by HIF. In renal cell carcinoma, the constitutive expression of HIF due to VHL deficiency may link this regulation of miR-23b* with VHL. The fact that HIF-1 negatively regulates mitochondrial biogenesis by inhibiting MYC activity in VHL-deficient renal carcinoma cells [187] further increases the possibility that miR-23b* could be regulated by VHL, HIF, thereby affecting the expression of PRODH/POX. These regulatory interactions are of great interest and worth to be pursued.

6. Regulation of proline metabolism by MYC

6.1. MYC suppresses PRODH/POX primarily through miR-23b*

In view of the above findings, it is not surprising that MYC suppresses the expression of PRODH/POX through upregulating miR-23b*. First, PRODH/POX protein increased in a time-dependent fashion with diminished MYC expression and then decreased on MYC recovery in P493 cells. PRODH/POX mRNA expression also showed a significant increase with suppressed MYC expression, but the increase was far less than that of protein levels, raising the likelihood that miRNA mediates the effect of MYC on PRODH/POX at the post-transcriptional level. MYC knockdown in PC3 prostate cancer cells by siRNA resulted in the inhibition of PRODH/POX expression with a pattern similar to the P493 cells. Secondly, the inhibition of miR-23b* by its antagomirs in the P493 cells with MYC overexpression increased PRODH/POX protein level [30]. By contrast, the transfection of mimic miR-23b* into the P493 cells under MYC inhibition by tetracycline resulted in a marked decrease of PRODH/POX protein expression. However, the decrease of PRODH/POX still was not comparable with that without tetracycline treatment, indicating that MYC could suppress PRODH/POX expression through pathways other than miRNA, such as the regulation at the transcriptional level, which also is supported by the decrease of PRODH/POX mRNA by MYC. Thirdly, the luciferase assays in PC cells showed that knockdown of MYC increased the luciferase activity of the luciferase reporter containing POX 3′UTR with the binding site of miR-23b*, indicating the decrease of miR-23b* by siMYC. Without MYC knockdown, the luciferase activity of this reporter was much lower than that of the original reporter without POX 3′UTR, due to high levels of miR-23b* binding to PRODH/POX mRNA 3′UTR, thereby suppressing luciferase expression.

By transfecting the PRODH promoter/luciferase reporter construct containing PRODH promoter region in PC3 prostate cancer cells, knockdown of MYC resulted in the increase of PRODH promoter activity, which confirmed that MYC regulates PRODH/POX at the transcriptional level [41]. Analysis of PRODH promoter nucleotide sequence revealed one canonical MYC binding site 5′-CACGTG-3′ (E-box) and one noncanonical binding site (5′-ACGGTG-3′) at -2808 to -2813bp and -637 to -642bp of the PRODH promoter region, respectively. However, ChIP assay showed none of these PRODH promoter regions had significant PCR amplification, suggesting that MYC does not directly interact with the

PRODH gene, and the decreased PRODH/POX mRNA expression may be mediated through other transcription factors regulated by MYC [30].

6.2. Suppression of proline catabolism is essential for MYC-mediated cancer cell proliferation and survival

In addition to PRODH/POX, MYC also inhibits the expression of another enzyme in proline catabolism, P5CDH [30], but the mechanism remains unclear. However, the suppression of proline catabolism reflected by PRODH/POX inhibition by MYC has been shown to be essential for MYC-induced proliferation and cell survival. First, knockdown of PRODH/POX in P493 cells with MYC suppressed by tetracycline consistently reduced the production of ROS at different time points [30], although the suppression of MYC itself by tetracycline also decreased the accumulation of ROS at late stage which implicates the different effects of various MYC regulated genes on ROS production at various stages [188-190]. Correspondingly, the apoptosis assay by flow cytometry showed that PRODH/POX knockdown decreased the percentage of apoptotic and dead cells occurring with MYC suppression. In contrast, PRODH/POX siRNA significantly rescued 30~40% of the diminished growth rates resulting from MYC suppression by tetracycline [30]. These results indicated that PRODH/POX suppression is critical for MYC-mediated cancer cell proliferation and survival. The same assays performed in PC3 prostate cancer cells confirmed these results [30].

To summarize, oncogenic transcription factor MYC inhibits PRODH/POX expression and thereby inhibits its tumor suppressor function. When MYC is suppressed, the increase of PRODH/POX promotes proline catabolism to generate ROS, leading to the initiation of apoptosis and the decrease of cell proliferation and growth. MYC-induced suppression of PRODH/POX contributes to MYC-mediated changes of cell behavior including proliferation and metabolic reprogramming, which in turn may contribute to tumorigenesis and tumor progression. These findings further indicate the critical roles of proline catabolism catalyzed by PRODH/POX in human cancers.

6.3. MYC increases the biosynthesis of proline from glutamine

Since MYC plays an important role in glutamine metabolism which is closely related with proline metabolism due to the interconversion of proline and glutamate, we not only investigated the effect of MYC on proline catabolism catalyzed by PRODH/POX as shown above, but also examined proline biosynthesis, especially from glutamine. Western blots showed that MYC robustly increased the expression of GLS, P5CS and PYCR1 in the pathway from glutamine to proline biosynthesis [30]. PC3 prostate cancer cells displayed the same correlation between MYC and glutamine and proline metabolism. The measurement of the intracellular proline levels showed that MYC dramatically increased the intracellular levels of proline. Consistently, using [^{13}C,^{15}N]-Glutamine as a tracer, the direct production of proline from glutamine induced by MYC was confirmed by GC-MS and NMR analysis [30]. Thus, MYC not only suppresses proline catabolism and stimulates glutamine oxidation to glutamate, but also markedly enhances proline biosynthesis from glutamate.

Both normal and tumor cells depend on glucose and glutamine consumption as sources of metabolic energy, and as precursors for biosynthesis of macromolecules [6, 191]. *MYC* oncogene is considered a master regulator of tumor cell metabolism and proliferation. It not only promotes glucose uptake and induces aerobic glycolysis, but also enhances glutamine uptake and stimulates glutamine catabolism. Although glutamine catabolism is linked to biosynthesis of protein, nucleotides and lipids, redox homeostasis and energy metabolism, the report from Wise *et al*. suggests that little of the glutamine uptake stimulated by MYC is used for macromolecular synthesis [6]. MYC-induced glutamine catabolism is involved in reprogramming mitochondrial metabolism to sustain cellular viability and TCA cycle anapleurosis [6]. More recent findings reported by Le *et al*. [192] and Wang *et al*. [193] emphasized the metabolic reprogramming controlled by MYC in tumor cells and activated T cells. The latter showed that glutamine catabolism driven by MYC coupled with multiple biosynthetic pathways, especially ornithine and polyamine biosynthesis [193]. However, the importance of the biosynthesis of the ornithine and polyamine from glutamine is understood only in part. Similarly, the metabolic advantage afforded by the increased conversion of glutamine to proline and how biosynthetic pathway fits into the MYC-driven metabolic reprogramming also remain unclear. The connection between the conversion of P5C to proline, the last step of proline biosynthesis and pentose phosphate pathway through the oxidation-reduction reactions of NADPH and $NADP^+$ [8, 14, 15] provides us a clue to understand the importance of proline biosynthesis induced by MYC in cancer, since proline synthesis from P5C could also oxidize NADH to NAD^+ to maintain glucose metabolism, glycolysis. In fact, our unpublished data showed that the blockade of proline biosynthesis by knocking down P5CS or PYCR1 markedly decreased glycolysis, which supports our hypothesis.

It's noteworthy that glutamine may be not the only source of proline biosynthesis promoted by MYC, since the increase of PYCR1 is much greater than that of P5CS and GLS [30], and ornithine could also be converted to proline by ornithine aminotransferase and PYCR1 (see Figure 1). This possibility and its importance in MYC-induced metabolic reprogramming are also worth pursuing.

7. Conclusion

Proline, the unique proteinogenic secondary amino acid, is metabolized by its own family of enzymes. Early studies showed that proline metabolism is linked with TCA cycle, pentose phosphate pathway and urea cycle. During the conversion of proline to P5C, the central enzyme of proline metabolism, PRODH/POX, donates electron to ETC to generate ROS or ATP depending on context. As a tumor suppressor, PRODH/POX is induced by p53, PPARγ and its ligands, and contributes to the initiation of apoptosis and the inhibition of tumor growth through ROS generation (Figure 2). On the other hand, PRODH/POX is suppressed by miR-23b* and oncogene MYC. MYC not only suppresses proline catabolism, but increases proline biosynthesis from glutamine (Figure 3). Thus, these recent studies reveal a new link in human cancer between MYC, miRNA regulation, proline metabolism, glutamine metabolism, TCA cycle, and even glycolysis. These metabolic links emphasizes the complexity of tumor metabolism. Further studies of proline metabolism in tumor microenvironment will provide a deeper understanding of tumor metabolism and novel therapeutic strategies in cancer.

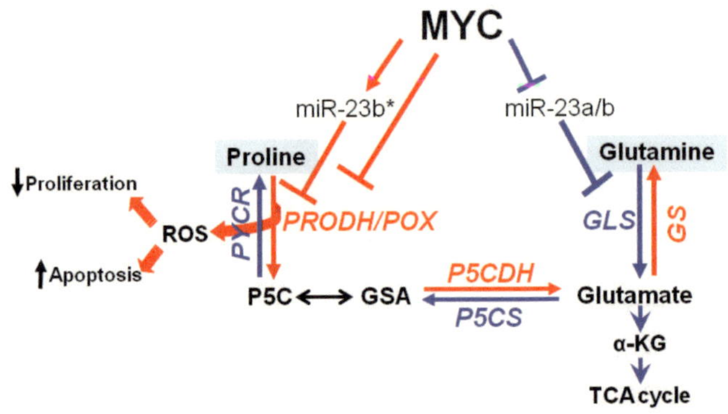

Figure 3. MYC regulation of proline and glutamine metabolism. MYC suppresses proline catabolism through its inhibition of the expression of PRODH/POX and P5CDH. MYC inhibits the expression of PRODH/POX at both transcriptional and post-transcriptional levels (upregulation of miR-23b*), which is essential for MYC-induced proliferation and cell survival. On the other hand, MYC stimulates glutamine catabolism through miR-23a/b-mediated glutaminase (GLS) upregulation. Furthermore, MYC not only suppresses proline catabolism, but also enhances proline biosynthesis from glutamine. Proline and glutamine metabolism are connected by MYC and miRNA regulation.

Author details

Wei Liu and James M. Phang*
Metabolism and Cancer Susceptibility Section, Basic Research Laboratory, Frederick National Laboratory for Cancer Research, NIH. Frederick, MD

Acknowledgement

The work was supported by the Intramural Research Program of the NIH, National Cancer Institute, Center for Cancer Research. This project also has been funded in part with Federal funds from the National Cancer Institute, NIH, under contract no. HHSN27612080001. The content of this review does not necessarily reflect the views or policies of the Department of Health and Human Services, nor does mention of trade names, commercial products, or organizations imply endorsement by the U.S. government. We thank Dr. Ziqiang Zhu for his reading of the manuscript.

8. References

[1] Warburg O (1956) On the origin of cancer cells, Science 123, 309-314.

* Corresponding Author

[2] Vander Heiden MG, Cantley LC, & Thompson CB (2009) Understanding the Warburg effect: the metabolic requirements of cell proliferation, Science 324, 1029-1033.

[3] Fogal V, Richardson AD, Karmali PP, Scheffler IE, Smith JW, & Ruoslahti E (2010) Mitochondrial p32 protein is a critical regulator of tumor metabolism via maintenance of oxidative phosphorylation, Mol Cell Biol 30, 1303-1318.

[4] Dang CV (2010) Rethinking the Warburg effect with Myc micromanaging glutamine metabolism, Cancer Res 70, 859-862.

[5] Gao P, Tchernyshyov I, Chang TC, Lee YS, Kita K, Ochi T, *et al.* (2009) c-Myc suppression of miR-23a/b enhances mitochondrial glutaminase expression and glutamine metabolism, Nature 458, 762-765.

[6] Wise DR, DeBerardinis RJ, Mancuso A, Sayed N, Zhang XY, Pfeiffer HK, *et al.* (2008) Myc regulates a transcriptional program that stimulates mitochondrial glutaminolysis and leads to glutamine addiction, Proc Natl Acad Sci U S A 105, 18782-18787.

[7] Adams E (1970) Metabolism of proline and of hydroxyproline, Int Rev Connect Tissue Res 5, 1-91.

[8] Phang JM (1985) The regulatory functions of proline and pyrroline-5-carboxylic acid, Curr Top Cell Regul 25, 91-132.

[9] Phang JM, Liu W, & Zabirnyk O (2010) Proline metabolism and microenvironmental stress, Annu Rev Nutr 30, 441-463.

[10] Phang JM & Liu W (2012) Proline metabolism and cancer, Front Biosci 17, 1835-1845.

[11] Phang JM, Hu CA, & Valle D (2001) Disorders of proline and hydroxyproline metabolism. In: Scriver CR, Beaudet AL, Sly WS, Valle D, editors. In Metabolic and Molecular Bases of Inherited Disease, New York: McGraw-Hill. pp. 1821-1838.

[12] Adams E & Frank L (1980) Metabolism of proline and the hydroxyprolines, Annu Rev Biochem 49, 1005-1061.

[13] Liu Y, Borchert GL, Donald SP, Surazynski A, Hu CA, Weydert CJ, *et al.* (2005) MnSOD inhibits proline oxidase-induced apoptosis in colorectal cancer cells, Carcinogenesis 26, 1335-1342.

[14] Phang JM, Downing SJ, Yeh GC, Smith RJ, Williams JA, & Hagedorn CH (1982) Stimulation of the hexosemonophosphate-pentose pathway by pyrroline-5-carboxylate in cultured cells, J Cell Physiol 110, 255-261

[15] Yeh GC, Roth EF, Jr., Phang JM, Harris SC, Nagel RL, & Rinaldi A (1984) The effect of pyrroline-5-carboxylic acid on nucleotide metabolism in erythrocytes from normal and glucose-6-phosphate dehydrogenase-deficient subjects, J Biol Chem 259, 5454-5458.

[16] Hu CA, Bart Williams D, Zhaorigetu S, Khalil S, Wan G, & Valle D (2008) Functional genomics and SNP analysis of human genes encoding proline metabolic enzymes, Amino Acids 35, 655-664.

[17] Schafer IA, Scriver CR, & Efron ML (1962) Familial hyperprolinemia, cerebral dysfunction and renal anomalies occuring in a family with hereditary nephropathy and deafness, N Engl J Med 267, 51-60.

[18] Willis A, Bender HU, Steel G, & Valle D (2008) PRODH variants and risk for schizophrenia, Amino Acids 35, 673-679.

[19] Bender HU, Almashanu S, Steel G, Hu CA, Lin WW, Willis A, *et al.* (2005) Functional consequences of PRODH missense mutations, Am J Hum Genet 76, 409-420.

[20] Reversade B, Escande-Beillard N, Dimopoulou A, Fischer B, Chng SC, Li Y, *et al.* (2009) Mutations in PYCR1 cause cutis laxa with progeroid features, Nat Genet 41, 1016-1021.

[21] Baumgartner MR, Hu CA, Almashanu S, Steel G, Obie C, Aral B, *et al.* (2000) Hyperammonemia with reduced ornithine, citrulline, arginine and proline: a new inborn error caused by a mutation in the gene encoding delta(1)-pyrroline-5-carboxylate synthase, Hum Mol Genet 9, 2853-2858.

[22] Baumgartner MR, Rabier D, Nassogne MC, Dufier JL, Padovani JP, Kamoun P, *et al.* (2005) Delta1-pyrroline-5-carboxylate synthase deficiency: neurodegeneration, cataracts and connective tissue manifestations combined with hyperammonaemia and reduced ornithine, citrulline, arginine and proline, Eur J Pediatr 164, 31-36.

[23] Dixit SN, Seyer JM, & Kang AH (1977) Covalent structure of collagen: amino-acid sequence of chymotryptic peptides from the carboxyl-terminal region of alpha2-CB3 of chick-skin collagen, Eur J Biochem 81, 599-607.

[24] Stallings-Mann M & Radisky D (2007) Matrix metalloproteinase-induced malignancy in mammary epithelial cells, Cells Tissues Organs 185, 104-110.

[25] Deryugina EI & Quigley JP (2006) Matrix metalloproteinases and tumor metastasis, Cancer Metastasis Rev 25, 9-34.

[26] Kakkad SM, Solaiyappan M, O'Rourke B, Stasinopoulos I, Ackerstaff E, Raman V, *et al.* (2010) Hypoxic tumor microenvironments reduce collagen I fiber density, Neoplasia 12, 608-617.

[27] Pandhare J, Donald SP, Cooper SK, & Phang JM (2009) Regulation and function of proline oxidase under nutrient stress, J Cell Biochem 107, 759-768.

[28] Klionsky DJ (2007) Autophagy: from phenomenology to molecular understanding in less than a decade, Nat Rev Mol Cell Biol 8, 931-937.

[29] Mathew R, Karantza-Wadsworth V, & White E (2007) Role of autophagy in cancer, Nat Rev Cancer 7, 961-967.

[30] Liu W, Le A, Hancock C, Lane AN, Dang CV, Fan TW, *et al.* (2012) Reprogramming of proline and glutamine metabolism contributes to the proliferative and metabolic responses regulated by oncogenic transcription factor c-MYC, Proc Natl Acad Sci U S A 109, 8983-8988.

[31] Polyak K, Xia Y, Zweier JL, Kinzler KW, & Vogelstein B (1997) A model for p53-induced apoptosis, Nature 389, 300-305.

[32] Rivera A & Maxwell SA (2005) The p53-induced gene-6 (proline oxidase) mediates apoptosis through a calcineurin-dependent pathway, J Biol Chem 280, 29346-29354.

[33] Donald SP, Sun XY, Hu CA, Yu J, Mei JM, Valle D, *et al.* (2001) Proline oxidase, encoded by p53-induced gene-6, catalyzes the generation of proline-dependent reactive oxygen species, Cancer Res 61, 1810-1815.

[34] Simon HU, Haj-Yehia A, & Levi-Schaffer F (2000) Role of reactive oxygen species (ROS) in apoptosis induction, Apoptosis 5, 415-418.

[35] Hu CA, Donald SP, Yu J, Lin WW, Liu Z, Steel G, *et al.* (2007) Overexpression of proline oxidase induces proline-dependent and mitochondria-mediated apoptosis, Mol Cell Biochem 295, 85-92.

[36] Liu Y, Borchert GL, Surazynski A, Hu CA, & Phang JM (2006) Proline oxidase activates both intrinsic and extrinsic pathways for apoptosis: the role of ROS/superoxides, NFAT and MEK/ERK signaling, Oncogene 25, 5640-5647.

[37] Willson TM, Brown PJ, Sternbach DD, & Henke BR (2000) The PPARs: from orphan receptors to drug discovery, J Med Chem 43, 527-550.

[38] Robbins GT & Nie D (2012) PPAR gamma, bioactive lipids, and cancer progression, Front Biosci 17, 1816-1834.

[39] Reka AK, Goswami MT, Krishnapuram R, Standiford TJ, & Keshamouni VG (2011) Molecular cross-regulation between PPAR-gamma and other signaling pathways: implications for lung cancer therapy, Lung Cancer 72, 154-159.

[40] Phang JM, Pandhare J, Zabirnyk O, & Liu Y (2008) PPARgamma and Proline Oxidase in Cancer, PPAR Res 2008, 542694.

[41] Pandhare J, Cooper SK, & Phang JM (2006) Proline oxidase, a proapoptotic gene, is induced by troglitazone: evidence for both peroxisome proliferator-activated receptor gamma-dependent and -independent mechanisms, J Biol Chem 281, 2044-2052.

[42] Kim KY, Ahn JH, & Cheon HG (2007) Apoptotic action of peroxisome proliferator-activated receptor-gamma activation in human non small-cell lung cancer is mediated via proline oxidase-induced reactive oxygen species formation, Mol Pharmacol 72, 674-685.

[43] Liu W, Glunde K, Bhujwalla ZM, Raman V, Sharma A, & Phang JM (2012) Proline oxidase promotes tumor cell survival in hypoxic tumor microenvironments, Cancer Res 72, 3677-3686.

[44] Zabirnyk O, Liu W, Khalil S, Sharma A, & Phang JM (2010) Oxidized low-density lipoproteins upregulate proline oxidase to initiate ROS-dependent autophagy, Carcinogenesis 31, 446-454.

[45] Smith ML & Kumar MA (2010) The "Two faces" of Tumor Suppressor p53-revisited, Mol Cell Pharmacol 2, 117-119.

[46] Liu Y, Borchert GL, Donald SP, Diwan BA, Anver M, & Phang JM (2009) Proline Oxidase Functions as a Mitochondrial Tumor Suppressor in Human Cancers, Cancer Res 69, 6414-6422.

[47] Liu Y, Borchert GL, Surazynski A, & Phang JM (2008) Proline oxidase, a p53-induced gene, targets COX-2/PGE2 signaling to induce apoptosis and inhibit tumor growth in colorectal cancers, Oncogene 27, 6729-6737.

[48] Greenhough A, Smartt HJ, Moore AE, Roberts HR, Williams AC, Paraskeva C, *et al.* (2009) The COX-2/PGE2 pathway: key roles in the hallmarks of cancer and adaptation to the tumour microenvironment, Carcinogenesis 30, 377-386.

[49] Brown JR & DuBois RN (2004) Cyclooxygenase as a target in lung cancer, Clin Cancer Res 10, 4266s-4269s.

[50] Arun B & Goss P (2004) The role of COX-2 inhibition in breast cancer treatment and prevention, Semin Oncol 31, 22-29.

[51] Henson ES & Gibson SB (2006) Surviving cell death through epidermal growth factor (EGF) signal transduction pathways: implications for cancer therapy, Cell Signal 18, 2089-2097.

[52] Yao H, Ashihara E, & Maekawa T (2011) Targeting the Wnt/beta-catenin signaling pathway in human cancers, Expert Opin Ther Targets 15, 873-887.

[53] Zhu W, Chen Y, & Dutta A (2004) Rereplication by depletion of geminin is seen regardless of p53 status and activates a G2/M checkpoint, Mol Cell Biol 24, 7140-7150.

[54] Stark GR & Taylor WR (2006) Control of the G2/M transition, Mol Biotechnol 32, 227-248.

[55] Liebermann DA & Hoffman B (2008) Gadd45 in stress signaling, J Mol Signal 3, 15.

[56] Gottlieb E & Tomlinson IP (2005) Mitochondrial tumour suppressors: a genetic and biochemical update, Nat Rev Cancer 5, 857-866.

[57] Yamakuchi M, Lotterman CD, Bao C, Hruban RH, Karim B, Mendell JT, *et al.* (2010) P53-induced microRNA-107 inhibits HIF-1 and tumor angiogenesis, Proc Natl Acad Sci U S A 107, 6334-6339.

[58] Verma A (2006) Oxygen-sensing in tumors, Curr Opin Clin Nutr Metab Care 9, 366-378.

[59] Hewitson KS, Lienard BM, McDonough MA, Clifton IJ, Butler D, Soares AS, *et al.* (2007) Structural and mechanistic studies on the inhibition of the hypoxia-inducible transcription factor hydroxylases by tricarboxylic acid cycle intermediates, J Biol Chem 282, 3293-3301.

[60] Koivunen P, Hirsila M, Remes AM, Hassinen IE, Kivirikko KI, & Myllyharju J (2007) Inhibition of hypoxia-inducible factor (HIF) hydroxylases by citric acid cycle intermediates: possible links between cell metabolism and stabilization of HIF, J Biol Chem 282, 4524-4532.

[61] Lu H, Dalgard CL, Mohyeldin A, McFate T, Tait AS, & Verma A (2005) Reversible inactivation of HIF-1 prolyl hydroxylases allows cell metabolism to control basal HIF-1, J Biol Chem 280, 41928-41939.

[62] Liu W, Zabirnyk O, Wang H, Shiao YH, Nickerson ML, Khalil S, *et al.* (2010) miR-23b targets proline oxidase, a novel tumor suppressor protein in renal cancer, Oncogene 29, 4914-4924.

[63] Lee RC, Feinbaum RL, & Ambros V (1993) The C. elegans heterochronic gene lin-4 encodes small RNAs with antisense complementarity to lin-14, Cell 75, 843-854.

[64] Wightman B, Ha I, & Ruvkun G (1993) Posttranscriptional regulation of the heterochronic gene lin-14 by lin-4 mediates temporal pattern formation in C. elegans, Cell 75, 855-862.

[65] Reinhart BJ, Slack FJ, Basson M, Pasquinelli AE, Bettinger JC, Rougvie AE, *et al.* (2000) The 21-nucleotide let-7 RNA regulates developmental timing in Caenorhabditis elegans, Nature 403, 901-906.

[66] Lee Y, Kim M, Han J, Yeom KH, Lee S, Baek SH, *et al.* (2004) MicroRNA genes are transcribed by RNA polymerase II, EMBO J 23, 4051-4060.

[67] Lee Y, Ahn C, Han J, Choi H, Kim J, Yim J, *et al.* (2003) The nuclear RNase III Drosha initiates microRNA processing, Nature 425, 415-419.

[68] Denli AM, Tops BB, Plasterk RH, Ketting RF, & Hannon GJ (2004) Processing of primary microRNAs by the Microprocessor complex, Nature 432, 231-235.

[69] Yi R, Qin Y, Macara IG, & Cullen BR (2003) Exportin-5 mediates the nuclear export of pre-microRNAs and short hairpin RNAs, Genes Dev 17, 3011-3016.

[70] Bohnsack MT, Czaplinski K, & Gorlich D (2004) Exportin 5 is a RanGTP-dependent dsRNA-binding protein that mediates nuclear export of pre-miRNAs, RNA 10, 185-191.

[71] Lund E, Guttinger S, Calado A, Dahlberg JE, & Kutay U (2004) Nuclear export of microRNA precursors, Science 303, 95-98.

[72] Lund E & Dahlberg JE (2006) Substrate selectivity of exportin 5 and Dicer in the biogenesis of microRNAs, Cold Spring Harb Symp Quant Biol 71, 59-66.

[73] Khvorova A, Reynolds A, & Jayasena SD (2003) Functional siRNAs and miRNAs exhibit strand bias, Cell 115, 209-216.

[74] Schwarz DS, Hutvagner G, Du T, Xu Z, Aronin N, & Zamore PD (2003) Asymmetry in the assembly of the RNAi enzyme complex, Cell 115, 199-208.

[75] Lin SL, Chang D, & Ying SY (2005) Asymmetry of intronic pre-miRNA structures in functional RISC assembly, Gene 356, 32-38.

[76] Kim S, Lee UJ, Kim MN, Lee EJ, Kim JY, Lee MY, *et al.* (2008) MicroRNA miR-199a* regulates the MET proto-oncogene and the downstream extracellular signal-regulated kinase 2 (ERK2), J Biol Chem 283, 18158-18166.

[77] Nass D, Rosenwald S, Meiri E, Gilad S, Tabibian-Keissar H, Schlosberg A, *et al.* (2009) MiR-92b and miR-9/9* are specifically expressed in brain primary tumors and can be used to differentiate primary from metastatic brain tumors, Brain Pathol 19, 375-383.

[78] Okamura K, Chung WJ, & Lai EC (2008) The long and short of inverted repeat genes in animals: microRNAs, mirtrons and hairpin RNAs, Cell Cycle 7, 2840-2845.

[79] Carmell MA, Xuan Z, Zhang MQ, & Hannon GJ (2002) The Argonaute family: tentacles that reach into RNAi, developmental control, stem cell maintenance, and tumorigenesis, Genes Dev 16, 2733-2742.

[80] Song JJ, Liu J, Tolia NH, Schneiderman J, Smith SK, Martienssen RA, *et al.* (2003) The crystal structure of the Argonaute2 PAZ domain reveals an RNA binding motif in RNAi effector complexes, Nat Struct Biol 10, 1026-1032.

[81] Ma JB, Ye K, & Patel DJ (2004) Structural basis for overhang-specific small interfering RNA recognition by the PAZ domain, Nature 429, 318-322.

[82] Lingel A & Sattler M (2005) Novel modes of protein-RNA recognition in the RNAi pathway, Curr Opin Struct Biol 15, 107-115.

[83] Okamura K, Ishizuka A, Siomi H, & Siomi MC (2004) Distinct roles for Argonaute proteins in small RNA-directed RNA cleavage pathways, Genes Dev 18, 1655-1666.

[84] Liu J, Carmell MA, Rivas FV, Marsden CG, Thomson JM, Song JJ, *et al.* (2004) Argonaute2 is the catalytic engine of mammalian RNAi, Science 305, 1437-1441.

[85] Meister G, Landthaler M, Patkaniowska A, Dorsett Y, Teng G, & Tuschl T (2004) Human Argonaute2 mediates RNA cleavage targeted by miRNAs and siRNAs, Mol Cell 15, 185-197.

[86] van Kouwenhove M, Kedde M, & Agami R (2011) MicroRNA regulation by RNA-binding proteins and its implications for cancer, Nat Rev Cancer 11, 644-656.

[87] Melo SA, Ropero S, Moutinho C, Aaltonen LA, Yamamoto H, Calin GA, *et al.* (2009) A TARBP2 mutation in human cancer impairs microRNA processing and DICER1 function, Nat Genet 41, 365-370.

[88] Hill DA, Ivanovich J, Priest JR, Gurnett CA, Dehner LP, Desruisseau D, *et al.* (2009) DICER1 mutations in familial pleuropulmonary blastoma, Science 325, 965.

[89] MacRae IJ, Ma E, Zhou M, Robinson CV, & Doudna JA (2008) In vitro reconstitution of the human RISC-loading complex, Proc Natl Acad Sci U S A 105, 512-517.

[90] Murchison EP & Hannon GJ (2004) miRNAs on the move: miRNA biogenesis and the RNAi machinery, Curr Opin Cell Biol 16, 223-229.

[91] Mourelatos Z, Dostie J, Paushkin S, Sharma A, Charroux B, Abel L, *et al.* (2002) miRNPs: a novel class of ribonucleoproteins containing numerous microRNAs, Genes Dev 16, 720-728.

[92] Caudy AA, Myers M, Hannon GJ, & Hammond SM (2002) Fragile X-related protein and VIG associate with the RNA interference machinery, Genes Dev 16, 2491-2496.

[93] Winter J & Diederichs S (2011) Argonaute proteins regulate microRNA stability: Increased microRNA abundance by Argonaute proteins is due to microRNA stabilization, RNA Biol 8, 1149-1157.

[94] Diederichs S & Haber DA (2007) Dual role for argonautes in microRNA processing and posttranscriptional regulation of microRNA expression, Cell 131, 1097-1108.

[95] O'Carroll D, Mecklenbrauker I, Das PP, Santana A, Koenig U, Enright AJ, *et al.* (2007) A Slicer-independent role for Argonaute 2 in hematopoiesis and the microRNA pathway, Genes Dev 21, 1999-2004.

[96] Zhang X, Graves PR, & Zeng Y (2009) Stable Argonaute2 overexpression differentially regulates microRNA production, Biochim Biophys Acta 1789, 153-159.

[97] Kai ZS & Pasquinelli AE (2010) MicroRNA assassins: factors that regulate the disappearance of miRNAs, Nat Struct Mol Biol 17, 5-10.

[98] Azuma-Mukai A, Oguri H, Mituyama T, Qian ZR, Asai K, Siomi H, *et al.* (2008) Characterization of endogenous human Argonautes and their miRNA partners in RNA silencing, Proc Natl Acad Sci U S A 105, 7964-7969.

[99] Yu B, Yang Z, Li J, Minakhina S, Yang M, Padgett RW, *et al.* (2005) Methylation as a crucial step in plant microRNA biogenesis, Science 307, 932-935.

[100] Li J, Yang Z, Yu B, Liu J, & Chen X (2005) Methylation protects miRNAs and siRNAs from a 3'-end uridylation activity in Arabidopsis, Curr Biol 15, 1501-1507.

[101] Landgraf P, Rusu M, Sheridan R, Sewer A, Iovino N, Aravin A, *et al.* (2007) A mammalian microRNA expression atlas based on small RNA library sequencing, Cell 129, 1401-1414.

[102] Lu S, Sun YH, & Chiang VL (2009) Adenylation of plant miRNAs, Nucleic Acids Res 37, 1878-1885.

[103] Reid JG, Nagaraja AK, Lynn FC, Drabek RB, Muzny DM, Shaw CA, *et al.* (2008) Mouse let-7 miRNA populations exhibit RNA editing that is constrained in the 5'-seed/ cleavage/anchor regions and stabilize predicted mmu-let-7a:mRNA duplexes, Genome Res 18, 1571-1581.

[104] Katoh T, Sakaguchi Y, Miyauchi K, Suzuki T, Kashiwabara S, & Baba T (2009) Selective stabilization of mammalian microRNAs by 3' adenylation mediated by the cytoplasmic poly(A) polymerase GLD-2, Genes Dev 23, 433-438.

[105] Valencia-Sanchez MA, Liu J, Hannon GJ, & Parker R (2006) Control of translation and mRNA degradation by miRNAs and siRNAs, Genes Dev 20, 515-524.

[106] Billeter AT, Druen D, Kanaan ZM, & Polk HC, Jr. (2012) MicroRNAs: new helpers for surgeons?, Surgery 151, 1-5.

[107] Lewis BP, Burge CB, & Bartel DP (2005) Conserved seed pairing, often flanked by adenosines, indicates that thousands of human genes are microRNA targets, Cell 120, 15-20.

[108] Mallory AC, Reinhart BJ, Jones-Rhoades MW, Tang G, Zamore PD, Barton MK, *et al.* (2004) MicroRNA control of PHABULOSA in leaf development: importance of pairing to the microRNA 5' region, EMBO J 23, 3356-3364.

[109] Yekta S, Shih IH, & Bartel DP (2004) MicroRNA-directed cleavage of HOXB8 mRNA, Science 304, 594-596.

[110] Bartel DP (2004) MicroRNAs: genomics, biogenesis, mechanism, and function, Cell 116, 281-297.

[111] Pillai RS, Bhattacharyya SN, Artus CG, Zoller T, Cougot N, Basyuk E, *et al.* (2005) Inhibition of translational initiation by Let-7 MicroRNA in human cells, Science 309, 1573-1576.

[112] Cimmino A, Calin GA, Fabbri M, Iorio MV, Ferracin M, Shimizu M, *et al.* (2005) miR-15 and miR-16 induce apoptosis by targeting BCL2, Proc Natl Acad Sci U S A 102, 13944-13949.

[113] Williams AE (2008) Functional aspects of animal microRNAs, Cell Mol Life Sci 65, 545-562.

[114] Zeng Y, Yi R, & Cullen BR (2003) MicroRNAs and small interfering RNAs can inhibit mRNA expression by similar mechanisms, Proc Natl Acad Sci U S A 100, 9779-9784.

[115] Kiriakidou M, Nelson PT, Kouranov A, Fitziev P, Bouyioukos C, Mourelatos Z, *et al.* (2004) A combined computational-experimental approach predicts human microRNA targets, Genes Dev 18, 1165-1178.

[116] Bartel DP & Chen CZ (2004) Micromanagers of gene expression: the potentially widespread influence of metazoan microRNAs, Nat Rev Genet 5, 396-400.

[117] Eulalio A, Huntzinger E, & Izaurralde E (2008) GW182 interaction with Argonaute is essential for miRNA-mediated translational repression and mRNA decay, Nat Struct Mol Biol 15, 346-353.

[118] Behm-Ansmant I, Rehwinkel J, & Izaurralde E (2006) MicroRNAs silence gene expression by repressing protein expression and/or by promoting mRNA decay, Cold Spring Harb Symp Quant Biol 71, 523-530.

[119] Miranda KC, Huynh T, Tay Y, Ang YS, Tam WL, Thomson AM, *et al.* (2006) A pattern-based method for the identification of MicroRNA binding sites and their corresponding heteroduplexes, Cell 126, 1203-1217.

[120] Calin GA, Dumitru CD, Shimizu M, Bichi R, Zupo S, Noch E, *et al.* (2002) Frequent deletions and down-regulation of micro- RNA genes miR15 and miR16 at 13q14 in chronic lymphocytic leukemia, Proc Natl Acad Sci U S A 99, 15524-15529.
[121] Caldas C & Brenton JD (2005) Sizing up miRNAs as cancer genes, Nat Med 11, 712-714.
[122] Calin GA & Croce CM (2006) MicroRNAs and chromosomal abnormalities in cancer cells, Oncogene 25, 6202-6210.
[123] Lu J, Getz G, Miska EA, Alvarez-Saavedra E, Lamb J, Peck D, *et al.* (2005) MicroRNA expression profiles classify human cancers, Nature 435, 834-838.
[124] Sandhu S & Garzon R (2011) Potential applications of microRNAs in cancer diagnosis, prognosis, and treatment, Semin Oncol 38, 781-787.
[125] Croce CM (2009) Causes and consequences of microRNA dysregulation in cancer, Nat Rev Genet 10, 704-714.
[126] Nicoloso MS, Spizzo R, Shimizu M, Rossi S, & Calin GA (2009) MicroRNAs--the micro steering wheel of tumour metastases, Nat Rev Cancer 9, 293-302.
[127] Lujambio A & Lowe SW (2012) The microcosmos of cancer, Nature 482, 347-355.
[128] Volinia S, Calin GA, Liu CG, Ambs S, Cimmino A, Petrocca F, *et al.* (2006) A microRNA expression signature of human solid tumors defines cancer gene targets, Proc Natl Acad Sci U S A 103, 2257-2261.
[129] Xiao C, Srinivasan L, Calado DP, Patterson HC, Zhang B, Wang J, *et al.* (2008) Lymphoproliferative disease and autoimmunity in mice with increased miR-17-92 expression in lymphocytes, Nat Immunol 9, 405-414.
[130] Ventura A, Young AG, Winslow MM, Lintault L, Meissner A, Erkeland SJ, *et al.* (2008) Targeted deletion reveals essential and overlapping functions of the miR-17 through 92 family of miRNA clusters, Cell 132, 875-886.
[131] He L, Thomson JM, Hemann MT, Hernando-Monge E, Mu D, Goodson S, *et al.* (2005) A microRNA polycistron as a potential human oncogene, Nature 435, 828-833.
[132] Diosdado B, van de Wiel MA, Terhaar Sive Droste JS, Mongera S, Postma C, Meijerink WJ, *et al.* (2009) MiR-17-92 cluster is associated with 13q gain and c-myc expression during colorectal adenoma to adenocarcinoma progression, Br J Cancer 101, 707-714.
[133] Mu P, Han YC, Betel D, Yao E, Squatrito M, Ogrodowski P, *et al.* (2009) Genetic dissection of the miR-17~92 cluster of microRNAs in Myc-induced B-cell lymphomas, Genes Dev 23, 2806-2811.
[134] Petrocca F, Visone R, Onelli MR, Shah MH, Nicoloso MS, de Martino I, *et al.* (2008) E2F1-regulated microRNAs impair TGFbeta-dependent cell-cycle arrest and apoptosis in gastric cancer, Cancer Cell 13, 272-286.
[135] Mendell JT (2008) miRiad roles for the miR-17-92 cluster in development and disease, Cell 133, 217-222.
[136] Garofalo M, Di Leva G, Romano G, Nuovo G, Suh SS, Ngankeu A, *et al.* (2009) miR-221&222 regulate TRAIL resistance and enhance tumorigenicity through PTEN and TIMP3 downregulation, Cancer Cell 16, 498-509.

[137] Di Leva G, Gasparini P, Piovan C, Ngankeu A, Garofalo M, Taccioli C, *et al.* (2010) MicroRNA cluster 221-222 and estrogen receptor alpha interactions in breast cancer, J Natl Cancer Inst 102, 706-721.

[138] Hu W, Chan CS, Wu R, Zhang C, Sun Y, Song JS, *et al.* (2010) Negative regulation of tumor suppressor p53 by microRNA miR-504, Mol Cell 38, 689-699.

[139] Roush S & Slack FJ (2008) The let-7 family of microRNAs, Trends Cell Biol 18, 505-516.

[140] Bueno MJ, Gomez de Cedron M, Gomez-Lopez G, Perez de Castro I, Di Lisio L, Montes-Moreno S, *et al.* (2011) Combinatorial effects of microRNAs to suppress the Myc oncogenic pathway, Blood 117, 6255-6266.

[141] Calin GA, Cimmino A, Fabbri M, Ferracin M, Wojcik SE, Shimizu M, *et al.* (2008) MiR-15a and miR-16-1 cluster functions in human leukemia, Proc Natl Acad Sci U S A 105, 5166-5171.

[142] Bonci D, Coppola V, Musumeci M, Addario A, Giuffrida R, Memeo L, *et al.* (2008) The miR-15a-miR-16-1 cluster controls prostate cancer by targeting multiple oncogenic activities, Nat Med 14, 1271-1277.

[143] Kota J, Chivukula RR, O'Donnell KA, Wentzel EA, Montgomery CL, Hwang HW, *et al.* (2009) Therapeutic microRNA delivery suppresses tumorigenesis in a murine liver cancer model, Cell 137, 1005-1017.

[144] Garzon R, Marcucci G, & Croce CM (2010) Targeting microRNAs in cancer: rationale, strategies and challenges, Nat Rev Drug Discov 9, 775-789.

[145] Dang CV (1999) c-Myc target genes involved in cell growth, apoptosis, and metabolism, Mol Cell Biol 19, 1-11.

[146] Eilers M & Eisenman RN (2008) Myc's broad reach, Genes Dev 22, 2755-2766.

[147] Dang CV, Le A, & Gao P (2009) MYC-induced cancer cell energy metabolism and therapeutic opportunities, Clin Cancer Res 15, 6479-6483.

[148] Dews M, Homayouni A, Yu D, Murphy D, Sevignani C, Wentzel E, *et al.* (2006) Augmentation of tumor angiogenesis by a Myc-activated microRNA cluster, Nat Genet 38, 1060-1065.

[149] O'Donnell KA, Wentzel EA, Zeller KI, Dang CV, & Mendell JT (2005) c-Myc-regulated microRNAs modulate E2F1 expression, Nature 435, 839-843.

[150] Ma L, Young J, Prabhala H, Pan E, Mestdagh P, Muth D, *et al.* (2010) miR-9, a MYC/MYCN-activated microRNA, regulates E-cadherin and cancer metastasis, Nat Cell Biol 12, 247-256.

[151] Chang TC, Yu D, Lee YS, Wentzel EA, Arking DE, West KM, *et al.* (2008) Widespread microRNA repression by Myc contributes to tumorigenesis, Nat Genet 40, 43-50.

[152] Bui TV & Mendell JT (2010) Myc: Maestro of MicroRNAs, Genes Cancer 1, 568-575.

[153] Klein U, Lia M, Crespo M, Siegel R, Shen Q, Mo T, *et al.* (2010) The DLEU2/miR-15a/16-1 cluster controls B cell proliferation and its deletion leads to chronic lymphocytic leukemia, Cancer Cell 17, 28-40.

[154] Cairo S, Wang Y, de Reynies A, Duroure K, Dahan J, Redon MJ, *et al.* (2010) Stem cell-like micro-RNA signature driven by Myc in aggressive liver cancer, Proc Natl Acad Sci U S A 107, 20471-20476.

[155] Linsley PS, Schelter J, Burchard J, Kibukawa M, Martin MM, Bartz SR, *et al.* (2007) Transcripts targeted by the microRNA-16 family cooperatively regulate cell cycle progression, Mol Cell Biol 27, 2240-2252.

[156] Chang TC, Zeitels LR, Hwang HW, Chivukula RR, Wentzel EA, Dews M, *et al.* (2009) Lin-28B transactivation is necessary for Myc-mediated let-7 repression and proliferation, Proc Natl Acad Sci U S A 106, 3384-3389.

[157] Newman MA, Thomson JM, & Hammond SM (2008) Lin-28 interaction with the Let-7 precursor loop mediates regulated microRNA processing, RNA 14, 1539-1549.

[158] Hagan JP, Piskounova E, & Gregory RI (2009) Lin28 recruits the TUTase Zcchc11 to inhibit let-7 maturation in mouse embryonic stem cells, Nat Struct Mol Biol 16, 1021-1025.

[159] Heo I, Joo C, Kim YK, Ha M, Yoon MJ, Cho J, *et al.* (2009) TUT4 in concert with Lin28 suppresses microRNA biogenesis through pre-microRNA uridylation, Cell 138, 696-708.

[160] Feng Z, Zhang C, Wu R, & Hu W (2011) Tumor suppressor p53 meets microRNAs, J Mol Cell Biol 3, 44-50.

[161] He L, He X, Lim LP, de Stanchina E, Xuan Z, Liang Y, *et al.* (2007) A microRNA component of the p53 tumour suppressor network, Nature 447, 1130-1134.

[162] Raver-Shapira N, Marciano E, Meiri E, Spector Y, Rosenfeld N, Moskovits N, *et al.* (2007) Transcriptional activation of miR-34a contributes to p53-mediated apoptosis, Mol Cell 26, 731-743.

[163] Jin L, Hu WL, Jiang CC, Wang JX, Han CC, Chu P, *et al.* (2011) MicroRNA-149*, a p53-responsive microRNA, functions as an oncogenic regulator in human melanoma, Proc Natl Acad Sci U S A 108, 15840-15845.

[164] Sachdeva M, Zhu S, Wu F, Wu H, Walia V, Kumar S, *et al.* (2009) p53 represses c-Myc through induction of the tumor suppressor miR-145, Proc Natl Acad Sci U S A 106, 3207-3212.

[165] Georges SA, Biery MC, Kim SY, Schelter JM, Guo J, Chang AN, *et al.* (2008) Coordinated regulation of cell cycle transcripts by p53-Inducible microRNAs, miR-192 and miR-215, Cancer Res 68, 10105-10112.

[166] Suzuki HI, Yamagata K, Sugimoto K, Iwamoto T, Kato S, & Miyazono K (2009) Modulation of microRNA processing by p53, Nature 460, 529-533.

[167] Kulshreshtha R, Ferracin M, Wojcik SE, Garzon R, Alder H, Agosto-Perez FJ, *et al.* (2007) A microRNA signature of hypoxia, Mol Cell Biol 27, 1859-1867.

[168] Mutharasan RK, Nagpal V, Ichikawa Y, & Ardehali H (2011) microRNA-210 is upregulated in hypoxic cardiomyocytes through Akt- and p53-dependent pathways and exerts cytoprotective effects, Am J Physiol Heart Circ Physiol 301, H1519-1530.

[169] Hu S, Huang M, Li Z, Jia F, Ghosh Z, Lijkwan MA, *et al.* (2010) MicroRNA-210 as a novel therapy for treatment of ischemic heart disease, Circulation 122, S124-131.

[170] Camps C, Buffa FM, Colella S, Moore J, Sotiriou C, Sheldon H, *et al.* (2008) hsa-miR-210 Is induced by hypoxia and is an independent prognostic factor in breast cancer, Clin Cancer Res 14, 1340-1348.

[171] Fasanaro P, D'Alessandra Y, Di Stefano V, Melchionna R, Romani S, Pompilio G, *et al.* (2008) MicroRNA-210 modulates endothelial cell response to hypoxia and inhibits the receptor tyrosine kinase ligand Ephrin-A3, J Biol Chem 283, 15878-15883.

[172] Kim HW, Haider HK, Jiang S, & Ashraf M (2009) Ischemic preconditioning augments survival of stem cells via miR-210 expression by targeting caspase-8-associated protein 2, J Biol Chem 284, 33161-33168.

[173] Zhang Z, Sun H, Dai H, Walsh RM, Imakura M, Schelter J, *et al.* (2009) MicroRNA miR-210 modulates cellular response to hypoxia through the MYC antagonist MNT, Cell Cycle 8, 2756-2768.

[174] Kent OA, Chivukula RR, Mullendore M, Wentzel EA, Feldmann G, Lee KH, *et al.* (2010) Repression of the miR-143/145 cluster by oncogenic Ras initiates a tumor-promoting feed-forward pathway, Genes Dev 24, 2754-2759.

[175] Calin GA, Sevignani C, Dumitru CD, Hyslop T, Noch E, Yendamuri S, *et al.* (2004) Human microRNA genes are frequently located at fragile sites and genomic regions involved in cancers, Proc Natl Acad Sci U S A 101, 2999-3004.

[176] Zhang L, Huang J, Yang N, Greshock J, Megraw MS, Giannakakis A, *et al.* (2006) microRNAs exhibit high frequency genomic alterations in human cancer, Proc Natl Acad Sci U S A 103, 9136-9141.

[177] Mayr C, Hemann MT, & Bartel DP (2007) Disrupting the pairing between let-7 and Hmga2 enhances oncogenic transformation, Science 315, 1576-1579.

[178] Veronese A, Visone R, Consiglio J, Acunzo M, Lupini L, Kim T, *et al.* (2011) Mutated beta-catenin evades a microRNA-dependent regulatory loop, Proc Natl Acad Sci U S A 108, 4840-4845.

[179] Saito Y, Liang G, Egger G, Friedman JM, Chuang JC, Coetzee GA, *et al.* (2006) Specific activation of microRNA-127 with downregulation of the proto-oncogene BCL6 by chromatin-modifying drugs in human cancer cells, Cancer Cell 9, 435-443.

[180] Cao Q, Mani RS, Ateeq B, Dhanasekaran SM, Asangani IA, Prensner JR, *et al.* (2011) Coordinated regulation of polycomb group complexes through microRNAs in cancer, Cancer Cell 20, 187-199.

[181] Davalos V, Moutinho C, Villanueva A, Boque R, Silva P, Carneiro F, *et al.* (2011) Dynamic epigenetic regulation of the microRNA-200 family mediates epithelial and mesenchymal transitions in human tumorigenesis, Oncogene doi: 10.1038/onc.2011.383.

[182] Guo QM, Malek RL, Kim S, Chiao C, He M, Ruffy M, *et al.* (2000) Identification of c-myc responsive genes using rat cDNA microarray, Cancer Res 60, 5922-5928.

[183] Li Z, Van Calcar S, Qu C, Cavenee WK, Zhang MQ, & Ren B (2003) A global transcriptional regulatory role for c-Myc in Burkitt's lymphoma cells, Proc Natl Acad Sci U S A 100, 8164-8169.

[184] Maxwell SA & Rivera A (2003) Proline oxidase induces apoptosis in tumor cells, and its expression is frequently absent or reduced in renal carcinomas, J Biol Chem 278, 9784-9789.

[185] Kulshreshtha R, Davuluri RV, Calin GA, & Ivan M (2008) A microRNA component of the hypoxic response, Cell Death Differ 15, 667-671.

[186] Guimbellot JS, Erickson SW, Mehta T, Wen H, Page GP, Sorscher EJ, *et al.* (2009) Correlation of microRNA levels during hypoxia with predicted target mRNAs through genome-wide microarray analysis, BMC Med Genomics 2, 15.

[187] Zhang H, Gao P, Fukuda R, Kumar G, Krishnamachary B, Zeller KI, *et al.* (2007) HIF-1 inhibits mitochondrial biogenesis and cellular respiration in VHL-deficient renal cell carcinoma by repression of C-MYC activity, Cancer Cell 11, 407-420.

[188] Vafa O, Wade M, Kern S, Beeche M, Pandita TK, Hampton GM, *et al.* (2002) c-Myc can induce DNA damage, increase reactive oxygen species, and mitigate p53 function: a mechanism for oncogene-induced genetic instability, Mol Cell 9, 1031-1044.

[189] DeNicola GM, Karreth FA, Humpton TJ, Gopinathan A, Wei C, Frese K, *et al.* (2011) Oncogene-induced Nrf2 transcription promotes ROS detoxification and tumorigenesis, Nature 475, 106-109.

[190] Wonsey DR, Zeller KI, & Dang CV (2002) The c-Myc target gene PRDX3 is required for mitochondrial homeostasis and neoplastic transformation, Proc Natl Acad Sci U S A 99, 6649-6654.

[191] Fan TW, Tan JL, McKinney MM, & Lane AN (2011) Stable isotope resolved metabolomics analysis of ribonucleotide and RNA metabolism in human lung cancer cells Metabolomics doi:10.1007/s11306-011-0337-9.

[192] Le A, Lane AN, Hamaker M, Bose S, Gouw A, Barbi J, *et al.* (2012) Glucose-Independent Glutamine Metabolism via TCA Cycling for Proliferation and Survival in B Cells, Cell Metab 15, 110-121.

[193] Wang R, Dillon CP, Shi LZ, Milasta S, Carter R, Finkelstein D, *et al.* (2011) The transcription factor Myc controls metabolic reprogramming upon T lymphocyte activation, Immunity 35, 871-882.

Chapter 16

microRNA: New Players in Metastatic Process

Tiziana Triulzi, Marilena V. Iorio, Elda Tagliabue and Patrizia Casalini

Additional information is available at the end of the chapter

http://dx.doi.org/10.5772/55583

1. Introduction

In the last years new players have been revealed in cancer biology: microRNA (miRNAs or miRs) a class of small non coding RNAs (19-22 nts) able to regulate gene expression at post-transcriptional level, binding through partial sequence homology mainly the 3' UTR of target mRNAs, and causing block of translation and/or mRNA degradation.

miRNAs are generated by an endogenous transcript, they represent approximately 1% of the genome of different species, and each of them has hundreds of different conserved or non conserved targets: it has been estimated that about 30% of the genes are regulated by at least one miRNA. miRNA genes, expressed in several organisms, including *Homo Sapiens*, are highly conserved across different species [1].

This discovery resulted in a pattern shift in our understanding of gene regulation because miRNAs are now known to repress thousands of target genes and coordinate normal processes, including cellular proliferation, differentiation and apoptosis. They are highly specific for tissue and developmental stage, and play crucial functions in the regulation of important processes, such as development, and stress response. In the last few years, miRNAs have indeed taken their place in the complex circuitry of cell biology, revealing a key role as regulators of gene expression.

In 2002, Croce and colleagues first demonstrated that a miRNA cluster was frequently deleted or downregulated in chronic lymphocytic leukemia. This discovery suggested that non coding genes were contributing to the development of cancer, and paved the way for a closer investigation of miRNA loss or amplification in tumors.

miRNAs expression profiling has indeed provided evidence of the association of these tiny molecules with tumor development, progression and response to therapy, suggesting their possible use as diagnostic, prognostic and predictive biomarkers. It has been demonstrated that miRNAs can act either as oncogenes or tumor suppressors, and more recently it has been demonstrated that a miRNAs can exploit both functions according to the cellular context of their target genes. Another important issue concerns the role of miRNAs in regulating the interaction between cancer cells and the microenvironment with respect to neo-angiogenesis or tissue invasion and metastasis.

Outgrowths of disseminated metastases remain the primary cause of mortality in cancer patients, but the molecular and cellular mechanisms regulating metastatic spread remain largely unknown. Metastatic processes involve multiple steps, including detachment from primary tumors, crossing the basement membrane barriers and extracellular matrix, intravasation into the circulation, survival within the vasculature, extravasation into distant tissues, and finally, establishment of secondary tumors [2] . These processes rely on coordinated spatio-temporal expression of various genes and finely regulated protein products, which govern the ability of tumor cells to successfully complete the intricate task, and the pivotal role of miRNAs in metastasis has emerged only recently.

2. miRNAs biogenesis and mechanism of action

miRNAs are generated by endonucleolytic cleavage of hairpin precursor transcripts by Dicer ribonuclease (RNase) III–like proteins and can direct the cleavage of target transcripts by Argonaute RNAse H–like proteins in a sequence-specific manner. miRNAs can also inhibit translation of target mRNAs.

miRNAs are transcribed for the most part by RNA Polimerase II as long primary transcripts characterized by hairpin structures (pri-microRNAs), and part of them are transcribed as distinct transcriptional units. 50% of known miRNA genes are located nearby other microRNAs, supporting the hypothesis that clustered miRNAs, representing miRNA families which are commonly related in sequence and function, can be transcribed from their own promoters as polycistronic pri-microRNAs.

According to their genomic localization, microRNAs can be classified in:

a) exonic microRNAs located in non coding transcripts, b) intronic microRNAs located in non coding transcripts and microRNA located in protein-coding trancripts, c) mixed miRNA genes that can be assigned to one of the above groups depending on the given splicing pattern. Exonic microRNAs are transcribed within the pri-miR (up to 1 kb long) containing both the 5′-cap and the 3′-poly-A tail. The miRNAs localized within introns of protein-encoding or -non-encoding genes have been denominated "miRtrons". miRtrons are regulatory RNAs transcribed within the mRNA of the host gene generating a hairpin structure, recognized and cleaved by the spliceosome machinery without Drosha-mediated cleavage.

The initial step in pri-miRNA processing (Figure 1) is performed in the nucleus by the enzymatic activity of an RNAse III-type protein called Drosha. Drosha is a highly conserved 160 kDa protein containing two RNAse III domains and one double-strand RNA-binding domain. Drosha forms a huge complex, 500 kDa in *D. melanogaster* and 650 kDA in *H. sapiens*, known as Microprocessor complex, which generates a ~70-nucleotides precursor miRNA (pre-miRNA) and contains the co-factor Di George syndrome critical region 8 (DGCR8), also known as Pasha in *D. melanogaster* and *C. elegans*.

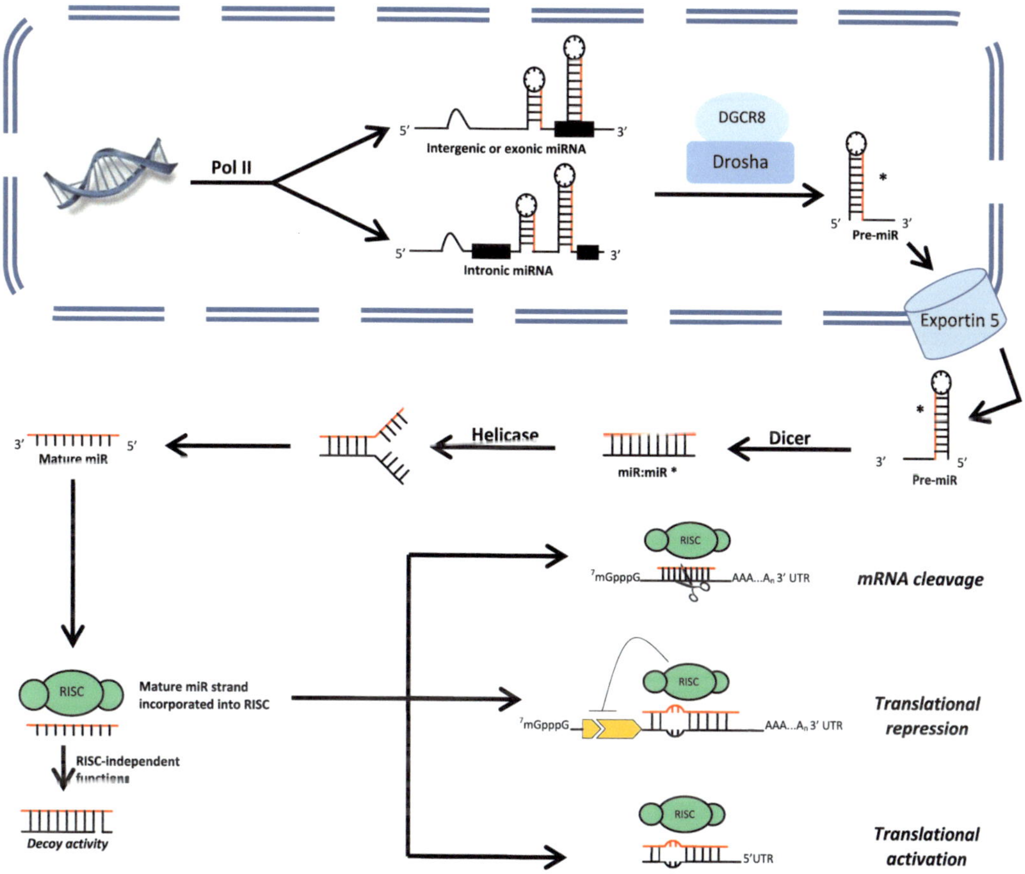

Figure 1. An overview of microRNAs biogenesis and mechanism of action.

The originated precursor molecules are then actively exported by a Ran-GTP and Exportin 5-mediated mechanism to the cytoplasm, where the second step of pre-miRNA processing (dicing) is mediated by the RNAse III Dicer (~200 kDa), which acts in complex with the transactivating response RNA-binding protein (TRBP), or PACT (also known as PRKRA), and Argonaute (AGO1-4), generating a dsRNA of approximately 22 nucleotides, named miR:miR*. This dsRNA includes the mature miRNA guide, and the complementary passenger strand, the miRNA* (star miRNA) (many publications refer to the two strand pair as miR-3p/miR-5p, referring to the direction of the functional miRNA). Whereas one of the two strands is selected as guide strand according to thermodynamic properties, the complementary one is usually subjected to degradation. The so called miRNA* was initially thought to be the strand subjected to degradation, instead more recent evidence suggests that it does not simply represent a non-functional bioproduct of miRNA biogenesis, but it can be selected as a functional strand and play significant biological roles [3] .

More in details, guided by the sequence complementarity between the small RNA and the target mRNA, miRNA-RISC-mediated gene inhibition is commonly divided into three processes: (i) site-specific cleavage, (ii) enhanced mRNA degradation and (iii) translational inhibition. The first process, commonly defined as RNA interference (RNAi) and restricted to miRNAs with a perfect or near-perfect match to the target RNA, is a very rare event in mammals, where it is carried out exclusively by Ago2. By contrast, the other two processes are more commonly associated with mismatched miRNA/target sequences, which is the most likely scenario in mammals. The combination of these two processes is commonly defined as a non-cleavage repression, and can be carried out by any of the four mammalian Ago proteins [4] . However, the exact mechanism through which miRNAs can impair translation is still debated.

Moreover, even though it is known that microRNAs mainly recognize complementary sequences in the 3′ untraslated regions (UTRs) of their target mRNAs, more recent studies have reported that they can also bind to the 5′UTR or the ORF [5-8] and, even more surprisingly, they can upregulate translation upon growth arrest conditions [9] .

Finally, whereas the 5′ end of the microRNA (the so called "seed site") has always been considered the most important for the binding to the mRNA, recently the target sites have been further divided into three main classes, according to grade and localization of the complementarity [10] : the dominant seed site targets (5′ seed-only), the 5′ dominant canonical seed site targets (5′ dominant) and the 3′ complementary seed site targets (3′ canonical).

Considering the different rules regulating the interaction between a microRNA and its target mRNA, it is not surprising that each miRNA has the potential to target a large number of genes [11-14]. Conversely, an estimated 60% of the mRNAs have one or more evolutionarily conserved sequences that are predicted to interact with miRNAs. Bioinformatical analysis predicts that the 3′ UTR of a single gene is frequently targeted by several different miRNAs [11] . Many of these predictions have been validated experimentally, suggesting that miRNAs might cooperate to regulate gene expression (a list of computational tools for miRNA target prediction is reported in Table 1).

name	website
miRNA map	http://mirnamap.mbc.nctu.edu.tw/
miRBASE	http://mirbase.org/
microRNA	http://www.microrna.org/microrna/home.do
coGemiR	http://www.cogemir.tigem.it/
miRGEN	http://www.diana.pcbi.upenn.edu/miRGen.html
deepBase	http://www.deepbase.sysu.edu.cn

Table 1. miRNA databases.

To complicate the already intricate scenario, it has been recently reported that miRNAs can bind to ribonucleoproteins in a seed sequence and a RISC-independent manner and then interfere with their RNA binding functions (decoy activity) [15] . Three studies have reported that miRNAs can also regulate gene expression at the transcriptional level by direct binding to the DNA [16-18].

Overall, these data show the complexity and widespread regulation of gene expression by miRNAs that should be taken into consideration when developing miRNA-based therapies.

3. Metastasis

The most deleterious effect of cancer is metastases development, indeed tumor metastasis is the primary cause of death in cancer patients. The ability to metastasize is a hallmark of malignant tumors [19] . Metastases represent the end point of a multi-step process that consists of local invasion through surrounding extracellular matrix and stromal cells, intravasation into the blood vessels, survival in the circulation, extravasation, and colonization of distant tissues [20]. Each step in this process represents a physiological barrier that must be overcome by the tumor cell to successfully metastasize. Malignant cells overcome these barriers through the accumulation of genetic and epigenetic changes, including modifications in microRNA expression profiles. Despite great improvement in the knowledge of metastasis biology, the molecular mechanisms which underlie this intricate process are still not completely understood.

Tumor cells can invade surrounding tissues as cohesive multicellular units or as individual cells, and individual cells can invade through the 'amoeboid invasion' or the 'mesenchymal invasion' programs [21] . Amoeboid movement depends mainly from Rho/ROCK expression, and is independent from adhesion and proteolytic degradation of ECM [22,23]. On the contrary, mesenchymal motility depends upon interaction of carcinoma cells with the extracellular matrix through integrin recruitment and upon pericellular ECM proteolysis of the moving cells. Cells that use this program to invade are characterized by an elongated and polarized morphology, achievable with an epithelial to mesenchymal transition (EMT). EMT, first described as typical of embryonic development, generates cells with mesenchymal features phenotypically similar to invading cells. The EMT transcriptional programme has been associated with activation of several key transcriptions factors, including Snail1 and Snail2 (Slug), Twist, ZEB-1-2, etc, which lead to the regulation of a series of proteins causing decrease of E-cadherin for disruption of adherent junctions, increase in N-cadherin and Met proto oncogene to drive motility, as well as increase in MMPs and urokinase–type plasminogen activator/urokinase–type plasminogen receptor (uPA/uPAR) proteolytic systems to degrade 3D barriers [24,25].

The overexpression of many of these EMT regulators have been shown to correlate with disease relapse and decreased survival in patients with breast, colorectal, and ovarian carcinomas, suggesting that the induction of EMT leads to more aggressive tumors and poorer clinical outcomes.

Once tumor cells have invaded local microenvironment, they should intravasate, survive in the circulation and extravasate at distant sites. To successfully perform these steps, they have to cross the pericyte and endothelial cell barriers that form the walls of microvessels. In order to overcome physical barriers which represent an obstacle to extravasation in tissues with low intrinsic microvessel permeability, primary tumors are capable of secreting factors that perturb these distant microenvironments and induce vascular hyperpermeability. The ability of the cancer cell to develop into a metastatic lesion at distant sites is the most limiting step in cancer metastasis formation. Indeed, the disseminated tumor cells may stay in a quiescent state for long time, probably due to incompatibilities with the foreign microenvironments that surround them [2]. Some have proposed that carcinoma cells can address the problem of an incompatible microenvironment at the metastatic site via the establishment of a "premetastatic niche" [26].

4. miRNAs and metastasis

Remarkably, a regulatory role for miRNAs in metastasis has been recognized, and the term "metastamir" has been coined by Welch and colleagues to refer to those regulatory miRNAs not just involved in tumorigenesis, but specific in the promotion or suppression of various steps of metastasis [27]. To date, microRNAs have mostly been found to influence the initial stages of metastasis, affecting cell migration and invasion (Figure 2). Although a particular miRNA that specifically regulates cancer cell intravasation and extravasation has not yet been identified, it is still believed that these steps may also be regulated by miRNAs.

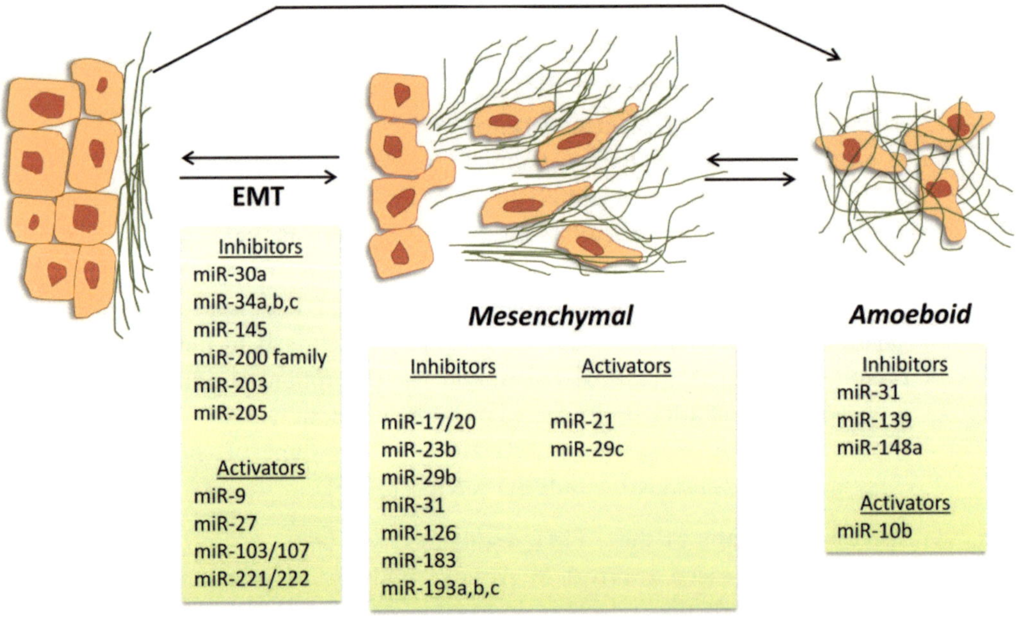

Figure 2. microRNAs implicated in the regulation of EMT and cell migration.

Several miRNAs have been found to regulate the EMT process, and the most well-known among them is the miR-200 family, which includes miR-200a, miR-200b, miR-200c, miR-141 and miR-429.

miR-200 family is recognized as a master regulator of the epithelial phenotype by post transcriptionally suppression of the expression of the ZEB1 and ZEB2 EMT-inducing transcription factors in breast [28] and gastric cancer [29]. Acting in the opposite direction, ZEB1 and ZEB2, which promote not only tumor cell dissemination, but also the tumor-initiating capacity, has been shown to transcriptionally repress miR-200 family members, thereby establishing a double negative feedback loop that causes the reinforcement of cells in either the mesenchymal or epithelial state [25]. This miR family, as others able to control epithelial–mesenchymal plasticity, is likely to also affect events at metastatic sites. Recently, the putative DNA methylation-associated inactivation of various miR-200 members has been described in cancer. miR-200 epigenetic silencing resulted to be not a static and fixed process, instead there can be a shift to hypermethylated or unmethylated 5'-CpG island status corresponding to the EMT and mesenchymal-epithelial-transition (MET) phenotypes, respectively. In fact, careful laser microdissection in human colon revealed that in normal colon mucosa crypts (epithelia) and stroma (mesenchyma) 5'-CpG island status are unmethylated and methylated at these loci, respectively, and that the colorectal tumors undergo selective miR-200 hypermethylation of their epithelial component. These findings indicate that the epigenetic silencing plasticity of the miR-200 family contributes to the evolving and adapting phenotypes of human tumors [30].

Unexpectedly, it was reported that overexpression of miR-200 enhances macroscopic metastases in mouse breast cancer models. These findings were surprising but provide yet another example of the opposing activities of some miRNAs [31]. miR-200 levels are indirectly downregulated by miR-103/107 that target Dicer, a key component of the miRNA processing machinery. Accordingly, miR-103/107 are associated with metastasis and poor outcome in human breast cancer [32].

The transcription factor ZEB1 can also repress the expression of stemness-inhibiting miR 203 [33] Recently, miR-203 was reported as a metastasis suppressor miRNA, targeting Slug [34] and Snail1 [35] and is often silenced in different malignancies including hepatocellular carcinoma, prostate cancer, oral cancer, breast cancer and hematopoietic malignancy Snail1 and Slug play a key role during the early step of EMT, activating expression of ZEB factors in a context-dependent manner. Functionally, ectopic expression of miR-203 in BT549 and MDA MB-231 breast cancer cell lines caused cell cycle arrest and apoptosis and inhibited cell invasion and migration *in vitro*. Thus the miR-203 and miR-200 feedback loops control cell plasticity in epithelial homeostasis. Snail1 is also regulated by miR-30a in non-small cell lung cancer (NSCLC), where it is dowmodulated [36].

Opposite to miR-200 family, miR-221/222 family promotes a poorly differentiated mesenchymal-like phenotype in breast cancer, and is highly expressed in triple negative breast cancers that basally expressed EMT markers. Increasing miR-221 or miR-222 can affect various characteristics associated with EMT, including increased invasive capacity,

[37,38], and anoikis resistance [39]. Forced expression of miR-221/222 in luminal breast cancer cells causes a decrease in E-cadherin and an increase in the mesenchymal marker vimentin [40]. Luminal cells expressing miR-221/222 gained a more mesenchymal morphology and had increased migratory and invasive capacity [41]. Furthermore, miR-221 and miR-222 can regulate angiogenesis, repressing the proliferative and angiogenic properties of c-Kit in endothelial cells [42]. In addition other miRNAs can manage EMT, such as the ZEB1- and ZEB2-suppressing miR-205 [28], which has also been shown to exert an oncosuppressive activity in breast cancer [43,44] prostate cancer [45] and melanoma [46]; and miR-27, which promotes EMT in gastric cancer cell directly targeting APC gene and activating the Wnt pathway [47].

Recently, the inhibition of EMT by p53 has been described as a new mode of tumor suppression which presumably prevents metastasis. p53 activation down-regulates Snail via induction of the miR-34a/b/c genes, which directly target Snail transcription factor. Ectopic miR-34a expression caused down-regulation of Slug and ZEB1, as well as the stemness factors BMI1, CD44, CD133, OLFM4 and c-MYC, thus provoking MET. Conversely, the transcription factors Snail and ZEB1 repress miR-34a and miR-34b/c expression [48]. Recently it has been described that miR-34 suppress also c-MET in hepatocellular carcinoma [49] and in osteosarcoma cells [50].

EMT is characterized by cadherin switching (from E-cadherin to N-cadherin), that correlates with a profound change in cell phenotype and behavior. miR-9, identified as a new "metastomiR" and activated by MYC and MYCN, directly targets CDH1, the E-cadherin-encoding messenger RNA, leading to increased cell motility and invasiveness, activation of β-catenin signaling and upregulation of VEGF. Moreover, overexpression of miR-9 in non-metastatic breast tumor cells enables these cells to form pulmonary micrometastases in mice, and in colorectal cancer cells it promotes cell motility [51]. Conversely, inhibition of miR-9 in highly malignant cells impairs metastasis formation [52].

N-cadherin (CDH2) was proved to be a direct target of miR-145 by Gao P and coworkers [53]. miR-145, suppressing N-cadherin protein translation and indirectly downregulating also its downstream effector matrix metallopeptidase 9 (MMP9), suppresses metastases. It has been reported that miR-145 exerts its anti metastatic role by directly targeting also the metastatic gene *mucin 1* [54] in breast cancer and VEGF in osteosarcoma cells [55]. Moreover, suppression of Mucin1 by miR-145 causes a reduction of β-catenin as well as the oncogenic Cadherin 11 [54]. Accordingly miR-145, acting as a metastasis suppressor, is stepwise downregulated in normal gastric mucosa, primary gastric cancers and their secondary metastases [53] , and in osteosarcoma in comparison to normal tissues [55].

Several miRNAs such as miR-34a [56], miR-373 and miR-520c [57] and mir-328 [58] have been reported to regulate the cell-surface glycoprotein encoding gene CD44 (cell surface receptor for hyaluronan). Cell lines with high CD44+/CD24− cell numbers are basal/mesenchymal or myoepithelial types and are more invasive than other cell lines [59]. miR-520/373 has been also reported to directly target TGFBR2 and to induce the suppression of Smad-dependent expression of the metastasis-promoting genes parathyroid hormone-related protein, plasminogen activator inhibitor-1 and angiopoietin-like 4, thus impairing tumor cell invasion, *in vitro* and *in vivo*. Remarkably, decreased expression of miR-520c correlated with lymph node metastasis specifically in ER negative breast tumors [60].

Recently Han M and coworkers [61] demonstrated that miR-21 regulates epithelial-mesenchymal transition phenotype and hypoxia-inducible factor-1α (HIF-1α) expression in sphere forming breast cancer stem cells (CSC). Indeed inhibition of miR-21 by antagomir led to reversal of EMT, down-expression of HIF-1α, as well as suppression of invasion and migration, which indicates a key role of miR-21 in regulating CSC-associated features.

EMT is a profound change in cell phenotype that causes immotile epithelial cells to acquire traits such as motility, invasiveness, anoikis and the ability to adapt to environmental changes to continue to invade successfully. Mesenchymal motility program is characterised by elongated and polarized cell morphology and depends upon ECM proteolysis of the moving cells and from integrin interaction with the extracellular matrix.

Urokinase, a serin protease, activating plasmin triggers a proteolysis cascade that, depending on the physiological environment, participates in extracellular matrix degradation. miR-193a/b overexpression in MDA-MB-231 and MDA-MB-435 breast carcinoma cells significantly reduced its direct target uPA protein amounts and inhibited cell invasion [62]. In an immunodeficient mouse model, miR-193b significantly inhibited the growth and dissemination of xenografted tumors [63]. The expression of miR-193b is downregulated in metastatic breast cancer, and this microRNA is in turn able to upregulate uPA expression and to contribute to the progression of breast cancer. Recently, miR-23b was reported to directly target uPA and c-MET and to decrease migration and proliferation of human hepatocellular carcinoma cells [64]. Plasminogen activation can be regulated also indirectly by mir-17/20 expression, which is usually downregulated in highly invasive breast cancer cell lines and node-positive breast cancer specimens [65]. microRNA17/20 directly repressed IL-8 by targeting its 3' UTR, and inhibited cytokeratin 8 via the cell cycle control protein cyclin D1, a secreted plasminogen activator. Indeed cell-conditioned medium from microRNA17/20-overexpressing non invasive breast cancer cell MCF7 was sufficient to inhibit MDA-MB-231 cell migration and invasion [65]. The invasion-related urokinase receptor is also indirectly regulated by a miRNA. Indeed, oncogenic miR-21, elevated in different tumor types, included colorectal cancer [66] melanoma and breast cancer [67], post-transcriptionally regulates PDCD4, that can suppress invasion and intravasation, at least in part by inhibiting expression of uPAR gene via the transcription factors Sp1/Sp3. Thus, miR-21 is able to enhance cancer cell intravasation, extravasation and metastasis in addition to cell proliferation.

The restoration in hepatocellular carcinoma cells of miR-122 that exerts some of its action via regulation of ADAM17 caused a dramatic reduction of *in vitro* migration, invasion, *in vivo* tumorigenesis, angiogenesis, and local invasion in the liver of nude mice [68]. Under the transcriptional control of HNF1A, HNF3A and HNF3B, miR-122 is specifically repressed in a subset of primary tumors that are characterized by poor prognosis [69].

ADAM9 is directly target by miR-126, which expression is reduced in invasive ductal adenocarcinoma (IDA) and pancreatic cancer cell lines. Re-expression of miR-126 and siRNA-based knockdown of ADAM9 in pancreatic cancer cells resulted in reduced cellular migration, invasion, and induction of epithelial marker E-cadherin [70]. It also directly regulates the adaptor protein Crk that binds to several tyrosine-phosphorylated proteins, inhibiting cell growth by inducing cell cycle arrest in G0/G1 phase, migration and invasion *in vitro* as well as tumorigenicity and metastasis *in vivo* in gastric cancer [71].

Matrix metalloproteinase-2 (MMP2), involved in matrix degradation and involved in angiogenesis, is directly regulated by miR-29b, whose down modulation promotes angiogenesis, invasion, and metastasis of hepatocellular carcinomas [72]. MMP2 was confirmed to be a miR-29b target apart from Mcl-1, COL1A1, and COL4A1 also in prostate cancer cells [73].

miR-29c-targeted genes identified in nasopharyngeal carcinomas (NPC) encode extracellular matrix proteins, including multiple collagens and Laminin $\gamma 1$, that are associated with tumor cell invasiveness in culture and increased metastasis in animal models and multiple human solid tumors as well as fibrillin SPARC [74]. Interestingly, introduction of miR-29c led to a reduced transcription of these genes in cultured cells, and the down-regulation of mir-29c level in NPC human cancer correlated with increase of target mRNAs, which could facilitate rapid matrix generation and renewal during tumor growth and the acquisition of tumor motility.

It was demonstrated that miR-183 targets ezrin, an intermediate between the plasma membrane and the actin cytoskeleton involved, together with radixin, in epithelial cell morphogenesis and adhesion [75], and may play a central role in the regulation of migration and metastasis in breast cancer [76], osteosarcoma [77] and lung cancer [78]. miR-183 is markedly down-regulated in osteosarcoma cells and tissues compared with matching normal bone tissues and its expression levels significantly correlated with lung metastasis as well as with local recurrence of osteosarcoma [77].

miR-223 is overexpressed in metastatic gastric cancer cells and stimulates non metastatic gastric cancer cells to migrate and to invade. Mechanistically, miR-223, induced by the transcription factor Twist, post transcriptionally downregulates EPB41L3 expression, thought to be involved in tethering the F-actin cytoskeleton to membrane proteins. Another functional downstream target of miR-223 is FBXW7, shown to have important roles in regulating the stability of multiple oncoprotein substrates, including Cyclin E, c-MYC, Notch, c-Jun, and Mcl-1. Overexpression of miR-223 is associated with poor metastasis-free survival in primary gastric carcinomas [79], with lymph node metastasis in gastric cancer, and poorer prognosis in oesophageal squamous cell carcinoma patients [80].

Cells can move also through an "amoeboid invasion" program. This motility style is largely independent from cell-ECM contact and from proteolytic degradation of ECM from MMPs. Furthermore, cell-ECM attachments of amoeboid moving cells are not organized in large focal adhesions but are very diffuse, and much weaker cell-ECM attachments are required, indeed, amoeboid movement cannot be blocked by inhibition of integrin function. The amoeboid invasion depends from Rho/ROCK expression, and their expression can be regulated also by miRNAs.

miR-10b, the first miRNA described to be pro-metastatic by Ma and colleagues in 2007 [81], inhibits the translation of mRNA encoding HOXD10, increasing the expression of Rho C, and thus leading to tumor cell invasion and metastasis. Ectopic expression of this miRNA endowed non-aggressive human breast cancer cells with the capacity to become invasive, as well as seed distant micrometastases when implanted as xenografts in immunodeficient mice. miR-10b was down-regulated in most breast cancers in comparison with normal mammary tissues, whereas it was highly expressed in about 50% of breast metastatic tumors. Induced by transcription factor Twist, miR-10b function as a metastasis driver in different types of cancer: i.e pancreatic [82], gastric [83] and colorectal [84] cancers.

RhoA, another member of Ras homolog gene family, was described also as a target for miR-155, a Smad4 regulated miR in breast cancer [85].

Mir 31 is able to inhibit multiple steps in the metastatic process: local invasion, one or more early post-intravasation events (intraluminal viability, extravasation efficiency and/or capacity to initially survive in the lung parenchyma), and metastatic colonization. MiR-31 carries out its anti-metastatic function regulating three genes: Rho A, Integrin $\alpha5$ and Radixin. Via suppression of Rho A, it is able to inhibit *in vitro* invasiveness [86,87]. Notably it also reduces Integrin $\alpha5$, a key effector of the mesenchymal invasion program, causing concomitant inhibition of both single-cell invasion programs. Controlling expression of Radixin, miR-31 causes anoikis-mediated cell death. In agreement with these data, miR-31 expression has been found to be attenuated in human breast [88-90], prostate [91], ovary [92], stomach [93,94] and bladder cancer [95]. Moreover miR-31 levels in primary human breast tumors were inversely associated with distant metastases [86]. Paradoxically, upregulation of miR-31 in human colorectal [96,97], liver [98] and head-and-neck tumors [99,100], as well as squamous cell carcinomas of the tongue [101] has also been observed [102] .

ROCK1 and ROCK2, the downstream targets of Rho A and Rho C, are regulated by miR 148a [103] and by miR-139 [104], respectively, which all behave as anti-metastatic miRNAs. Overexpression of miR-148a in gastric cancer cells [103] as well as in head and neck cancer cells [105], and of miR-139 in hepatocellular carcinoma cells (HCC) [104], suppressed cell migration and invasion *in vitro* and lung metastasis formation *in vivo*. Accordingly, miR-148a expression was suppressed in gastric cancer compared with their corresponding non tumor tissues, and the downregulated miR-148a was significantly associated with tumor node metastasis and miR-139 expression is reduced in metastatic HCC tumors compared with primary tumors.

In addition, others miRNAs with prominent roles in breast cancer metastasis have been reported.

The c-MYC regulated miR-17-92 cluster, which targets the connective tissue growth factor (CTGF) and the anti-angiogenic adhesive glycoprotein Thrombospondin 1 (TSP1) is shown to be elevated in metastatic breast cancer cells compared with nonmetastatic cells. miRNAs belonging to this cluster, attenuating also the TGFβ signaling pathway, indirectly shut down clusterin and angiopoietin-like 4 expressions, thereby stimulating angiogenesis and tumor cell growth [106]. Accordingly, blockade of miR-17 is shown to decrease breast cancer cell invasion/migration *in vitro* and metastasis *in vivo* [107]. Furthermore miR-17 and miR-20a were found to be significantly associated with reduced progression free survival in gastrointestinal cancer patients [108] .

The team led by Joan Massague [109] found that miR-335, miR-126, and miR-206 are metastasis-suppressors. Authors performed array-based miRNA profiling in MDA-MB-231 breast cancer cell derivatives (LM2) highly breast cancer cell derivatives highly metastatic to bone and lung, and found a signature of six genes (miR-335, miR-126, miR-206, miR-122a, miR-199a*, and miR-489) whose expression was highly decreased in metastatic cells. Restoring the expression of miR-335, miR-126 or miR-206 in LM2 cells decreased the lung colonizing activity of these cells by more than fivefold. They found that miR-335 suppresses metastasis and migration by targeting the progenitor cell transcription factor SOX4 and TNC messenger RNAs. Consequently, loss of miR-335 leads to the activation of SRY-box containing SOX4 and TNC, which are responsible for the acquisition of metastatic properties. Notably, knockdown of SOX4 and TNC using RNA interference diminished *in vitro* invasive ability and *in vivo* metastatic potential, evidencing that both genes are key effectors of metastasis [110]. miR-126, has recently been described to suppress metastatic endothelial recruitment, metastatic angiogenesis and metastatic colonization through coordinate targeting of IGFBP2, PITPNC1 and MERTK, novel pro-angiogenic genes and biomarkers of human metastasis through the IGFBP2/IGF1/IGF1R and GAS6/MERTK signaling pathways [111]. In addition, low expression of miR-335 or miR-126 in primary tumors from patients was associated with poor distal metastasis-free survival.

IGF1R was identified as a direct target of miR-493 that has been described as a metastasis inhibitor. Indeed, high levels of miR-493 and miR-493(*), but not pri-miR-493, in primary colon cancer were inversely related to the presence of liver metastasis, and attributed to an increase of miR-493 expression during carcinogenesis [112].

Raf kinase inhibitor protein (RKIP) represses breast tumour cell intravasation and bone metastasis through inhibition of MAPK leading to decreased transcription of LIN28 by Myc. Suppression of LIN28 enables enhanced let-7 processing in breast cancer cells. let-7 appears to play a major role in regulating stemness however elevated let-7 expression inhibits HMGA2, a chromatin remodelling protein that activates pro-invasive and pro-metastatic genes, including Snail. LIN28 depletion and let-7 expression suppress bone metastasis, and LIN28 restores bone metastasis in mice bearing RKIP-expressing breast tumour cells [113].

miR-146a is very similar to miR-146b, which is encoded by a different gene, but differs by only two bases and appears to function redundantly in many systems as mediators of inflammatory signaling, influencing differentiation, proliferation and apoptosis. They are pleiotropic regulators of tumorigenesis, as altered expression of both miR-146a/b have been linked with cancer risk, tumor histogenesis and invasive and metastatic capacity in diverse cancers [114]. In fact Hurst and coworkers [27], showed that breast cancer metastasis suppressor 1 (BRMS1), a protein that regulates expression of multiple genes [115] leading to suppression of metastasis, significantly up-regulates miR-146a and miR-146b in metastatic breast cancer cells. Transduction of miR-146a or miR-146b into MDA-MB-231 inhibited invasion and migration *in vitro*, and suppressed experimental lung metastasis. Bhaumik et al. confirmed that expression of miR-146a/b in MDA-MB-231 cells, impaired invasion and migration capacity by suppressing NF-κB activity [116]. In Table 2 both suppressing and promoting metastasis related miRNAs are summarized.

miRNA	Target
Suppressing miRNAs	
miR-17/20	IL8, Cyclin D1
miR-23b	c-MET, uPA
miR-29b	COL1A1,COL4A1, MMP-2
miR-29c	Laminin γ1, collagens
miR-30a	Snail
miR-31	Integrin α5, Radixin, Rho A
miR-34a	Snail, CD44, c-MET
miR-122	ADAM17
miR-126	ADAM9, Crk, IGFBP2, PTPNC1, MERTK
miR-139	ROCK2
miR-145	Mucin 1, N-cadherin, VEGF
miR-146a,b	NF-κB
miR-148a	ROCK
miR-155	Rho A
miR-183	Ezrin
miR-193a,b	uPA
miR-203	Slug, Snail1
miR-205	ZEB1, ZEB2
miR-335	SOX4, TNC
let-7	HMGA2, RAS
miR-200 family	ZEB1, ZEB2
miR 328	CD44
miR-373/520c	CD44, TGFBR2
miR-493	IGF1R
Promoting miRNAs	
miR-9	E-cadherin
miR-10b	HOXD10
miR-17-92	CTGF, TSP1
miR-21	PDCD4
miR-27	APC
miR-103/107	Dicer
miR-221/222	TRPS1
miR-223	EPB41L3, FBXW7

Table 2. microRNAs and their targets relevant in metastasis.

5. miRNAs as prognostic biomarkers

After early studies indicating the role of microRNA genes in the pathogenesis of human cancer, platforms to assess the global expression of microRNA genes in normal and diseased tissues have been developed. Gene expression profiling has already demonstrated its effectiveness at subtyping various cancers, however miRNA profiles are equally discriminatory and can even be more informative, as changes in their expression can provide insights into the myriad of gene permutations observed in various cancer subtypes: links have indeed been made between misregulated miRNAs and the target genes that are affected, thus unraveling some of the unique gene networks involved [117]. miRNA profiles may identify cancer-specific signatures distinguishing between normal and cancerous tissue [118-121], but they can also discriminate different subtypes of a particular cancer [119,122,123].

To discover microRNAs regulating the critical transition from ductal carcinoma in situ to invasive ductal carcinoma, a key event in breast cancer progression, Volinia et al. [124] performed a microRNA profile on 80 biopsies from invasive ductal carcinoma, 8 from ductal carcinoma in situ, and 6 from normal breast selected from a recently published deep-sequencing dataset [125]. They found that the microRNA profile established for the normal breast to ductal carcinoma in situ transition was largely maintained in the in situ to invasive ductal carcinoma transition. Nevertheless, a nine-microRNA signature that differentiated invasive from in situ carcinoma was identified. Specifically, let-7d, miR-210, and -221 were down-regulated in the in situ and up-regulated in the invasive transition, thus featuring an expression reversal along the cancer progression path. Additionally, they identified microRNAs for overall survival and time to metastasis. Five noncoding genes were associated with both prognostic signatures miR-210, -21, -106b*, -197, and let-7i, with miR-210 the only one also involved in the invasive transition.

Concerning the possibility to use miRNAs as prognostic markers to predict outcome, several groups have successfully addressed this issue [123,126-130] and in particular, concerning involvement of microRNAs in metastatic disease. For example several studies conducted on samples from patient with lung cancer assessed the involvement of metastamiRs: Landi et al [122] analyzed 107 male with early-stage squamous cell lung cancers (SQ) and found 5 miRNAs (miR-25, -34c-5p, -191, let- 7e, miR-34a) whose high expression strongly predicted longer SQ survival [122]. In another study, based on miRNA expression profiling of lung adenocarcinoma and SQ, ten miRNAs (hsa-miR-450b-3p, hsa-miR-29c*, hsa-miR-145*, hsa-miR-148a*, hsa-miR-1, hsa-miR-30d, hsa-miR-187, hsa-miR-218, hsa-miR-708* and hsa-miR-375) associated with brain metastasis were identified including miR-145*, which inhibit cell invasion and metastasis. Two miRNA signatures that are highly predictive of recurrence free survival of 357 stage I NSCLC were also identified, one independent of cancer subtype, the other specific for adenocarcinoma or SQ subtype [131]. From a small cohort of 20 NSCLC patients, Donnem and co-workers [132] in addition to miR differentially expressed between NSCLC tumors and normal control, found 37 miRs up/down regulated in tumors derived from patients with short versus long disease specific survival (DSS) including upregulated miR-31, miR-183, let-7a, miR-193b and downregulated miR-205, miR-378, miR-708 and miR-

29c. A further analysis comparing short versus long DSS patients tumors identified significantly altered angiogenesis-related miRs (miR-21, miR-106a, miR-126, miR-155, miR-182, miR-210 and miR-424) [123], on the basis of a small number of cases, found that the reduced expression of miR-17-5p and -30c in malignant mesothelioma correlated with better survival in patients with the sarcomatoid subtype.

Studies relative to tumors in other body districts have been carried out to determine the involvement of miRs in metastatic disease. Heinzelman et al, analysed miRNA expression of 30 human clear cell renal carcinoma (ccRCC) including 10 non-metastatic tumors, 4 tumors with metastasis after 3 years or later and 4 tumors with primary metastasis. They detected a miRNA signature that distinguishes between metastatic and non-metastatic ccRCC, including miR-451, miR-221, miR-30a, miR-10b and miR-29a. Furthermore, the authors identified a group of 12 miRNAs, such as let-7 family, miR-30c, miR-26a, which are decreased in highly aggressive primary metastatic tumours. They found also correlations between expression levels of specific miRNAs with progression-free survival and overall survival [133].

Veerla et al [95], by miRNA expression analysis of 34 cases of urothelial carcinomas identified 51 miRNAs that discriminated the 3 pathological subtypes Ta, T1 and T2-T3. A score based on the expression levels of the 51 miRNAs, identified muscle invasive tumors with high precision and sensitivity. miRNAs showing high expression in muscle invasive tumors included miR-222 and miR-125b and in Ta tumors miR-10a. Moreover authors identified 2 miRNAs, miR-452 and miR-452*, associated with metastases in the lymph nodes and with a strong prognostic impact on death as endpoint.

353 gastric samples from two independent subsets of patients from Japan were analysed by Ueda et al [119], with the aim to assess the relation between microRNA expression and prognosis of gastric cancer. They found a progression-related signature including miR-125b, miR-199a, and miR-100 as the most important microRNAs involved. Moreover they found that low expression of let-7g and miR-433 and high expression of miR-214 were associated with unfavourable outcome in overall survival independent of clinical covariates, including depth of invasion, lymph-node metastasis, and stage.

6. Conclusion

Although miRs that have been demonstrated to be implicated in the metastatic process might represent a possible therapeutic tool, there have been so far few reported successes in the development of miRNAs for use in therapy. There are two main strategies to target miRNAs expression in cancer. Direct strategies involve the use of oligonucleotides or virus-based constructs to either block the expression of an oncogenic miRNA or to reintroduce a tumor suppressor miRNA lost in cancer. The indirect strategy involves the use of drugs to modulate miRNAs expression by targeting their transcription and their processing. Indeed, even though a number of reports have described the possibility to reintroduce or inhibit microRNAs (reviewed by Iorio and Croce, [134]), there are still many issues that need to be addressed for an effective translation in clinics, as the development of efficient methods of a specific drug delivery, and the accurate prevision of putative unwanted off target effects.

Nevertheless, the results obtained up to date seem quite promising and encouraging, and even though we still have to improve the knowledge in microRNA field to even think of future therapeutic applications, we might be not so far from there.

Author details

Tiziana Triulzi, Elda Tagliabue* and Patrizia Casalini
Molecular Targeting Unit, Department of Experimental Oncology and Molecular Medicine, Fondazione IRCCS , Istituto Nazionale dei Tumori, Milan; Italy

Marilena V. Iorio
Start-Up Unit, Department of Experimental Oncology and Molecular Medicine, Fondazione IRCCS , Istituto Nazionale dei Tumori, Milan; Italy

Acknowledgement

Authors gratefully acknowledge Dr. Viola Regondi for figures preparation.

7. References

[1] Bartel DP. MicroRNAs: genomics, biogenesis, mechanism, and function. Cell 2004 Jan 23;116:281-97.
[2] Chambers AF, Groom AC, MacDonald IC. Dissemination and growth of cancer cells in metastatic sites. Nat Rev Cancer 2002 Aug;2:563-72.
[3] Bhayani MK, Calin GA, Lai SY. Functional relevance of miRNA sequences in human disease. Mutat Res 2012 Mar 1;731(1-2):14-9.
[4] Su H, Trombly MI, Chen J, Wang X. Essential and overlapping functions for mammalian Argonautes in microRNA silencing. Genes Dev 2009 Feb 1;23(3):304-17.
[5] Orom UA, Nielsen FC, Lund AH. MicroRNA-10a binds the 5'UTR of ribosomal protein mRNAs and enhances their translation. Mol Cell 2008 May 23;30(4):460-71.
[6] Lytle JR, Yario TA, Steitz JA. Target mRNAs are repressed as efficiently by microRNA-binding sites in the 5' UTR as in the 3' UTR. Proc Natl Acad Sci U S A 2007 Jun 5;104(23):9667-72.
[7] Moretti F, Thermann R, Hentze MW. Mechanism of translational regulation by miR-2 from sites in the 5' untranslated region or the open reading frame. RNA 2010 Dec;16(12):2493-502.
[8] Qin W, Shi Y, Zhao B, Yao C, Jin L, Ma J, et al. miR-24 regulates apoptosis by targeting the open reading frame (ORF) region of FAF1 in cancer cells. PLoS One 2010 Feb 25;5(2):e9429.
[9] Vasudevan S, Tong Y, Steitz JA. Switching from repression to activation: microRNAs can up-regulate translation. Science 2007 Dec 21;318(5858):1931-4.

* Corresponding Author

[10] Brennecke J, Stark A, Russell RB, Cohen SM. Principles of microRNA-target recognition. PLoS Biol 2005 Mar;3(3):e85.

[11] Lewis BP, Burge CB, Bartel DP. Conserved seed pairing, often flanked by adenosines, indicates that thousands of human genes are microRNA targets. Cell 2005 Jan 14;120(1):15-20.

[12] Krek A, Grun D, Poy MN, Wolf R, Rosenberg L, Epstein EJ, et al. Combinatorial microRNA target predictions. Nat Genet 2005 May;37(5):495-500.

[13] Betel D, Wilson M, Gabow A, Marks DS, Sander C. The microRNA.org resource: targets and expression. Nucleic Acids Res 2008 Jan;36(Database issue):D149-D153.

[14] Friedman RC, Farh KK, Burge CB, Bartel DP. Most mammalian mRNAs are conserved targets of microRNAs. Genome Res 2009 Jan;19(1):92-105.

[15] Beitzinger M, Meister G. Preview. MicroRNAs: from decay to decoy. Cell 2010 Mar 5;140(5):612-4.

[16] Khraiwesh B, Arif MA, Seumel GI, Ossowski S, Weigel D, Reski R, et al. Transcriptional control of gene expression by microRNAs. Cell 2010 Jan 8;140(1):111-22.

[17] Gonzalez S, Pisano DG, Serrano M. Mechanistic principles of chromatin remodeling guided by siRNAs and miRNAs. Cell Cycle 2008 Aug 15;7(16):2601-8.

[18] Kim DH, Saetrom P, Snove O, Jr., Rossi JJ. MicroRNA-directed transcriptional gene silencing in mammalian cells. Proc Natl Acad Sci U S A 2008 Oct 21;105(42):16230-5.

[19] Hanahan D, Weinberg RA. The hallmarks of cancer. Cell 2000;100:57-70.

[20] Gupta GP, Massague J. Cancer metastasis: building a framework. Cell 2006 Nov 17;127(4):679-95.

[21] Friedl P, Wolf K. Tumour-cell invasion and migration: diversity and escape mechanisms. Nat Rev Cancer 2003 May;3(5):362-74.

[22] Friedl P, Wolf K. Plasticity of cell migration: a multiscale tuning model. J Cell Biol 2010 Jan 11;188(1):11-9.

[23] Wolf K, Mazo I, Leung H, Engelke K, von Andrian UH, Deryugina EI, et al. Compensation mechanism in tumor cell migration: mesenchymal-amoeboid transition after blocking of pericellular proteolysis. J Cell Biol 2003 Jan;%20;160(2):267-77.

[24] Kalluri R. EMT: when epithelial cells decide to become mesenchymal-like cells. J Clin Invest 2009 Jun;119(6):1417-9.

[25] Thiery JP. Epithelial-mesenchymal transitions in development and pathologies. Curr Opin Cell Biol 2003 Dec;15:740-6.

[26] Psaila B, Lyden D. The metastatic niche: adapting the foreign soil. Nat Rev Cancer 2009 Apr;9(4):285-93.

[27] Hurst DR, Edmonds MD, Welch DR. Metastamir: the field of metastasis-regulatory microRNA is spreading. Cancer Res 2009 Oct 1;69(19):7495-8.

[28] Gregory PA, Bert AG, Paterson EL, Barry SC, Tsykin A, Farshid G, et al. The miR-200 family and miR-205 regulate epithelial to mesenchymal transition by targeting ZEB1 and SIP1. Nat Cell Biol 2008 May;10(5):593-601.

[29] Kurashige J, Kamohara H, Watanabe M, Hiyoshi Y, Iwatsuki M, Tanaka Y, et al. MicroRNA-200b Regulates Cell Proliferation, Invasion, and Migration by Directly Targeting ZEB2 in Gastric Carcinoma. Ann Surg Oncol 2012 Feb 4.

[30] Davalos V, Moutinho C, Villanueva A, Boque R, Silva P, Carneiro F, et al. Dynamic epigenetic regulation of the microRNA-200 family mediates epithelial and mesenchymal transitions in human tumorigenesis. Oncogene 2011 Aug 29;10.

[31] Korpal M, Ell BJ, Buffa FM, Ibrahim T, Blanco MA, Celia-Terrassa T, et al. Direct targeting of Sec23a by miR-200s influences cancer cell secretome and promotes metastatic colonization. Nat Med 2011 Aug 7;17(9):1101-8.

[32] Martello G, Rosato A, Ferrari F, Manfrin A, Cordenonsi M, Dupont S, et al. A MicroRNA targeting dicer for metastasis control. Cell 2010 Jun 25;141:1195-207.

[33] Wellner U, Schubert J, Burk UC, Schmalhofer O, Zhu F, Sonntag A, et al. The EMT-activator ZEB1 promotes tumorigenicity by repressing stemness-inhibiting microRNAs. Nat Cell Biol 2009 Dec;11(12):1487-95.

[34] Zhang Z, Zhang B, Li W, Fu L, Fu L, Zhu Z, et al. Epigenetic Silencing of miR-203 Upregulates SNAI2 and Contributes to the Invasiveness of Malignant Breast Cancer Cells. Genes Cancer 2011 Aug;2(8):782-91.

[35] Moes M, Le BA, Crespo I, Laurini C, Halavatyi A, Vetter G, et al. A Novel Network Integrating a miRNA-203/SNAI1 Feedback Loop which Regulates Epithelial to Mesenchymal Transition. PLoS One 2012;7(4):e35440.

[36] Kumarswamy R, Mudduluru G, Ceppi P, Muppala S, Kozlowski M, Niklinski J, et al. MicroRNA-30a inhibits epithelial-to-mesenchymal transition by targeting Snai1 and is downregulated in non-small cell lung cancer. Int J Cancer 2012 May 1;130(9):2044-53.

[37] Zheng C, Yinghao S, Li J. MiR-221 expression affects invasion potential of human prostate carcinoma cell lines by targeting DVL2. Med Oncol 2011 Apr 13.

[38] Guttilla IK, Phoenix KN, Hong X, Tirnauer JS, Claffey KP, White BA. Prolonged mammosphere culture of MCF-7 cells induces an EMT and repression of the estrogen receptor by microRNAs. Breast Cancer Res Treat 2012 Feb;132(1):75-85.

[39] Gramantieri L, Fornari F, Ferracin M, Veronese A, Sabbioni S, Calin GA, et al. MicroRNA-221 targets Bmf in hepatocellular carcinoma and correlates with tumor multifocality. Clin Cancer Res 2009 Aug 15;15(16):5073-81.

[40] Stinson S, Lackner MR, Adai AT, Yu N, Kim HJ, O'Brien C, et al. TRPS1 targeting by miR-221/222 promotes the epithelial-to-mesenchymal transition in breast cancer. Sci Signal 2011 Jun 14;4(177):ra41.

[41] Howe EN, Cochrane DR, Richer JK. The miR-200 and miR-221/222 microRNA Families: Opposing Effects on Epithelial Identity. J Mammary Gland Biol Neoplasia 2012 Mar;17(1):65-77.

[42] Poliseno L, Tuccoli A, Mariani L, Evangelista M, Citti L, Woods K, et al. MicroRNAs modulate the angiogenic properties of HUVECs. Blood 2006 Nov 1;108(9):3068-71.

[43] Iorio MV, Casalini P, Piovan C, Di Leva G, Merlo A, Triulzi T, et al. microRNA-205 regulates HER3 in human breast cancer. Cancer Res 2009 Mar 15;69:2195-200.

[44] Piovan C, Palmieri D, Di Leva G, Braccioli L, Casalini P, Tortoreto M, et al. Oncosuppressive role of p53-induced miR-205 in triple negative breast cancer. Mol Oncol 2012;In press.

[45] Gandellini P, Folini M, Longoni N, Pennati M, Binda M, Colecchia M, et al. miR-205 Exerts tumor-suppressive functions in human prostate through down-regulation of protein kinase Cepsilon. Cancer Res 2009 Mar 15;69:2287-95.

[46] Dar AA, Majid S, de SD, Nosrati M, Bezrookove V, Kashani-Sabet M. miRNA-205 suppresses melanoma cell proliferation and induces senescence via regulation of E2F1 protein. J Biol Chem 2011 May 13;286(19):16606-14.
[47] Zhang Z, Liu S, Shi R, Zhao G. miR-27 promotes human gastric cancer cell metastasis by inducing epithelial-to-mesenchymal transition. Cancer Genet 2011 Sep;204(9):486-91.
[48] Siemens H, Jackstadt R, Hunten S, Kaller M, Menssen A, Gotz U, et al. miR-34 and SNAIL form a double-negative feedback loop to regulate epithelial-mesenchymal transitions. Cell Cycle 2011 Dec 15;10(24):4256-71.
[49] Li N, Fu H, Tie Y, Hu Z, Kong W, Wu Y, et al. miR-34a inhibits migration and invasion by down-regulation of c-Met expression in human hepatocellular carcinoma cells. Cancer Lett 2009 Mar 8;275:44-53.
[50] Yan K, Gao J, Yang T, Ma Q, Qiu X, Fan Q, et al. MicroRNA-34a Inhibits the Proliferation and Metastasis of Osteosarcoma Cells Both In Vitro and In Vivo. PLoS One 2012;7(3):e33778.
[51] Zhu L, Chen H, Zhou D, Li D, Bai R, Zheng S, et al. MicroRNA-9 up-regulation is involved in colorectal cancer metastasis via promoting cell motility. Med Oncol 2011 May 12.
[52] Ma L, Reinhardt F, Pan E, Soutschek J, Bhat B, Marcusson EG, et al. Therapeutic silencing of miR-10b inhibits metastasis in a mouse mammary tumor model. Nat Biotechnol 2010 Apr;28:341-7.
[53] Gao P, Xing AY, Zhou GY, Zhang TG, Zhang JP, Gao C, et al. The molecular mechanism of microRNA-145 to suppress invasion-metastasis cascade in gastric cancer. Oncogene 2012 Feb 27;10.
[54] Sachdeva M, Mo YY. MicroRNA-145 suppresses cell invasion and metastasis by directly targeting mucin 1. Cancer Res 2010 Jan 1;70:378-87.
[55] Fan L, Wu Q, Xing X, Wei Y, Shao Z. MicroRNA-145 targets vascular endothelial growth factor and inhibits invasion and metastasis of osteosarcoma cells. Acta Biochim Biophys Sin (Shanghai) 2012 May;44(5):407-14.
[56] Liu C, Kelnar K, Liu B, Chen X, Calhoun-Davis T, Li H, et al. The microRNA miR-34a inhibits prostate cancer stem cells and metastasis by directly repressing CD44. Nat Med 2011 Feb;17(2):211-5.
[57] Huang Q, Gumireddy K, Schrier M, le SC, Nagel R, Nair S, et al. The microRNAs miR-373 and miR-520c promote tumour invasion and metastasis. Nat Cell Biol 2008 Feb;10:202-10.
[58] Wang CH, Lee DY, Deng Z, Jeyapalan Z, Lee SC, Kahai S, et al. MicroRNA miR-328 regulates zonation morphogenesis by targeting CD44 expression. PLoS One 2008 Jun 18;3(6):e2420.
[59] Li F, Tiede B, Massague J, Kang Y. Beyond tumorigenesis: cancer stem cells in metastasis. Cell Res 2007 Jan;17(1):3-14.
[60] Keklikoglou I, Koerner C, Schmidt C, Zhang JD, Heckmann D, Shavinskaya A, et al. MicroRNA-520/373 family functions as a tumor suppressor in estrogen receptor negative breast cancer by targeting NF-kappaB and TGF-beta signaling pathways. Oncogene 2011 Dec 12;10.

[61] Han M, Wang Y, Liu M, Bi X, Bao J, Zeng N, et al. MiR-21 regulates EMT phenotype and HIF-1alpha expression in third-sphereforming breast cancer stem cell-like cells. Cancer Sci 2012 Mar 21;10-7006.

[62] Noh H, Hong S, Dong Z, Pan ZK, Jing Q, Huang S. Impaired MicroRNA Processing Facilitates Breast Cancer Cell Invasion by Upregulating Urokinase-Type Plasminogen Activator Expression. Genes Cancer 2011 Feb;2(2):140-50.

[63] Li XF, Yan PJ, Shao ZM. Downregulation of miR-193b contributes to enhance urokinase-type plasminogen activator (uPA) expression and tumor progression and invasion in human breast cancer. Oncogene 2009 Nov 5;28(44):3937-48.

[64] Salvi A, Sabelli C, Moncini S, Venturin M, Arici B, Riva P, et al. MicroRNA-23b mediates urokinase and c-met downmodulation and a decreased migration of human hepatocellular carcinoma cells. FEBS J 2009 Jun;276(11):2966-82.

[65] Yu Z, Willmarth NE, Zhou J, Katiyar S, Wang M, Liu Y, et al. microRNA 17/20 inhibits cellular invasion and tumor metastasis in breast cancer by heterotypic signaling. Proc Natl Acad Sci U S A 2010 May 4;107(18):8231-6.

[66] Asangani IA, Rasheed SA, Nikolova DA, Leupold JH, Colburn NH, Post S, et al. MicroRNA-21 (miR-21) post-transcriptionally downregulates tumor suppressor Pdcd4 and stimulates invasion, intravasation and metastasis in colorectal cancer. Oncogene 2008 Apr 3;27:2128-36.

[67] Zhu S, Wu H, Wu F, Nie D, Sheng S, Mo YY. MicroRNA-21 targets tumor suppressor genes in invasion and metastasis. Cell Res 2008 Mar;18:350-9.

[68] Tsai WC, Hsu PW, Lai TC, Chau GY, Lin CW, Chen CM, et al. MicroRNA-122, a tumor suppressor microRNA that regulates intrahepatic metastasis of hepatocellular carcinoma. Hepatology 2009 May;49(5):1571-82.

[69] Coulouarn C, Factor VM, Andersen JB, Durkin ME, Thorgeirsson SS. Loss of miR-122 expression in liver cancer correlates with suppression of the hepatic phenotype and gain of metastatic properties. Oncogene 2009 Oct 8;28(40):3526-36.

[70] Hamada S, Satoh K, Fujibuchi W, Hirota M, Kanno A, Unno J, et al. MiR-126 acts as a tumor suppressor in pancreatic cancer cells via the regulation of ADAM9. Mol Cancer Res 2012 Jan;10(1):3-10.

[71] Feng R, Chen X, Yu Y, Su L, Yu B, Li J, et al. miR-126 functions as a tumour suppressor in human gastric cancer. Cancer Lett 2010 Dec 1;298(1):50-63.

[72] Fang JH, Zhou HC, Zeng C, Yang J, Liu Y, Huang X, et al. MicroRNA-29b suppresses tumor angiogenesis, invasion, and metastasis by regulating matrix metalloproteinase 2 expression. Hepatology 2011 Nov;54(5):1729-40.

[73] Steele R, Mott JL, Ray RB. MBP-1 upregulates miR-29b that represses Mcl-1, collagens, and matrix-metalloproteinase-2 in prostate cancer cells. Genes Cancer 2010 Apr 1;1(4):381-7.

[74] Sengupta S, den Boon JA, Chen IH, Newton MA, Stanhope SA, Cheng YJ, et al. MicroRNA 29c is down-regulated in nasopharyngeal carcinomas, up-regulating mRNAs encoding extracellular matrix proteins. Proc Natl Acad Sci U S A 2008 Apr 15;105(15):5874-8.

[75] Pujuguet P, Del ML, Gautreau A, Louvard D, Arpin M. Ezrin regulates E-cadherin-dependent adherens junction assembly through Rac1 activation. Mol Biol Cell 2003 May;14(5):2181-91.

[76] Lowery AJ, Miller N, Dwyer RM, Kerin MJ. Dysregulated miR-183 inhibits migration in breast cancer cells. BMC Cancer 2010 Sep 21;10:502.:502.

[77] Zhu J, Feng Y, Ke Z, Yang Z, Zhou J, Huang X, et al. Down-Regulation of miR-183 Promotes Migration and Invasion of Osteosarcoma by Targeting Ezrin. Am J Pathol 2012 Apr;%20.

[78] Wang G, Mao W, Zheng S. MicroRNA-183 regulates Ezrin expression in lung cancer cells. FEBS Lett 2008 Oct 29;582(25-26):3663-8.

[79] Li X, Zhang Y, Zhang H, Liu X, Gong T, Li M, et al. miRNA-223 promotes gastric cancer invasion and metastasis by targeting tumor suppressor EPB41L3. Mol Cancer Res 2011 Jul;9(7):824-33.

[80] Kurashige J, Watanabe M, Iwatsuki M, Kinoshita K, Saito S, Hiyoshi Y, et al. Overexpression of microRNA-223 regulates the ubiquitin ligase FBXW7 in oesophageal squamous cell carcinoma. Br J Cancer 2012 Jan 3;106(1):182-8.

[81] Ma L, Teruya-Feldstein J, Weinberg RA. Tumour invasion and metastasis initiated by microRNA-10b in breast cancer. Nature 2007 Oct 11;449:682-8.

[82] Nakata K, Ohuchida K, Mizumoto K, Kayashima T, Ikenaga N, Sakai H, et al. MicroRNA-10b is overexpressed in pancreatic cancer, promotes its invasiveness, and correlates with a poor prognosis. Surgery 2011 Nov;150(5):916-22.

[83] Liu Z, Zhu J, Cao H, Ren H, Fang X. miR-10b promotes cell invasion through RhoC-AKT signaling pathway by targeting HOXD10 in gastric cancer. Int J Oncol 2012 May;40(5):1553-60.

[84] Nishida N, Yamashita S, Mimori K, Sudo T, Tanaka F, Shibata K, et al. MicroRNA-10b is a Prognostic Indicator in Colorectal Cancer and Confers Resistance to the Chemotherapeutic Agent 5-Fluorouracil in Colorectal Cancer Cells. Ann Surg Oncol 2012 Feb 10.

[85] Kong W, Yang H, He L, Zhao JJ, Coppola D, Dalton WS, et al. MicroRNA-155 is regulated by the transforming growth factor beta/Smad pathway and contributes to epithelial cell plasticity by targeting RhoA. Mol Cell Biol 2008 Nov;28(22):6773-84

[86] Valastyan S, Reinhardt F, Benaich N, Calogrias D, Szasz AM, Wang ZC, et al. A pleiotropically acting microRNA, miR-31, inhibits breast cancer metastasis. Cell 2009 Jun 12;137(6):1032-46.

[87] Valastyan S, Chang A, Benaich N, Reinhardt F, Weinberg RA. Activation of miR-31 function in already-established metastases elicits metastatic regression. Genes Dev 2011 Mar 15;25(6):646-59.

[88] Calin GA, Sevignani C, Dumitru CD, Hyslop T, Noch E, Yendamuri S, et al. Human microRNA genes are frequently located at fragile sites and genomic regions involved in cancers. Proc Natl Acad Sci U S A 2004 Mar 2;101:2999-3004.

[89] Zhang L, Huang J, Yang N, Greshock J, Megraw MS, Giannakakis A, et al. microRNAs exhibit high frequency genomic alterations in human cancer. Proc Natl Acad Sci USA 2006 Jun 13;103:9136-41.

[90] Yan LX, Huang XF, Shao Q, Huang MY, Deng L, Wu QL, et al. MicroRNA miR-21 overexpression in human breast cancer is associated with advanced clinical stage, lymph node metastasis and patient poor prognosis. RNA 2008 Nov;14:2348-60.

[91] Schaefer A, Jung M, Mollenkopf HJ, Wagner I, Stephan C, Jentzmik F, et al. Diagnostic and prognostic implications of microRNA profiling in prostate carcinoma. Int J Cancer 2010 Mar 1;126(5):1166-76.

[92] Creighton CJ, Fountain MD, Yu Z, Nagaraja AK, Zhu H, Khan M, et al. Molecular profiling uncovers a p53-associated role for microRNA-31 in inhibiting the proliferation of serous ovarian carcinomas and other cancers. Cancer Res 2010 Mar 1;70(5):1906-15.

[93] Guo J, Miao Y, Xiao B, Huan R, Jiang Z, Meng D, et al. Differential expression of microRNA species in human gastric cancer versus non-tumorous tissues. J Gastroenterol Hepatol 2009 Apr;24(4):652-7.

[94] Zhang Y, Guo J, Li D, Xiao B, Miao Y, Jiang Z, et al. Down-regulation of miR-31 expression in gastric cancer tissues and its clinical significance. Med Oncol 2010 Sep;27(3):685-9.

[95] Veerla S, Lindgren D, Kvist A, Frigyesi A, Staaf J, Persson H, et al. MiRNA expression in urothelial carcinomas: important roles of miR-10a, miR-222, miR-125b, miR-7 and miR-452 for tumor stage and metastasis, and frequent homozygous losses of miR-31. Int J Cancer 2009 May 1;124(9):2236-42.

[96] Bandres E, Cubedo E, Agirre X, Malumbres R, Zarate R, Ramirez N, et al. Identification by Real-time PCR of 13 mature microRNAs differentially expressed in colorectal cancer and non-tumoral tissues. Mol Cancer 2006 Jul;%19;5:29.:29.

[97] Motoyama K, Inoue H, Takatsuno Y, Tanaka F, Mimori K, Uetake H, et al. Over- and under-expressed microRNAs in human colorectal cancer. Int J Oncol 2009 Apr;34(4):1069-75.

[98] Wong QW, Lung RW, Law PT, Lai PB, Chan KY, To KF, et al. MicroRNA-223 is commonly repressed in hepatocellular carcinoma and potentiates expression of Stathmin1. Gastroenterology 2008 Jul;135(1):257-69.

[99] Liu X, Chen Z, Yu J, Xia J, Zhou X. MicroRNA profiling and head and neck cancer. Comp Funct Genomics 2009.

[100] Liu CJ, Tsai MM, Hung PS, Kao SY, Liu TY, Wu KJ, et al. miR-31 ablates expression of the HIF regulatory factor FIH to activate the HIF pathway in head and neck carcinoma. Cancer Res 2010 Feb 15;70(4):1635-44.

[101] Wong TS, Liu XB, Wong BY, Ng RW, Yuen AP, Wei WI. Mature miR-184 as Potential Oncogenic microRNA of Squamous Cell Carcinoma of Tongue. Clin Cancer Res 2008 May 1;14(9):2588-92.

[102] Valastyan S, Weinberg RA. Tumor metastasis: molecular insights and evolving paradigms. Cell 2011 Oct 14;147(2):275-92.

[103] Zheng B, Liang L, Wang C, Huang S, Cao X, Zha R, et al. MicroRNA-148a suppresses tumor cell invasion and metastasis by downregulating ROCK1 in gastric cancer. Clin Cancer Res 2011 Dec 15;17(24):7574-83.

[104] Wong CC, Wong CM, Tung EK, Au SL, Lee JM, Poon RT, et al. The microRNA miR-139 suppresses metastasis and progression of hepatocellular carcinoma by down-regulating Rho-kinase 2. Gastroenterology 2011 Jan;140(1):322-31.

[105] Lujambio A, Calin GA, Villanueva A, Ropero S, Sanchez-Cespedes M, Blanco D, et al. A microRNA DNA methylation signature for human cancer metastasis. Proc Natl Acad Sci U S A 2008 Sep 9;105(36):13556-61.

[106] Dews M, Fox JL, Hultine S, Sundaram P, Wang W, Liu YY, et al. The myc-miR-17~92 axis blunts TGF{beta} signaling and production of multiple TGF{beta}-dependent antiangiogenic factors. Cancer Res 2010 Oct 15;70(20):8233-46.

[107] Liu S, Goldstein RH, Scepansky EM, Rosenblatt M. Inhibition of rho-associated kinase signaling prevents breast cancer metastasis to human bone. Cancer Res 2009 Nov 15;69(22):8742-51.

[108] Valladares-Ayerbes M, Blanco M, Haz M, Medina V, Iglesias-Diaz P, Lorenzo-Patino MJ, et al. Prognostic impact of disseminated tumor cells and microRNA-17-92 cluster deregulation in gastrointestinal cancer. Int J Oncol 2011 Nov;39(5):1253-64.

[109] Oskarsson T, Acharyya S, Zhang XH, Vanharanta S, Tavazoie SF, Morris PG, et al. Breast cancer cells produce tenascin C as a metastatic niche component to colonize the lungs. Nat Med 2011 Jun 26;17(7):867-74.

[110] Tavazoie SF, Alarcon C, Oskarsson T, Padua D, Wang Q, Bos PD, et al. Endogenous human microRNAs that suppress breast cancer metastasis. Nature 2008 Jan 10;451:147-52.

[111] Png KJ, Halberg N, Yoshida M, Tavazoie SF. A microRNA regulon that mediates endothelial recruitment and metastasis by cancer cells. Nature 2011 Dec 14;481(7380):190-4.

[112] Okamoto K, Ishiguro T, Midorikawa Y, Ohata H, Izumiya M, Tsuchiya N, et al. miR-493 induction during carcinogenesis blocks metastatic settlement of colon cancer cells in liver. EMBO J 2012 Feb 28;31(7):1752-63.

[113] Dangi-Garimella S, Yun J, Eves EM, Newman M, Erkeland SJ, Hammond SM, et al. Raf kinase inhibitory protein suppresses a metastasis signalling cascade involving LIN28 and let-7. EMBO J 2009 Feb 18;28(4):347-58.

[114] Elsarraj HS, Stecklein SR, Valdez K, Behbod F. Emerging Functions of microRNA-146a/b in Development and Breast Cancer : MicroRNA-146a/b in Development and Breast Cancer. J Mammary Gland Biol Neoplasia 2012 Mar;17(1):79-87.

[115] Hurst DR, Welch DR. Unraveling the enigmatic complexities of BRMS1-mediated metastasis suppression. FEBS Lett 2011 Oct;%20;585(20):3185-90.

[116] Bhaumik D, Scott GK, Schokrpur S, Patil CK, Campisi J, Benz CC. Expression of microRNA-146 suppresses NF-kappaB activity with reduction of metastatic potential in breast cancer cells. Oncogene 2008 Sep 18;27(42):5643-7.

[117] O'Day E, Lal A. MicroRNAs and their target gene networks in breast cancer. Breast Cancer Res 2010;12(2):201.

[118] Piepoli A, Tavano F, Copetti M, Mazza T, Palumbo O, Panza A, et al. Mirna expression profiles identify drivers in colorectal and pancreatic cancers. PLoS One 2012;7(3):e33663.

[119] Ueda T, Volinia S, Okumura H, Shimizu M, Taccioli C, Rossi S, et al. Relation between microRNA expression and progression and prognosis of gastric cancer: a microRNA expression analysis. Lancet Oncol 2010 Feb;11(2):136-46.

[120] Martens-Uzunova ES, Jalava SE, Dits NF, van Leenders GJ, Moller S, Trapman J, et al. Diagnostic and prognostic signatures from the small non-coding RNA transcriptome in prostate cancer. Oncogene 2012 Feb 23;31(8):978-91.

[121] Schaefer A, Jung M, Miller K, Lein M, Kristiansen G, Erbersdobler A, et al. Suitable reference genes for relative quantification of miRNA expression in prostate cancer. Exp Mol Med 2010 Nov 30;42(11):749-58.

[122] Landi MT, Zhao Y, Rotunno M, Koshiol J, Liu H, Bergen AW, et al. MicroRNA expression differentiates histology and predicts survival of lung cancer. Clin Cancer Res 2010 Jan 15;16(2):430-41.

[123] Busacca S, Germano S, De CL, Rinaldi M, Comoglio F, Favero F, et al. MicroRNA signature of malignant mesothelioma with potential diagnostic and prognostic implications. Am J Respir Cell Mol Biol 2010 Mar;42(3):312-9.

[124] Volinia S, Galasso M, Sana ME, Wise TF, Palatini J, Huebner K, et al. Breast cancer signatures for invasiveness and prognosis defined by deep sequencing of microRNA. Proc Natl Acad Sci U S A 2012 Feb 21;109(8):3024-9.

[125] Farazi TA, Horlings HM, Ten Hoeve JJ, Mihailovic A, Halfwerk H, Morozov P, et al. MicroRNA sequence and expression analysis in breast tumors by deep sequencing. Cancer Res 2011 Jul 1;71(13):4443-53.

[126] du Rieu MC, Torrisani J, Selves J, Al ST, Souque A, Dufresne M, et al. MicroRNA-21 is induced early in pancreatic ductal adenocarcinoma precursor lesions. Clin Chem 2010 Apr;56(4):603-12.

[127] Heneghan HM, Miller N, Kerin MJ. Circulating miRNA signatures: promising prognostic tools for cancer. J Clin Oncol 2010 Oct 10;28:e573-e574.

[128] Huang Z, Huang D, Ni S, Peng Z, Sheng W, Du X. Plasma microRNAs are promising novel biomarkers for early detection of colorectal cancer. Int J Cancer 2010 Jul 1;127(1):118-26.

[129] Xing L, Todd NW, Yu L, Fang H, Jiang F. Early detection of squamous cell lung cancer in sputum by a panel of microRNA markers. Mod Pathol 2010 Aug;23(8):1157-64.

[130] Boeri M, Verri C, Conte D, Roz L, Modena P, Facchinetti F, et al. MicroRNA signatures in tissues and plasma predict development and prognosis of computed tomography detected lung cancer. Proc Natl Acad Sci USA 2011 Mar 1;108:3713-8.

[131] Lu Y, Govindan R, Wang L, Liu PY, Goodgame B, Wen W, et al. MicroRNA profiling and prediction of recurrence/relapse-free survival in stage I lung cancer. Carcinogenesis 2012 May;33(5):1046-54.

[132] Donnem T, Fenton CG, Lonvik K, Berg T, Eklo K, Andersen S, et al. MicroRNA signatures in tumor tissue related to angiogenesis in non-small cell lung cancer. PLoS One 2012;7(1):e29671.

[133] Heinzelmann J, Henning B, Sanjmyatav J, Posorski N, Steiner T, Wunderlich H, et al. Specific miRNA signatures are associated with metastasis and poor prognosis in clear cell renal cell carcinoma. World J Urol 2011 Jun;29(3):367-73.

[134] Iorio MV, Croce CM. MicroRNA dysregulation in cancer: diagnostics, monitoring and therapeutics. A comprehensive review. EMBO Mol Med 2012 Mar;4(3):143-59.

Chapter 17

Is *CCDC26* a Novel Cancer-Associated Long-Chain Non-Coding RNA?

Tetsuo Hirano

Additional information is available at the end of the chapter

http://dx.doi.org/10.5772/54966

1. Introduction

Large-scale analysis of total genome transcripts (transcriptome) in organisms including human and mouse has revealed that many RNAs are transcribed from genomic regions that encode no proteins (referred to as ncRNA) (1-5). Among such ncRNAs, microRNAs (miRNAs), small molecule RNAs 18-28 bases long, have been extensively studied over the past decade, and a gene regulatory system called "RNA silencing" has been revealed. In humans, more than 400 miRNAs are known to regulate at least one-third of protein-encoding genes (6-10). Most miRNAs are generated by processing of long miRNA precursors (pri-miRNAs) (6, 9). Pri-miRNAs are transcribed by RNA polymerase II and 5′ cap structures and poly A tails are added, similarly to protein-encoding mRNAs. Pri-miRNAs are further processed in the nucleus into pre-miRNAs with an approximately 70 base hairpin structure and are then exported to the cytoplasm. pre-miRNAs are finally processed into mature miRNAs by the enzyme, Dicer. It is noteworthy that miRNAs are sometimes encoded in the introns of other genes. A mature miRNA is incorporated into the RNA-induced silencing complex to act on its target mRNA. Broadly speaking, miRNAs can act on mRNAs in two ways. If there is limited homology between an miRNA and a target mRNA, the miRNA suppresses translation of the mRNA. However, if the miRNA has complete or nearly complete homology with a target mRNA, the mRNA is rapidly degraded. In animal cells, the former scenario usually occurs (7, 10-12). Many miRNAs have been reported to be associated with tumors, including AML and glioma; however, it is still unclear how predominant miRNAs are in tumorigenesis.

Relatively large ncRNAs of over several hundred bases, which are longer than pri-miRNAs whose length is usually 200-300 bases, are called long-chain non-coding RNAs (lncRNAs). Despite their somewhat unclear definition and their largely undetermined functions (13), the public databases for lncRNAs, for example, lncRNAdb (http://www.lncrnadb.org/) (14)

or NONCODE (http://www.noncode.org) (15), contain several hundred mammalian lncRNAs, including more than 100 from human (16). The RNAs included are heterologous; some localize in the nucleus to form certain structures, others interact with chromatin modifying enzymes such as p300, while others function in the cytoplasm (Fig. 1).

Both miRNAs and lncRNAs are physiologically important in many biological processes, including development and cell differentiation. Their association with disease, especially cancers, is of great interest (5). Association of miRNAs with various tumors, including different types of leukemia (Table 1) and glioma (Table 2), has been demonstrated. They sometimes act as tumor-promoting factors and sometimes as tumor suppressors. Expression of many lncRNAs, including *NDM29* (neuroblastoma) (17, 18) and *MALAT-1* (lung cancer) (19) are correlated with tumor progression, while *MEG3* (pituitary tumor) (20, 21), *HOTAIR* (breast carcinoma) (22), *H19* (Wilms' tumor) (23), *AK023948* (papillary thyroid tumor) (24) and *LOC285194* (osteosarcoma) (25) are putative tumor suppressors (Table 3). These lncRNAs seem to control cancer cell growth by regulating other genes (*NDM29*, *HOTAIR*, *H19*) or by adjusting the mRNA splicing mechanism (*MALAT-1*) (Fig. 1) (14).

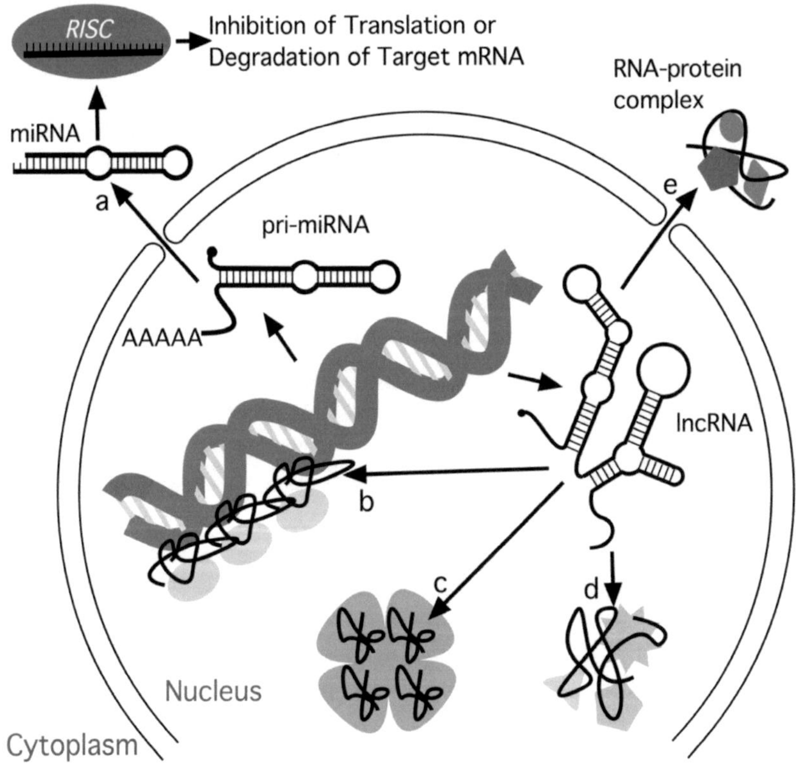

Figure 1. Classification of ncRNAs. (a) Pri-miRNAs are synthesized and processed in the nucleus, then exported to the cytoplasm. They are incorporated in the RISC complex to degrade or inhibit transcription of target mRNAs. However, some synthesized lncRNAs associate with chromatin (b) to silence certain genes. Some lncRNAs are incorporated in intranuclear bodies (c) or make complexes with specific proteins (d). Some are exported to the cytoplasm to work in the RNA-protein complex (e).

Name	Loci	Name	Loci
Oncogenic or Increased Expression in AML		*Tumor Suppressive or Decreased Expression in AML*	
let-7b	*22q13.31*	let-7	*9q22.32*
let-7e	*19q13.41*	let-7b	*22q13.31*
miR-10a	*17q21.32*	miR-9*	*1q22*
miR-10b	*2q31.1*	miR-15a	*13q14.2*
miR-27a	*19p13.13*	miR-15b	*3q25.33*
miR-30d	*8q24.22*	miR-16	*13q14.2*
miR-126	*9q34.3*	miR-19a	*13q31.3*
miR-129-5p	*7q32.1*	miR-20a	*13q31.3*
miR-130b	*22*	miR-26a	*3p22.2*
miR-142-5p	*17q22*	miR-29a	*7q32.3*
miR-155	*21q21.3*	miR-29b	*7q32.3*
miR-181a	*1q31.3/9q33.3*	miR-29c	*1q32.2*
miR-181b	*1q31.3/9q33.3*	miR-30a-3p	*6q13*
miR-181c	*19p13.13*	miR-34b	*11q23.1*
miR-181d	*19p13.13*	miR-34c	*11q23.1*
miR-195	*17p13.1*	miR-124	*8p23.1*
miR-221	*Xp11.3*	miR-128-1	*2q21.3*
miR-223	*Xq12*	miR-145	*5q32*
miR-221/222	*Xp11.3*	miR-147	*9q33.2*
miR-324-5p	*17p13.1*	miR-148a	*7p15.2*
miR-326	*11q13.4*	miR-151	*8q24.3*
miR-328	*16q22.1*	miR-181a	*1q31.3/9q33.3*
miR-331	*12q22*	miR-181b	*1q31.3/9q33.3*
miR-340	*5q35.3*	miR-182	*7q32.2*
miR-374	*Xq13.2*	miR-184	*15q25.1*
miR-424	*Xq26.3*	miR-194	*1q41*
		miR-196a	*17q21.32*
		miR-196a	*17q21.32*
		miR-199a	*19p13.2*
		miR-204	*9q21.12*
		miR-219-5p	*6q21.32*
		miR-220a	*Xq25*
		miR-302b*	*4q25*
		miR-302d	*4q25*
		miR-320	*8q21.3*
		miR-320	*8q21.3*
		miR-325	*Xq21.1*

Data are chosen from references 54, 55, 62, 63, 65, 66. Data confined to cytogenetically normal AML where possible. Note some miRNA appeared both oncogenic and tumor-suppressive.

Table 1. Examples of miRNAs associated with AML that change expression level

Name	Genetic Locus	Name	Genetic Locus
Oncogenic or Increased Expression in Glioma		*Tumor Suppressive or Decreased Expression in Glioma*	
miR-9*	*1q22*	let-7 family	*9q22.32*
miR-10a*	*17q21.32*	miR-7	*9q21.32*
miR-10b	*2q31.1*	miR-15b	*3q25.33*
miR-17/92 cluster	*13q31.3*	miR-17	*13q31.3*
miR-21	*17q23.1*	miR-26b	*2q35*
miR-25	*7q22.1*	miR-29b	*7q32.3*
miR-26a	*3p22.2*	miR-34a	*1p36.22*
miR-93	*7q22.1*	miR-101	*1p31.3*
miR-125b	*11q24.1*	miR-106a	*Xq26.2*
miR-182	*7q32.2*	miR-124	*8p23.1*
miR-195	*17p13.1*	miR-125a	*19q13.41*
miR-196a	*17q21.32*	miR-128	*2q21.3*
miR-196b	*7p15.2*	miR-137	*1p21.3*
miR-221/222	*Xp11.3*	miR-146b/146b-5p	*10q24.32*
miR-296	*20q13.32*	miR-153	*2q35*
miR-381	*14q32.31*	miR-181	*1q31.3/9q33.3*
miR-455-3p	*9q32*	miR-184	*15q25.1*
miR-486	*8p11.21*	miR-195	*17p13.1*
		miR-199b-5p	*9q34.11*
		miR-218	*4p15.31*
		miR-326	*11q13.4*
		miR-451	*17q11.2*

Data are chosen from references 67 and 68. Data confined to cases of low grade gliomas but exclusion of data from high grade glioblastoma is not necessarily complete. Note some miRNAs appeared both oncogenic and tumor-suppressive.

Table 2. miRNAs that show altered expression levels in glioma cells

Name	Alias	Mouse Homolog	Genetic Locus	Product Length (bp)	Tumor	Function	Refs
Tumor promoting or Increased Expression							
AIRN		*Airn*	*6q26*	NA	Wilms' tumor	NA	(59)
BC200	*BCYRN1*	*Bc1*	*2p21*	200	Breast cancer	Regulation of protein biosynthesis	(70)
HIF1A-AS2	*aHIF*	NA	*14q23.2*	2051	Multiple cancers	Decoy of mRNA	(71)
HOTAIR	*Gm16258*	*Hotair*	*12q13.3*	2364	Multiple cancers	Epigenetic silencing of HOXD gene through histoneH3K27 methylation	(72)
HULC		NA	*6p24.3*	500	Hepatocellular carcinoma	Post-transcriptional regulation	(73)
IGF2AS	*PEG8*	*Igh2as*	*11p15.5*	2091	Wilms' tumor	NA	(74)
KRASP1		NA	*6p12-p11*	5178	Prostate cancer	Decoy of miRNA	(75)
L1PA16		*VL30-1*[a)]	*3q26.3*	833	Many tumor cell lines	Activation of proto-oncogene	(76)
MALAT1	*Neat2*	*Malat1*	*11q13.1*	8708	Multiple cancer	Control of RNA procession	(19, 77)
MER11C	*HERVK11*	*VL30-1*[a)]	*11p11.1*	1060	Many tumor cell lines	Activation of proto-oncogene	(76)
PCA3	*DD3*	NA	*9q21-q22*	3735	Prostate cancer	NA	(78)
PCGEM1		NA	*2q32*	1603	Prostate cancer	NA	(79)
PRNCR1		NA	*8q24*	>12756	Prostate cancer	NA	(80)
SRA1		*Sra1*	*5q31.3*	1955	Breast cancer	Activation of nuclear receptors	(81)
TERC		*Terc*	*3q26*	451	Multiple cancer	Telomere template	(82)
UCA1	*CUDR*	NA	*19p13.12*	1591	Bladder cancer	Regulation of cell cycle	(83)
WT1-AS	*WIT1*	NA	*11p13*	1333	Wilms' tumor AML	Downregulation of WT1, tumor suppressor	(84)
XIST		*Xist*	*Xq13.2*	19271	Multiple cancers	Xinactivation	(56, 85)
Tumor Suppressing or Decreased Expression in Tumor							
AK023948		NA	*8q24*	2807	Papillary thyroid carcinoma	NA	(24)
ANRIL	*CDK2BAS, p15AS*	NA	*9q21*	941	Prostate cancer, breast cancer, melanoma, and other tumors	Regulation of epigenetic transcriptional repression	(58)
BC040587		NA	*3q13.31*	NA	Osteosarcoma	NA	(25)
DLEU2		*Dleu2*	*13q14.3*	2768	Chronic lymphocytic leukemia	pri-miRNA for miR15a and miR16	(86)

Name	Alias	Mouse Homolog	Genetic Locus	Product Length (bp)	Tumor	Function	Refs
GAS5		*Gas5*	*1q25.1*	651	Breast cancer	Decoy of glucocorticoid receptor	(87)
H19		*H19*	*11p15.5*	2322	Wilms' tumor	Epigenetic regulation through DNA methylation	(88)
KCNQ1OT1	*LIT1, KvLQT1-AS, KvLQT1OT1*	*Kcnq1ot1*	*11p15*	91671	Embryonal cancer associated with Beckwith-Wiedemann syndrome	Epigenetic imprinting through H3K27 methylation	(57)
LOC285194		NA	*3q13.31*	NA	Osteosarcoma	NA	(25)
MEG3	*Gtl2*	*Meg3*	*14q32*	1595	Glioma, pituitary adenoma and other tumor	Regulation of p53 target proteins	(89)
NDM29	*29A*	NA	*11p15.3*	131	Neuroblastoma	Induction the appearance of neuronal-like properties	(18)
p53 mRNA		*Tp53*	*17p13.1*	19144	Multiple cancer	RNA protein binding, MDM3	(90)
PTENP1		NA	*9p21*	3932	Prostate cancer	Decoy for PTEN-targeting miRNAs	(75)
RMRP		*Rmrp*	*9p21-p12*	267	Leukemia and lymphoma	Mitochondrial RNA processing endoribonuclease, hTERT-dependent	(91)
TERRA		*TelRNAs*	telomere repeats	NA	Many cancer cell lines	Interaction with the TRF1	(92)
vtRNA2-1		NA	*5q31.1*	100	AML, papillary thyroid cancer	Regulation of RNA dependent protein kinase (pPKR)	(93)
ZNFX1-AS1	*Zfas1*	*1500012 F01Rik*	*20q13.13*	1020	Breast cancer	NA	(94)

(a) no homologous RNA but binds to PSF, a transcriptional repressor. NA, not available.

Table 3. Human lncRNAs associated with tumors described in public data bases.

2. Genetic abnormality observed in acute myeloid leukemia (AML)

AML, which comprises approximately 25% of hematopoietic malignancies, has heterogeneous clinical features and variable responses to contemporary therapy (26). Genetic alterations are often observed in AML cells and the clinical heterogeneity of the disease is considered to reflect the genetic diversity of these cells (27, 28). It is very important to study the genetic mutations in AML cells to fully understand the cause of the disease. However, genetic lesion(s) responsible for AML, such as the loss or gain of a certain gene, have not yet been fully elucidated. Indeed, the complex features of AML suggest that the genetic cause of this disease is multifactorial (29). Several protein-encoding genes have been identified that are useful for indicating the prognosis of the disease (30-32). These include *RUNX1* (*AML1*)-*RUNX1T1* (*ETO*) and *CBFB-MYH11*, which are associated with specific chromosomal mutations, *t(8;21)(q22;q22)* and *inv(16)(p13;q12)/t(16;16)(p13;q22)*, respectively. AML with these cytogenetic features (singly or together) represents about 15% of *de novo* AML. The patients with these diagnostic criteria are classified in the favorable clinical outcome group (standard-risk group). Several other chromosomal abnormalities have been recurrently observed, as described in the WHO classification. AML with balanced or unbalanced translocations involving the *MLL* gene located on chromosome 11 are also well documented and are mostly classified in the intermediate-risk group. Meanwhile, AML patients with a normal karyotype and no cytological abnormality include cases classified in the unfavorable (adverse-risk) or intermediate-risk group. Moreover, a genetic abnormality of the *FL3* gene (internal tandem repeat) is found in many AML subtypes and, in combination with a wild-type *NPM* gene, contributes to poor prognosis (31). Recently, Paschka and colleagues have revealed that the genes encoding the metabolic enzymes, isocitrate dehydrogenase 1 and 2 (*IDH1/2*) are important for diagnosis and prognosis prediction of AML patients (33). These mutations of *IDH1/2* change the activity of the enzymes to reduce α-ketoglutarate levels and to elevate 2-hydroxyglutarate levels. This results in changes to chromatin structure and destabilization of certain gene-regulatory proteins, including *HIF-1* (34). While cytogenetically normal AML patients with an *NPM* mutation and a normal *FL3* gene tend to show favorable outcomes, AML patients with the same genetic profile but also with *IDH1/2* mutation showed adverse prognosis with poorer remission. *IDH1/2* mutation was also found in several other tumors, including glioma (35). Therefore, a combination of genetic alterations resulting in mutation of specific genes as well as cytogenetically apparent chromosomal changes are important for AML malignancy.

3. AML and *CCDC26*

In HL-60 cells derived from AML, a small part of chromosome 8 is excised and amplified as an extrachromosomal element, or double minute chromosome (dmin). Dmin is a cytogenetic abnormality infrequently observed in AML. The dmin of HL-60 cells consists of several repeats of an amplification unit (referred as amplicon) of about 2 million base pairs. The amplicon, which is derived from several areas of an approximately 4.6 million base pair region of chromosome *8q24*, contains an intact *MYC* oncogene. Besides *MYC*, several other genes, including *CCDC26* and tribbles homolog 1 (*TRIB1*), are also encoded on the amplicon (Fig. 2). All are actively transcribed in HL-60 cells. The drug-induced differentiation of HL-60 cells suppressed the expression of all these genes, indicating that they might be related to the cancerous nature of the cells. Some types of cancer cell respond to the anticancer drug hydroxyurea by excluding unstable extrachromosomal elements, which then lose their proliferative nature. In HL-60 cells, the original *MYC* genetic locus remained intact after dmin was excluded, but was no longer transcribed (36). These observations suggest that the expression of genes from dmin, with its altered DNA structure, and from the intact chromosome are different, and can be interpreted as being due to aberrant gene expression from dmin (including the *MYC* oncogene). Interestingly, in HL-60 cells, the *CCDC26* gene on dmin is rearranged as a result of chromosomal rejoining and is amplified in an incomplete form to produce abnormal transcripts (37).

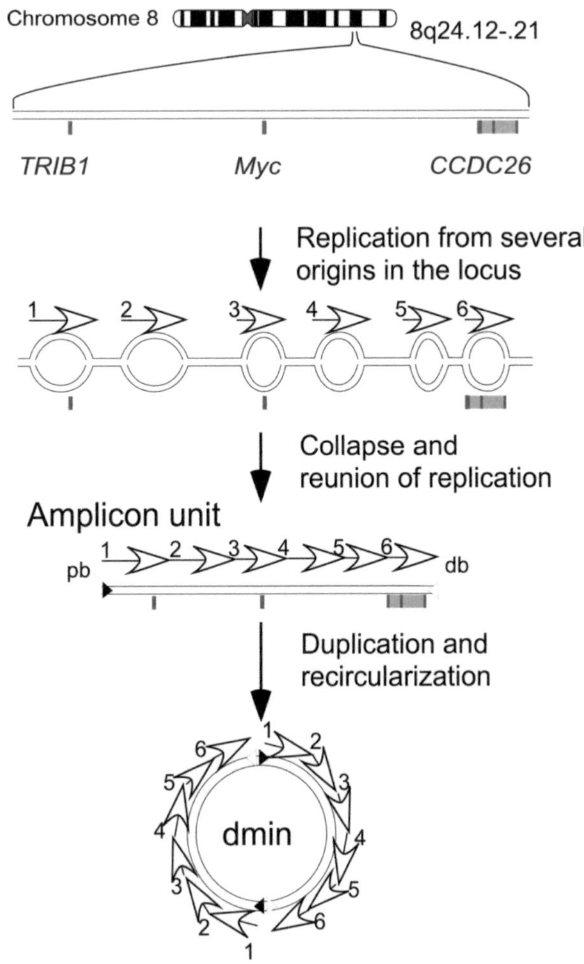

Figure 2. Depiction of the generation of the discontinuous amplicon unit of dmin in HL-60 cells. Several replication initiation bubbles collapse and "corrupted" bubbles reunite to form an amplicon unit. Excision of an initial large amplicon (possibly as an episome) might precede replication. The arrows numbered 1 through 6 indicate regions reunited in the amplicon. Note that the lengths of the various regions are not to scale. Once the amplicon unit has formed, its multimerization results in a dmin.

A common change occurs at the *CCDC26* locus in cytologically dmin-positive AML patients. This chromosomal change occurs at a position consistent with the amplified region observed in HL-60 cells (38, 39). Furthermore, destruction of the internal structure of the *CCDC26* gene seems to underlie the common mechanism behind the generation of dmin-positive AML cells.

A comprehensive genome-wide study of a group of childhood AML patients revealed that *CCDC26* was one of the genes with the highest increase in copy number in AML cells. Radtke and colleagues investigated chromosome number alteration (CNA) in pediatric AML using a comprehensive single nucleotide polymorphism (SNP) array analysis. They found the most common CNA, in 14% (15 in 111) of pediatric AML patients, to be in chromosome band 8q24 with a low-burden copy number increase (2.83-3.77 copies) (40). These included cases of trisomy 8, which frequently occurs in AML (41). The minimum altered region common in all 15 of these patients was located in a 20-megabase region of *8q24*, which contains *CCDC26*.

Originally, *CCDC26* was reported as a gene associated with differentiation and apoptosis of PLB985 cells (an HL-60 subclone) following induction by treatment with retinoic acid (*CCDC26* is also known as *RAM*, retinoic acid modifying). In cells that have become resistant to differentiation and apoptosis after infection of retrovirus, the viral genome was seen to be inserted in the intron of *CCDC26*. Retinoic acid promotes differentiation and apoptosis of not only many leukemia cells but also of neuroblastoma and glioblastoma cells through transcriptional regulation of many other genes. *CCDC26* may have a role with retinoic acid in differentiation and growth arrest of these cells (42).

4. Glioma and *CCDC26*

Primary brain tumor (PBT) is a disease with an incidence of 12 in 100,000 per year. Glioma accounts for a major part of PBT, and contains cases with different grades of malignancy, namely (I) benign glioma, (II) diffuse astrocytoma, (III) anaplastic astrocytoma and (IV) glioblastoma (43). Although many genetic abnormalities have been reported in gliomas, a single critical lesion responsible for tumorigenesis has not been found. Among these abnormalities, mutations occur in genes for DNA repair enzymes, including *PRKDC, XRCC, PARP1, MGMT, ERCC1, ERCC2*, epidermal growth factor and the inflammatory cytokine, *IL-13*. Furthermore, over-expression or amplification of the epidermal growth factor receptor gene and deletion of *p16INK* are correlated with poor survival (43). A genome wide association study using SNPs revealed the association of several genes with glioma, including telomerase regulating gene *TERT, RTEL1*, tumor suppressor gene *CDKN2A/2B*, pleckstrin homology-like domain family B member 1 (a protein with unknown function) and *CCDC26* (44). The *CCDC26* gene locus was strongly linked with this glioma by several SNPs, including rs4295627, rs16904140, rs6470745, rs891835, and rs10464870 (see Fig. 3a). A different SNP in the intergenic region bordering *CCDC26*, rs987525, was linked to cleft palate (45). Notably, cleft palate is also a risk factor of PBT. *CCDC26* is, therefore, a potential common factor of both conditions. *CCDC26* is just one of the risk factors for glioma and other genetic risk factors increase glioma incidence cumulatively. Therefore, there might be a synergistic effect with other genetic risk factors (46). *CCDC26* is not necessarily a risk factor of high grade (III-IV) glioma (47). Interestingly, in concordance with the situation for AML, the *CCDC26* genotype is associated with *IDH1/2* mutation in low grade glioma. Considering the synergy of *CCDC26* with *IDH1/2*, *CCDC26* may have linkage to a subpopulation of gliomas with relatively lower grade (46, 48).

The Gene Expression Omnibus database (GEO; http://www.ncbi.nlm.nih.gov/geo/) (49) contains data showing altered *CCDC26* expression between normal and tumorigenic cells. Expression of *CCDC26* is higher in myeloid leukemia cell lines, namely KG-1, THP-1 and U937, compared with normal monocytes (GEO dataset accession ID; GDS2251), and is higher in sporadic basal-like cancer compared with normal cells (GD2250). On the other

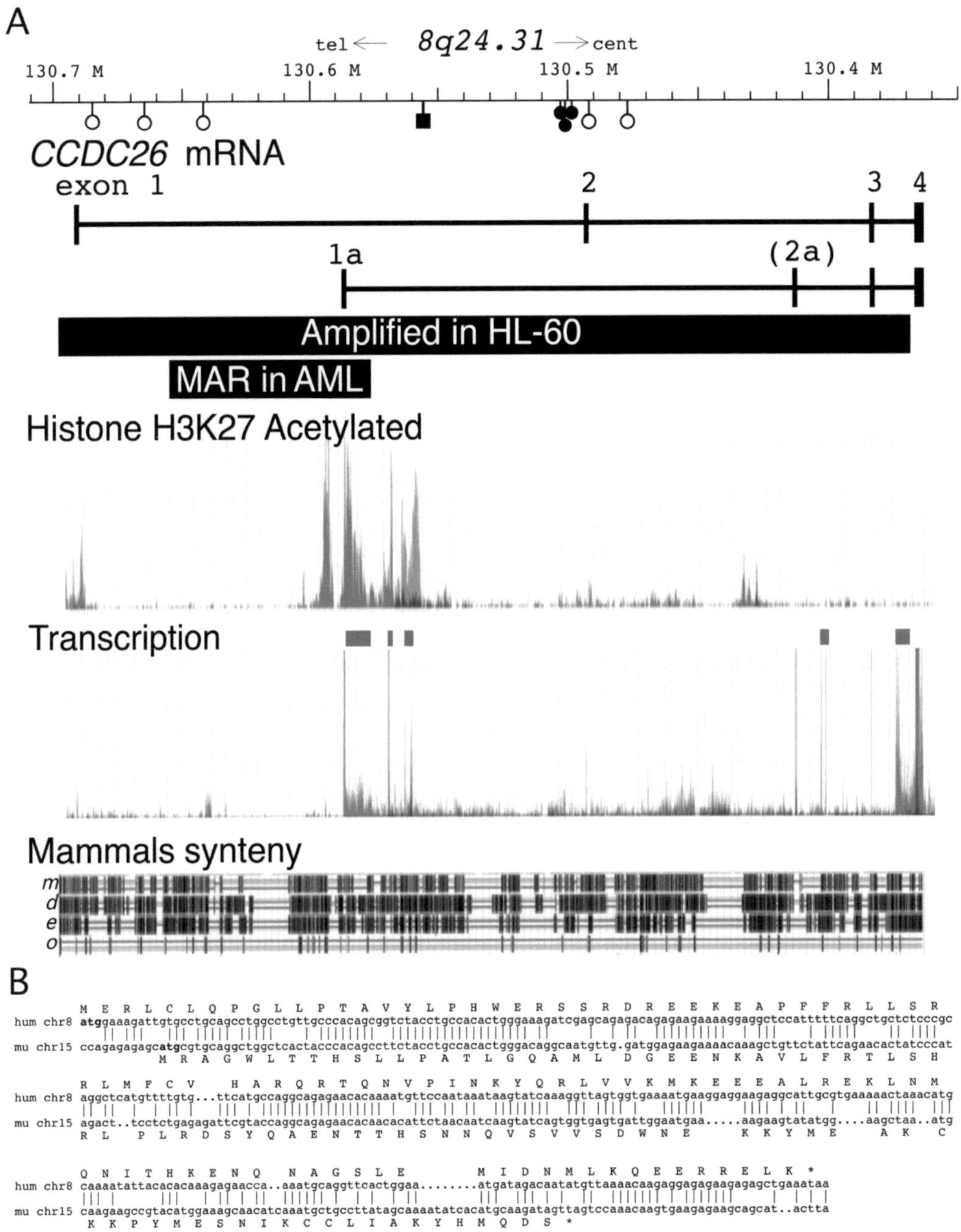

Figure 3. (A) Summary of genetic locus 8q24.31. The scale indicates the region 8q24.31 (130.35 Mb to 130.71 Mb; numbering is based on human genome assembly 37.1). Marks on the scale indicate the locations of five SNPs that are linked to glioma (open circles; rs4295627, rs16904140, rs6470745, rs891835 and rs10464870, left to right), three miRNAs registered in the public database (filled circles; mir-3669, mir-3673 and mir-3686, left to right) and a retrovirus insertion site (filled square) within the introns of *CCDC26*. Below the scale, which covers a 350-kb region, major variants of *CCDC26* mRNA (long and

short) are shown. The long transcript consists of four (1-2-3-4) exons, and the short transcripts consist of three (1a-3-4) or four (1a-2a-3-4) exons. All variants share exon 3 and 4, in which the hypothetical open reading frame is encoded. Locations of the amplified region in HL-60 cells and the commonly amplified region (MAR) in childhood AML are shown with filled rectangles. The hypothetical open reading frame encoded in exons 3 and 4 is not included in the region amplified in HL-60 cells. The pattern of histone H3K27 acetylation, activity of transcription in leukemia cell lines, and bar plots for conserved synteny between human and each organism (m: mouse, d: dog, e: elephant and o: opossum) obtained from the UCSC Genome Browser (95) are shown. Actively transcribed regions that are not the major exons of *CCDC26* mRNA are indicated by grey rectangles. (B) Optimal alignment of the *CCDC26* exon 3-4 encoded ORF and the region of conserved synteny on mouse chromosome 15. A possible ORF (94 amino acids) in the mouse sequence is totally mismatched with that of human by frameshift changes.

hand, *CCDC26* expression is decreased in hyperplastic enlarged lobular units considered as the earliest precursors of breast cancer compared with normal units (GDS2739). Increased *CCDC26* expression is associated with malignancy progression in some cancerous cells. *CCDC26* expression was increased in CD133 positive neurosphere-like glioma cell lines compared with CD133 negative adherent glioma cell lines (GDS2728), and was increased in alveolar macrophages of cigarette smokers comparison with macrophages of non-smokers (GDS3496). Increased expression of *CCDC26* might mean this gene is tumorigenic or oncogenic. However, the relationship of altered *CCDC26* expression to malignancy is still ambiguous.

5. Overview of the *CCDC26* genetic locus

As described in the previous section, all SNPs associated with glioma, and a retrovirus insertion site where virus insertion makes AML cells resistant to retinoic acid (42) are located in the intron of *CCDC26* (Fig. 3a). Exon 4, which encodes the majority of a hypothetical open reading frame (ORF), is not amplified in pediatric AML or in AML-derived HL-60 cells. The exonic sequence of *CCDC26* is not well conserved in other species, including mouse, and an ORF has no homology with known proteins. These data strongly suggest that *CCDC26* does not function as a protein-encoding RNA; rather it functions as a ncRNA. Highly conserved regions in the intron sequence of *CCDC26* suggest the existence of another intronic ncRNA. As mentioned above, the *CCDC26* locus is rearranged in the genome of HL-60 cells. It is plausible that the ncRNA encoded by this locus is important for the growth of these cells.

A short putative ORF encoding a protein or with a length of 109 amino acids is present in the *CCDC26* exons; there is no other ORF of more than 50 amino acids. This actual protein, however, has not been observed. Moreover, orthologous proteins are not found in any other organism. For example, a loosely homologous sequence of human exon 4, found in the mouse chromosome 15 region of conserved synteny, with an ORF of 94 amino acids is actively transcribed in mouse leukemia cells (T. Hirano unpublished observation). However, this ORF is completely different from the human sequence and even contains frame shift alterations (Fig. 3b). This indicates that the putative protein encoded by *CCDC26* has no conserved function among species. Although this ORF may be coincidental due to the absence of stop codons, an interesting possibility is that this unique protein has newly emerged during human evolution. mRNA stability is influenced by whether an ORF is encoded because nonsense mediated RNA decay, a mechanism associated with quality control of mRNA, rapidly degrades mRNAs that are not useful as templates for protein synthesis. Absence of an ORF in an mRNA promotes degradation by this mechanism, however, the existence of a *CCDC26* protein will prolong the lifetime of *CCDC26* mRNA and may maintain the function (if any) of the RNA itself.

Because of the considerable length of the *CCDC26* intron (330 kbp versus 1200 bp exons), it is very difficult to ignore the possibility that there is another transcript(s) within this intron with important function. Possible encoded ncRNAs within the *CCDC26* exon-intron region are summarized in Fig. 4 and include, mRNA (a), intronic encoded ncRNA (b), intronic lariat RNA (c-d) and miRNA independently transcribed or processed from the precursor of the *CCDC26* mRNA (e). Actually there are several regions in the *CCDC26* intron where nucleosomal histones undergo high levels of methylation and acetylation, meaning that these locations may be actively transcribed (Fig.3a). Furthermore, most of these regions are

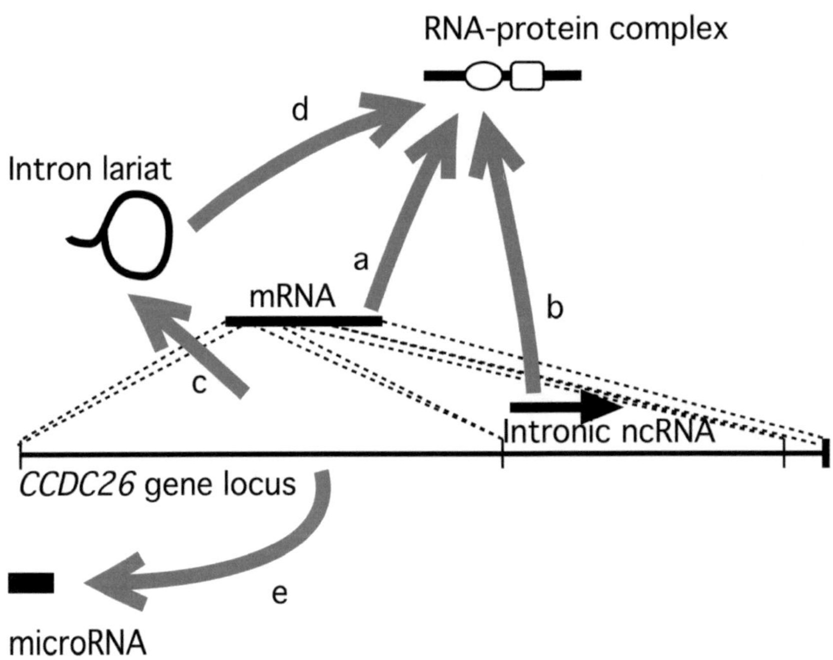

Figure 4. A possible function of *CCDC26*. The 330-kb precursor RNA transcribed from the gene is processed into mature mRNA. It then forms a complex with proteins to perform its biological function, for example, silencing a certain genetic locus (a). Alternatively, the ncRNA independently encoded in the intronic region (b) or the processed intron lariat (c-d) could have biological functions. The intronic microRNA could be transcribed directly from the genome using its own promoter or processed from the precursor of the *CCDC26* mRNA(e). Note that lengths of nucleic acid chains are not to scale. Length of the precursor RNA is approximately 330 kb; *CCDC26* mRNA is 1.3 kb; the spliced lariat is more than 100 kb; intronic microRNA is 18-23 bases.

highly conserved among mammals, suggesting that function is encoded. Also, expressed sequence tags other than known spliced *CCDC26* mRNAs have been reported in the intron. There are three miRNAs (miR-3669, 3673 and 3686) in the intron of *CCDC26* that are registered in the miRNA database (miRBase; http://www.mirbase.org/)(50). Although their functions are unknown, they may act as oncogenic or tumor suppressive ncRNAs.

6. Hypothetical function of *CCDC26* as a non-coding RNA

Although many ncRNAs are registered in databases, only a few have clearly demonstrated functions and detailed mechanisms of action. *CCDC26* might be a new ncRNA that is associated with cancer, including AML. Interestingly, expression of an miRNA, miR-21, is observed in many malignant cells, including AML cells (51). Also phorbol ester-induced differentiation of HL-60 cells into macrophage-like cells is accompanied by up-regulation of miR-21 (52). There are several reports suggesting that miRNAs act as oncogenic or tumor suppressive miRNAs in AML, as reviewed in (53, 54). Recently, Marcucci and colleagues used 305 different probes to search for miRNA expression in favorable and adverse-risk groups of normal karyotype AML (monocytic leukemia). They then used these data to link expression profiles with the cohort analysis of the patients. They identified a certain pattern of miRNA expression in the adverse-risk group and linked the expression level of eight types of miRNA to AML prognosis (55). It is possible that an unknown miRNA in the *CCDC26* locus affects cancer malignancy through the regulation of other genes. But all miRNAs described so far in the *CCDC26* locus (mir-3669, mir-3673 and mir-3686) show no expression in leukemia cells and no conservation among mammals in contrast to other oncogenic miRNAs; for example miR21 and let7, are actively transcribed and strongly conserved.

Within the CCDC26 intronic region, there are some long regions (>10 kb) that are actively transcribed in leukemia cells (Fig. 3a). They seem to be too long for pri-miRNAs but could encode lncRNAs. Indeed, active transcription occurs in the *CCDC26* region in cells derived from AML (T. Hirano unpublished observation), meaning that these transcripts might function as a tumor promoting or oncogenic lncRNAs. In contrast, if the original function of *CCDC26*, or of lncRNAs associated with *CCDC26*, was lost by chromosomal abnormality (for example in dmin of HL-60 cells), then they might function naturally as tumor suppressors. Some lncRNAs including *XIST* (56), *KCNQ1OT1* (57), *ANRIL* (58) and *AIRN* (59) are known to suppress (in cis) the expression of neighboring gene. It is well known that genes located in extrachromosomal elements such as dmin are actively transcribed, but the mechanism behind this phenomenon is not well understood (60, 61). Differences between dmin and an intact chromosome are caused by differences in chromatin structure, which is indicated by differences in DNase I hypersensitivity (36). Similarly to other gene silencing lncRNAs, an ncRNA encoded by the *CCDC26* locus might suppress the expression of other nearby genes. The hypothesis that neighboring genes, including the *MYC* oncogene, are activated when the normal *CCDC26* locus structure is destroyed by a chromosomal abnormality could explain the high transcriptional activity of genes in extrachromosomal elements (Fig.5). Further evidence is needed to determine whether *CCDC26* mRNA and/or its transcripts encoded in its intron are oncogenic or tumor suppressive.

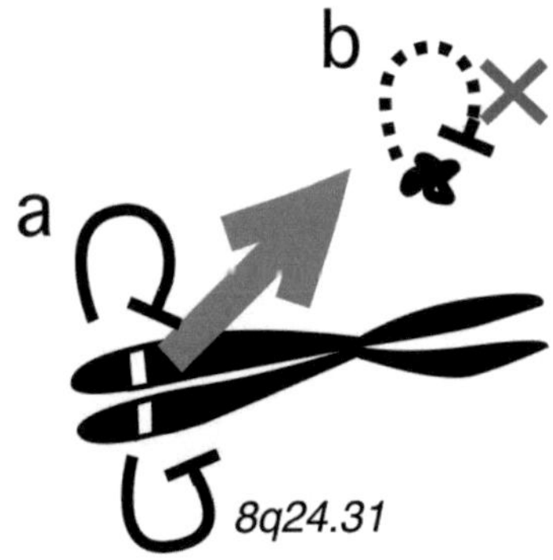

Figure 5. Hypothetical mechanism by which an oncogene (for example *MYC*) is inactivated in an intact chromosome (a) by *CCDC26* regulation. This suppression does not function on extrachromosomal chromatin (b).

7. Future perspectives

The size of the *CCDC26* locus, spanning over 330,000 base pairs, makes it difficult to study. If the ORF of the gene is not functional then it is unclear which part(s) of the locus are functional. Therefore, to study this gene, it is first necessary to determine all transcripts produced by the *CCDC26* locus and then to analyze their function. Comprehensive analysis of transcriptome of the relevant region using tiling microarray analysis is needed. Although lncRNA orthologs are frequently not found between species, homology analysis of this region between human and mouse could be helpful to identify functional sequences. Once transcripts are identified, we will be able to perform *in situ* hybridization to determine subcellular localization. Knock-down of transcripts will be useful to investigate their functions. Proteins interacting with the RNA transcripts will be identifiable by pull-down assays and mass spectrometry analysis. Finally, gene targeting should be used to investigate the effects of disruption of the region encoding the transcript. It will be of special interest if transcription of neighboring genes is activated or inactivated (in particular *MYC*), suggesting a regulatory function of the ncRNA encoded in the *CCDC26* locus. If an ortholog of the gene is found in mice, making a knock-out mouse of the ncRNA or a transgenic mouse with forced expression of the ncRNA will help to demonstrate its relationship to disease.

8. Conclusion

As a conclusion, the *CCDC26* locus is considered to encode an lncRNA involved in tumorigenesis. *CCDC26* itself might be an lncRNA or its intron might contain a functional miRNA or lncRNA. The study of this gene will bring new knowledge to gene regulation and to cancer treatment strategies targeting lncRNAs. Further *in vitro* and *in vivo* study is needed to prove the relationship between transcripts from the locus and disease, such as leukemia and glioma.

Author details

Tetsuo Hirano
Life Science Group, Graduate School of Integrated Arts and Sciences, Hiroshima University, Kagamiyama, Higashihiroshima, Hiroshima, Japan

9. References

[1] Wilusz JE, Sunwoo H, Spector DL. Long noncoding RNAs: functional surprises from the RNA world. Genes Dev. 2009;23:1494-504.

[2] Mattick JS. The genetic signatures of noncoding RNAs. PLoS Genet. 2009;5:e1000459.

[3] Alexander RP, Fang G, Rozowsky J, Snyder M, Gerstein MB. Annotating non-coding regions of the genome. Nat Rev Genet. 2010;11:559-71.

[4] Chen L-L, Carmichael GG. Decoding the function of nuclear long non-coding RNAs. Curr Opin Cell Biol. 2010;22:357-64.

[5] Wapinski O, Chang HY. Long noncoding RNAs and human disease. Trends in Cell Biol. 2011;21:354-61

[6] Liu N, Okamura K, Tyler DM, Phillips MD, Chung W-j, Lai EC. The evolution and functional diversification of animal microRNA genes. Cell Res. 2008;18:985-96.

[7] Kutter C, Svoboda P. miRNA, siRNA, piRNA. RNA Biology. 2008;5:181-8.

[8] Vaz C, Ahmad HM, Sharma P, Gupta R, Kumar L, Kulshreshtha R, et al. Analysis of microRNA transcriptome by deep sequencing of small RNA libraries of peripheral blood. BMC Genomics. 2010;11:288.

[9] Czech B, Hannon GJ. Small RNA sorting: matchmaking for Argonautes. Nat Rev Genet. 2011;12:19-31.

[10] Varol N, Konac E, Gurocak OS, Sozen S. The realm of microRNAs in cancers. Mol Biol Rep. 2011;38:1079-89.

[11] Valeri N, Vannini I, Fanini F, Calore F, Adair B, Fabbri M. Epigenetics, miRNAs, and human cancer: a new chapter in human gene regulation. Mammalian Genome. 2009;20:573-80.

[12] Lujambio A, Lowe SW. The microcosmos of cancer. Nature. 2012;482:347-55

[13] Brosnan CA, Voinnet O. The long and the short of noncoding RNAs. Curr Opin Cell Biol. 2009;21:416-25.

[14] Amaral PP, Clark MB, Gascoigne DK, Dinger ME, Mattick JS. lncRNAdb: a reference database for long noncoding RNAs. Nucleic Acids Res. 2011;39:D146-51.

[15] Bu D, Yu K, Sun S, Xie C, Skogerbø G, Miao R, et al. NONCODE v3.0: integrative annotation of long noncoding RNAs. Nucleic Acids Res. 2012;40:D210-5.

[16] Spizzo R, Almeida MI, Colombatti A, Calin Ga. Long non-coding RNAs and cancer: a new frontier of translational research? Oncogene. 2012:1-11.

[17] Castelnuovo M, Massone S, Tasso R, Fiorino G, Gatti M, Robello M, et al. An Alu-like RNA promotes cell differentiation and reduces malignancy of human neuroblastoma cells. FASEB J. 2010;24:4033-46.

[18] Gavazzo P, Vella S, Marchetti C, Nizzari M, Cancedda R, Pagano A. Acquisition of neuron-like electrophysiological properties in neuroblastoma cells by controlled expression of NDM29 ncRNA. J Neurochem. 2011;119:989-1001.

[19] Bernard D, Prasanth KV, Tripathi V, Colasse S, Nakamura T, Xuan Z, et al. A long nuclear-retained non-coding RNA regulates synaptogenesis by modulating gene expression. The EMBO J. 2010;29:3082-93.

[20] Zhang X, Gejman R, Mahta A, Zhong Y, Rice Ka, Zhou Y, et al. Maternally expressed gene 3, an imprinted noncoding RNA gene, is associated with meningioma pathogenesis and progression. Cancer Res. 2010;70:2350-8.

[21] Zhou Y, Zhang X, Klibanski A. MEG3 non-coding RNA: a tumor suppressor. J Mol Endocrinol. 2012:45-53.

[22] Gupta Ra, Shah N, Wang KC, Kim J, Horlings HM, Wong DJ, et al. Long non-coding RNA HOTAIR reprograms chromatin state to promote cancer metastasis. Nature. 2010;464:1071-6.

[23] Yoshimizu T, Miroglio A, Ripoche M-A, Gabory A, Vernucci M, Riccio A, et al. The H19 locus acts in vivo as a tumor suppressor. Proc Natl Acad Sci USA. 2008;105:12417-22.

[24] He H, Nagy R, Liyanarachchi S, Jiao H, Li W, Suster S, et al. A susceptibility locus for papillary thyroid carcinoma on chromosome 8q24. Cancer Res. 2009;69:625-31.

[25] Pasic I, Shlien A, Durbin AD, Stavropoulos DJ, Baskin B, Ray PN, et al. Recurrent focal copy-number changes and loss of heterozygosity implicate two noncoding RNAs and one tumor suppressor gene at chromosome 3q13.31 in osteosarcoma. Cancer Res. 2010;70:160-71.

[26] Estey E, Döhner H. Acute myeloid leukaemia. Lancet. 2006;368:1894-907.

[27] Walter MJ, Payton JE, Ries RE, Shannon WD, Deshmukh H, Zhao Y, et al. Acquired copy number alterations in adult acute myeloid leukemia genomes. Proc Natl Acad Sci USA. 2009;106:12950-5.

[28] Akagi T, Ogawa S, Dugas M, Kawamata N, Yamamoto G, Nannya Y, et al. Frequent genomic abnormalities in acute myeloid leukemia/myelodysplastic syndrome with normal karyotype. Haematologica. 2009;94:213-23.

[29] Renneville A, Roumier C, Biggio V, Nibourel O, Boissel N, Fenaux P, et al. Cooperating gene mutations in acute myeloid leukemia: a review of the literature. Leukemia. 2008;22:915-31.

[30] Vardiman JW, Thiele J, Arber Da, Brunning RD, Borowitz MJ, Porwit A, et al. The 2008 revision of the World Health Organization (WHO) classification of myeloid neoplasms and acute leukemia: rationale and important changes. Blood. 2009;114:937-51.

[31] Mrózek K, Radmacher MD, Bloomfield CD, Marcucci G. Molecular signatures in acute myeloid leukemia. Curr Opin Hematol. 2009;16:64-9.

[32] Döhner H, Estey EH, Amadori S, Appelbaum FR, Büchner T, Burnett AK, et al. Diagnosis and management of acute myeloid leukemia in adults: recommendations from an international expert panel, on behalf of the European LeukemiaNet. Blood. 2010;115:453-74.

[33] Paschka P, Schlenk RF, Gaidzik VI, Habdank M, Krönke J, Bullinger L, et al. IDH1 and IDH2 mutations are frequent genetic alterations in acute myeloid leukemia and confer

adverse prognosis in cytogenetically normal acute myeloid leukemia with NPM1 mutation without FLT3 internal tandem duplication. J Clin Oncol. 2010;28:3636-43.

[34] Xu W, Yang H, Liu Y, Yang Y, Wang P, Kim S-H, et al. Oncometabolite 2-hydroxyglutarate is a competitive inhibitor of α-ketoglutarate-dependent dioxygenases. Cancer Cell. 2011;19:17-30.

[35] Dang L, Jin S, Su SM. IDH mutations in glioma and acute myeloid leukemia. Trends Mol Med. 2010;16:387-97.

[36] Kitajima K, Haque M, Nakamura H, Hirano T, Utiyama H. Loss of irreversibility of granulocytic differentiation induced by dimethyl sulfoxide in HL-60 sublines with a homogeneously staining region. Biochem Biophys Res Commun. 2001;288:1182-7.

[37] Hirano T, Ike F, Murata T, Obata Y, Utiyama H, Yokoyama KK. Genes encoded within 8q24 on the amplicon of a large extrachromosomal element are selectively repressed during the terminal differentiation of HL-60 cells. Mutat Res. 2008;640:97-106.

[38] Storlazzi CT, Fioretos T, Paulsson K, Strömbeck B, Lassen C, Ahlgren T, et al. Identification of a commonly amplified 4.3 Mb region with overexpression of C8FW, but not MYC in MYC-containing double minutes in myeloid malignancies. Hum Mol Genet. 2004;13:1479-85.

[39] Storlazzi CT, Fioretos T, Surace C, Lonoce A, Mastrorilli A, Strömbeck B, et al. MYC-containing double minutes in hematologic malignancies: evidence in favor of the episome model and exclusion of MYC as the target gene. Hum Mol Genet. 2006;15:933-42.

[40] Radtke I, Mullighan CG, Ishii M, Su X, Cheng J, Ma J, et al. Genomic analysis reveals few genetic alterations in pediatric acute myeloid leukemia. Proc Natl Acad Sci USA. 2009;106:12944-9.

[41] Paulsson K, Johansson B. Trisomy 8 as the sole chromosomal aberration in acute myeloid leukemia and myelodysplastic syndromes. Pathologie-biologie. 2007;55:37-48.

[42] Yin W, Rossin A, Clifford JL, Gronemeyer H. Co-resistance to retinoic acid and TRAIL by insertion mutagenesis into RAM. Oncogene. 2006;25:3735-44.

[43] Liu Y, Shete S, Hosking F, Robertson L, Houlston R, Bondy M. Genetic advances in glioma: susceptibility genes and networks. Curr Opin Genet Dev. 2010;20:239-44.

[44] Shete S, Hosking FJ, Robertson LB, Dobbins SE, Sanson M, Malmer B, et al. Genome-wide association study identifies five susceptibility loci for glioma. Nat Genet. 2009;41:899-904.

[45] Boehringer S, van der Lijn F, Liu F, Günther M, Sinigerova S, Nowak S, et al. Genetic determination of human facial morphology: links between cleft-lips and normal variation. Eu J Hum Genet. 2011;19:1192-7.

[46] Lasho TL, Tefferi A, Pardanani A, Finke CM, Fink SR, Caron aa, et al. Differential distribution of CCDC26 glioma-risk alleles in myeloid malignancies with mutant IDH1 compared with their IDH2R140-mutated or IDH-unmutated counterparts. Leukemia. 2012;26:1406-7.

[47] Wrensch M, Jenkins RB, Chang JS, Yeh R-f, Xiao Y, Decker PA, et al. Variants in the CDKN2B and RTEL1 regions are associated with high-grade glioma susceptibility. Nat Genet. 2009;41:905-8.

[48] Melin B. Genetic causes of glioma: new leads in the labyrinth. Curr Opin Oncol. 2011;23:643-7.

[49] Barrett T, Troup DB, Wilhite SE, Ledoux P, Evangelista C, Kim IF, et al. NCBI GEO: archive for functional genomics data sets--10 years on. Nucleic Acids Res. 2011;39:D1005-10.

[50] Kozomara A, Griffiths-Jones S. miRBase: integrating microRNA annotation and deep-sequencing data. Nucleic Acids Res. 2011;39:D152-7.

[51] Volinia S, Calin Ga, Liu C-G, Ambs S, Cimmino A, Petrocca F, et al. A microRNA expression signature of human solid tumors defines cancer gene targets. Proc Natl Acad Sci USA. 2006;103:2257-61.

[52] Fujita S, Ito T, Mizutani T, Minoguchi S, Yamamichi N, Sakurai K, et al. miR-21 Gene expression triggered by AP-1 is sustained through a double-negative feedback mechanism. J Mol Biol. 2008;378:492-504.

[53] Havelange V, Garzon R, Croce CM. MicroRNAs: new players in acute myeloid leukaemia. Br J Cancer. 2009;101:743-8.

[54] Larson RA. Micro-RNAs and copy number changes: new levels of gene regulation in acute myeloid leukemia. Chem Biol Interact. 2010;184:21-5.

[55] Marcucci G, Radmacher MD, Maharry K, Mrózek K, Ruppert AS, Paschka P, et al. MicroRNA expression in cytogenetically normal acute myeloid leukemia. New Eng J Med. 2008;358:1919-28.

[56] Agrelo R, Wutz A. X inactivation and disease. Semin Cell Dev Biol. 2010;21:194-200.

[57] DeBaun MR, Niemitz EL, McNeil DE, Brandenburg Sa, Lee MP, Feinberg AP. Epigenetic alterations of H19 and LIT1 distinguish patients with Beckwith-Wiedemann syndrome with cancer and birth defects. Am J Hum Genet. 2002;70:604-11.

[58] Aguilo F, Zhou M-M, Walsh MJ. Long noncoding RNA, polycomb, and the ghosts haunting INK4b-ARF-INK4a expression. Cancer Res. 2011;71:5365-9.

[59] Yotova IY, Vlatkovic IM, Pauler FM, Warczok KE, Ambros PF, Oshimura M, et al. Identification of the human homolog of the imprinted mouse Air non-coding RNA. Genomics. 2008;92:464-73.

[60] Haque MM, Hirano T, Itoh N, Utiyama H. Evolution of large extrachromosomal elements in HL-60 cells during culture and the associated phenotype alterations. Biochem Biophys Res Commun. 2001;288:592-6.

[61] Haque MM, Hirano T, Nakamura H, Utiyama H. Granulocytic differentiation of HL-60 cells, both spontaneous and drug-induced, might require loss of extrachromosomal DNA encoding a gene(s) not c-MYC. Biochem Biophys Res Commun. 2001;288:586-91.

[62] Garzon R, Garofalo M, Martelli MP, Briesewitz R, Wang L, Fernandez-Cymering C, et al. Distinctive microRNA signature of acute myeloid leukemia bearing cytoplasmic mutated nucleophosmin. Proc Natl Acad Sci USA. 2008;105:3945-50.

[63] Dixon-McIver A, East P, Mein CA, Cazier J-b, Molloy G, Chaplin T, et al. Distinctive patterns of microRNA expression associated with karyotype in acute myeloid leukaemia. PloS One. 2008;3:e2141.

[64] Langer C, Marcucci G, Holland KB, Radmacher MD, Maharry K, Paschka P, et al. Prognostic importance of MN1 transcript levels, and biologic insights from MN1-

associated gene and microRNA expression signatures in cytogenetically normal acute myeloid leukemia: a cancer and leukemia group B study. J Clin Oncol. 2009;27:3198-204.
[65] Zhao H, Wang D, Du W, Gu D, Yang R. MicroRNA and leukemia: tiny molecule, great function. Crit Rev Oncol Hematol. 2010;74:149-55.
[66] Marcucci G, Radmacher MD, Mrózek K, Bloomfield CD. MicroRNA expression in acute myeloid leukemia. Cur Hematol Malignancy Reports. 2009;4:83-8.
[67] Chistiakov Da, Chekhonin VP. Contribution of microRNAs to radio- and chemoresistance of brain tumors and their therapeutic potential. Eur J Pharmacol. 2012.
[68] Zhang X, Yang H, Lee JJ, Kim E, Lippman SM, Khuri FR, et al. MicroRNA-related genetic variations as predictors for risk of second primary tumor and/or recurrence in patients with early-stage head and neck cancer. Carcinogenesis. 2010;31:2118-23.
[69] Hummel R, Maurer J, Haier J. MicroRNAs in brain tumors : a new diagnostic and therapeutic perspective? Mol Neurobiol. 2011;44:223-34.
[70] Iacoangeli A, Lin Y, Morley EJ, Muslimov Ia, Bianchi R, Reilly J, et al. BC200 RNA in invasive and preinvasive breast cancer. Carcinogenesis. 2004;25:2125-33.
[71] Bertozzi D, Iurlaro R, Sordet O, Marinello J, Zaffaroni N, Capranico G. Characterization of novel antisense HIF-1 α transcripts in human cancers. Cell Cycle. 2011;10:3189-97.
[72] Niinuma T, Suzuki H, Nojima M, Nosho K, Yamamoto H, Takamaru H, et al. Upregulation of miR-196a and HOTAIR Drive Malignant Character in Gastrointestinal Stromal Tumors. Cancer Res. 2012;72:1126-36.
[73] Panzitt K, Tschernatsch MMO, Guelly C, Moustafa T, Stradner M, Strohmaier HM, et al. Characterization of HULC, a novel gene with striking up-regulation in hepatocellular carcinoma, as noncoding RNA. Gastroenterol. 2007;132:330-42.
[74] Vu TH, Chuyen NV, Li T. Loss of Imprinting of IGF2 Sense and Antisense Transcripts in Wilms ' Tumor. Cancer Res. 2003;63:1900-5.
[75] Poliseno L, Salmena L, Zhang J, Carver B, Haveman WJ, Pandolfi PP. A coding-independent function of gene and pseudogene mRNAs regulates tumour biology. Nature. 2010;465:1033-8.
[76] Li L, Feng T, Lian Y, Zhang G, Garen A, Song X. Role of human noncoding RNAs in the control of tumorigenesis. Proc Natl Acad Sci USA. 2009;106:12956-61.
[77] Zong X, Tripathi V, Prasanth KV. RNA splicing control: yet another gene regulatory role for long nuclear noncoding RNAs. RNA Biology. 2011;8:968-77.
[78] Schalken Ja. Towards Early and More Specific Diagnosis of Prostate Cancer? Beyond PSA: New Biomarkers Ready for Prime Time. Eur Urol Supple. 2009;8:97-102.
[79] Srikantan V, Zou Z, Petrovics G, Xu L, Augustus M, Davis L, et al. PCGEM1, a prostate-specific gene, is overexpressed in prostate cancer. Proc Natl Acad Sci USA. 2000;97:12216-21.
[80] Chung S, Nakagawa H, Uemura M, Piao L, Ashikawa K, Hosono N, et al. Association of a novel long non-coding RNA in 8q24 with prostate cancer susceptibility. Cancer Science. 2011;102:245-52.
[81] Cooper C, Guo J, Yan Y, Chooniedass-Kothari S, Hube F, Hamedani MK, et al. Increasing the relative expression of endogenous non-coding Steroid Receptor RNA

Activator (SRA) in human breast cancer cells using modified oligonucleotides. Nucleic Acids Res. 2009;37:4518-31.

[82] Cao Y, Bryan TM, Reddel RR. Increased copy number of the TERT and TERC telomerase subunit genes in cancer cells. Cancer Science. 2008;99:1092-9.

[83] Yang C, Li X, Wang Y, Zhao L, Chen W. Long non-coding RNA UCA1 regulated cell cycle distribution via CREB through PI3-K dependent pathway in bladder carcinoma cells. Gene. 2012;496:8-16.

[84] Dallosso AR, Hancock AL, Malik S, Salpekar A, King-Underwood L, Pritchard-Jones K, et al. Alternately spliced WT1 antisense transcripts interact with WT1 sense RNA and show epigenetic and splicing defects in cancer. RNA. 2007;13:2287-99.

[85] Agrelo R, Wutz A. Cancer progenitors and epigenetic contexts: an Xisting connection. Epigenetics. 2009;4:568-70.

[86] Klein U, Lia M, Crespo M, Siegel R, Shen Q, Mo T, et al. The DLEU2/miR-15a/16-1 cluster controls B cell proliferation and its deletion leads to chronic lymphocytic leukemia. Cancer Cell. 2010;17:28-40.

[87] Mourtada-Maarabouni M, Pickard MR, Hedge VL, Farzaneh F, Williams GT. GAS5, a non-protein-coding RNA, controls apoptosis and is downregulated in breast cancer. Oncogene. 2009;28:195-208.

[88] Schofield PN, Joyce Ja, Lam WK, Grandjean V, Ferguson-Smith a, Reik W, et al. Genomic imprinting and cancer; new paradigms in the genetics of neoplasia. Toxicol Lett. 2001;120:151-60.

[89] Wang X-S, Gong J-N, Yu J, Wang F, Zhang X-H, Yin X-L, et al. MicroRNA-29a and microRNA-142-3p are regulators of myeloid differentiation and acute myeloid leukemia. Blood. 2012.

[90] Candeias MM, Malbert-Colas L, Powell DJ, Daskalogianni C, Maslon MM, Naski N, et al. P53 mRNA controls p53 activity by managing Mdm2 functions. Nat Cell Biol. 2008;10:1098-105.

[91] Maida Y, Yasukawa M, Furuuchi M, Lassmann T, Possemato R, Okamoto N, et al. An RNA-dependent RNA polymerase formed by TERT and the RMRP RNA. Nature. 2009;461:230-5.

[92] Azzalin CM, Reichenbach P, Khoriauli L, Giulotto E, Lingner J. Telomeric repeat containing RNA and RNA surveillance factors at mammalian chromosome ends. Science. 2007;318:798-801.

[93] Treppendahl MB, Qiu X, Søgaard A, Yang X, Nandrup-Bus C, Hother C, et al. Allelic methylation levels of the noncoding VTRNA2-1 located on chromosome 5q31.1 predict outcome in AML. Blood. 2012;119:206-16.

[94] Askarian-Amiri ME, Crawford J, French JD, Smart CE, Smith Ma, Clark MB, et al. SNORD-host RNA Zfas1 is a regulator of mammary development and a potential marker for breast cancer. RNA. 2011;17:878-91.

[95] Kent WJ, Sugnet CW, Furey TS, Roskin KM, Pringle TH, Zahler AM, et al. The human genome browser at UCSC. Genome Res. 2002;12:996-1006.

Section 6

Oncogenes for Transcription Factors

Chapter 18

The MYCN Oncogene

Leanna Cheung, Jayne E. Murray, Michelle Haber and Murray D. Norris

Additional information is available at the end of the chapter

http://dx.doi.org/10.5772/54813

1. Introduction

MYCN is a member of the *MYC* family of oncogenes, which also includes *c-MYC* and *MYCL*. Despite knowing about the existence of MYCN for nearly thirty years, the majority of functional studies involving MYC family members have focused on c-MYC due to the limited expression profile of MYCN in human cancers, and also in part due to the existence of highly conserved functional domains between c-MYC and MYCN [1]. MYCN is normally expressed during embryonal development and orchestrates cell proliferation and differentiation in the developing peripheral neural crest [2]. However, the deregulated expression of MYCN has been shown to contribute to tumorigenesis and neuronal transformation [3]. Thus, MYCN represents a highly desirable therapeutic target. Previous studies have shown that downregulating *MYCN* expression, via antisense oligonucleotides, resulted in lower tumour incidence and decreased tumour mass in a murine neuroblastoma tumour model [4]. However, to date, no molecularly targeted therapies have been developed that are able to mimic this response in the clinic, and further studies are required to help elucidate the mechanisms that drive *MYCN* tumour formation and progression.

2. The MYC family and the discovery of MYCN

The eventual discovery of *MYC* oncogenes arose from early pioneering work on the Rous sarcoma virus (RSV), a transforming retrovirus able to cause sarcomas in infected chicken cells. Using the information provided by RSV, hybridisation studies were performed on a specific group of avian tumours involving a retrovirus responsible for inducing myeloid leukaemia. This led to the identification of a sequence that was named *v-gag-myc*, or *v-myc* for myelocytomatosis (the leukaemia that is induced following the transduction of avian cells with this virus) and supported the idea that viral integration into a host genome could activate a nearby host oncogene [5, 6]. As it transpired, the human homologue of *v-myc*, termed *c-MYC* (cellular-*MYC*) was the first cellular oncogene whose overexpression was shown to be activated through retroviral insertional mutagenesis [7]. Deregulated expression of *c-MYC* has since been implicated in a range of cancers, and allowed the discovery of other important *MYC* family members including *MYCN* and *MYCL*.

Neuroblastoma is the most common extracranial solid tumour of early childhood and accounts for approximately 15% of all cancer related deaths in children. Aggressive drug refractory neuroblastoma cells have been frequently observed to contain genomic aberrations referred to as double-minute chromatin bodies and homogeneously staining regions. Both of these types of aberrations were found to contain multiple copies or amplification of specific genes, and in particular, the critical gene within these regions was later identified to be the *c-MYC*-related oncogene, *MYCN*, so-called because of its identification in neuroblastoma cells [8]. Amplification of the *MYCN* oncogene has also been demonstrated in retinoblastoma, glioblastoma, medulloblastoma, astrocytoma and small cell lung cancer cells [9]. In addition, another member of the *MYC*-oncogene family, *MYCL*, was identified in small cell lung cancer (SCLC), and demonstrated homology to a small region of both *c-MYC* and *MYCN*. Gene mapping studies assigned *MYCL* to human chromosome region 1p32, a location that is distinct from that of either *c-MYC* or *MYCN* (regions 8q24 and 2p24 respectively) but is also associated with cytogenetic abnormalities in certain human tumours such as thyroid cancer and lung cancer [10, 11]. *MYCL* was found to be amplified in some SCLC cells [12]. In mammals, a fourth member of the *MYC* family, *s-Myc* has been identified, however only *c-MYC, MYCN* and *MYCL* have been implicated in the tumorigenesis of specific human cancers [13].

All three tumour-associated *MYC* genes have the same characteristic three-exon structure with the major polypeptide open reading frame residing in the second and third exons. The first exon is not conserved between the genes, but rather possesses regulatory functions, whereas the two coding exons produce highly homologous sections of amino acids interspersed with areas of diminished conservation, leading to the suggestion that individual MYC polypeptides have discrete, independent, functional domains [14]. In tumour biology, many cancers have been shown to exhibit increased levels of MYC protein in tumour tissue relative to the surrounding normal tissues, and this has been shown to contribute to the aggressiveness of the tumour [15]. Importantly, the MYC family of proteins share functionally similar roles, acting as transcription factors to drive cellular proliferation and vasculogenesis, promote metastasis and genomic instability, as well as inhibit cell differentiation and reduce cell adhesion [13, 16]. However, recent findings have also raised the possibility of transcriptionally-independent functions of the MYC proteins [17].

3. The functional activity of MYCN

MYC proteins are well established as nuclear phosphoproteins that act as regulators of transcription, and can both activate and repress the expression of its target genes [16]. *MYCN* encodes a 60kDa protein that has affinity for and binds to DNA, and is phosphorylated by casein kinase II [18, 19]. Phosphorylation is important for the transforming abilities of MYC family members and also for the regulation of MYC protein stability and activity [20]. The affinity of MYCN protein for DNA relies on the presence of certain motifs, comprising a basic DNA binding region, an α-helical protein-protein interaction domain or helix-loop-helix (HLH), and a leucine zipper motif (Zip) encompassing the bHLH-Zip domain at the carboxy or C-terminus of the protein [9]. The mechanism that mediates the DNA-binding capacity of MYC proteins was confirmed via the identification of MAX, also a bHLH-Zip protein [21]. MYCN and MAX (Figure 1) interact to form a complex that binds to DNA in a sequence specific manner [22]. MYCN binds to MAX protein via its bHLH-LZ region. Several other proteins have also been shown to interact with the C-terminus of MYCN, including YY-1, AP-2, TFII-I and BRCA1 [23], or with the central region of MYCN such as NMi [24], all of which are associated with MYCN's function as a transcriptional regulator.

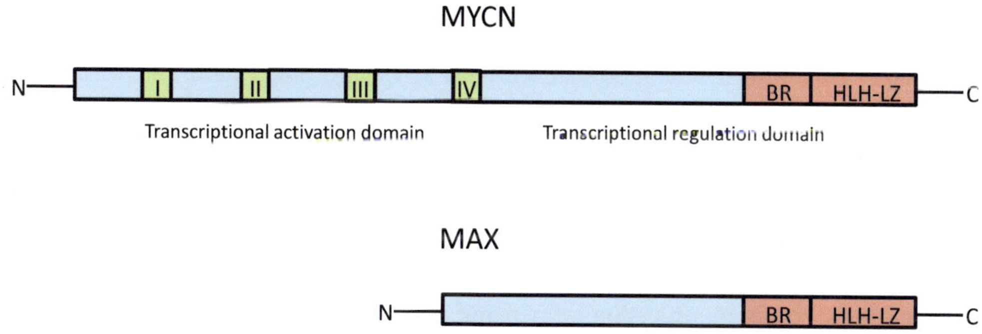

Figure 1. Domains of the MYCN and MAX proteins. The N-terminus of MYCN has three elements, known as MYC homology boxes I-III, which are highly conserved in MYC proteins. The C-terminus contains the basic-region/helix-loop-helix/leucine-zipper that is responsible for interaction with the MAX protein.

The amino or N-terminus of MYCN acts as a transactivation domain that contains two highly conserved regions called Myc Homology Boxes I and II (MBI and MBII) [1]. This region has been shown to bind to nuclear cofactors, including TRRAP, p107, BIN1, MM-1, AMY-1, PAM, α-Tubulin, TIP48 and TIP49, to assist the targeting of protein to specific gene promoters [23, 25]. Another protein YAF2, has been demonstrated to bind to the central region of MYCN to further stimulate transcription upon MYCN-MAX transactivation [26]. All of these interacting proteins are a part of a transcription factor complex by which target genes are activated. Myc Homology Box III (MBIII) is conserved only within c-MYC and MYCN, but not MYCL, and is necessary for cellular transformation [27]. A fourth Myc Homology Box (MBIV) is also necessary for MYC transforming activity [28].

Recent studies have provided evidence of a function of MYCN that is independent from its role as a classical transcription factor. MYCN was shown to remodel large domains of euchromatin, regions of lightly packaged chromatin that contain active, functioning genes, by regulating histone acetylation [29, 30]. Two possibilities have been suggested for this role. The first is that MYCN maintains the activity of euchromatin, whilst the second is that MYCN maintains euchromatin at remote sites to act as an enhancer and regulator of genes at a distance. Novel functions of other MYC proteins have been identified through mutational analyses that have uncoupled the transforming ability of c-MYC from its role as a transcription factor [28, 31]. c-MYC was found to increase the translation of specific mRNAs by promoting the methylation of the 5′ mRNA guanine "cap", including mRNAs encoding cyclin T1 and CDK9 [31]. A role for c-MYC has also been described in the initiation of DNA replication by binding to various components of the pre-replicative complex and localising to early sites of DNA replication [32]. These observations suggest that c-MYC may play a role in controlling initiation of the S phase of the cell cycle and contribute to replicative stress and genomic instability, to further accelerate tumorigenesis [17]. Even though the evidence has yet to be provided, given the high level of homology between c-MYC and MYCN, the described transcription-independent roles of c-MYC suggest similar roles will be identified for MYCN in contributing to tumour cell biology.

4. MYCN as a transcriptional activator

As indicated above, MYCN heterodimerises with MAX and binds with high affinity to a CACA/GTG E-box sequence found upstream of promoter target sequences [13]. The MYCN-MAX heterodimer activates transcription via several mechanisms. TRRAP (or TRansactivation/tRansformation Associated Protein) binds to the N-terminal region of MYCN and is essential for MYCN transformation. Through TRRAP, MYCN recruits histone acetylation (HAT) complexes to chromatin, including the 1.8 megaDalton SAGA complex (SPT/ADA/GCN5/Acetyltransferase) [33]. Histone acetylation is associated with gene activation by chromatin modification influencing histone-DNA and histone-histone contact [34]. TRRAP is involved with another HAT complex, TIP60, an H2A/H4 acetylase [35]. Interestingly, *in vivo* acetylation of histone H4 is highly associated with MYC target gene activation [36]. Two other proteins, TIP48 and TIP49 that are found in the TIP60 complex also bind to the N-terminus of MYCN [25]. Both proteins are highly conserved hexameric ATPases that are involved in chromatin remodelling involving the movement or displacement of nucleosomes, as opposed to chromatin modification [37].

The MYC family represents a particularly unusual set of transcription factors in that they can bind to and regulate approximately 10-15% of the entire genome [14]. Some MYCN target genes have been shown to be activated independently of TRRAP and HAT complexes. Investigation into HAT independent activation has revealed the involvement of RNA polymerase II at the promoter regions of target genes. c-MYC protein binding has been shown to stimulate the clearance of RNA polymerase II from the promoter region to allow for efficient transcription elongation by the RNA pol II kinases, TFIIH and positive transcription elongation factor b (PTEFb) [38]. c-MYC also regulates RNA pol II promoter clearance by controlling the expression of RNA pol II kinases via mRNA cap methylation, polysome loading, and the rate of translation [31].

5. MYCN as a transcriptional repressor

Most studies have focused on the role of MYC proteins as transcriptional activators. However, cells transformed by constitutive expression of c-MYC are characterised by the loss of expression of numerous genes such as those involved in cell adhesion and cell cycle regulation, and even loss of *c-MYC* itself [39-41]. An early indicator of the transcriptional repressor role of MYC proteins was the involvement of c-MYC in a negative feedback loop, where the introduction of ectopic c-MYC or MYCN was able to downregulate endogenous expression of c-MYC in mouse fibroblast cells [42]. Structure and function analyses found that the regions of c-MYC that are required for transformation are also required for negative autoregulation [43] and led to the idea that the repression of target genes by MYC proteins could also contribute to transformation.

The understanding of transcriptional repression by MYC proteins was greatly advanced via the identification of repressed target genes such as *transglutaminase-2* (*TG2*) and *interleukin-6* (*IL-6*) [44]. Genomic studies have now revealed that MYC proteins repress as many targets as they activate, emphasising the role of gene repression by these oncoproteins during cellular transformation [14]. One recent example is the identification of *TG2* repression by MYCN in neuroblastoma, which occurs via the interaction between MYCN with Specificity Protein I (SP1) [45]. *TG2* is a multifunctional enzyme that catalyses the transamidation and multimerisation of proteins, but also promotes programmed cell death and induces neuritic differentiation in neuroblastoma cells [46]. Hence downregulation of *TG2* by MYCN would allow neuroblastoma cells to overcome apoptosis and continue to proliferate. Similarly, MYCN has been shown to interact with SP1 to downregulate the expression of *MRP3* (also known as *ABCC3*), the gene encoding an intermembrane transporter which is involved in the transport of organic anions, prostaglandins, leukotrienes and selected chemotherapeutics [47-49]. Another important gene that is downregulated by MYCN is *IL-6*, which has been shown to play an important anti-angiogenic role by inhibiting vascular endothelial cell proliferation [50]. The transcriptional repression by MYCN is also supported by the interaction between MYC proteins and another transcription factor MIZ-1 (Myc-interacting zinc finger protein-1) [51]. MIZ-1 is a POZ/BTB (poxvirus and zinc finger/bric-a-brac, tramtrack and broad complex) domain protein that transactivates genes involved in cell cycle regulation as well as tumour suppressor genes via the recruitment of the p300 histone acetyltransferase [52]. Interestingly, high-level MIZ-1 expression is associated with a favourable disease outcome of neuroblastoma [53]. MIZ-1 interacts with the carboxy-terminal HLH region of c-MYC and MYCN, where the binding of the MYC-MAX heterodimer to MIZ-1 disrupts the interaction between MIZ-1 and p300, causing the transcriptional repression of tumour suppressor genes [54]. MYC has also been shown to recruit a DNA methyltransferase, DNMT3a to the MYC-MIZ-1 complex, suggesting that repression can be mediated by the methylation of target gene promoters [55].

6. Mechanisms of regulating MYCN expression

Due to the gross transforming ability of deregulated expression of MYC proteins, the expression of these protooncogenes is tightly regulated in normal cells at both the transcriptional and protein level. For example, MYC mRNA transcripts and proteins have very short half-lives and are expressed at constant levels as cells enter the cell cycle [56, 57]. Furthermore, anti-proliferative signals trigger rapid down-regulation in expression, and the phosphorylation patterns of MYC proteins are known to influence their stability. In addition to these mechanisms, expression of MYCN is particularly tightly regulated with regards to timing and tissue specificity. Thus, MYCN is normally expressed during embryonal development of the peripheral nervous system in neural crest cells [2]. Neural crest cells migrate during mid-gestation to populate the entire peripheral nervous system, including autonomic and peripheral ganglia and the adrenal gland. These migrating progenitor cells represent a highly proliferative population, and during normal development exit the cell-cycle and undergo differentiation following the colonisation to the ganglia and spinal cord area. This event is orchestrated by extracellular signalling molecules such as mitogens and cytokines and coincides with decreased expression of MYCN [56, 58]. Without this strict control, dysregulated MYCN expression impairs the ability of progenitor cells to undergo differentiation. Studies which sustained MYCN expression in murine neural crest cells under the control of a tyrosine hydroxylase promoter, demonstrated the capacity to cause neuroblastoma in transgenic mice [3]. Despite this transforming ability, MYCN is vital for normal embryonic development, and murine embryos lacking MYCN exhibit profound hypoplasia, particularly in the central and peripheral nervous system, disorganized architecture of the brain, defective heart development and defects in the lung, genitourinary system, stomach, intestines and limb buds [59].

In order to understand how extracellular stimuli controlled MYC expression in cells, gene mapping studies in association with *MYC* transcription studies were undertaken, and these identified response elements within the *MYC* transcript as well as their regulators. In neuronal cells, *MYCN* has been shown to be regulated in its promoter region as well as in an enhancer region upstream of the coding region. The elongation transcription factor, E2F binds to the promoter region of *MYCN* in response to different mitogenic signals [60]. The promoter region also contains positive transcription factor binding sites for SP1, SP3 and TGFβ [61]. However, the presence of a retinoic acid response element (RARE) within this region allows for negative regulation of *MYCN* by retinoic acid [62].

A key finding was made in 1986 which identified *c-MYC* as the first eukaryotic gene to be negatively regulated by transcriptional elongation control, where a block in the elongation of mRNA during transcription occurred during cellular differentiation [63]. This finding was later confirmed in *MYCN* studies where transcription elongation pausing sites were identified in exon 1 and intron 1 of human *MYCN* [64, 65]. Furthermore, there is *in vivo* evidence that the downregulation of *MYCN* during mouse embryogenesis is partly regulated by the control of transcriptional elongation [66].

Transcription alone cannot account for the large difference in mRNA levels following the introduction of proliferative or anti-proliferative stimuli. The rapid turnover of mRNA was also associated with the discovery of two distinct mechanisms of *MYC* mRNA decay. The first involves a translation-independent mechanism involving poly(A) tail shortening of the untranslated region of the transcript, while the second represents a translation-dependent mechanism that is regulated by a region of mRNA which corresponds to the C-terminus of the protein, called the coding region determinant [67-69]. This region is bound to a 75kDa protein that protects the region of mRNA from endonuclease attack, in response to growth signals that induce c-MYC stabilisation. In the case of *MYCN*, RNA stability factors have also been identified which bind to the untranslated region of *MYCN* mRNA. In addition, an internal ribosomal entry segment (IRES) in the transcript acts to enhance neuronal specific translation [70, 71].

7. Regulation of MYCN protein expression

The regulation of MYCN protein levels has also been investigated and phosphopeptide analysis has revealed that specific serine and threonine residues of MYCN are phosphorylated *in vivo*. Two residues in particular, Threonine 58 (Thr58) and Serine 62 (Ser62) have been demonstrated as important determinants of transformation and MYCN protein stability and activity [20]. Proliferative stimuli activate phosphorylation of Ser62 by cyclin B and Cdk1 during prophase to increase MYCN protein stability [72]. Phospho-ser62 via a feedback mechanism, then serves as a platform for the phosphorylation of Thr58 by glycogen synthase kinase 3 (GSK3), allowing the tumour suppressor FBW7 to bind and recruit a ubiquitylation complex, directing MYCN protein for degradation. Mitotic degradation of MYCN in the absence of growth factor-dependent signals allows cell cycle exit and the commencement of differentiation [73]. Another kinase, Aurora A, has recently been identified and shown to inhibit degradation of ubiquitinated MYCN by supporting the synthesis of non-degradable ubiquitin chains [74].

8. MYCN downstream target genes

The first transcriptional target for a MYC protein was discovered ten years after the identification of human *c-MYC*. The development of a conditionally expressed *c-MYC* construct, via the fusion of human *c-MYC* to the hormone-binding domain of the oestrogen receptor, led to the identification of a downstream target involved in cell cycle progression, α-prothymosin [75]. This approach was then used to identify additional targets including ornithine decarboxylase 1 (ODC1), the rate-limiting enzyme involved in polyamine synthesis [76]. A different method of identifying MYC targets utilised *MYC*-null models to determine whether the regulation of expression of genes was dependent on the presence of a *MYC* oncogene. Such examples of labour-intensive techniques were invaluable in determining single *bona fide* MYC targets, however recent advances in technology have allowed for large-scale analyses of MYC-regulated genes [77, 78].

Expression microarrays and chromatin immunoprecipitation assays (ChIP) have helped researchers identify MYC-regulated targets as well as link MYC-target expression to functional cellular pathways which are associated with transformation [79, 80]. MYC and MYCN-regulated targets have since been linked to a number of transforming activities involving the cell cycle (eg. cyclin D2, CDK4, p21), cell proliferation (e.g. MDM2), growth, metabolism (e.g. ribosomal proteins, proteins involved in nucleotide biosynthesis such as thymidylate synthase and ODC1), cell adhesion and migration (e.g. integrins) and angiogenesis (e.g. thrombospondin) [81-86]. Indeed, the activation and repression of MYC target genes is a well-coordinated event. Time course studies using microarray have identified differences between early and delayed gene expression responses, following MYC activation in a MYC-inducible cell system [87]. Early-response MYC target genes are primarily involved in MAPK signalling, RNA metabolism and transcription factors, which suggests a program that prepares cells for entry into the S phase. On the other hand, delayed-response MYC target genes are involved in ribosomal biogenesis, nucleotide metabolism and energy metabolism, suggesting subsequent maintenance of cells during the S phase. Finally, late steady-state MYC-mediated transcription involved genes that regulate the cell cycle, nucleotide metabolism and DNA replication. Most genes that were activated in the early response were then repressed during this late steady-state phase. Furthermore, sustained MYC activation led to the silencing of differentiation-related genes and upregulation of genes that are involved cell proliferation.

During tumorigenesis, MYCN promotes cell cycle progression by the activation of cyclins (such as cyclin D1 and D2) as well as cyclin-dependent kinase 4 (CDK4), and represses the expression of mediators of cell cycle arrest such as p21 [73]. One important MYCN-regulated metabolic pathway involves the synthesis of polyamines, which are organic cations that enhance transcription, translation and replication [88]. *MYCN* expression is strongly correlated with *ODC1* expression in neuroblastoma, and the high levels of *ODC1* expression that are driven by *MYCN*-amplification and over-expression are strongly associated with poor clinical outcome of this disease [89].

Another gene whose expression is strongly correlated with *MYCN* expression in neuroblastoma is that encoding the multidrug resistance-associated protein, MRP1, a glycoprotein that belongs to the superfamily of ATP-binding cassette (ABC) transmembrane transporters [90-92]. MRP1, also known as ABCC1, is able to confer resistance to a broad range of structurally unrelated chemotherapeutic drugs [93]. MRP1 has since been shown to be a downstream transcriptional target of MYCN in neuroblastoma, whose expression is highly predictive of outcome in this disease [91, 94, 95]. The expression of another gene that is also a member of the ABC family of transporters, *MRP4* (or *ABCC4*), has also been demonstrated to be positively correlated to *MYCN* expression in neuroblastoma and like *MRP1*, its over-expression is a prognostic indicator of neuroblastoma outcome [95, 96]. In fact, it has recently been shown that MYCN can coordinate the transcription of a large set of *ABC* genes, and the expression profiles of these genes correlate with MYCN function [48].

9. MYCN tumorigenesis

The evidence for a clinical role of MYCN in the tumorigenesis of neuroblastoma was first recognised when the amplification of the *MYCN* oncogene was identified in 24 out of 63 primary untreated neuroblastoma tumour samples and appeared to correlate with more advanced stage of disease [97]. *MYCN*-amplification was subsequently associated with rapid disease progression as well as poor patient outcome in this disease [98]. Importantly, the progression-free survival of neuroblastoma patients was then shown to be dose-dependent on *MYCN* where higher copy number resulted in lower survival. This association was independent of patient age and disease stage. *MYCN*-amplification was later confirmed in numerous studies to be a powerful prognostic marker for predicting neuroblastoma patient outcome, independent of other clinical variables [99-102]. Determination of *MYCN* amplification status is now routinely determined in primary neuroblastomas and is one of the most powerful prognostic markers yet identified for this disease.

The *MYCN* oncogene is normally located on the distal short arm of chromosome 2 (2p24). This region was found to be amplified across a panel of neuroblastoma cell lines [8], and although the exact mechanism by which this occurs is unknown, the process of amplification usually results in 50 to 400 copies of the gene per cell, leading to the production of abnormally high levels of *MYCN* RNA and protein, presumably conferring a selective advantage to the tumour cell [103].

The potent transforming ability of MYCN has been demonstrated by several studies, while *MYCN* transfection studies have demonstrated that the oncoprotein plays a crucial role in neuroblastoma progression [104, 105]. Conditional overexpression of *MYCN* in neuroblastoma cell lines was shown to dramatically increase the growth rates and metastatic ability of these tumour cells, increase DNA synthesis, and inhibit exit from the cell cycle and neuronal differentiation [106, 107]. Furthermore, targeted expression of the *MYCN* oncogene in neuroectodermal cells of transgenic mice resulted in the development of neuroblastoma [3]. In these animals, human *MYCN* (*hMYCN*) oncogene expression was targeted to neural crest cells via an upstream rat tyrosine hydroxylase promoter. Tyrosine hydroxylase is the first and rate-limiting step in catecholamine synthesis. In contrast, reduction in the *MYCN* RNA levels via introduction of *MYCN* antisense oligonucleotides *in vitro* as well as *in vivo* led to reduced rates of growth and of tumorigenicity [4, 108, 109].

Whilst *MYCN*-amplification has been shown to be associated with a highly malignant neuroblastoma phenotype, the precise role of this oncogene in non-amplified tumours remains controversial. Approximately 40% of those neuroblastomas that lack *MYCN*-amplification are nevertheless still clinically aggressive, and the clinical significance of *MYCN* expression in the absence of *MYCN*-amplification, remains elusive with evidence both for and against an association with adverse outcome [110, 111]. One study that analysed both *MYCN* mRNA and protein levels in a cohort of non-amplified tumours, found no prognostic significance attributable to expression of this oncogene [110]. Rather, since the survival rates for older children with or without high MYCN expression were poor, the results suggested that additional factors contribute to tumour aggressiveness in this subgroup. Furthermore, in a more recent study involving 91 neuroblastoma patients, high *MYCN* expression was found to be associated with a favourable outcome in neuroblastomas lacking *MYCN*-amplification [111]. Interestingly, in this study, the forced expression of *MYCN* significantly suppressed growth of non-amplified neuroblastoma cells by inducing apoptosis. It is possible that the prognostic value of *MYCN* gene expression in neuroblastoma may be an artefact of the different biology of neuroblastoma in infants compared to older children, and further well-controlled, large cohort studies will be needed in order to clarify the precise role of MYCN in non-amplified neuroblastoma.

Although the majority of the literature investigating *MYCN* in cancer comes from studies on neuroblastoma, this oncogene has also been shown to play a role in the tumorigenesis of other cancers, both adult and paediatric. For example, *MYCN* amplification and/or overexpression has been observed in high grade C5 serous ovarian tumours, small cell lung cancer, rhabdomyosarcoma and neuroendocrine prostate cancer [112-115], while gain of 2p (and *MYCN*) plays a role in chronic lymphocytic leukaemia [116]. In childhood medulloblastoma, MYCN, c-MYC, and to a lesser extent MYCL, appear to be involved in the biology of this disease [117]. *MYCN* amplification occurs in up to 10% of medulloblastoma patients and is associated with poor clinical outcome, and like neuroblastoma, the risk of death increases with increasing copy number [117]. Furthermore, *MYCN* expression was found to be high in foetal cerebella, with the levels decreasing to almost absent in adult cerebella, suggesting that MYCN is essential to normal foetal development [118]. Interestingly, in this study, *MYCN* expression was absent from the medulloblastoma cell lines tested, which differed from the expression pattern observed in the primary tumours [118]. Finally, as with neuroblastoma, the association of *MYCN* mRNA levels with clinical outcome remains unclear [119] and it has been postulated that mRNA levels of both *c-MYC* and *MYCN* may only be clinically relevant in subgroups of medulloblastoma [117].

The most compelling evidence for a role of MYCN in the biology of medulloblastoma comes from two mouse models of this disease. Firstly, targeted expression of MYCN to the cerebellum in transgenic mice has demonstrated the importance of MYCN in contributing to the initiation and progression of medulloblastoma and also in the metastatic spread of disease to the spinal and paraspinal tissues via cerebral spinal fluid. Furthermore, the MYCN downstream targets Odc1, MDM2 and Fb1 were upregulated and correlated with *MYCN* mRNA levels [118]. The second model used targeted Smoothened (SmoA1) to the cerebella of transgenic mice, which were then crossed with mice harbouring conditional knock-out of MYCN, to demonstrate that MYCN was essential for medulloblastoma tumorigenesis [120]. These two models thus serve to demonstrate the importance of MYCN in the initiation and progression of this disease.

10. Molecular targeting of MYCN for therapeutic benefit

Molecular targeted therapy involves targeting malignant cell growth by directly inhibiting the function of specific molecules within a cell, namely those that are responsible for driving cancer progression. Such agents aim to block or exploit various aspects of cancer biology, such as genetic instability, proliferative signal transduction, aberrant cell cycle control, deregulated survival, angiogenesis and metastasis [121]. Numerous methods of molecular targeted therapy have been investigated, including antisense oligonucleotides (ASOs) that hybridise to and inhibit the mRNA of a specific gene; peptide nucleic acids (PNAs), which are DNA analogues that specifically hybridise to DNA and/or RNA in a complementary manner to inhibit transcription/translation of a target gene; and small interfering RNA (siRNA), which silences gene expression by inducing the sequence specific degradation of complementary mRNA or by inhibiting translation [122]. However, such technologies although useful in the laboratory, have had limited success in the clinic due to problems associated with their delivery.

Immunotherapy has also generated interest, and utilises the body's immune system to target and remove cancer cells by the recognition of certain molecular markers, or block specific cell receptor pathways. Another approach to molecular targeting, involves the development of synthetic small molecule inhibitors which potentially have the ability to interfere with a molecular target at multiple levels [122]. These small molecules may diffuse into cells to act directly on intracellular targets, such as inhibiting the expression of a target gene at the transcriptional or translational level, or inhibiting the function of a protein by directly binding to the protein and inducing conformational changes that prevent its interaction with other factors [123]. Synthetic small molecules are generally defined by a molecular weight cut-off of <500Da. They are favoured by the pharmaceutical industry because of their attractive pharmacokinetic properties, especially tumour cell penetration, and their relative ease of development and pharmaceutical production [123]. At present, strategies to develop novel small molecule inhibitors as viable therapies are aimed at using these technologies in combination with other cytotoxic drugs, with the hope of reducing drug dosages, and thus overcoming drug resistance associated with intensive chemotherapy, and reducing drug-related toxicity and side effects.

A number of molecular mechanisms have been identified as possible targets for the treatment of neuroblastoma. However, the prominent deregulated expression and amplification of *MYCN* suggests that this oncogene represents an ideal target for therapeutic inhibition [124]. In addition, normal MYCN expression is restricted to the early stages of embryonic development and is virtually undetectable in normal post-natal tissues, therefore weighing in its favour as a target for inhibition. Inhibition of *MYCN* expression by antisense treatment against *MYCN* mRNA or by retinoic acid has been demonstrated to decrease proliferation and induce neuronal differentiation in neuroblastoma cells [125-127]. Furthermore, the introduction of *MYCN* antisense oligonucleotides in the human *MYCN* (*hMYCN*) trangenic mouse model led to reduced rates of tumour growth in these animals [4, 108, 109].

Inhibition of MYCN protein through its protein-protein interactions and protein-DNA interactions was previously seen as too difficult to target by small molecules [128]. However, it has been reported that small-molecule antagonists of MYC/MAX dimerisation interfered with c-MYC-induced oncogenic transformation of chicken embryo fibroblasts *in vitro* [129]. In addition, a number of endogenous MYCN/MAX antagonists such as MAX/MAX have been found to compete for binding to E-box sequences and repress transcription [130], causing cell cycle arrest, terminal differentiation or apoptosis. More recently, inhibition of c-MYC transcription via a Bromodomain and Extra Terminal Domain (BET) inhibitor, JQ1, has been described [131]. This inhibitor has been shown to disrupt c-MYC mRNA synthesis by preventing the recruitment of coactivator proteins required for c-MYC transcriptional initiation and mRNA elongation [131]. Furthermore, this molecule was able to decrease the tumour burden in an orthotopic mouse model of multiple myeloma. Treatment of several MYCN-amplified neuroblastoma cell lines with JQ1, resulted in a decrease in MYCN expression, although this effect was far less dramatic that that observed in a c-MYC driven cell line [132]. Despite promising evidence for targeting MYCN as a therapeutic strategy, no MYC or MYCN inhibitors have yet entered clinical trial, and further studies are required to develop effective MYCN inhibitors.

11. Future perspectives

The validity for targeting MYCN for therapeutic benefit relies on the gross transforming ability of this transcription factor. MYCN represents a particularly attractive target due to its lack of expression in adult and normal paediatric tissues. Although MYCN, and MYC proteins in general are commonly viewed as "undruggable" due to the nature of these proteins, MYCN offers potential advantages at a number of levels for therapeutic inhibition, either upstream, or downstream along the MYCN transcriptional pathway. If clinically useful MYCN inhibitors can be successfully developed, they are likely to find application in combination therapies involving conventional chemotherapeutic drugs and be used as an improved approach to target aggressive cancers that are driven by this oncoprotein.

Author details

Leanna Cheung, Jayne E. Murray, Michelle Haber and Murray D. Norris
Children's Cancer Institute Australia for Medical Research, Lowy Cancer Research Centre, UNSW, Sydney, Australia

12. References

[1] Cowling, V.H. and M.D. Cole, *Mechanism of transcriptional activation by the Myc oncoproteins.* Semin Cancer Biol, 2006. 16(4): p. 242-52.
[2] Grimmer, M.R. and W.A. Weiss, *Childhood tumors of the nervous system as disorders of normal development.* Curr Opin Pediatr, 2006. 18(6): p. 634-8.
[3] Weiss, W.A., et al., *Targeted expression of MYCN causes neuroblastoma in transgenic mice.* EMBO J, 1997. 16(11): p. 2985-95.
[4] Burkhart, C.A., et al., *Effects of MYCN antisense oligonucleotide administration on tumorigenesis in a murine model of neuroblastoma.* J Natl Cancer Inst, 2003. 95(18): p. 1394-403.
[5] Varmus, H.E., *The molecular genetics of cellular oncogenes.* Annu Rev Genet, 1984. 18: p. 553-612.
[6] Hayward, W.S., B.G. Neel, and S.M. Astrin, *Activation of a cellular onc gene by promoter insertion in ALV-induced lymphoid leukosis.* Nature, 1981. 290(5806): p. 475-80.
[7] Payne, G.S., J.M. Bishop, and H.E. Varmus, *Multiple arrangements of viral DNA and an activated host oncogene in bursal lymphomas.* Nature, 1982. 295(5846): p. 209-14.
[8] Schwab, M., et al., *Amplified DNA with limited homology to myc cellular oncogene is shared by human neuroblastoma cell lines and a neuroblastoma tumour.* Nature, 1983. 305(5931): p. 245-8.
[9] Schwab, M., *MYCN in neuronal tumours.* Cancer Lett, 2004. 204(2): p. 179-87.
[10] Yaylim-Eraltan, I., et al., *L-myc gene polymorphism and risk of thyroid cancer.* Exp Oncol, 2008. 30(2): p. 117-20.
[11] Kumimoto, H., et al., *L-myc genotype is associated with different susceptibility to lung cancer in smokers.* Jpn J Cancer Res, 2002. 93(1): p. 1-5.
[12] Nau, M.M., et al., *L-myc, a new myc-related gene amplified and expressed in human small cell lung cancer.* Nature, 1985. 318(6041): p. 69-73.

[13] Adhikary, S. and M. Eilers, *Transcriptional regulation and transformation by Myc proteins.* Nat Rev Mol Cell Biol, 2005. 6(8): p. 635-45.

[14] Meyer, N. and L.Z. Penn, *Reflecting on 25 years with MYC.* Nat Rev Cancer, 2008. 8(12): p. 976-90.

[15] Pelengaris, S., M. Khan, and G.I. Evan, *Suppression of Myc-induced apoptosis in beta cells exposes multiple oncogenic properties of Myc and triggers carcinogenic progression.* Cell, 2002. 109(3): p. 321-34.

[16] Marcu, K.B., S.A. Bossone, and A.J. Patel, *myc function and regulation.* Annu Rev Biochem, 1992. 61: p. 809-60.

[17] Cole, M.D. and V.H. Cowling, *Transcription-independent functions of MYC: regulation of translation and DNA replication.* Nat Rev Mol Cell Biol, 2008. 9(10): p. 810-5.

[18] Ramsay, G., et al., *Human proto-oncogene N-myc encodes nuclear proteins that bind DNA.* Mol Cell Biol, 1986. 6(12): p. 4450-7.

[19] Hamann, U., et al., *The MYCN protein of human neuroblastoma cells is phosphorylated by casein kinase II in the central region and at serine 367.* Oncogene, 1991. 6(10): p. 1745-51.

[20] Vervoorts, J., J. Luscher-Firzlaff, and B. Luscher, *The ins and outs of MYC regulation by posttranslational mechanisms.* J Biol Chem, 2006. 281(46): p. 34725-9.

[21] Blackwood, E.M. and R.N. Eisenman, *Max: a helix-loop-helix zipper protein that forms a sequence-specific DNA-binding complex with Myc.* Science, 1991. 251(4998): p. 1211-7.

[22] Wenzel, A., et al., *The N-Myc oncoprotein is associated in vivo with the phosphoprotein Max(p20/22) in human neuroblastoma cells.* EMBO J, 1991. 10(12): p. 3703-12.

[23] Sakamuro, D. and G.C. Prendergast, *New Myc-interacting proteins: a second Myc network emerges.* Oncogene, 1999. 18(19): p. 2942-54.

[24] Bannasch, D., I. Weis, and M. Schwab, *Nmi protein interacts with regions that differ between MycN and Myc and is localized in the cytoplasm of neuroblastoma cells in contrast to nuclear MycN.* Oncogene, 1999. 18(48): p. 6810-7.

[25] Wood, M.A., S.B. McMahon, and M.D. Cole, *An ATPase/helicase complex is an essential cofactor for oncogenic transformation by c-Myc.* Mol Cell, 2000. 5(2): p. 321-30.

[26] Bannasch, D., B. Madge, and M. Schwab, *Functional interaction of Yaf2 with the central region of MycN.* Oncogene, 2001. 20(41): p. 5913-9.

[27] Herbst, A., et al., *A conserved element in Myc that negatively regulates its proapoptotic activity.* EMBO Rep, 2005. 6(2): p. 177-83.

[28] Cowling, V.H., et al., *A conserved Myc protein domain, MBIV, regulates DNA binding, apoptosis, transformation, and G2 arrest.* Mol Cell Biol, 2006. 26(11): p. 4226-39.

[29] Cotterman, R., et al., *N-Myc regulates a widespread euchromatic program in the human genome partially independent of its role as a classical transcription factor.* Cancer Res, 2008. 68(23): p. 9654-62.

[30] Knoepfler, P.S., *Myc goes global: new tricks for an old oncogene.* Cancer Res, 2007. 67(11): p. 5061-3.

[31] Cowling, V.H. and M.D. Cole, *The Myc transactivation domain promotes global phosphorylation of the RNA polymerase II carboxy-terminal domain independently of direct DNA binding.* Mol Cell Biol, 2007. 27(6): p. 2059-73.

[32] Dominguez-Sola, D., et al., *Non-transcriptional control of DNA replication by c-Myc.* Nature, 2007. 448(7152): p. 445-51.

[33] McMahon, S.B., M.A. Wood, and M.D. Cole, *The essential cofactor TRRAP recruits the histone acetyltransferase hGCN5 to c-Myc.* Mol Cell Biol, 2000. 20(2): p. 556-62.

[34] Strahl, B.D. and C.D. Allis, *The language of covalent histone modifications.* Nature, 2000. 403(6765): p. 41-5.

[35] Ikura, T., et al., *Involvement of the TIP60 histone acetylase complex in DNA repair and apoptosis.* Cell, 2000. 102(4): p. 463-73.

[36] Frank, S.R., et al., *Binding of c-Myc to chromatin mediates mitogen-induced acetylation of histone H4 and gene activation.* Genes Dev, 2001. 15(16): p. 2069-82.

[37] Shen, X., et al., *A chromatin remodelling complex involved in transcription and DNA processing.* Nature, 2000. 406(6795): p. 541-4.

[38] Eberhardy, S.R. and P.J. Farnham, *Myc recruits P-TEFb to mediate the final step in the transcriptional activation of the cad promoter.* J Biol Chem, 2002. 277(42): p. 40156-62.

[39] Marhin, W.W., et al., *Myc represses the growth arrest gene gadd45.* Oncogene, 1997. 14(23): p. 2825-34.

[40] Wu, S., et al., *Myc represses differentiation-induced p21CIP1 expression via Miz-1-dependent interaction with the p21 core promoter.* Oncogene, 2003. 22(3): p. 351-60.

[41] Judware, R. and L.A. Culp, *Over-expression of transfected N-myc oncogene in human SKNSH neuroblastoma cells down-regulates expression of beta 1 integrin subunit.* Oncogene, 1995. 11(12): p. 2599-607.

[42] Cleveland, J.L., et al., *Negative regulation of c-myc transcription involves myc family proteins.* Oncogene Res, 1988. 3(4): p. 357-75.

[43] Grignani, F., et al., *Negative autoregulation of c-myc gene expression is inactivated in transformed cells.* EMBO J, 1990. 9(12): p. 3913-22.

[44] Bell, E., et al., *MYCN oncoprotein targets and their therapeutic potential.* Cancer Lett, 2010. 293(2): p. 144-57.

[45] Liu, T., et al., *Activation of tissue transglutaminase transcription by histone deacetylase inhibition as a therapeutic approach for Myc oncogenesis.* Proc Natl Acad Sci U S A, 2007. 104(47): p. 18682-7.

[46] Tucholski, J., M. Lesort, and G.V. Johnson, *Tissue transglutaminase is essential for neurite outgrowth in human neuroblastoma SH-SY5Y cells.* Neuroscience, 2001. 102(2): p. 481-91.

[47] Zeng, H., et al., *Transport of amphipathic anions by human multidrug resistance protein 3.* Cancer Res, 2000. 60(17): p. 4779-84.

[48] Porro, A., et al., *Direct and coordinate regulation of ATP-binding cassette transporter genes by Myc factors generates specific transcription signatures that significantly affect the chemoresistance phenotype of cancer cells.* J Biol Chem, 2010. 285(25): p. 19532-43.

[49] Paumi, C.M., et al., *Multidrug resistance protein (MRP) 1 and MRP3 attenuate cytotoxic and transactivating effects of the cyclopentenone prostaglandin, 15-deoxy-Delta(12,14)prostaglandin J2 in MCF7 breast cancer cells.* Biochemistry, 2003. 42(18): p. 5429-37.

[50] Hatzi, E., et al., *N-myc oncogene overexpression down-regulates IL-6; evidence that IL-6 inhibits angiogenesis and suppresses neuroblastoma tumor growth.* Oncogene, 2002. 21(22): p. 3552-61.

[51] Schneider, A., et al., *Association of Myc with the zinc-finger protein Miz-1 defines a novel pathway for gene regulation by Myc.* Curr Top Microbiol Immunol, 1997. 224: p. 137-46.

[52] Peukert, K., et al., *An alternative pathway for gene regulation by Myc.* EMBO J, 1997. 16(18): p. 5672-86.

[53] Ikegaki, N., et al., *De novo identification of MIZ-1 (ZBTB17) encoding a MYC-interacting zinc-finger protein as a new favorable neuroblastoma gene.* Clin Cancer Res, 2007. 13(20): p. 6001-9.

[54] Wanzel, M., S. Herold, and M. Eilers, *Transcriptional repression by Myc.* Trends Cell Biol, 2003. 13(3): p. 146-50.

[55] Brenner, C., et al., *Myc represses transcription through recruitment of DNA methyltransferase corepressor.* EMBO J, 2005. 24(2): p. 336-46.

[56] Schwab, M., *Human neuroblastoma: from basic science to clinical debut of cellular oncogenes.* Naturwissenschaften, 1999. 86(2): p. 71-8.

[57] Laird-Offringa, I.A., *What determines the instability of c-myc proto-oncogene mRNA?* Bioessays, 1992. 14(2): p. 119-24.

[58] Mirsky, R., et al., *Novel signals controlling embryonic Schwann cell development, myelination and dedifferentiation.* J Peripher Nerv Syst, 2008. 13(2): p. 122-35.

[59] Stanton, B.R., et al., *Loss of N-myc function results in embryonic lethality and failure of the epithelial component of the embryo to develop.* Genes Dev, 1992. 6(12A): p. 2235-47.

[60] Strieder, V. and W. Lutz, *E2F proteins regulate MYCN expression in neuroblastomas.* J Biol Chem, 2003. 278(5): p. 2983-9.

[61] Morrow, M.A., et al., *Interleukin-7 induces N-myc and c-myc expression in normal precursor B lymphocytes.* Genes Dev, 1992. 6(1): p. 61-70.

[62] Wada, R.K., et al., *Cell type-specific expression and negative regulation by retinoic acid of the human N-myc promoter in neuroblastoma cells.* Oncogene, 1992. 7(4): p. 711-7.

[63] Bentley, D.L. and M. Groudine, *A block to elongation is largely responsible for decreased transcription of c-myc in differentiated HL60 cells.* Nature, 1986. 321(6071): p. 702-6.

[64] Sivak, L.E., et al., *A novel intron element operates posttranscriptionally To regulate human N-myc expression.* Mol Cell Biol, 1999. 19(1): p. 155-63.

[65] Keene, R.G., et al., *Transcriptional pause, arrest and termination sites for RNA polymerase II in mammalian N- and c-myc genes.* Nucleic Acids Res, 1999. 27(15): p. 3173-82.

[66] Xu, L., S.D. Morgenbesser, and R.A. DePinho, *Complex transcriptional regulation of myc family gene expression in the developing mouse brain and liver.* Mol Cell Biol, 1991. 11(12): p. 6007-15.

[67] Brewer, G. and J. Ross, *Poly(A) shortening and degradation of the 3′ A+U-rich sequences of human c-myc mRNA in a cell-free system.* Mol Cell Biol, 1988. 8(4): p. 1697-708.

[68] Ross, J., *mRNA stability in mammalian cells.* Microbiol Rev, 1995. 59(3): p. 423-50.

[69] Bernstein, P.L., et al., *Control of c-myc mRNA half-life in vitro by a protein capable of binding to a coding region stability determinant.* Genes Dev, 1992. 6(4): p. 642-54.

[70] Chagnovich, D. and S.L. Cohn, *Activity of a 40 kDa RNA-binding protein correlates with MYCN and c-fos mRNA stability in human neuroblastoma.* Eur J Cancer, 1997. 33(12): p. 2064-7.

[71] Jopling, C.L. and A.E. Willis, *N-myc translation is initiated via an internal ribosome entry segment that displays enhanced activity in neuronal cells.* Oncogene, 2001. 20(21): p. 2664-70.

[72] Sjostrom, S.K., et al., *The Cdk1 complex plays a prime role in regulating N-myc phosphorylation and turnover in neural precursors.* Dev Cell, 2005. 9(3): p. 327-38.

[73] Knoepfler, P.S., P.F. Cheng, and R.N. Eisenman, *N-myc is essential during neurogenesis for the rapid expansion of progenitor cell populations and the inhibition of neuronal differentiation.* Genes Dev, 2002. 16(20): p. 2699-712.

[74] Kim, H.T., et al., *Certain pairs of ubiquitin-conjugating enzymes (E2s) and ubiquitin-protein ligases (E3s) synthesize nondegradable forked ubiquitin chains containing all possible isopeptide linkages.* J Biol Chem, 2007. 282(24): p. 17375-86.
[75] Eilers, M., S. Schirm, and J.M. Bishop, *The MYC protein activates transcription of the alpha-prothymosin gene.* EMBO J, 1991. 10(1): p. 133-41.
[76] Bello-Fernandez, C., G. Packham, and J.L. Cleveland, *The ornithine decarboxylase gene is a transcriptional target of c-Myc.* Proc Natl Acad Sci U S A, 1993. 90(16): p. 7804-8.
[77] Grandori, C. and R.N. Eisenman, *Myc target genes.* Trends Biochem Sci, 1997. 22(5): p. 177-81.
[78] Cole, M.D. and S.B. McMahon, *The Myc oncoprotein: a critical evaluation of transactivation and target gene regulation.* Oncogene, 1999. 18(19): p. 2916-24.
[79] Zeller, K.I., et al., *An integrated database of genes responsive to the Myc oncogenic transcription factor: identification of direct genomic targets.* Genome Biol, 2003. 4(10): p. R69.
[80] Guccione, E., et al., *Myc-binding-site recognition in the human genome is determined by chromatin context.* Nat Cell Biol, 2006. 8(7): p. 764-70.
[81] McMahon, S.B., *Control of nucleotide biosynthesis by the MYC oncoprotein.* Cell Cycle, 2008. 7(15): p. 2275-6.
[82] Bell, E., J. Lunec, and D.A. Tweddle, *Cell cycle regulation targets of MYCN identified by gene expression microarrays.* Cell Cycle, 2007. 6(10): p. 1249-56.
[83] Lastowska, M., et al., *Identification of candidate genes involved in neuroblastoma progression by combining genomic and expression microarrays with survival data.* Oncogene, 2007. 26(53): p. 7432-44.
[84] Dang, C.V., et al., *The c-Myc target gene network.* Semin Cancer Biol, 2006. 16(4): p. 253-64.
[85] Nesbit, C.E., J.M. Tersak, and E.V. Prochownik, *MYC oncogenes and human neoplastic disease.* Oncogene, 1999. 18(19): p. 3004-16.
[86] Slack, A., G. Lozano, and J.M. Shohet, *MDM2 as MYCN transcriptional target: implications for neuroblastoma pathogenesis.* Cancer Lett, 2005. 228(1-2): p. 21-7.
[87] Fan, J., et al., *Time-dependent c-Myc transactomes mapped by Array-based nuclear run-on reveal transcriptional modules in human B cells.* PLoS One, 2010. 5(3): p. e9691.
[88] Pegg, A.E., *Polyamine metabolism and its importance in neoplastic growth and a target for chemotherapy.* Cancer Res, 1988. 48(4): p. 759-74.
[89] Hogarty, M.D., et al., *ODC1 is a critical determinant of MYCN oncogenesis and a therapeutic target in neuroblastoma.* Cancer Res, 2008. 68(23): p. 9735-45.
[90] Bordow, S.B., et al., *Expression of the multidrug resistance-associated protein (MRP) gene correlates with amplification and overexpression of the N-myc oncogene in childhood neuroblastoma.* Cancer Res, 1994. 54(19): p. 5036-40.
[91] Norris, M.D., et al., *Expression of the gene for multidrug-resistance-associated protein and outcome in patients with neuroblastoma.* N Engl J Med, 1996. 334(4): p. 231-8.
[92] Haber, M., et al., *Altered expression of the MYCN oncogene modulates MRP gene expression and response to cytotoxic drugs in neuroblastoma cells.* Oncogene, 1999. 18(17): p. 2777-82.
[93] Munoz, M., et al., *Role of the MRP1/ABCC1 multidrug transporter protein in cancer.* IUBMB Life, 2007. 59(12): p. 752-7.
[94] Manohar, C.F., et al., *MYCN-mediated regulation of the MRP1 promoter in human neuroblastoma.* Oncogene, 2004. 23(3): p. 753-62.

[95] Henderson, M.J., et al., *ABCC multidrug transporters in childhood neuroblastoma: clinical and biological effects independent of cytotoxic drug efflux.* J Natl Cancer Inst, 2011. 103(16): p. 1236-51.

[96] Norris, M.D., et al., *Expression of multidrug transporter MRP4/ABCC4 is a marker of poor prognosis in neuroblastoma and confers resistance to irinotecan in vitro.* Mol Cancer Ther, 2005. 4(4): p. 547-53.

[97] Brodeur, G.M., et al., *Amplification of N-myc in untreated human neuroblastomas correlates with advanced disease stage.* Science, 1984. 224(4653): p. 1121-4.

[98] Seeger, R.C., et al., *Association of multiple copies of the N-myc oncogene with rapid progression of neuroblastomas.* N Engl J Med, 1985. 313(18): p. 1111-6.

[99] Bartram, C.R. and F. Berthold, *Amplification and expression of the N-myc gene in neuroblastoma.* Eur J Pediatr, 1987. 146(2): p. 162-5.

[100] Nakagawara, A., et al., *Amplification of N-myc oncogene in stage II and IVS neuroblastomas may be a prognostic indicator.* J Pediatr Surg, 1987. 22(5): p. 415-8.

[101] Brodeur, G.M., et al., *International criteria for diagnosis, staging, and response to treatment in patients with neuroblastoma.* J Clin Oncol, 1988. 6(12): p. 1874-81.

[102] Brodeur, G.M. and C.T. Fong, *Molecular biology and genetics of human neuroblastoma.* Cancer Genet Cytogenet, 1989. 41(2): p. 153-74.

[103] Amler, L.C. and M. Schwab, *Multiple amplicons of discrete sizes encompassing N-myc in neuroblastoma cells evolve through differential recombination from a large precursor DNA.* Oncogene, 1992. 7(4): p. 807-9.

[104] Brodeur, G.M., *Neuroblastoma: clinical significance of genetic abnormalities.* Cancer Surv, 1990. 9(4): p. 673-88.

[105] Xu, L., et al., *Loss of transcriptional attenuation in N-myc is associated with progression towards a more malignant phenotype.* Oncogene, 1995. 11(9): p. 1865-72.

[106] Bogenmann, E., M. Torres, and H. Matsushima, *Constitutive N-myc gene expression inhibits trkA mediated neuronal differentiation.* Oncogene, 1995. 10(10): p. 1915-25.

[107] Lutz, W., et al., *Conditional expression of N-myc in human neuroblastoma cells increases expression of alpha-prothymosin and ornithine decarboxylase and accelerates progression into S-phase early after mitogenic stimulation of quiescent cells.* Oncogene, 1996. 13(4): p. 803-12.

[108] Whitesell, L., A. Rosolen, and L.M. Neckers, *Antisense suppression of N-myc expression inhibits the transdifferentiation of neuroectoderm tumor cell lines.* Prog Clin Biol Res, 1991. 366: p. 45-54.

[109] Whitesell, L., A. Rosolen, and L.M. Neckers, *In vivo modulation of N-myc expression by continuous perfusion with an antisense oligonucleotide.* Antisense Res Dev, 1991. 1(4): p. 343-50.

[110] Cohn, S.L., et al., *MYCN expression is not prognostic of adverse outcome in advanced-stage neuroblastoma with nonamplified MYCN.* J Clin Oncol, 2000. 18(21): p. 3604-13.

[111] Tang, X.X., et al., *The MYCN enigma: significance of MYCN expression in neuroblastoma.* Cancer Res, 2006. 66(5): p. 2826-33.

[112] Tonelli, R., et al., *Antitumor activity of sustained N-myc reduction in rhabdomyosarcomas and transcriptional block by antigene therapy.* Clin Cancer Res, 2012. 18(3): p. 796-807.

[113] Helland, A., et al., *Deregulation of MYCN, LIN28B and LET7 in a molecular subtype of aggressive high-grade serous ovarian cancers.* PLoS One, 2011. 6(4): p. e18064.

[114] Kim, Y.H., et al., *Combined microarray analysis of small cell lung cancer reveals altered apoptotic balance and distinct expression signatures of MYC family gene amplification.* Oncogene, 2006. 25(1): p. 130-8.

[115] Beltran, H., et al., *Molecular Characterization of Neuroendocrine Prostate Cancer and Identification of New Drug Targets.* Cancer Discov, 2011. 1(6): p. 487-495.

[116] Ma, D., et al., *Array Comparative Genomic Hybridization Analysis Identifies Recurrent Gain of Chromosome 2p25.3 Involving the ACP1 and MYCN Genes in Chronic Lymphocytic Leukemia.* Clinical Lymphoma Myeloma and Leukemia, 2011. 11, Supplement 1(0): p. S17-S24.

[117] Ryan, S.L., et al., *MYC family amplification and clinical risk-factors interact to predict an extremely poor prognosis in childhood medulloblastoma.* Acta Neuropathol, 2012. 123(4): p. 501-13.

[118] Swartling, F.J., et al., *Pleiotropic role for MYCN in medulloblastoma.* Genes Dev, 2010. 24(10): p. 1059-72.

[119] Eberhart, C.G., et al., *Histopathological and molecular prognostic markers in medulloblastoma: c-myc, N-myc, TrkC, and anaplasia.* J Neuropathol Exp Neurol, 2004. 63(5): p. 441-9.

[120] Hatton, B.A., et al., *N-myc is an essential downstream effector of Shh signaling during both normal and neoplastic cerebellar growth.* Cancer Res, 2006. 66(17): p. 8655-61.

[121] Garrett, M.D. and P. Workman, *Discovering novel chemotherapeutic drugs for the third millennium.* Eur J Cancer, 1999. 35(14): p. 2010-30.

[122] Vita, M. and M. Henriksson, *The Myc oncoprotein as a therapeutic target for human cancer.* Semin Cancer Biol, 2006. 16(4): p. 318-30.

[123] Jain, R.K., *Delivery of novel therapeutic agents in tumors: physiological barriers and strategies.* J Natl Cancer Inst, 1989. 81(8): p. 570-6.

[124] Lu, X., A. Pearson, and J. Lunec, *The MYCN oncoprotein as a drug development target.* Cancer Lett, 2003. 197(1-2): p. 125-30.

[125] Negroni, A., et al., *Decrease of proliferation rate and induction of differentiation by a MYCN antisense DNA oligomer in a human neuroblastoma cell line.* Cell Growth Differ, 1991. 2(10): p. 511-8.

[126] Marshall, G.M., et al., *Increased retinoic acid receptor gamma expression suppresses the malignant phenotype and alters the differentiation potential of human neuroblastoma cells.* Oncogene, 1995. 11(3): p. 485-91.

[127] Thiele, C.J., C.P. Reynolds, and M.A. Israel, *Decreased expression of N-myc precedes retinoic acid-induced morphological differentiation of human neuroblastoma.* Nature, 1985. 313(6001): p. 404-6.

[128] Soucek, L., et al., *Modelling Myc inhibition as a cancer therapy.* Nature, 2008. 455(7213): p. 679-83.

[129] Berg, T., et al., *Small-molecule antagonists of Myc/Max dimerization inhibit Myc-induced transformation of chicken embryo fibroblasts.* Proc Natl Acad Sci U S A, 2002. 99(6): p. 3830-5.

[130] Facchini, L.M. and L.Z. Penn, *The molecular role of Myc in growth and transformation: recent discoveries lead to new insights.* FASEB J, 1998. 12(9): p. 633-51.

[131] Delmore, J.E., et al., *BET bromodomain inhibition as a therapeutic strategy to target c-Myc.* Cell, 2011. 146(6): p. 904-17.

[132] Mertz, J.A., et al., *Targeting MYC dependence in cancer by inhibiting BET bromodomains.* Proc Natl Acad Sci U S A, 2011. 108(40): p. 16669-74.

Chapter 19

STAT Transcription Factors in Tumor Development and Targeted Therapy of Malignancies

Gordana Konjević, Sandra Radenković, Ana Vuletić,
Katarina Mirjačić Martinović, Vladimir Jurišić and Tatjana Srdić

Additional information is available at the end of the chapter

http://dx.doi.org/10.5772/54893

1. Introduction

The signal transducers and activators of transcription, STAT proteins, were originally discovered in interferon (IFN)-regulated gene transcription in the early 1990's. Since then, a number of cytokines have been recognized to activate various STAT proteins. STATs constitute a family of seven transcription factors, STAT1α/β, STAT2, STAT3α/β, STAT4, STAT5A, STAT5B and STAT6, that transduce signals from a variety of extracellular stimuli initiated by different cytokine families that aside from interferons (interferon α, β and γ) include gp130 cytokines, i.e., IL-6, IL-12, IL-23 and γC cytokines that include IL-2, IL-15 and IL-21 [1].

Although structurally similar, the seven STAT family members possess diverse biological roles and are engaged in numerous processes from embryonic development, organogenesis, cell differentiation to regulation of immune processes. Awareness of their important role in regulation of cell proliferation, differentiation and survival has spurred interest in investigation of their activity in malignant transformation [2]. Evidence has now accumulated that confirms their role in pathogenesis of leukemias and numerous solid tumors [3] (Table1).

Aside from cytokine receptors, STATs are also activated by receptors for growth factors (family of tyrosine kinase receptors) that include receptors for epidermal growth factor - EGFR, platelet-derived growth factor - PDGF, hepatocyte growth factor - HGF and colony-stimulating factor 1- CSF-1 receptors that possess an intrinsic tyrosine kinase activity [4]. These receptors may activate STAT proteins either directly or indirectly by means of JAK kinase proteins. Also, free intracellular enzymes, i.e., non-receptor tyrosine kinases that include oncogenes *src* and *bcr-abl* activate various STATs [5].

Different biological processes regulated by STAT proteins
Embryonic development
Organogenesis and function
Cells proliferation
Cell differentiation, growth and apoptosis
Innate and adoptive immunity
Inflammation
Angiogenesis
Wound healing
Malignant transformation

Table 1. Role of STATs in the organism

Interaction of cytokines and their specific receptors directly activates free intracellular non-receptor enzymes, Janus kinases, and subsequently, latent STAT transcription factors that through the JAK/STAT signaling pathway lead to the expression of numerous genes that regulate important cellular processes. It is of importance that numerous cytokines, growth factors in different cell types activate STAT1, STAT3 and STAT5 and mediate broadly diverse biologic processes that control cell homeostasis. On the other hand, STATs such as STAT4 and STAT6 have a more specific role and they are engaged in T helper cell differentiation and maintenance of equilibrium between Th1 and Th2 immune response [6]. Defects in STAT molecules can lead to serious defects in development and to fetal death indicating the importance of JAK/STAT pathway in normal cell development. Defects in the JAK/STAT signaling pathway are often encountered in primary malignant tumors, as well as in peripheral blood lymphocytes [7,8,9] and STAT3 has been the first to be identified as a potential oncogene [2] (Fig.1).

Given the critical roles of STAT proteins such as activation of pro-inflammatory and anti-proliferative processes by STAT1 and control of cell-cycle progression and apoptosis by STAT3 and STAT5 it has been established in many studies that their dysregulation can contribute to oncogenesis [10] by increasing proliferation and slowing-down apoptosis. In this sense, studies show that STAT3 is activated in a majority of breast and prostate cancers, and that STAT3 inhibition using RNA interference or a dominant negative genotype leads to reduced cell proliferation, survival, and induces wound healing. Further, blocking STAT3 interaction with EGFR using peptide aptamers has been shown to reduce tumor growth. On the other hand, STAT1 has been primarily defined as a tumor suppressor gene and its inactivation was associated with malignant transformation. Initially STAT proteins were extensively studied in leukemias, but later their role in the development of different solid tumors has been shown.

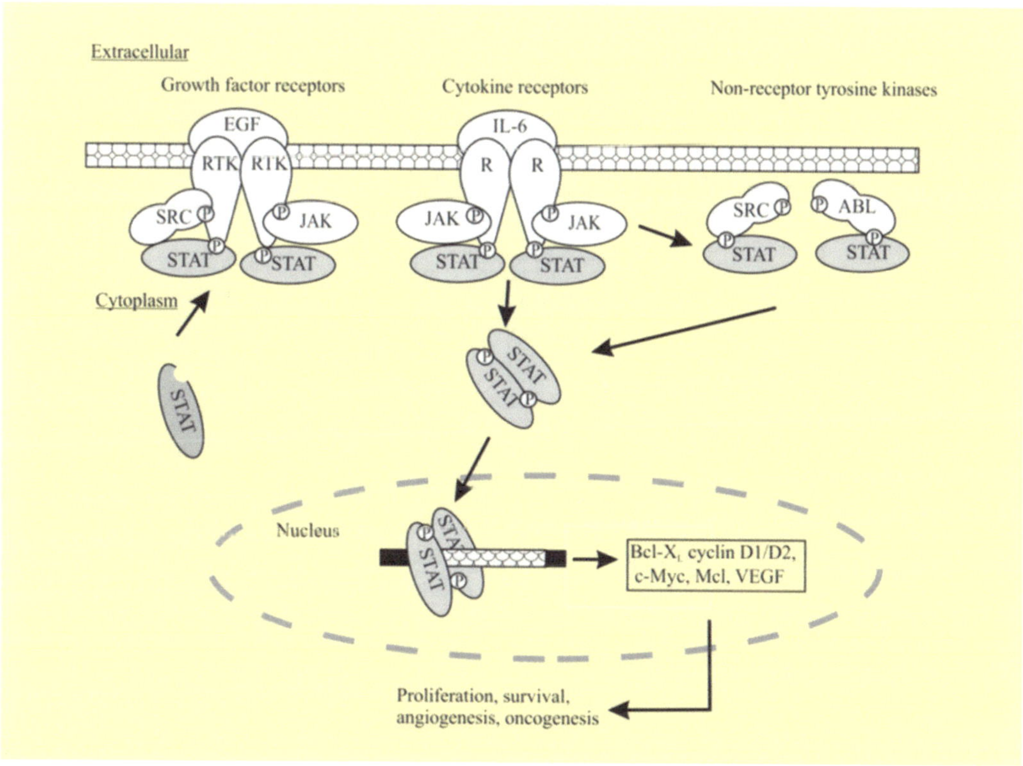

Figure 1. Mechanisms of STAT signaling upon activation of different tyrosine kinase (TK) signaling pathways that can induce activation of STAT proteins. In the case of growth factors like EGF that bind to receptor tyrosine kinases (RTKs), the receptor can directly phosphorylate STATs and/or indirectly induce STAT phosphorylation. Also, cytokines, like IL-6, that bind to cytokine receptors lacking intrinsic TK activity undergo ligand-induced dimerization of the receptor that results in phosphorylation of receptor-associated JAK kinases. JAKs in turn phosphorylate the receptor cytoplasmic tails on tyrosine, providing "docking sites" for recruitment of monomeric STATs. JAKs then phosphorylate the recruited STAT proteins on tyrosine, inducing dimerization, nuclear translocation, and DNA-binding activity. Other non-receptor bound free intracellular enzymes named non receptor TKs such as SRC family kinases are also involved and can directly induce STAT activation. Once in the nucleus, activated STAT proteins bind to specific DNA sequences in the promoters of genes and induce their expression. In the context of oncogenesis, constitutive activation of TK-STAT signaling pathways induces elevated expression of genes involved in controlling cellular processes such as cell proliferation and survival.

Aside from their role in the development of tumors STAT1,3 and 5 can be considered as molecular markers for early detection of certain types of tumors, as well as prognostic factors for determining tumor aggressiveness and predictors of response to various types of therapy. Novel data also indicate functional interplay between several activated STATs and association of STAT5 with certain well differentiated tumors with favorable prognosis [11].Based on numerous new data it appears that dysregulation of STAT signaling pathway may serve as a basis for designing novel targeted molecular therapeutic strategies that hold great potential for the treatment of solid tumors and leukemias.

1.1. Structural and functional characteristics of STATs

STATs share structurally and functionally conserved domains that include the amino-terminal domain (NH2), the coiled-coiled domain (CCD), the DNA binding domain (DBD), the linker domain and the SH2/tyrosine activation domain [12]. In contrast, the carboxyl-terminal transcriptional activation domain (TAD) is quite divergent and contributes to STAT specificity (Table 2).

Functionally, the amino-terminal domain of STAT molecules is the oligomerization domain that interacts with other proteins and mediates oligomerization of STAT dimers to form tetramers [13]. The DNA binding domain defines the DNA-binding specificity to tandem GAS elements and each STAT component of the dimer recognizes bases in the most proximal half of GAS and mediates distinct signals for specific ligands.

SH2 domain, located near the C-terminal domain, plays an important role in signaling through its capacity to bind to specific phosphotyrosine motifs and to mediate specific interactions. Consistent with this, it is the most highly conserved STAT domain. The ability of this SH2 domain to recognize specific phosphotyrosine motifs plays an essential role in three STAT signaling events that include recruitment to the phosphorylated cytokine receptor through recognition of specific receptor phosphotyrosine motifs, association with the activating JAKs, as well as STAT homo- or heterodimerization [14].

Domain	Role
NH2-terminal domain Oligomerization domain	Interacts with other proteins and mediates oligomerization of STAT dimers to form tetramers
DNA binding domain	Defines the DNA-binding specificity and mediates distinct signals for specific ligands
SH2 domain	Mediates specific interactions between STAT and receptors, STAT and JAK and STAT homo or hetero dimerization
COOH-terminal domain Transcription activation domain (TAD)	TAD regulates the transcriptional activity of STATs and provides specificity
Tyrosine residue	Phosphorylation site in the COOH-terminal domain that regulates the DNA-binding activity of all STATs. On phosphorylation mediates STAT dimerization
Serine residue	A second phosphorylation site in the C-terminal domain

Table 2. STAT structure

Close to the SH2 domain the critical tyrosine residue is located that is required for SH-phosphotyrosine interaction and thus STAT activation. This tyrosine residue is then rapidly phosphorylated by the active JAK determining STAT dimerization by binding to the SH2 domain of the reciprocal STAT molecule.

A conserved serine residue in the C-terminal domain of STAT1,3, and 5 is a second phosphorylation site that enhances DNA binding affinity and transcriptional activity [15]. It has been determined that the transcriptional activity of several STATs can be modulated through serine phosphorylation. Serine phosphorylation appears to enhance the transcription of some, but not all target genes. It has been suggested that serine phosphorylation may alter the affinity for other transcriptional regulators like minichromosome maintenance complex component 5 (MCM5) and BRCA1 [12].

C-terminal domain also encodes transcriptional activation domain (TAD) that contributes to STAT specificity and is thought to be involved in communication with transcriptional complexes, to regulate the transcriptional activity of STATs and provide functional specificity. Altered serine phosphorylation site associated with the c-terminal transactivation domain truncation of STAT1 and STAT3 reduces their transcriptional capacity by 20% [16]. Moreover, a c-TAD truncation leads to the α and β isoforms of STAT proteins that are biologically significant and appear to affect the cell's fate [13].

1.2. Mechanism and regulation of STAT protein function

When ligands bind to their receptors they initiate a cascade of intracellular phosphorylation events. However, members of the hematopoietin receptor family possess no catalytic kinase activity. Rather, they rely on members of the JAK family of tyrosine kinases to provide this activity. JAKs are constitutively associated with a proline-rich domain of these receptors [17]. Upon ligand stimulation, receptors undergo the conformational changes that bring JAKs into proximity of each other, enabling activation by trans-phosphorylation [18]. Once activated, JAKs mediate the described signal transduction. Several studies have also suggested that JAKs associate with the receptor tyrosine kinases [12]. The phosphorylated JAKs, in turn, mediate phosphorylation at the specific receptor tyrosine residues, which then serve as docking sites for STATs and other signaling molecules. Once recruited to the receptor, STATs also become phosphorylated by JAKs, on a single tyrosine residue. The position of these tyrosines in STAT molecule is specific for each member of STAT family of proteins, such as Tyr 701 for STAT1, Tyr690 for STAT2, Tyr 705 for STAT3, Tyr 693 for STAT4, Tyr 694 for STAT5, and Tyr 641 for STAT6. Their phosphorylation mediates STAT dimerization which occurs by binding of the SH2 domain of one molecule with the domain containing the phosphotyrosine of another STAT molecule [19], so the resulting dimers are thus stabilized by bivalent bonds. STAT2 is the only STAT representative that does not act as a homodimer, forming instead a complex with STAT1 and p48. As a response to several cytokines, the heterodimers STAT1-2, STAT1-3 STAT5A-5B are formed, while no heterodimers with STAT 4 and STAT6 have been identified [20] (Table 3).

Activated STATs dissociate from the receptor, dimerize, translocate to the nucleus and bind to members of the GAS (gamma activated site) family of enhancers. There are several more recent developments regarding STAT signaling, structural studies, nuclear as well as mitochondrial translocation, gene targeting and newly identified regulatory molecules.

Classical activation of STATs occurs after cytokine binding to cell-surface receptors that initiates a cascade of intracellular phosphorylation events. The phosphorylation of STATs is essential not only for dimerization, but also for the concomitant translocation of the dimers into the nucleus. Binding of STAT1 and STAT5B to importin-α5, a part of the nucleocytoplasmic transport machinery, has been described [21].

Considering that a second phosphorylation site is serine residue in the c-terminal domain, STATs, in addition to tyrosine phosphorylation can be serine phosphorylated by various serine kinases [22] that regulate and increase STAT1,3 and 5 transcriptional activity. It is of interest that one of the kinases responsible for the phosphorylation of this serine in STAT1 and STAT3, belongs to the MAP kinases family (ERKs, JNK and p38) which emphasizes the important "cross-talk" occurring between the two transductional pathways [23]. Furthermore, there is also evidence of the activity of ERK-independent serine kinases [24], such as the role of protein kinase C (PKC) in serine phosphorylation of STATs [25] and mTOR of the PKI2 pathway. The relative contribution of each of these serine kinases to STAT signaling in vivo would depend on cell-type specific expression of kinases [22]. Therefore, STATs can be phosphorylated in great many serine/threonine residues, which may modulate DNA binding and/or their transcriptional activity [26].

One can envision a negative feedback mechanism in which serine phosphorylation of STATs promotes the induction of physiologic inhibitors of STAT signaling, such as those of the suppressor of cytokine signaling (SOCS) family that inhibit at the level of JAKs [27]. Assumingly dual functional role is thus implied for STAT serine phosphorylation events, whereby the same serine kinases can apparently both enhance and repress STAT signaling, the indirect negative effect being due to preferential association of STAT proteins with the serine kinases, precluding interaction with tyrosine kinases [2, 25].

In addition to classical, canonical activation by tyrosine phosphorylation, the noncanonical STAT activation includes, besides serine phosphorylation, other, phosphorylation-independent modifications that regulate their activity. In this sense, it has been shown that following stimulation of cells with IL-1 plus IL-6 unphosphorylated STAT3 affects gene expression in the nucleus through binding to NF-κB that mediates its nuclear import [28]. Furthermore, the classical IL-6 mediated activation of STAT3 induces tyrosine-phosphorylation of STAT3 and activates many genes, including the STAT3 gene itself that results in STAT3 synthesis that in its unphosphorylated form can induce not only the synthesis of IL-6 but also the expression of other genes such as *RANTES, IL-8, Met,* and *MRAS.*

Aside from this, the noncanonical STAT activation includes acetylation of lysine 685 in the SH2 STAT domain [29] that occurs in IL-6-induced acute phase reactions [30]. Novel findings indicate that acetylation of STAT3 is an important regulatory modification that influences protein–protein interaction and its transcriptional activity. Moreover, in oncogenesis new data regarding transmembrane glycoprotein CD44 [31], a marker of tumor metastatic phenotype, translocates into the nucleus in association with acetylated STAT3 and by regulating transcription of cyclin D enhances cell proliferation [32] (Fig. 2).

Also, many more posttranslational STAT modifications such as isgylation [33], sumoylation [34] and ubiquitination [35] are being explored in STAT-dependent tumor formation and metastasis. These noncanonical pathways include the many roles of nontyrosine phosphorylated STATs, which alter their stability, dimerization, nuclear localization, transcriptional activation function, and association with histone acetyltransferases (HAT), and histone deacetylases (HDAC) [36] (Fig. 2).

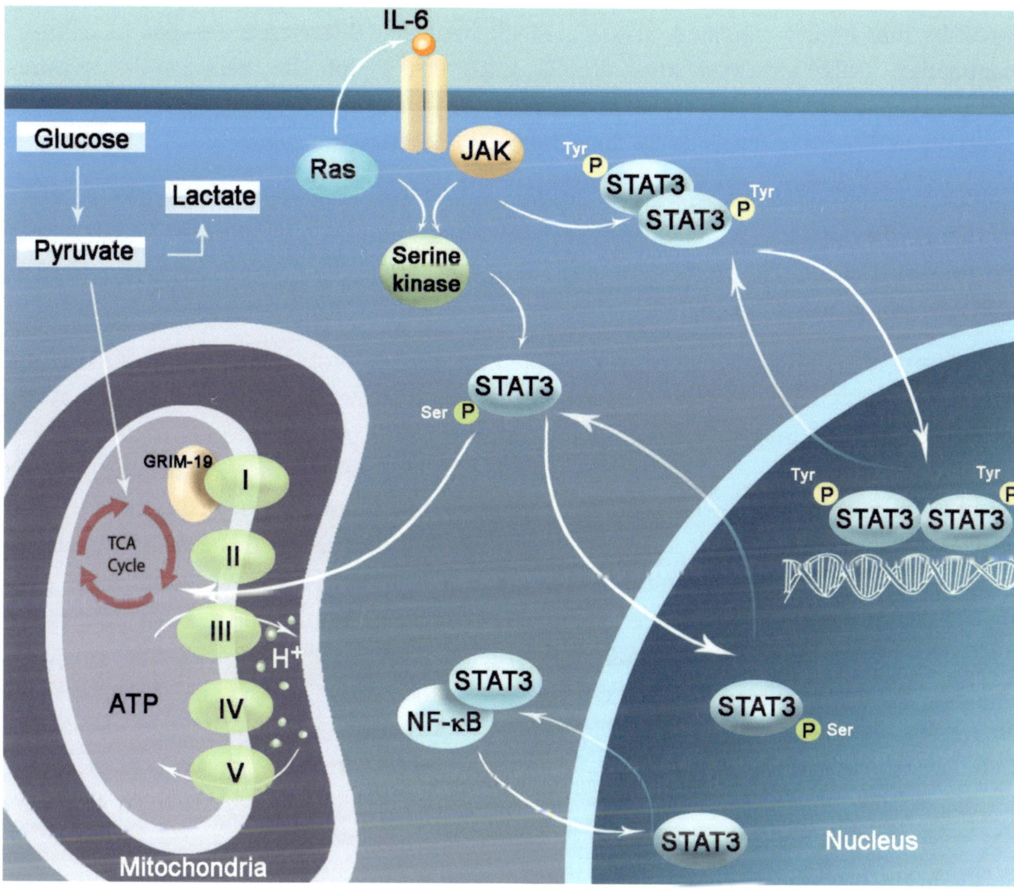

Figure 2. Different signaling pathways initiated by phosphorylation of STAT3 on tyrosine or serine residues. STAT3 is constitutively imported into and exported from the nucleus independent of its phosphorylation status. Oncogenic Ras can stimulate the autocrine production of IL-6, and the resulting phosphorylation of STAT3 Tyr705 promotes dimerization and the ability to bind specific DNA target sequences. STAT3 can also be phosphorylated on Ser727 and can mediate nuclear import of the NF-κB transcription factor. Serine phosphorylated STAT3 stimulates the electron transport chain in mitochondria and augments transformation by oncogenic Ras.

The duration of STATs activation is a temporary process, thus within hours the activating signals decay and the STATs are exported back to the cytoplasm. Negative nuclear regulators of STATs are nuclear tyrosine phosphatases that induce STAT dephosphorylation in the nucleus important for its export back to the cytoplasm. There is evidence that a specific nuclear tyrosine phosphatase (TC45), is a phosphatase relevant for STAT1 and STAT3 [37]. In addition, it has been reported that cells lacking this enzyme retain tyrosine phosphorylated STAT1 for much longer than normal cells, and overexpression of TC45 leads to dephosphorylation of STAT5 [38]. However, TC45 has also been implicated in regulating cytoplasmic dephosphorylation of JAK1 and JAK3 [39].

Recently, the negative activity on STAT protein of a group of nuclear proteins termed "proteins that inhibit activated STATs" (PIAS) has been discovered. Studies in cultured mammalian cells indicated that PIAS1 and PIAS3 interact only with tyrosine-phosphorylated STAT1 and STAT3, respectively [40]. PIAS prevents their binding to DNA, especially of STAT1, or it speeds-up their degradation in the proteasome.

Besides nuclear, other phosphatases in the cytoplasm also represent negative STAT regulators, they include phosphatases such as SH2-containing phosphatase-1 (SH1), SH2, and protein-tyrosine-phosphatase-1B (PTP1B) implicated as cytoplasmic regulators of JAKs or STATs' phosphorylation [38].

The activity of STAT proteins is also regulated by the inhibitors of the suppressors of the cytokine signal (SOCS) family, responsible for modulating the JAK-STAT pathway by acting on the JAK kinases. These cytokine-induced SOCS proteins are recruited to active receptor complexes to cause inhibition, and can also cause protein turnover of the receptor through a process of proteolytic degradation ubiquitine-proteasome mediated [41]. As SOCS belong to the family of target STAT genes they constitute with them a classical negative feedback mechanism [12] that can negatively regulate their own phosphorylation state [42]. Several members of this family have been identified, SOCS1,2,3,4,5,6 and 7. These regulatory proteins have an indirect negative effect on STATs by inhibiting their activating enzymes, especially Janus kinases (JAK1, JAK2, JAK3 and Tyk2), as well as, upstream receptors for growth factors [43]. Considering their negative regulatory role, SOCS proteins represent an important intracellular mechanism for limiting the potentially adverse effects of cytokines in immune reactions [44].

Aside from these mechanisms, mutations that augment the function of their activators or decreases the function of their inhibitors may lead to STAT hyperactivity and their engagement in malignant transformation.

Moreover, due to alternate splicing of STAT gene the short forms of STATs, i.e., inactive STATβ form, can potentially act as dominant-negative protein and by competitive inhibition occupy DNA as non-functional protein without transcriptional capability or by binding to wild-type STATs form [45] competitive inhibition, prevent binding of the STATα isoform and transcription of target genes. Aside from that, the truncated STATγ isoform of this molecule that is created by proteolysis, also competitively inhibits transcription mediated by the active α form (Table 3).

Positive regulation of STATs	Effects	
Canonical regulation of STATs		
Phosphorylation of tyrosine	STAT1 - Tyr 701 STAT2 - Tyr690 STAT3 - Tyr 705	STAT4 - Tyr 693 STAT5 - Tyr 694 STAT6 - Tyr 641
Noncannonical regulation of STATs		
Phosphorylation of serine	STAT3 - Ser727 STAT4 - Ser721 STAT5 - Ser725/730	
Unphosphorylated STAT	IL-6 gene dependant expression IL-6 mediated acute phase reactions	
NFκB	Nuclear import of CD44	
Acetylation		
Isgylation		
Sumoylation		
Genetic regulation		
Mutations		
Hypermorphic allele of STAT3	Increased transcription	
Epigenetic regulation		
Histone acetyl transferase (HAT)		

Negative regulation of STATs	
Negative cytoplasmic regulators	
Tyrosine phosphatase (SHP1,2)	Dephosphorylation
Protein-tyrosine-phosphatase-1B	
Suppressors of cytokine signals (SOCS1-7)	Inhibit JAK degrade receptors
Proteases	STAT inactive forms (β and γ)
Negative nuclear regulators	
Nuclear tyrosine phosphatase	Dephosphorylation
Proteins that inhibit activated STATs (PIAS1-3)	Inhibits STAT1-3 DNA binding Proteasome degradation
DNA methyltransferase (DNMT)	Decreased transcription
Ubiquitination	Degradation

Table 3. Regulation of STAT activity

2. STAT proteins in carcinogenesis

Aside from their essential role in mediating the effect of cytokines, it has been shown that STATs can have a significant role in tumor development and they are being considered as potential oncogenes. In normal cells, the activation of STAT proteins is transient, ranging from between a few minutes to a few hours. However, in a large group of different tumors constitutive activation of STAT family, especially STAT3 and STAT5 members, as well as the loss of

STAT1 signaling, has been detected [3, 46]. Novel results indicate that STAT proteins regulate numerous pathways that participate in oncogenesis, such as cell cycle progression, apoptosis, angiogenesis, tumor invasiveness, metastasis, and immune response evasion. Based on this STAT proteins have become significant target molecules in novel therapeutic approaches in oncology as blocking of these molecules, directly or indirectly, may arrest the malignant process [47].

Gough et al. [48] provide evidence that STAT3 has joined a set of transcription factors that in mitochondria exhibit noncanonical roles independent of classical STAT3-mediated transcription in the nucleus. In this sense, mitochondria have become important in cancer research because they regulate proapoptotic and antiapoptotic factors.

It is also of importance that according to their general principle of action STAT proteins may be divided into two groups that differ greatly. The group that comprises STAT2, STAT4 and STAT6 is activated by a limited number of cytokines and it is engaged in T cell development and the effect of interferons, while the other group that is comprised of STAT1, STAT3 and STAT5 is activated in numerous tissues and cell types by great many cytokines, different hormones and growth factors and aside from mediating immune reactions, regulates many important general processes such as cell proliferation, differentiation and survival in embryogenesis, as well as breast development [49]. In that sense, this second group of STAT proteins is of importance in malignant transformation. Aside from that, earlier results indicated that active STAT1 protein has tumor-suppressor characteristics as it down-regulates cell proliferation and induces apoptosis, so that its decreased activity is associated with numerous neoplasias. On the other hand, it has been shown for STAT3 and STAT5 that they are proto-oncogenes that activate oncogenes, *c-myc*, *cyklin D* and antiapoptotic Bcl-XL protein, facilitate passage through G1/S check-point and in that sense, aside from down-regulating apoptosis, enhance cell proliferation and transformation [12].

It has been shown that STAT3 is frequently activated in hematological and epithelial malignancies. Constitutive activation of STAT3 leads to proliferation of tumor cells and prevents apoptosis, down-regulates the production of numerous proinflamatory cytokines and chemokines and leads to secretion of factors that prevent dendritic cell (DC) maturation that suppresses adaptive antitumor immunity establishment. Aside from the disturbance of the JAK/STAT signaling pathway in primary tumors, a similar finding is frequently found in peripheral blood lymphocytes of patients with malignancies [3].

2.1. Constitutively activated STATs affect tumor microenvironment

It is known that invasive tumors need to modulate gene expression in a manner that impairs the activity of innate and adaptive immunity in immune surveillance [50, 51]. STAT3 positive tumors achieve this by preventing the production of proinflamatory cytokines, i.e., "danger signals". Activation of the transcription factor STAT3 in the tumor and adjacent immune cells, including tumor associated macrophages (TAMs),T regulatory cells (Treg cells), DCs, Th1 cells, Th2 cells, B regulatory cells (Bregs), myeloid derived suppressor cells (MDSCs), Th17 cells, as well as, normal epithelial cells, lead to production of cytokines IL-1β, IL-6, IL-10, IL-17, as well as VEGF creating a feedback loop that promotes tumor growth, angiogenesis, evasion of immune surveillance and metastasis [52].

It has been shown that especially tumor produced IL-6 through JAKs/STAT3 signaling has an important role in modulating the tumor-associated immune microenvironment. IL-6 has pleiotropic functions by activating numerous cell types expressing membrane-bound gp130 IL-6 receptor, i.e., classical IL-6 signaling, as well as, by soluble form of the IL-6 receptor (sIL-6 receptor) that after binding IL-6 and interaction with gp130 in the form of IL-6 *trans*-signaling modulates a broad spectrum of target cells including epithelial cells, neutrophils, macrophages, and T cells [53]. Upregulated STAT3 in TAM has been shown to enhance the expression of IL-23 that leads to the expansion of Tregs, while conversely, transcriptionally repressing IL-12 that supports proinflamatory cytokines and antitumor immune reactions within the tumor milieu [54]. Also, tumor-evoked Bregs express activated STAT3 and induce TGFβ conversion of Tregs from resting T cells [55] (Fig.3). Therefore, the production

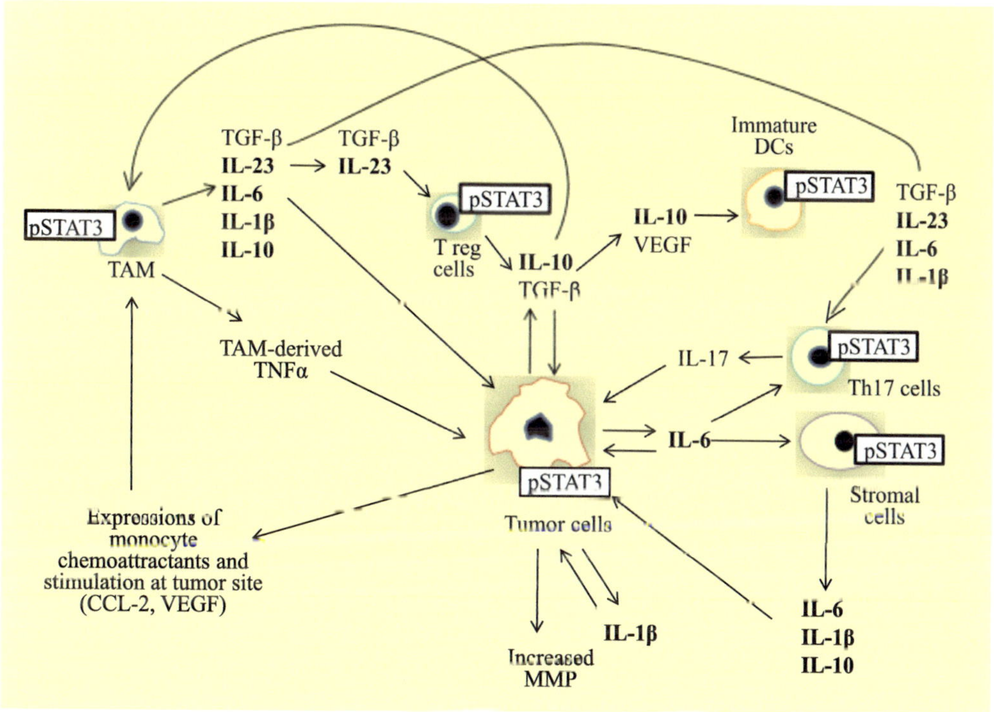

Figure 3. Interaction between tumor cells and tumor microenvironment mediated by cytokines. Tumor cells and different immune cells including TAMs, Treg cells, DC, Th17 cells, and non-tumor (normal epithelial) cells undergo STAT3 activation under the effect of various cytokines, and in turn produce more cytokines forming a feedback loop. STAT3 also regulates cell proliferation, cell cycle progression, apoptosis, angiogenesis together with immune evasion. Inhibition of STAT signaling could eliminate tumor cells while exerting minimal effect on the normal cells. Preclinical models have validated STAT3 as a target for cancer therapy, although only indirect JAK inhibitors have advanced to clinical trials (Cytokines that induce STAT3 activation are written in bold letters).

and release of various survival factors, including IL-6 as a major activator of STAT3, also serve to block apoptosis in cells during the inflammatory process, keeping them alive in very toxic environments. Unfortunately, at the same time these same pathways serve to maintain cells progressing towards neoplastic growth, protecting them from cellular apoptotic deletion and chemotherapeutic drugs.

It is of importance that activation of STAT3 within tumors is heterogeneous and it has been found that pSTAT3 are highest on the leading edge of tumors and that this is associated with stromal, immune, and endothelial cells. This follows from IL-6 from cancer-associated fibroblasts or myeloid cells that in a feedback loop induces autocrine production of IL-6 and pSTAT3 expression in tumor cells, thus also leading to heterogeneous levels of pSTAT3 [56].

Therefore tumor STAT3 activity can mediate tumor immune evasion and induce tolerance rather than immunity by blocking both the production and sensing of inflammatory signals by components of the innate and adaptive immune systems that have been recently defined as "extrinsic tumor suppressors" [57].

Regarding tumor microenvironment, in physiological conditions the activation of STAT3 is of paramount importance during tissue remodeling in the process of „wound healing" [58]. As tumor growth also includes tissue damage, the dysregulation of STAT3 in the context of tumor microenvironment has a detrimental effect that instead of wound healing leads to further tissue destruction, together with evasion of immune response.

2.2. STATs support oncogene-dependent cellular transformation

Oncogenes can only transform cells that have been immortalized by carcinogens or other oncogenes exemplifying the paradigm of multistep carcinogenesis. In this sense, mammal cells transformed by oncogenic *src* show constitutively active STAT3 and negative-dominant forms of STAT3 block the transforming ability of *src*, demonstrating a close correlation between STAT3 activation and the oncogenic transformation by this oncogene [59].

Moreover, recent studies have shown that constitutive activation of STAT3 in human breast cancer cells correlates with EGFR family kinase signaling and also with aberrant JAK and Src activity [60]. In addition to Src, many other transforming tyrosine kinases, such as Eyk, Ros and Lck, constitutively activate STAT3 in the context of oncogenesis. Another example of tumorigenic stimuli known to activate STAT proteins is Abl that may constitutively activate STAT3 and STAT5, whereas the fusion protein, Bcr-Abl, may activate them in the absence of constitutive JAK activation, showing that the presence of the JAK kinases is not always essential for STAT activation [2] (Table 4).

In addition to its previously characterized nuclear roles, transformation specific function for mitochondrial STAT3 has now been shown. Although previous data implicated a Ras-STAT3 axis in transformation, those cases were in the context of activated tyrosine kinases, such as NPM-ALK [61], RET [62], or autocrine cytokine signaling requiring STAT3 function in the nucleus. However, it has now been shown that for cellular transformation and anchorage-independent growth induced by activated H-, N- or K-Ras, STAT3 phosporylated on Serine727 and expressed exclusively in mitochondria was required. In contrast, recent findings also show that mitochondrially restricted STAT3 did not support *src*-driven anchorage-independent growth, consistent with former data that *src* requires nuclear functions of STAT3 [63].

Cell type	Oncogene	Activated STATs
Fibroblasts	v-Src	STAT3
	c-Src	STAT3
	v-Sis	STAT3
	v-Ras	
	v-Raf	
	IGF-1 receptor	STAT3
Myeloid	v-Src	STAT1, STAT3, STAT5
T cell	Lck	STAT3, STAT5
Mammary/Lung epithelial	v-Src	STAT3
Gallbladder adenocarcinoma	v-Src	STAT3
Pre-B lymphocytes	v-Abl	STAT1, STAT5
Erythroleukemia/blast cells/ basophils/mast cells	Bcr-Abl	STAT1, STAT5
Primary bone marrow	Bcr-Abl	STAT5

Table 4. STAT activation by oncogenes

Mitochondrial STAT3 contributes to Ras-dependent cellular transformation by augmenting electron transport chain activity, particularly that of complexes II and V, accompanied by energy production to favor cytoplasmatic glycolysis that represents a hallmark of cancer formulated in the 1950's by Warburg [64]. Additional analyses are required to understand the connections between glycolysis and oxidative phosphorylation affected by STAT3 in the presence or absence of oncogenic Ras.

STAT3 apparently enters mitochondria associated with GRIM-19 that was identified as a subunit of the mitochondrial complex I and Ser727 appears to be needed for their interaction [65].

Therefore, the "metabolic shift" important for tumor growth mediated by mitochondrial STAT3 may reflect exploitation of a normal function and in this sense mitochondrial STAT3 function could provide a new target for therapeutic approaches to cancer [65].

2.3. Anti-oncogenic and oncogenic characteristics of STAT1

STAT1 has been considered to be an anti-oncogene, i.e., tumor-suppressor protein that blocks proliferation and induces apoptosis [66]. Moreover, it has been shown that its dysfunction leads to the loss of immune surveillance [67]. Loss of STAT1 supports angiogenesis and metastasis of tumors.

It has been established that STAT1, the first STAT to be discovered, is required for signaling by the IFNs which in addition to their role in innate immunity, serve as potent inhibitors of proliferation and promoters of apoptosis. The involvement of STAT1 in growth arrest and apoptosis in many cell types may be explained by its capacity to induce caspase and p21 expression [68] and reduce c-myc expression. Although, normally, high p21 expression is associated with cell growth arrest, p21 increase has also been observed in some human neoplasias. This contradiction has been explained by Bowman et al. (2000) [2] with the fact that p21 is also responsible for the correct association of the cyclin D1/CDK cyclin complex, and thus its increase may be necessary for cell-cycle progression. Interestingly, in mammary cells p21 upregulation by STAT1 appears to involve BRCA1, which is often lost in familial and other forms of breast cancer. Effective STAT1-BRCA1 binding is mediated by serine phosphorylation of STAT1. More recently besides its role as tumor suppressor, new evidence has shown that STAT1 can be activated in some malignancies such as breast, lung, head and neck cancer and brain tumors [46]. In this sense, STAT1 tyrosine 701 phosphorylation increase was demonstrated in human breast tumor cells with elevated levels of HER-2/Neu as well as in cell lines transfected with HER-2/Neu gene [70]. However, it is of interest that breast cancer patients with higher levels of phosphorylated and DNA-bound STAT1 show better prognosis and live longer.

Besides increased STAT activation, high expression of the unphosphorylated form of STAT1 was also found in cancer cells. Moreover, it has been also shown that recurrent tumors express higher levels of unphosphorylated STAT1 compared to the original tumors [72], as well as cancer cells resistant to ionizing radiation and anticancer agents [73]. Recently, functions of some STAT1-induced genes in cancer cells have been investigated, and some have been shown to have pro-metastatic, pro-proliferative, or antiapoptotic properties [74]. In this sense it has been found in melanoma cells that high levels of STAT1 expression inhibits caspase 3/7 activation in response to doxorubicin which contributes to patients' resistance to this chemotherapeutic agent [75]. It has also been shown by Khodarev et al. (2007) [76] that ectopically increased expression of STAT1 can induce a radiation-resistant phenotype.

Both type I and type II IFNs increase STAT1 expression in many cell types, including normal fibroblasts and mammary epithelial cells, and the newly synthesized STAT1 protein persists for many days after IFN stimulation in unphosphorylated form [77]. Certain types of human tumors are unresponsive to IFNs due to defects in the STAT1 activation pathway.

Contrary to these findings, recent data states that the expression level of STAT1 does not influence the response to IFN adjuvant therapy in cancer [72] and that the overexpression of STAT1 in recurrent tumors might be caused by IFN treatment. In these tumor cells the found increase in STAT1 level does not result in enhanced anticancer effects of STAT1 as many IFN-induced pro-apoptotic and antiproliferative proteins as APO2L/TRAIL and IRF1 [78] are not upregulated in resistant cells. This strongly indicates that IFN signaling is not responsible for STAT1 upregulation in cancer cells. It has also been found that high level of unphosphorylated STAT1 in tumors protects cancer cells from DNA damage [79].

These observations suggest that increased levels of unphsphorylated STAT1 might participate in oncogenesis as well as resistance to cell death by inducing target genes that increase proliferation, decrease cell death, or increase repair of DNA damage. Increased DNA damage in cancer is due to oncogene-induced damage, chromosome instability, and other causes that are intrinsic to tumorigenesis. Therefore, evolving cancer cells must learn to resist the consequences of DNA damage, avoiding normal cellular responses such as cell cycle arrest or apoptosis, thus relying on support mechanisms that are characteristic for the tumor "stress phenotype". A working hypothesis that is now being formulated is that the increase in STAT1 expression in cancers is due to processes intrinsic to tumorogenesis [77].

2.4. Oncogenic characteristics of STAT3 and STAT5

Although STAT3 was originally identified as an acute phase response factor that is activated after stimulation by interleukin-6 (IL-6) [65], the biological functions of STAT3 are diverse, in part stemming from the activation of STAT3 by a wide range of cytokines, growth factors, as well as oncogenes. Among its many effects, it is now known to promote oncogenesis, while a hypermorphic allele of STAT3 can function as an oncogene [10].

It is established that the basic role of STAT3 in tumors is the prevention of apoptosis that is achieved by increased expression of antiapoptotic molecule, Bcl-2, or by affecting cell cycle progression by increased expression of c-myc and cyclin D1 engaged in the transition through G1/S check point. This is a characteristic of tumor cell lines with deleted STAT3 gene (STAT3 -,-) where the lack of STAT3 activity leads to the appearance of apoptosis due to an increase in the level of caspases, and a decrease in the level of Bcl-2, while down-regulated proliferation follows from decreased level of cycline D i c myc oncogenes.

In contrast to normal cells, in which STAT tyrosine phosphorylation occurs transiently, it has been determined that STATs 1, 3, and 5 are persistently tyrosine phosphorylated in most malignancies (particularly STAT3) [2, 46]. The mechanisms by which STAT3 is persistently or constitutively tyrosine phosphorylated in cancers include increased production of cytokines and cytokine receptors, which is initiated by tumor cells in an autocrine, and by tumor microenvironment in a paracrine manner, by a decrease in the expression of the SOCS proteins through gene promoter methylation, as well as loss of tyrosine phosphatase activity [11].

Most of the described oncogenic functions of STAT3 depend on the phosphorylation status of Tyr705, however, another role of STAT3 is independent of tyrosine phosphorylation, as unphosphorylated STAT3 can also affect gene expression in the nucleus, one mechanism is through binding to NF-κB and mediating its nuclear import [80].

STAT3 has been directly linked to human cancer as it is required for cell transformation by the *src* oncogene [81], as well as in promoting cellular transformation by the *H-ras* oncogene. This function, which is dependent on the noncanonical serine phosphorylation of STAT3, takes place in mitochondria.

Unlike another member of STAT family, STAT1, that is imported in the nucleus only in phosphorylated form, STAT3 dynamically shuttles in and out of the nucleus independent of its tyrosine phosphorylation status [82, 83]. Nuclear import requires binding of STAT3 to an importin-α–importin-β dimer. On the other hand, mitochondrial import could be mediated in several ways, including by association with the cytosolic chaperones, heat shock proteins (Hsp70, Hsp90) [84] or associated with GRIM-19, a subunit of mitochondrial complex I of the electron transport chain [85] engaged in cell death processes in mitochondria that when overexpressed inhibits the activity of STAT3 by direct binding [86].

In light of this finding and the fact that STAT3 function has been linked to cancer, Gough et al. (2009) [48] evaluated the contribution of STAT3 to Ras oncogenic transformation. Ras protooncogenes become constitutively active oncogenes with the acquisition of specific point mutations [87], which stabilize Ras binding to guanosine 5′-triphosphate (GTP), thus allowing Ras in its GTP-bound state to stimulate numerous downstream effectors. However, Ras oncogenes can only transform cells that have been immortalized by carcinogens or other oncogenes, in the classical multistep carcinogenesis. Some of the signaling molecules activated in response to Ras can impact the STAT3 transcription factor. For example, mitogen-activated protein kinases (MAPKs) can phosphorylate STAT3 on Ser727 and downstream activation of the NF-κB transcription factor induces autocrine IL-6 production canonical tyrosine phosphorylation of STAT3 [88].

Cancer cells tend to have reduced oxidative phosphorylation in mitochondria, and have increased glycolysis in the cytoplasm leading to lactate production [89]. STAT3, inspite of its role in cellular transformation and cancer, promotes oxidative phosphorylation in mitochondria. New findings show that Ser727 phosphorylation of STAT3 contributed to oxidative phosphorylation in mitohondria. The effect of STAT3 on oxidative phosphorylation in mitochondria was investigated by comparing enzyme activity in STAT3+/+ to STAT3–/– cells [48]. Wegrzyn et al. (2009) [90] showed that STAT3+/+ cells had comparatively greater activity of electron transport complex I and complex II but no difference in the activities of complex III or complex VI. Comparing Ras-transformed STAT3+/+ and STAT3–/– cells revealed that, the presence of STAT3 increased activities of electron transport complex II and V. Analogous to cells that lack oncogenic Ras [90], STAT3 appears to stoke the powerhouse, i.e., mitochondria.

Unexpectedly, STAT3-expressing cells also had decreased mitochondrial membrane potential and increased lactate dehydrogenase production, indicating a shift to cytoplasmic glycolysis. Additional analyses are required to understand the complex connections between glycolysis and oxidative phosphorylation affected by STAT3 in the presence or absence of oncogenic Ras.

Originally, STAT5 was originally identified as a specific transcription factor that mediates the effects of prolactin [91]. STAT5A and STAT5B forms are 96% conserved at the protein level but they differ in their C terminal domain as STAT5A has 20 and STAT5B 8 unique amino acids in the C-terminus [92]. However, STAT5A transmits predominantly the signals initiated by the prolactin receptor, while STAT5B mediates the biological effects of growth hormone.

The most important role of STAT5A and STAT5B is in lymphoid, myeloid and erythroid cell development and function as they are activated by multiple cytokines, including IL-2, IL-3, IL-5, IL-7, IL-9, IL-15, GM-CSF and erythropoietin [93]. STAT5B serine 193 is a novel cytokine induced phospho-regulatory site that is constitutively activated in primary hematopoietic malignancies [94]. Following cytokine stimulation, human STAT5A and STAT5B are phosphorylated by JAK1, JAK2 or Tyk on the conserved tyrosine residues 694 and 699, respectively, which allows for their dissociation from the receptor complex, formation of hetero- or homo-dimers, and nuclear translocation to bind specific elements in the promoter of target genes and activate transcription [95]. While tyrosine phosphorylation is a part of activation signal, the serine 726 on STAT5A and 731 on STAT5B phosphorylation may abrogate the transcriptional activity of STAT5A/B [96].

In addition to the physiological role of STAT5 in hematopoietic cell development, dysregulation of the STAT5 signaling pathway plays a role in oncogenesis and leukemogenesis [97]. Specifically, STAT5 has been shown to be constitutively activated in several forms of lymphoid, myeloid and erythroid leukemia [98-100]. Persistent activation of STAT5 was found to be a result of deregulated cytokine signaling [101] or the presence of oncogenic tyrosine kinases. STAT5 proteins can activate many oncogenic tyrosine kinases, including Bcr-Abl, mutated forms of Flt-3 and Kit, and the JAK2 V617F mutant [102-104]. In acute promyelocytic leukemia (APL) beside the most common PML-RARα chromosomal translocation, RARα gene can be fused with STAT5B forming a fusion protein that blocks myeloid differentiation [105].

The most probable molecular mechanism by which STAT5 promotes tumorogenesis is upregulation of cyclin D and c-myc expression which promotes progression from the G1 to the S-phase of the cell cycle [2]. Aside from stimulating proliferation, STAT5 inhibits apoptosis by inducing the expression of anti-apoptotic Bcl-x_l protein and promotes survival of tumor cells [106].

In addition to several types of leukemia and hematopoietic disorders [8], active STAT5A/B is also frequently detected in solid tumors, such as prostate cancer, breast cancer, uterine cancer, squamous cell carcinoma of the head and neck [107].

STAT5A/B controls viability and growth of prostate and breast cancer. The expression of nuclear, active STAT5A/B is often associated with high grade prostate cancer, predicts early disease recurrence and promotes metastatic dissemination. In prostate cancer, active STAT5A/B signaling pathway increases transcriptional activity of androgen receptors. Androgen receptor, in turn, increases transcriptional activity of STAT5A/B. STAT5A/B potentially contributes to castration resistant growth of prostate cancer [108]. The molecular mechanisms underlying constitutive activation of STAT5 in primary and recurrent human prostate cancers are currently unclear, and may involve the autocrine prolactine–JAK2 pathway [109], Src kinases, or Rho GTPases.

In breast cancer, the role of STAT5A/B is more complex. In rodent model systems STAT5A/B may promote malignant transformation and enhance growth of breast tumors [110], while in contrast, STAT5A/B activation in established human breast cancer positively correlates with tumor differentiation [111], prevents metastatic dissemination, and predicts favorable clinical outcome [112] of node-negative breast cancer. In addition, active STAT5A/B, induced by Akt-1, positively correlated with mammary epithelial cell differentiation and possibly a better response to endocrine therapy [113]. Collectively, these studies suggest a dual role for STAT5A/B in the mammary gland as an initiator of tumor formation, as well as a promoter of differentiations of established tumors.

2.5. STAT dysfunction associated with different malignancies

In addition to individual roles of each STAT, they may be coactivated in cancers. In this sense, STATs 1, 3, and 5 are simultaneously tyrosine phosphorylated in a number of human cancers including breast, lung, and head and neck tumors (Table5). The presence of pSTAT5 in addition to pSTAT3 in head and neck tumors can enhance tumor growth and invasion and may contribute to resistance to EGFR inhibitors and chemotherapy [114].

The functional interplay between activated STAT3 and STAT5 has also been described in breast cancers. Considering that STAT3 is included in breast development in association with EGFR, it has been shown on breast cancer cell lines and primary tumors that EGFR mutations, as well as the activity of *src* proto-oncogene, lead to hyperactivity and STAT3 oncogenic properties [115]. JAK/STAT3 signaling pathway is required for growth of CD44+CD23- breast cancer stem cells in tumors [116]. It has been shown that STAT1 blocking by EGFR in this tumor, unlike inhibition of STAT3, does not show any influence on cell proliferation [117].

Activated STAT3 and IL-6 are preferentially found in triple-negative breast cancers or in high-grade tumors and are associated with poor response to chemotherapy [118]. In human tumors, however, the presence of pSTAT5 is found predominantly in well-differentiated estrogen receptor (ER)–positive tumors and is associated with favorable prognosis. Furthermore, the presence of pSTAT5 is a predictive factor for endocrine therapy response and strong prognostic molecular marker in ER-positive breast cancer. Tumors expressing both activated STAT3 and STAT5 were more likely to be ER positive and human EGFR2 negative and of a lower stage.

Aside from the detected STAT dysregulation in tumors, more recent data report STAT status in peripheral blood lymphocytes (PBL). Results of an investigation of STATs in PBL of patients with breast cancer indicates constitutive, as well as stage-dependent, decrease in STAT1, STAT3, STAT5 expression and impaired induction of these proteins by Th1 cytokines [119]. The commonly found dysfunction of NK cells in breast cancer patients [120-122] is probably the consequence of cytokine dysbalance due to the prevalence of immunosuppressive cytokines such as IL-10 and TGFβ [123], as well as tumor-produced inhibitory factors [124]. This finding is in concordance with the only previous study published for breast cancer patients [125] and also with several other investigations showing STAT dysregulation in PBL of melanoma and renal cell carcinoma patients [126,127]. Moreover, we showed that breast cancer patients' T and NK cell subsets have lower pSTAT1 level that could be a biomarker of decreased NK cell cytotoxicity and IFNγ production associated with progression of this disease [120, 128,129].

Constitutively active STAT3 present in breast cancer and many human solid tumors, is associated with immunosuppression of the host immune response. STAT3 expression promotes the production of IL-1β, IL-6, IL-10, TGFβ and VEGF by tumor cells [130] leading to STAT3 activation in immune cells and in turn production of more cytokines forming a feedback loop. These cytokines also inhibit dendritic cell maturation, exerting a pro-tumor response. In this sense, evaluation of STATs in PBL is of importance in predicting the possibility of immunomodulatory and antitumor effect of immunotherapy with cytokines in patients with malignancies.

Constitutive activation of STATs has been detected in human head and neck squamous carcinoma cells [131]. In these cells, activation of STATs is dependent on TGFα induced activation of EGFR and studies utilizing antisense oligonucleotides have demonstrated that STAT3 mediates oncogenic growth of these cells. Activation of STATs in non-small cell lung carcinoma (NSCLC) increased production of TGFα by activating EGFR tyrosine kinase [132] induces downstream STAT3 activation and engages it in the pathogenesis of this malignancy. EGFR constitutive activation of STATs has also been detected in prostate, renal cell, lung, ovarian, and pancreatic cancers, as well as melanomas.

In addition, activation of *src* also occurs with elevated frequency during progression of human breast, ovarian and prostate cancer, and EGFR and Src have been shown to cooperate in human breast cancer [133]. Aside from that, it is of importance that in prostate cancer cell lines the role of BRCA1 gene has been shown in forming of hyperactive STAT3 [134]. When castration resistant disease develops in androgen receptor (AR) positive prostate cancer, these tumors often express higher levels of AR, possibly through activated STAT3, which can transcriptionally regulate AR. Thus, combining antiandrogens with anti-STAT3 drugs should be considered, rather than with chemotherapy in hormone-refractory metastatic prostate cancer [11]. Also, in B16 mouse melanoma cell line hyperactive STAT3 has also been detected [135] (Table 5).

STAT hyperactivity has been demonstrated in lymphomas and leukemias. In acute myeloid leukemia (AML), characterized by the presence of immature myeloid cells in the bone marrow, STAT3 and STAT5 hyperactivity has been found. This may follow from an overproduction of hematopoietic cytokines by tumor cells [136]. An increased level of STAT3β isoform in leuekimic blasts in the bone marrow has been found in patients with this leukemia that have an overall shorter time of survival [137]. It is presumed that STAT5 in AML is activated by mutations in the *flt 3* gene. It has also been shown that hyperactive STAT3 induces increased production of VEGF in bone marrow of acute and chronic leukemia. This is in accord with the common finding of increased blood vessel density in bone marrow in these malignancies [138]. Constitutive activation of STATs 1 and 5 has been additionally detected in acute myelogenous leukemia (AML) and chronic myelogenous leukemia (CML) cells possessing the activated Bcr-Abl tyrosine kinase [139]. Moreover, T cell leukemia that arise in HIV infections, as well as Hodgkin's disease, express active STAT3.

Tumor type	Activated STAT proteins
Solid tumors	
Breast cancer	STAT1,STAT3, STAT5
Head and neck cancer	STAT1,STAT3, STAT5
Melanoma	STAT3
Lung cancer	STAT3,STAT5
Ovarian cancer	STAT3
Pancreatic cancer	STAT3
Prostate cancer	STAT3,STAT5
Hematological malignancies	
Acute myelogenous leukemia	STAT1,STAT3
HTLV-1 dependent leukemia	STAT3,STAT5
Multiple myeloma	STAT1,STAT3, STAT5
Acute lymphoblastic leukemia	STAT5
LGL leukemia	STAT3
Chronic myelogenous leukemia	STAT5
Lymphomas	
Cutaneous T cell lymphoma	STAT3
EBV-related and Burkitt's lymphoma	STAT3
B-cell non-Hodgkin's lymphoma	STAT3
Anaplastic LGL lymphoma	STAT3

Table 5. Activated STAT proteins found in various solid and hematologic tumors

The constitutive activation of STAT3 is more striking than STAT5 in ALK+ anaplastic large T-cell lymphoma (ALCL). In Sezary Syndrome, a leukaemic form of cutaneous T cell lymphoma (CTCL), the JAK3-STAT3 pathway is constitutively activated, while STAT5 activation is inducible [140]. In APL, aside from characteristic RARα - PML chimeric fusion protein, the novel translocation resulting in STAT5B - RARα is considered to be responsible for the lack of response to ATRA-mediated prodifferentiation therapy [141]. Moreover, inadequate activity of STAT4 leads to T helper 2 (Th2) cytokine (IL-4, IL-5 and IL-10) production and prevents adequate antitumor immune response.

3. STATs as therapeutic targets

As malignant tumors are now treated, aside from standard chemo and radiation therapy, by novel therapeutic approaches based on tumor molecular profile, therapy of different tumors now includes agents for specific targeted therapy designed to neutralize pathogenic mutations, a goal that is complex and in development. For this reason, novel therapy has extended to transcription factors, such as STATs, and agents have been designed that directly or indirectly block oncogenic STAT3 and STAT5 activity.

Following extensive cell-based screening systems for these agents in different normal, gene modified and malignant cell lines, as well as studies in experimental animals, it has been established that oncogenic STATs may be inhibited in a direct manner. One of the means is by decreasing STAT gene expression by antisense oligonucleotides (DNA and RNA) or by blocking STAT3 and STAT5 activity by small inhibitory molecules and peptide analogues. These STAT inhibitory agents have been most commonly designed to target the domains responsible for STAT dimerization , i.e., the N-terminus domain and the Src homology (SH2) domain, as well as the DNA-binding domain that makes physical contact with the STAT-responsive elements in the promoters of target genes [142] (Figure 4).

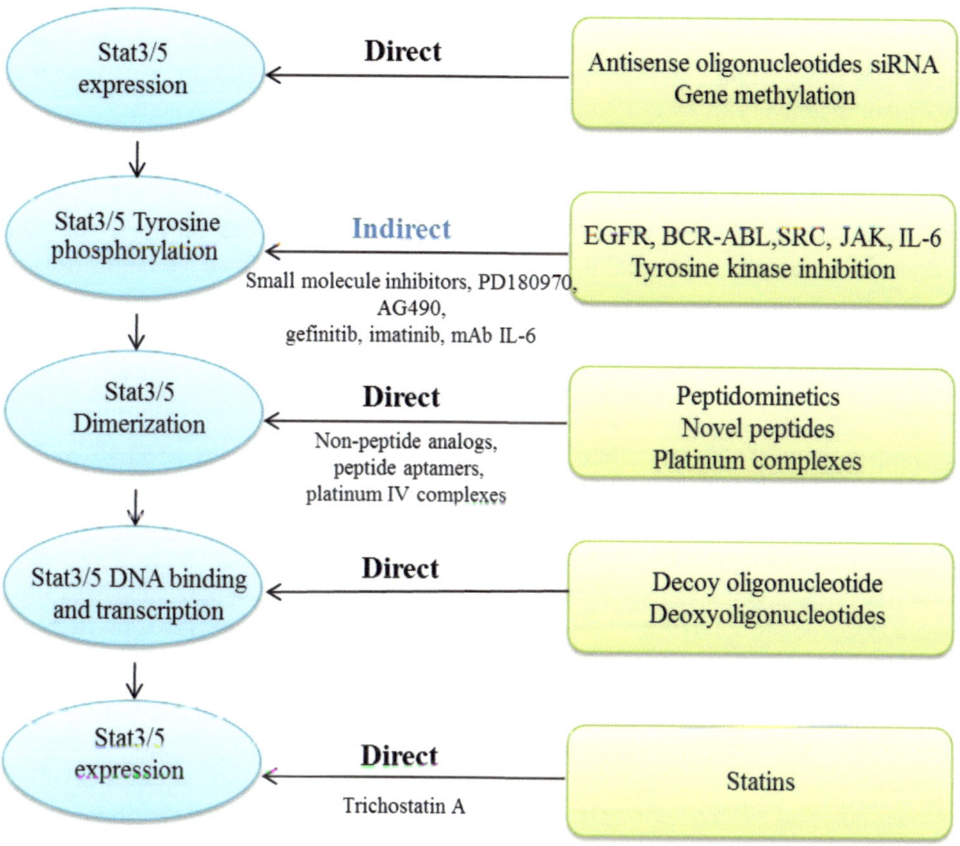

Figure 4. Available approaches and strategies to target STAT signaling pathways. These approaches target directly or indirectly STAT signaling in tumors and include interfering with STAT3 and/or STAT5 expression, phosphorylation, degradation, inhibition of receptor and non-receptor tyrosine kinases, direct interaction with STAT proteins intended to disrupt dimerization, and finally approaches to inhibit DNA-binding activity and gene transcription. These strategies should lead to a decrease in STAT signaling activity and even lower their level to normal values.

On the other hand, hyperactive STAT molecules can also be inhibited indirectly by inhibiting up-stream, either receptor or non-receptor tyrosine kinases that drive tyrosine phosphorylation and activate STATs leading to their hyperactive state [143]. In this sense, aside from JAK enzyme inhibitors, in use are also inhibitors of *src* oncogene and inhibitors of EGFR enzymatic activity, including tyrosine kinase inhibitor gefitinib, and imatinib, an inhibitor of *bcr-abl* oncogene characteristic for CML, as well as passive immunotherapy with antibody for IL-6 or its receptor [47].

JAK enzyme inhibitors, such as tyrphostine AG490, have been shown in clinical trials to be effective in the therapy of multiple myeloma and other hematological malignancies and solid tumors with aberrant activation of the JAK-STAT signaling pathway [144]. Other agents of this type, including ruxolitinib, by showing promising results in phase III clinical trials for myelofibrosis provide a basis for their study in solid tumors such as prostate cancer. In addition to improved outcome, many JAK inhibitors have been found to be tolerable with no adverse impact on the quality of life of patients possibly due to redundancies in signaling downstream of cytokine receptors, with STATs being only a part of the signaling network.

Considering both the crosstalk between STAT and other signaling pathways and activation of other pathways by STAT inhibiting agents, such as activation of Erk MAPK kinases during pimozide STAT5 inhibitor therapy, therapeutic modalities may include STAT inhibitors in combination with MEK inhibitors, an approach defined as complementary signaling pathway inhibition [145]. Although STAT inhibitors may decrease expression of pro-survival genes, this may not be sufficient to induce apoptosis, but may merely lower the threshold for apoptosis. In this sense, a STAT inhibitor may reduce resistance to cytotoxic agents or ionizing radiation and may best be used in combination with standard therapies.

Other indirect methods for inhibition include modulation of the activity of STAT molecule by using their natural negative regulators. Thus, the activity of these signaling molecules is suppressed by increased protease activity, especially for hyperactive STAT5, induction of nuclear and cytoplasmatic STAT inhibitory proteins, SOCS and PIAS, respectively, or up-regulation of tyrosine-phosphatases that dephosphorylate them [146]. Application of statins, as trichostatin A, leads to inhibition of enzyme histone deacetylase (HDAC) that by decreasing STAT transcriptional activity promotes apoptosis of malignant cells, whereas direct binding of statins to STATs leads to their covalent modification and enhanced degradation [147].

In this sense, different approaches in the context of modern targeted therapy of malignancies by decreasing expression, phosphorylation, dimerization or DNA binding of STATs can decrease the activity of these important signaling molecules or down-regulate them to almost normal level. Considering that inhibition of STAT3 and STAT5 leads to growth arrest and selective apoptosis of tumor cells, sparing benign cells, this approach may be of importance not only in the therapy, but also in chemoprevention of tumors. These aspects of molecular targeted therapy of cancer patients need to be validated in additional, properly designed clinical trials.

4. Conclusion

As STAT proteins are involved in regulating fundamental biological processes, including apoptosis and cell proliferation that are known to be dysregulated in tumors, it is not surprising to frequently find defects in STAT signaling pathways in malignancies. In the past few years advances have been made in understanding molecular mechanisms that are responsible for STAT protein dysregualtion in different malignant diseases. The critical role of constitutively active STAT3 and STAT5 in tumorogenesis has now been definitely established. Aside from that, STAT1, 3 and 5 can be considered as molecular markers for early detection of certain tumors, as well as prognostic parameters for evaluation of tumor aggressiveness and response to various types of therapies.

Obtained data that associate these molecules with tumor development support the use of STATs as molecular targets in the therapy and chemoprevention of malignancies. Inhibition of oncogenic STATs represents a comprehensive approach in tumor therapy that leads to decreased cell proliferation, survival, angiogenesis and evasion of immune response. Blocking of constitutively active STATs in tumors allows the destruction of tumor cells with minimal effect on normal cells. It is of importance that this type of molecular therapy that inhibits hyperactive STATs can potentiate response to chemo or radiation therapy and may have great potential in the therapy of solid tumors and leukemia. The efficacy of STAT inhibitors in oncological therapy remains still to be evaluated in numerous undergoing and future clinical trials.

Author details

Gordana Konjević
Institute of Oncology and Radiology of Serbia, Laboratory for Immunology
Medical Faculty, University of Belgrade, Serbia

Sandra Radenković, Ana Vuletić, Katarina Mirjačić Martinović and Tatjana Srdić
Institute of Oncology and Radiology of Serbia, Laboratory for Immunology

Vladimir Jurišić
Medical Faculty, University of Kragujevac, Serbia

Acknowledgement

This study was supported by the Ministry of Education, Science and Technological development of the Republic of Serbia through grants 41031 and 175056. The authors would like to thank Dr. Milica Apostolović Stojanović for excellent assistance in the preparation of this manuscript.

5. References

[1] Darnell JE Jr. STATs and gene regulation. Science 1997; 277(5332):1630-1635.

[2] Bowman T, Garcia R, Turkson J Jove R. STATs in oncogenesis. Oncogene 2000; 19(21):2474-2488.

[3] Konjević G, Jović V, Jurisić V Radulović S, Jelić S, Spuzić I. IL-2-mediated augmentation of NK-cell activity and activation antigen expression on NK- andT-cell subsets in

patients with metastatic melanoma treated with interferon-alphaand DTIC. Clin Exp Metastasis 2003; 20(7):647-655.
[4] Catlett-Falcone R, Dalton WS, Jove R. STAT proteins as novel targets for cancer therapy. Curr Opin Oncol. 1999; 11(6): 490–496.
[5] Quesnelle KM, Boehm AL, Grandis JR. STAT-mediated EGFR signaling in cancer. J Cell Biochem. 2007; 102(2): 311-319.
[6] Kaplan MH, Grusby MJ. Regulation of T helper cell differentiation by STAT molecules. J Leukoc Biol. 1998; 64(1): 2-5.
[7] Konjević G, Spuzić I. The possibilities of modulation of NK cell activity. Glas Srp Akad Nauka 2002; (47): 89-101.
[8] Konjević G, Mirjačić Martinović K, Vuletić A, Babović N. In-vitro IL-2 or IFN-α-induced NKG2D and CD161 NK cell receptor expression indicates novel aspects of NK cell activation in metastatic melanoma patients. Melanoma Res. 2010; 20(6): 459-467.
[9] Konjević G, Mirjačić Martinović K, Vuletić A, Radenković S. Novel aspects of in vitro IL-2 or IFN-α enhanced NK cytotoxicity of healthy individuals based on NKG2D and CD161 NK cell receptor induction. Biomed Pharmacother. 2010; 64(10): 663-671.
[10] Bromberg JF. Stat proteins and oncogenesis. J Clin Invest. 2002; 109(9): 1139–1142.
[11] Sansone P, Bromberg J. Targeting the interleukin-6/jak/stat pathway in human malignancies. J Clin Oncol. 2012; 30(9): 1005-1014.
[12] Kisseleva T, Bhattacharya S, Braunstein, Schindler CW. Signaling through the JAK/STAT pathway, recent advances and future challenges. Gene 2002; 285(1-2): 1-24.
[13] Benekli M, Baer MR, Baumann H, Wetzler M. Signal transducer and activator of transcription proteins in leukemias. Blood 2003; 101(8): 2940-2954.
[14] Gupta S, Yan H, Wong LH, Ralph S, Krolewski J, Schindler C. The SH2 domain of Stat1 and Stat2 mediate multiple interactions in the transduction of IFN alpha signals. EMBO J. 1996; 15(5): 1075-1084.
[15] Zhang X, Blenis J, Li HC, Schindler C, Chen-Kiang S. Requirement of serine phosphorylation for formation of STAT-promoter complexes. Science 1995; 267(5206): 1990-1994.
[16] Imada K, Leonard WJ. The Jak-STAT pathway. Mol Immunol. 2000; 37(1-2): 1-11.
[17] Ihle JN. The STAT family in cytokine signaling. Curr Opin Cell Biol. 2001; 13(2): 211–217.
[18] Remy I, Wilson IA, Michnick SW. Erythropoietin receptor activation by a ligand-induced conformation change. Science 1999; 283(2): 990-993.
[19] Chatterjee-Kishore M, Wright KL, Ting JP, Stark GR. How Stat1 mediates constitutive gene expression: A complex of unphosphorylated Stat1 and IRF1 supports transcription of LMP2 gene. EMBO J. 2000; 19(15): 4111–4122.
[20] Horvath CM. STAT proteins and transcriptional responses to extracellular signals. TIBS 2000; 25(10): 496–502.
[21] McBride KM, Banninger G, McDonald C, Reich NC. Regulated nuclear import of the STAT1 transcription factor by direct binding of importin-a. EMBO J. 2002; 219(7): 1754–1763.
[22] Decker T, Kovarik P. Serine phosphorylation of STATs. Oncogene 2000; 19(21): 2628–2637.

[23] Goh KC, Haque SJ, Williams BR. p38 MAP kinase is required for STAT1 serine phosphorylation and trascriptional activation induced by interferon. EMBO J. 1999; 18(20): 5601–5608.

[24] Ceresa BP, Pessin JE. Insulin stimulates the serine phosphorylation of the signal transducer and activator of transcription (STAT3) isoform. J Biol Chem. 1996; 271(21): 12121-12124.

[25] Jain N, Zhang T, Kee WH, Li W, Cao X. Protein kinase C delta associates with and phosphorylates Stat3 in an interleukin-6-dependent manner. J Biol Chem. 1999; 274: 24392-24400.

[26] Briscole J, Kohlhuber F, Muller M. JAKs and STATs branch out. Trends Cell Biol. 1996; 6(9): 336–340.

[27] Starr R, Willson TA, Viney EM, Murray LJ, Rayner JR, Jenkins BJ, et al. A family of cytokine-inducible inhibitors of signalling. Nature 1997; 387(6636):917-921.

[28] Hagihara K, Nishikawa T, Sugamata Y, Song J, Isobe T, Taga T et al. Essential role of STAT3 in cytokine-driven NF-_B-mediated serum amyloid A gene expression. Genes Cells. 2005; 10(11): 1051–1063.

[29] Yuan ZL. Guan YJ, Chatterjee D, Chin YE. Stat3 dimerization regulated by reversible acetylation of a single lysine residue. Science 2005; 307(5707): 269–273.

[30] Ray S, Sherman CT, Lu M, Brasier AR. Angiotensinogen gene expression is dependent on signal transducer and activator of transcription 3-mediated p300/cAMP response element binding protein-binding protein coactivator recruitment and histone acetyltransferase activity. Mol Endocrinol. 2002; 16(4): 824–836.

[31] Ponti D, Costa A, Zaffaroni N, Pratesi G, Petrangolini G, Coradini D et al. Isolation and in vitro propagation of tumorigenic breast cancer cells with stem/progenitor cellproperties. Cancer Res. 2005; 65(13): 5506–5511.

[32] Yang XJ, Seto E. HATs and HDACs: from structure, function and regulation to novel strategies for therapy and prevention. Oncogene 2007; 26(37): 5310-5318.

[33] Kim KI, Zhang DE. UBP43, an ISG15-specific deconjugating enzyme: expression, purification, and enzymatic assays. Methods Enzymol. 2005; 398 491-499.

[34] Zhao J. Sumoylation regulates diverse biological processes. Cell Mol Life Sci. 2007; 64(24): 3017–3033.

[35] Giandomenico V, Simonsson M, Gronroos E, Ericsson J. Coactivator dependent acetylation stabilizes members of the SREBP family of transcription factors. Mol Cell Biol. 2003; 23(7): 2587–2599.

[36] Lee JL, Wang MJ, Chen JY. Acetylation and activation of STAT3 mediated by nuclear translocation of CD44. J Cell Biol. 2009; 185(6): 949-957.

[37] Ibarra-Sanchez MJ, Simoncic PD, Nestel FR, Duplay P, Lapp WS, Tremblay ML. The T-cell protein tyrosine phosphatase. Semin Immunol. 2000; 12(4): 379–386.

[38] Aoki N, Matsuda TA. A nuclear protein tyrosine phosphatase TC-PTP is a potential negative regulator of the PRL-mediated signaling pathway; dephosphorilation and deactivation of signal trasducer and activator of transcription 5a and 5b by TC-PTP in nucleus. Mol Endocrinol. 2002; 16(1): 58–69.

[39] Simononic PD, Lee-Loy A, Barder DL, Tremblay ML, McGlade CJ. The T cell protein tyrosine phosphatase is a negative regulator of Janus family kinases 1 and 3. Curr Biol. 2002; 12(6): 446–453.

[40] Shuai K. Modulation of STAT signaling by STAT-interacting proteins. Oncogene. 2000; 19(21): 2638–2644.

[41] Krebs DL, Hilton DJ. SOCS proteins: Negative regulators of cytokine signaling. Stem Cells 2001; 19(5): 378–387.

[42] Starr R, Hilton DJ. Negative regulation of the JAK/STAT pathway. Bioessays 1999; 21(1): 47–52.

[43] Cooney RN. Suppressors of cytokine signaling (SOCS): inhibitors of the JAK/STAT pathway. Shock. 2002; 17(2): 83-90.

[44] Nicola NA, Greenhalgh CJ. The suppressors of cytokine signaling (SOCS) proteins: important feedback inhibitors of cytokine action. Exp Hematol. 2000; 28(10): 1105-1112.

[45] Yu CL, Jin YJ, Burakoff SJ. Cytosolic tyrosine dephosphorylation of STAT5.Potential role of SHP-2 in STAT5 regulation. J Biol Chem. 2000; 275(1):599-604.

[46] Calò V, Migliavacca M, Bazan V, Macaluso M, Buscemi M, Gebbia N, et al. STAT proteins: from normal control of cellular events to tumorigenesis. J Cell Physiol. 2003; 197(2):157-168.

[47] Haura EB, Turkson J, Jove R. Mechanisms of disease: Insights into the emerging role of signal transducers and activators of transcription in cancer. Nat Clin Pract Oncol. 2005; 2(6): 315-324.

[48] Gough DJ, Corlett A, Schlessinger K, Wegrzyn J, Larner AC, Levy DE. Mitochondrial STAT3 supports Ras-dependent oncogenic transformation. Science 2009; 324(5935): 1713-1716.

[49] Levy DE, Darnell JE Jr. STATs: Transcriptional control and biological impact. Nat Rev. 2002; 3(9): 651-662.

[50] Dunn GP, Bruce AT, Ikeda H, Old LJ, Schreiber RD. Cancer immunoediting: from immunosurveillance to tumor escape. Nat Immunol. 2002; 3(11): 991-998.

[51] Konjević G, Jović V, Vuletić A, Radulović S, Jelić S, Spuzić I. CD69 on CD56+ NK cells and response to chemoimmunotherapy in metastatic melanoma. Eur J Clin Invest. 2007; 37(11): 887-896.

[52] Jindal S, Borges VF. The emerging role of cytokines in breast cancer: from initiation to survivorship. CML-Breast Cancer 2011; 23(4): 113-126.

[53] Culig Z. Cytokine disbalance in common human cancers. Biochim Biochim Biophys Acta. 2011; 1813(2): 308-314.

[54] Kortylewski M, Xin H, Kujawski M, Lee H, Liu Y, Harris T, et al. Regulation of the IL-23 and IL-12 balance by Stat3 signaling in the tumor microenvironment. Cancer Cell. 2009; 15(2):114-23.

[55] Olkhanud PB, Damdinsuren B, Bodogai M, Gress RE, Sen R, Wejksza K et al. Tumor-evoked regulatory B cells promote breast cancer metastasis by converting resting CD4^{+} T cells to T-regulatory cells. Cancer Res. 2011; 71(10):3505-15.

[56] Grivennikov S, Karin E, Terzic J, Mucida D, Yu GY, Vallabhapurapu S et al.IL-6 and Stat3 are required for survival of intestinal epithelial cells and development of colitis-associated cancer. Cancer Cell. 2009; 15(2):103-13.

[57] Wang T, Niu G, Kortylewski M, Burdelya L, Shain K, Zhang S et al. Regulation of the innate and adaptive immune responses by Stat-3 signaling in tumor cells. Nat Med. 2004; 10(1): 48-54.

[58] Sano S, Itami S, Takeda K, Tarutani M, Yamaguchi Y, Miura H et al. Keratinocyte-specific ablation of Stat3 exhibits impaired skin remodeling, but does not affect skin morphogenesis. EMBO J. 1999; 18(17):4657-4668.

[59] Turkson J, Bowman T, Garcia R, Caldenhoven E, De Groot RP, Jove R. Stat3 activation by Src induces specific gene regulation and is required for cell transformation. Mol Cell Biol. 1998; 18(5): 2545-2552.

[60] Garcia R, Yu CL, Hudnall A, Catlett R, Nelson KL, Smithgall T et al. Dicer dependent microRNAs regulate gene expression and functions in human endothelial cells. Circ Res. 2007; 100(8):1164-1173.

[61] Suárez Y, Fernández-Hernando C, Pober JS, Sessa WC. Dicer dependent microRNAs regulate gene expression and functions in human endothelial cells. Circ Res. 2007;100(8):1164-73.

[62] Potente M, Ghaeni L, Baldessari D, Mostoslavsky R, Rossig L, Dequiedt F et al. SIRT1 controls endothelial angiogenic functions during vascular growth. Genes Dev. 2007; 21(20): 2644-2658.

[63] Kuehbacher A, Urbich C, Zeiher AM, Dimmeler S. Role of Dicer and Drosha for endothelial microRNA expression and angiogenesis. Circ Res. 2007; 101(1): 59-68.

[64] O. Warburg. Photosynthesis. Science 1958; 128(3315): 68-73.

[65] Reich NC. STAT3 revs up the powerhouse. Sci Signal. 2009;2 (90):pe61

[66] Lin TS, Mahajan S, Frank DA. Stat signaling in the pathogenesis and treatment of leukemias. Oncogene. 2000; 19(21): 2496-2504.

[67] Kaplan DH, Shankaran V, Dighe AS, Stockert E, Aguet M, Old LJ et al. Demonstration of an interferon gamma-dependent tumor surveillance system in immunocompetent mice. Proc Natl Acad Sci U S A. 1998; 95(13):7556-7561.

[68] Kumar A, Commane M, Flickinger TW, Horwath CM, Stark GR. Detective TNF-alpha-induced apoptosis in Stat1-null cells due to low costitutive levels of caspases. Science. 1997; 278(2543): 1630–1632.

[69] Ouchi T, Lee SW, Ouchi M, Aaroson SA, Horvath CM. Collaboration of signal transducer and activator of transcription 1 (STAT1) and BRCA1 in differential regulation of IFN-g target genes. Proc Natl Acad Sci USA. 2000; 97(10): 5208–5213.

[70] Raven JF, Williams V, Wang S, Tremblay ML, Muller WJ, Durbin JE et al. Stat1 is a suppressor of ErbB2/Neu-mediated cellular transformation and mouse mammary gland tumor formation. Cell Cycle. 2011; 10(5): 794-804.

[71] Widschwendter A, Tonko-Geymayer S, Welte T, Daxenbichler G, Marth C, Doppler W. Prognostic significance of signal transducer and activator of transcription 1 activation in breast cancer. Clin Cancer Res. 2002; 8(10): 3065–3074.

[72] Lesinski GB, Valentino D, Hade EM, Jones S, Magro C, Chaudhury AR et al. Expression of STAT1 and STAT2 in malignant melanoma does not correlate with response to interferon-alpha adjuvant therapy. Cancer Immunol Immunother. 2005; 54(9): 815–825.

[73] Khodarev NN, Beckett M, Labay E, Darga T, Roizman B, Weichselbaum RR. STAT1 is overexpressed in tumors selected for radioresistance and confers protection from radiation in transduced sensitive cells. Proc Natl Acad Sci USA. 2004; 101(6): 1714–1719.

[74] Cai D, Cao J, Li Z, Zheng X, Yao Y, Li W, et al. Upregulation of bone marrow stromal protein 2 (BST2) in breast cancer with bone metastasis. BMC Cancer. 2009; 9:102.

[75] Khodarev NN, Roach P, Pitroda SP, Golden DW, Bhayani M, Shao MY et al. STAT1 pathway mediates amplification of metastatic potential and resistance to therapy. PLoS One. 2009; 4: e5821.

[76] Khodarev NN, Minn AJ, Efimova EV, Darga TE, Labay E, Beckett M et al. Signal transducer and activator of transcription 1 regulates both cytotoxic and prosurvival functions in tumor cells. Cancer Res. 2007; 67(19): 9214–9220.

[77] Cheon H, Yang J, Stark GR. The functions of signal transducers and activators of transcriptions 1 and 3 as cytokine-inducible proteins. J Interferon Cytokine Res. 2011; 31(1): 33-40.

[78] Borden EC, Sen GC, Uze G, Silverman RH, Ransohoff RM, Foster GR et al. Interferons at age 50: past, current, and future impact on biomedicine. Nat Rev Drug Discov. 2007; 6(12): 975–990.

[79] Luszczek W, Cheriyath V, Mekhail TM, Borden EC. Combinations of DNA methyltransferase and histone deacetylase inhibitors induce DNA damage in small cell lung cancer cells: correlation of resistance with interferon stimulated gene expression. Mol Cancer Ther 2010;9(8):2309-2321.

[80] Yang J, Stark GR. Roles of unphosphorylated STATs in signaling. Cell Res 2008;18(4):443–451.

[81] Yu H, Jove R. The STATs of cancer-New molecular targets come of age. Nat. Rev Cancer 2004;4(2):97–105

[82] Reich NC, Liu L. Tracking STAT nuclear traffic. Nat Rev Immunol 2006;6(8):602–612.

[83] Liu L, McBride KM, Reich NC. STAT3 nuclear import is independent of tyrosine phosphorylation and mediated by importin-alpha3. Proc Natl Acad Sci. U.S.A 2005;102(23):8150–8155.

[84] Neupert W, Herrmann JM. Translocation of proteinsinto mitochondria. Annu Rev Biochem 2007;76: 723–749.

[85] Fearnley IM, Carroll J, Shannon RJ, Runswick MJ, Walker E, Hirst J. GRIM-19, a cell death regulatory gene product, is a subunit of bovine mitochondrial NADH:ubiquinone oxidoreductase (complex I). J Biol Chem 2001;276(42):38345–38348.

[86] Lufei C, Ma J, Huang G, Zhang T, Novotny- Diermayr V, Ong CT et al. GRIM-19, a deathregulatory gene product, suppresses Stat3 activity via functional interaction. EMBO J 2003;22(6):1325–1335.

[87] Karnoub AE, Weinberg RA. Ras oncogenes: Split personalities. Nat Rev Mol Cell Biol 2008;9(7):517–531.

[88] Faruqi TR, Gomez D, Bustelo XR, Bar-Sagi D, Reich NC. Rac1 mediates STAT3 activation by autocrine IL-6. Proc Natl Acad Sci. U.S.A 2001;98(16):9014–9019.

[89] Vander Heiden MG, Cantley LC, Thompson CB. Understanding the Warburg effect: The metabolic requirements of cell proliferation. Science 2009;324(5930): 1029–1033.

[90] Wegrzyn J, Potla R, Chwae YJ, Sepuri NB, Zhang Q, Koeck T et al. Function of mitochondrial Stat3 incellular respiration. Science 2009;323(5915):793–797.

[91] Wakao H, Gouilleux F, Groner B. Mammary gland factor (MGF) is a novel member of the cytokine regulated transcription factor gene family and confers the prolactin response. EMBO J 1994;13(9):2182–2191.

[92] Schindler CW. Series Introduction: Jak-STAT signaling in human disease. J Clin Invest 2002;109(9):1133–1137.

[93] Kirken RA, Rui H, Malabarba MG, Howard OM, Kawamura M, O'Shea JJ et al. Activation of JAK3, but not JAK1, is critical for IL-2-induced proliferation and STAT5 recruitment by a COOH-terminal region of the IL-2 receptor beta-chain. Cytokine 1995;7(7):689-700.

[94] Mitra A, Ross JA, Rodriguez G, Nagy ZS, Wilson HL, Kirken RA. Signal transducer and activator of transcription 5b (Stat5b) serine 193 is a novel cytokine induced phospho-regulatory site that is constitutively activated in primary hematopoietic malignancies. J Biol Chem 2012;287(20):16596-16608.

[95] Leonard WJ. Role of Jak kinases and STATs in cytokine signal transduction. Int J Hematol 2001;73(3):271-277.

[96] Yamashita H, Nevalainen MT, Xu J, LeBaron MJ, Wagner KU, Erwin RA et al. Role of serine phosphorylation of Stat5a in prolactin-stimulated beta-casein gene expression. Mol Cell Endocrinol 2001;183(1-2):151–163.

[97] Bunting KD. STAT5 signaling in normal and pathologic hematopoiesis. Front Biosci 2007;12:2807-2820.

[98] Chai SK, Nichols GL, Rothman P. Constitutive activation of JAKs and STATs in BCR-Abl-expressing cell lines and peripheral blood cells derived from leukemic patients. J Immunol 1997;159(10):4720-4728.

[99] Ho JM, Beattie BK, Squire JA, Frank DA, Barber DL. Fusion of the ets transcription factor TEL to Jak2 results in constitutive Jak-Stat signaling. Blood (1999);93(12):4354-4364.

[100] Ilaria RL Jr, Van Etten RA. P210 and P190 (BCR/ABL) induce the tyrosine phosphorylation and DNA binding activity of multiple specific STAT family members. J Biol Chem 1996;271(49): 31704-31710.

[101] Van Etten RA. Aberrant cytokine signaling in leukemia. Oncogene 2007;26(47):6738-6749.

[102] Carron C, Cormier F, Janin A, Lacronique V, Giovannini M, Daniel M et al. TEL JAK2 transgenic mice develop T-cell leukemia. Blood 2000;95(12):3891-3899.

[103] Nieborowska-Skorska M, Wasik MA, Slupianek A, Salomoni P, Kitamura T, Calabretta B et al. Signal transducer and activator of transcription (STAT)5 activation by BCR/ABL is dependent on intact Src homology (SH)3 and SH2 domains of BCR/ABL and is required for leukemogenesis. J Exp Med 1999;189(8):1229-1242.

[104] Mizuki M, Fenski R, Halfter H, Matsumura I, Schmid, R, Muller C et al. Flt3 mutations from patients with acute myeloid leukemia induce transformation of 32D cells mediated by the Ras and STAT5 pathways. Blood 2000;96(12):3907-3914.

[105] Maurer AB, Wichmann C, Gross A Kunkel H, Heinzel T, Ruthardt M et al. The Stat5-RARα fusion protein represses transcription and differentiation through interaction with a corepressor complex. Blood 2002;99(8):2647-2652.

[106] Buettner R, Mora LB, Jove R. Activated Stat signaling in human tumors provides novel molecular targets for therapeutic intervention. Clin Cancer Res 200;8(4):945–954.

[107] Nikitakis NG, Siavash H, Sauk JJ. Targeting the STAT pathway in head and neck cancer: recent advances and future prospects. Curr Cancer Drug Targets 2004;4(8):637-651.

[108] Tan SH, Dagvadorj A, Shen F, Gu L, Liao Z, Abdulghani J et al. Transcription factor Stat5 synergizes with androgen receptor in prostate cancer cells. Cancer Res 2008;68(1):236-248.

[109] Li H, Ahonen TJ, Alanen K, Xie J, LeBaron MJ, Pretlow TG et al. Activation of signal transducer and activator of transcription 5 in human prostate cancer is associated with high histological grade. Cancer Research 2004;64(14):4774–4782.

[110] Ren S, Cai HR, Li M, Furth PA. Loss of Stat5a delays mammary cancer progression in a mouse model. Oncogene 2002;21(27):4335–4339.

[111] Cotarla I, Ren S, Zhang Y, Gehan E, Singh B, Furth PA. Stat5a is tyrosine phosphorylatedand nuclear localized in a high proportion of human breast cancers. Int J Cancer 2004;108(5):665–671.

[112] Nevalainen MT, Xie J, Torhorst J, Bubendorf L, Haas P, Kononen J et al. Signal transducer and activator of transcription-5 activation and breast cancer prognosis. J Clin Oncol 2004;22(11):2053–2060.

[113] Creamer BA, Sakamoto K, Schmidt JW, Triplett AA, Moriggl R, Wagner KU. Stat5 promotes survival of mammary epithelial cells through transcriptional activation of a distinct promoter in Akt1. Mol Cell Biol 2010;30(12): 2957–2970.

[114] Koppikar P, Lui VW, Man D, Xi S, Chai RL, Nelson E et al. Constitutive activation of signal transducer and activator of transcription 5 contributes to tumor growth, epithelial-mesenchymal transition, and resistance to epidermal growth factor receptor targeting. Clin Cancer Res 2008;14(23):7682-7690.

[115] Garcia R, Yu CL, Hudnall A, Catlett R, Nelson KL, Smithgall T et al. Constitutive activation of Stat3 in fibroblasts transformed by diverse oncoproteins and in breast carcinoma cells. Cell Growth Differ 1997;8(12):1267-1276.

[116] Marotta LL, Almendro V, Marusyk A Shipitsin M, Schemme J, Walker SR et al. The JAK2/STAT3 signaling pathway is required for growth of CD44+CD24- stem cell-like breast cancer cells in human tumors. J Clin Invest 2011;121(7):2723-2735.

[117] Grandis JR, Grenning SD, Chakraborty A, Zhou MY, Zeng Q, Pitt AS et al. Requirement of Stat3 but not Stat1 activation for epidermel growth factor receptor-mediated cell growth in vitro. J Clin Invest 1998;102(7):1385-1392.

[118] Dolled-Filhart M, Camp RL, Kowalski DP, Smith BL, Rimm DL. Tissue microarray analysis of signal transducers and activators of transcription 3 (Stat3) and phospho-Stat3 (Tyr705) in node-negative breast cancer shows nuclear localization is associated with a better prognosis. Clin Cancer Res 2003;9(2):594-600.

[119] Shankaran V, Ikeda H, Bruce AT White JM, Swanson PE, Old LJ et al. IFNgamma and lymphocytes prevent primary tumor development and shape tumor immunogenicity. Nature 2001;410(6832):1107-1111.

[120] Konjević G, Jurisić V, Spuzić I. Association of NK cell dysfunction with changes in LDH characteristics of peripheral blood lymphocytes (PBL) in breast cancer patients. Breast Cancer Res Treat 2001;66(3):255-263.

[121] Konjevic G, Radenkovic S, Srdic T, Jurisic V, Stamatovic Lj, Milovic M. Association of decreased NK cell activity and IFNγ expression with pSTAT dysregulation in breast cancer patients. J BUON 2011;16(2):219-226.

[122] Konjevic G, Jurisic V, Jovic V, Vuletic A, Mirjacic Martinovic K, Radenkovic S et al. Investigation of NK cell function and their modulation in different malignancies. Immunol Res 2012;52(1-2):139-156.

[123] Jarnicki AG, Lysaght J, Todryk S, Mills KH. Suppression of antitumor immunity by IL-10 and TGF-beta-producing T cells infi ltrating the growing tumor: infl uence of tumor environment on the induction of CD4+ and CD8+ regulatory T cells. J Immunol 2006;177(2):896-904.

[124] Zwirner NW, Fuertes MB, Girart MV, Domaica CI, Rossi LE. Cytokine-driven regulation of NK cell functions in tumor immunity: role of the MICA-NKG2D system. Cytokine Growth Factor Rev 2007;18(1-2):159-170.

[125] Critchley-Thorne RJ, Simons DL, Yan N, Miyahira AK, Dirbas FM, Johnson DL et al. Impaired interferon signaling is a common immune defect in human cancer. Proc Natl Acad Sci USA 2009;106(22):9010-9015.

[126] Lesinski GB, Kondadasula SV, Crespin T, Shen L, Kendra K, Walker M et al. Multiparametric flowcytometric analysis of inter-patient variation in STAT1 phosphorylation following interferon alfa immunotherapy. J Natl Cancer Inst 2004;96(17):1331-1342.

[127] Varker KA, Kondadasula SV, Go MR Lesinski GB, Ghosh-Berkebile R, Lehman A et al. Multiparametric flow cytometric analysis of signal transducer and activator of transcription 5 phosphorylation in immune cell subsets in vitro and following interleukin-2 immunotherapy. Clin Cancer Res 2006;12(19):5850-5858.

[128] Konjević G, Spuzić I. Stage dependence of NK cell activity and its modulation by interleukin 2 in patients with breast cancer. Neoplasma 1993;40(2):81-85.

[129] Konjević G, Spuzić I. Evaluation of different effects of sera of breast cancer patients on the activity of natural killer cells. J Clin Lab Immunol 1992;38(2):83-93.

[130] Wang T, Niu G, Kortylewski M Burdelya L, Shain K, Zhang S et al. Regulation of the innate and adaptive immune responses by Stat-3 signaling in tumor cells. Nat Med 2004;10(1): 48–54.

[131] Grandis JR, Drenning SD, Chakraborty A, Zhou MY, Zeng Q, Pitt AS et al. Requirement of Stat3 but not Stat1 activation for epidermal growth factor receptor-mediated cell growth in vitro. J Clin Invest 1998;102(7):1385-1392.

[132] Fernandes A, Hamburger AW, Gerwin BI. ErbB-2 kinase is required for constitutive stat 3 activation in malignant human lung epithelial cells. Int J Cancer 1999;83(4):564-570.

[133] Reddy MVR, Chaturvedi P, Reddy EP. Src kinase mediated activation of STAT3 plays an essential role in the proliferation and oncogenicity of human breast, prostate and ovarian carcinomas. Proceeding in Abstract book: Proc Am Assoc Cancer Res 1999; 40: Abstract No.376.

[134] Gao B, Shen X, Kunos G Meng Q, Goldberg ID, Rosen EM et al. Constitutive activation of JAK-STAT3 signaling by BRCA1 in human prostate cancer cells. FEBS Lett 2001;488(3): 179-184.

[135] Niu G, Bowman T, Huang M Shivers S, Reintgen D, Daud A et al. Roles of activated Src and Stat3 signaling in melanoma tumor cell growth. Oncogene 2002;21(46):7001-7010.

[136] Lowenberg B, Touw IP. Hematopoietic growth factors and their receptors in acute leukemia. Blood 1993;81(2):281-292.

[137] Xia Z, Sait SN, Baer MR Barcos M, Donohue KA, Lawrence D et al. Truncated STAT proteins are prevalent at relapse of acute myeloid leukemia. Leuk Res 2001;25(6):473-482.

[138] Niu G, Wright KL, Huang M, Song L, Haura E, Turkson J et al. Constitutive STAT3 activity upregulates VEGF expression and tumor angiogenesis. Oncogene 2002;21(13): 2000-2008.

[139] Skorski T, Nieborowska-Skorska M, Wlodarski P, Wasik M, Trotta R, Kanakaraj P et al. The SH3 domain contributes to BCR/ABL-dependent leukemogenesis in vivo: role in adhesion, invasion, and homing. Blood 1998;91(2):406-418.

[140] Mitchell TJ, John S. Signal transducer and activator of transcription (STAT) signalling and T-cell lymphomas. Immunology 2005;114(3):301-312.

[141] Maurer AB, Wichmann C, Gross A, Kunkel H, Heinzel T, Ruthardt M et al. The Stat5-RARα fusion protein represses transcription and differentiation through interaction with a corepressor complex. Blood 2002;99(8):2647-2652.

[142] Yue P, Turkson J. Targeting STAT3 in cancer: how successful are we? Expert Opin Investig Drugs 2009;18(1):45-56.

[143] Walker SR, Frank DA. STAT Signaling in the Pathogenesis and Treatment of Cancer. In: Frank DA. (ed.) Signaling Pathways in Cancer Pathogenesis and Therapy. New York Dordrecht Heidelberg London: Springer; 2012. p95-108.

[144] Shodeinde AL, Barton BE. Potential use of STAT3 inhibitors in targeted prostate cancer therapy. Onco Targets and Therapy 2012;5:119-125.

[145] Nelson EA, Walker SR, Weisberg E, Bar-Natan M, Barrett R, Gashin LB et al. The STAT5 inhibitor pimozide decreases survival of chronic myelogenous leukemia cells resistant to kinase inhibitors. Blood 2011;117(12):3421–3429.

[146] Hendry L, John S. Regulation of STAT signalling by proteolytic processing. Eur J Biochem 2004;271(23-24):4613-4620.

[147] Chan KK, Oza AM, Siu LL. The statins as anticancer agents. Clin Cancer Res 2003;9(1):10-19.